Oxford Medical Publications

BRAIN, PERCEPTION, MEMORY

BRAIN, PERCEPTION, MEMORY

Advances in Cognitive Neuroscience

Edited by

Johan J. Bolhuis

Associate Professor of Behavioural Biology,
Institute of Evolutionary and Ecological Sciences,
Leiden University, The Netherlands

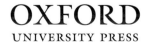

OXFORD

UNIVERSITY PRESS

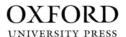

OXFORD
UNIVERSITY PRESS

Great Clarendon Street, Oxford OX2 6DP

Oxford University Press is a department of the University of Oxford.
It furthers the University's objective of excellence in research, scholarship,
and education by publishing worldwide in

Oxford New York

Athens Auckland Bangkok Bogotá Buenos Aires Calcutta
Cape Town Chennai Dar es Salaam Delhi Florence Hong Kong Istanbul
Karachi Kuala Lumpur Madrid Melbourne Mexico City Mumbai
Nairobi Paris São Paulo Singapore Taipei Tokyo Toronto Warsaw

with associated companies in
Berlin Ibadan

Oxford is a registered trade mark of Oxford University Press
in the UK and in certain other countries

Published in the United States
by Oxford University Press Inc., New York

A catalogue record for this title is available from the British Library

Library of Congress Cataloguing in Publication Data
(Data available)

ISBN 0 19 852483 8 (Hbk)
0 19 852482 X (Pbk)

Typeset by EXPO HOLDINGS, Malaysia

Printed in Great Britain on acid-free paper by
The Bath Press, Avon

CONTENTS

CONTRIBUTORS

Patrick Bateson
Sub-Department of Animal Behaviour, University of Cambridge, Madingley, Cambridge CB3 8AA, UK

Johan J. Bolhuis
Institute of Evolutionary and Ecological Sciences, Behavioural Biology, Leiden University, P.O. Box 9516, 2300 RA Leiden, The Netherlands

Peter A. Brennan
Sub-Department of Animal Behaviour, University of Cambridge, Madingley, Cambridge CB3 8AA, UK

Malcolm W. Brown
MRC Centre for Synaptic Plasticity, Department of Anatomy, University of Bristol, School of Medical Sciences, University Walk, Bristol BS8 1TD, UK

Mark J. Buckley
Department of Experimental Psychology, University of Oxford, South Parks Road, Oxford OX1 3UD, UK

Larry Cahill
Center for the Neurobiology of Learning and Memory and the Department of Neurobiology and Behavior, University of California, Irvine, CA 92697-3800, USA

David F. Clayton
Beckman Institute, University of Illinois at Urbana-Champaign, 405 North Mathews Avenue, Urbana, IL 61801, USA

Timothy J. DeVoogd
Department of Psychology, Cornell University, Uris Hall, Ithaca, NY 14853-7601, USA

Raymond J. Dolan
Wellcome Department of Cognitive Neurology, Institute of Neurology, University College London, 12 Queen Square, London WC1N 3BG, UK

Yadin Dudai
The Weizmann Institute of Science, Department of Neurobiology, Rehovot 76100, Israel.

John Duncan
MRC Cognition and Brain Sciences Unit, 15 Chaucer Road, Cambridge CB2 2EF, UK

Barbara Ferry
Center for the Neurobiology of Learning and Memory and the Department of Neurobiology and Behavior, University of California, Irvine, CA 92697-3800, USA

David Gaffan
Department of Experimental Psychology, University of Oxford, South Parks Road, Oxford OX1 3UD, UK

Michael S.A. Graziano
Department of Psychology, Princeton University, Green Hall, Princeton, NJ, 08544-1010, USA

Charles G. Gross
Department of Psychology, Princeton University, Green Hall, Princeton, NJ, 08544-1010, USA

Robert A. Hinde
St John's College, Cambridge CB2 1TP, UK

Gabriel Horn
Sub-Department of Animal Behaviour, University of Cambridge, Madingley, Cambridge CB3 8AA, UK

Mark H. Johnson
Centre for Brain and Cognitive Development, School of Psychology, Birkbeck College, University of London, Malet Street, London WC1E 7HX, UK

Eric R. Kandel
Center for Neurobiology and Behavior, Howard Hughes Medical Institute, Columbia University, 722 West 168 Street, New York, NY 10032, USA

Eric B. Keverne
Sub-Department of Animal Behaviour, University of Cambridge, Madingley, Cambridge CB3 8AA, UK

David A.T. King
Program for Neural, Informational, and Behavioral Sciences, University of Southern California, Hedco Neurosciences Building–HNB 122, University Park, Los Angeles, CA 90089-2520, USA

Joseph E. LeDoux
Center for Neural Science, New York University, 4 Washington Place, Room 1108A, New York, NY 10003, USA

James L. McGaugh
Center for the Neurobiology of Learning and Memory and the Department of Neurobiology and Behavior, University of California, Irvine, CA 92697-3800, USA

John G. McHaffie
Department of Neurobiology and Anatomy, Wake Forest University School of Medicine, Medical Center Blvd, Winston-Salem, NC 27157-1010, USA

Richard G.M. Morris
Department of Neuroscience, University of Edinburgh, 1 George Square, Edinburgh EH8 9JZ, UK

Karim Nader
Center for Neural Science, New York University, 4 Washington Place, Room 1108A, New York, NY 10003, USA

Benno Roozendaal
Center for the Neurobiology of Learning and Memory and the Department of Neurobiology and Behavior, University of California, Irvine, CA 92697-3800, USA

Wolf Singer
Max Planck Institute for Brain Research, Deutschordenstrasse 46, D-60528 Frankfurt/Main, Germany

Tom V. Smulders
Department of Physiology and Pharmacology, Wake Forest University School of Medicine, Medical Center Boulevard, Winston-Salem, NC 27157, USA

Terrence R. Stanford
Department of Neurobiology and Anatomy, Wake Forest University School of Medicine, Medical Center Blvd, Winston-Salem, NC 27157-1010, USA

Barry E. Stein
Department of Neurobiology and Anatomy, Wake Forest University School of Medicine, Medical Center Blvd, Winston-Salem, NC 27157-1010, USA

Richard F. Thompson
Program for Neural, Informational, and Behavioral Sciences, University of Southern California, Hedco Neurosciences Building–HNB 122, University Park, Los Angeles, CA 90089-2520, USA

Mark T. Wallace
Department of Neurobiology and Anatomy, Wake Forest University School of Medicine, Medical Center Blvd, Winston-Salem, NC 27157-1010, USA

Lawrence Weiskrantz
Department of Experimental Psychology, University of Oxford, South Parks Road, Oxford OX1 3UD, UK

Mary E. Wheeler
Department of Psychology, Princeton University, Green Hall, Princeton, NJ, 08544-1010, USA

Danny Winder
Department of Molecular Physiology and Biophysics, Vanderbilt University School of Medicine, Nashville, TN 37232-0615, USA

Dedicated to Gabriel Horn

FOREWORD

Robert A. Hinde

It is both a pleasure and an honour to contribute a Foreword to this collection of essays marking the achievements of Gabriel Horn. He has been a close personal friend and an inspiration to me for over 40 years.

What is especially remarkable about Gabriel's career to date is the number of different lines of research in which he has been ahead of the field. For instance, as an undergraduate, he, together with Eayrs, was the first to demonstrate that experimentally induced hypothyroidism in rats led to a reduction in the density of cortical neuropil (Eayrs and Horn, 1955). That work triggered an extensive field of study of the role of thyroid hormone in controlling neuronal growth (see Grave, 1978).

Gabriel later became interested in the mechanisms whereby we can attend selectively to some stimuli that impinge on our sense organs and ignore others. While working in this field (Horn, 1960), he wrote a review which was to be highly influential (Horn, 1965). His interest in attentive behavior led him to study the ways in which signals from two sensory modalities interact in the visual system. In pursuing this work, he and Hill were the first to demonstrate that the organization of receptive fields in the cat visual cortex is not static, and that tilting the cat altered the orientation of the line sensitivity of cortical neurons (Horn and Hill, 1969). Both of these findings were heretical at the time and both subsequently have been confirmed: receptive fields in the cat show striking changes over time (see DeAngelis *et al.*, 1995) and their orientation is affected by body tilt (Tomko *et al.*, 1981). There is now extensive evidence that, in other cortical areas, visual receptive fields move, sometimes with arm movements (Graziano *et al.*, 1994), sometimes before an eye movement (Duhamel *et al.*, 1992). Similar shifts occur also in the superior colliculus, as when auditory receptive fields shift with changes in eye position (Jay and Sparks, 1984). Horn was also ahead of the field in showing for the first time that neurons in the mammalian superior colliculus respond to auditory and to somatic sensory stimuli as well as to visual stimuli (Horn and Hill, 1964). These findings were soon followed up by others (e.g. Wickelgren, 1971; Drager and Hubel, 1975). He and Griffith were also the first to investigate quantitatively the functional coupling between cortical neurons (Griffith and Horn, 1963), an issue that is at the center of much current research (see Singer, Chapter 3).

In studying the superior colliculus, Horn and Hill (1964) noticed that an initially brisk neuronal response to a visual stimulus waned if the stimulus was presented repeatedly. They demonstrated that the properties of this neuronal habituation were closely similar to those of behavioral habituation. This study was probably the first to make this comparison. In relating these two levels of analysis, Horn suggested that the failure of synaptic transmission during habituation involved changes in the movement of calcium ions on the presynaptic side of the synapse. Horn's work on habituation involved a wide range of species, including cephalopods, insects and mammals.

By the 1950s, Lashley's failure to localize the engram provided a discouraging context for investigations of the basis of memory. In a chapter published in 1970, Horn remarked that progress in the understanding of forms of learning other than habituation was not encouraging, and ascribed it to the fact that 'no simple preparation has been found which exhibits at all rigorously properties similar to those of associative learning' (Horn, 1970, p. 601). Nearly all his work since then has resulted from his realization that the phenomenon of imprinting presented a unique opportunity for studying the neural basis of an example of vertebrate learning that clearly has considerable complexity. Originally seen as a special form of learning enabling nidifugous birds to learn the characteristics of their parents,

Horn and his colleagues (initially especially Bateson) refined techniques for its experimental analysis. Domestic chicks could be reared under controlled conditions, their stimulus preferences could be assessed quantitatively, electrodes could be implanted with precision, and in some experiments individual chicks could be used as their own controls by training the two halves of the brain independently.

Horn and his colleagues soon established that the neuronal changes underlying this form of learning are not widely distributed in the brain, but are subserved by at least three brain regions. The location of two of these are known—the left and right intermediate medial hyperstriatum ventrale (IMHV). The location of the third, which becomes functional about 6 h after training, is not yet known. Neuronal changes consequent upon training have been identified in the left and right IMHV, but are different in the two regions. As so often in the study of the brain, the situation is turning out to be even more complicated than could have been expected: Horn has been able to show that the changes which bring about strengthening of connections between specific groups of neurons in learning and memory are diverse, involve anatomical and biochemical changes, and occur with differing time courses.

Although this volume is concerned primarily with Horn's academic achievements, I must also mention his contribution as a teacher and administrator. He has held teaching appointments at the Universities of Cambridge and Bristol: at Bristol, he held the Chair of Anatomy from 1974 to 1977. At Cambridge, he was from 1956 to 1972 successively Demonstrator and Lecturer in Anatomy, and from 1972 to 1974 Reader in Neurobiology. After the period in Bristol, he returned to Cambridge in 1977, and was Professor of Zoology until 1995, being Head of Department for 15 of those years. The appointment of an anatomist to a Zoology Chair was in itself noteworthy, since Comparative Anatomy had become unfashionable; but Horn was not that sort of anatomist and had already worked on species ranging from insects to primates—a wider range than many zoologists achieve in a lifetime. He carried the Department through a difficult time, during which Governmental and University bureaucracy demanded far-reaching changes, with consummate skill. He earned gratitude, respect and, especially, affection not only from the academic but also from the technical and administrative staff. He was also Master of Sidney Sussex College, Cambridge, from 1992 to 1999, where his wise and friendly leadership earned him the gratitude of the Fellowship. For four of those years, he was Deputy Vice-Chancellor of the University. In addition, he has held Visiting Lectureships or Research Fellowships at Birmingham, McGill, Gif-sur-Yvette, Edinburgh and Leeds; and Visiting Professorships at Berkeley (twice), Ohio State, Makerere, Edmonton and Hong Kong. He has been a Fellow of the Royal Society since 1986, and a Foreign Fellow of the Academy of Sciences (Republic of Georgia) since 1996. A recognition that gave him particular pleasure was the award of an Honorary Degree from the University of Birmingham, where he had been an undergraduate. His contributions to the Committees of Research Councils and other bodies have been too numerous to list here.

In what some would erroneously call retirement, Gabriel is as hard at it as ever, and the productivity of his group continues unabated. Long may it continue.

REFERENCES

DeAngelis, G.C., Ohzawa, I. and Freeman, R.D. (1995) Receptive field dynamics in the central visual pathways. *Trends in Neurosciences*, 18, 451–458.

Drager, U.C. and Hubel, D.H. (1975) Physiology of visual cells in mouse superior colliculus and correlation with somatosensory and auditory input. *Nature*, 253, 203–204.

Duhamel, J.R., Colby, C.L. and Goldberg, M.E. (1992) The updating of the representation of visual space in parietal cortex by intended eye movements. *Science*, 255, 90–92.

Eayrs, J.T. and Horn, G. (1955) The development of cerebral cortex in hypothyroid and starved rats. *Anatomical Record*, 121, 53–62.

Grave, G.D. (ed.) (1978) *Thyriod Hormones and Brain Development*. Raven Press, New York.

Graziano, M.S.A., Yap, G.S. and Gross, C.G. (1994) Coding of visual space by premotor neurons. *Science*, 266, 1054–7.

Griffith, J.S. and Horn, G. (1963) Functional coupling between cells in the visual cortex of the unrestrained cat. *Nature*, 199, 893–895.

Horn, G. (1960) Electrical activity of the cerebral cortex of the unanaesthitized cat during attentive behaviour. *Brain*, 83, 57–76.

Horn, G. (1965) Physiological and psychological aspects of selective perception. In: Lehrman, D.S., Hinde, R.A. and Shaw, E. (eds), *Advances in the Study of Animal Behaviour*, Vol. 1. Academic Press, New York, pp. 155–215.

Horn, G. (1970) Changes in neuronal activity and their relationship to behaviour. In: Horn, G. and Hinde, R.A. (eds), *Short-term Changes in Neural Activity and Behaviour*. Cambridge University Press, Cambridge, pp. 567–606.

Horn, G. and Hill, R.M. (1964) Habituation of the response to sensory stimuli of neurones in the brain stem of rabbits. *Nature*, 202, 296–298.

Horn, G. and Hill, R.M. (1969) Modifications of receptive fields of cells in the visual cortex occurring spontaneously and associated with body tilt. *Nature*, 221, 186–188.

Jay, M.F. and Sparks, D.L. (1984) Auditory receptive fields in primate superior colliculus shift with changes in eye position. *Nature*, 309, 345–347.

Tomko, D.L., Barbaro, N.M. and Ali, F.N. (1981) Effect of body tilt on receptive field orientation of simple visual cortex neurons in unanaesthetized cats. *Experimental Brain Research*, 43, 309–314.

Wickelgren, B. (1971) Superior colliculus: some receptive field properties of bimodally responsive cells. *Science*, 173, 69–72.

PREFACE

This book is dedicated to Gabriel Horn, who in his distinguished career has achieved major advances in cognitive neuroscience investigating brain, perception and memory. Yet, it is not a *Festschrift* in the conventional sense, for two reasons. First, although officially retired as Professor of Zoology at Cambridge, Gabriel continues with his scientific work as before. Normally, a *Festschrift* is put together for a colleague who has left the field through retirement or otherwise, but that is clearly not the case for Gabriel. In fact, he has such a prominent position in the field that this book would have been incomplete without a chapter by him. Secondly, it is customary that a *Festschrift* consists of contributions from (former) students, close colleagues and collaborators. Again, the present volume is quite different: we have attempted to produce a comprehensive textbook with up to date reviews of the field, written by its leading proponents. Some of these have at some time collaborated with Gabriel, but most of them have not. Several of the contributors to Part one of the present volume came into the field of perception and attention some time after Gabriel Horn's classic work done in the 1960s and 1970s. Their immediate willingness to write a chapter for this book is a tribute to Gabriel's important contributions. Some of the contributors to Parts two and three might be considered representatives of rival paradigms in the competitive field of learning and memory. Without exception, they were keen to contribute to this book, which is testimony to the quality and importance of Horn's work, that transcends the sometimes strong controversies in the study of learning and memory. This is not to say that suddenly everyone agrees about everything: a certain amount of 'agreeing to disagree' is healthy, and will stimulate the growth of knowledge.

This book aims to give an overview of our current knowledge of the essential neural mechanisms of perception, learning and memory, but it also addresses some of the controversies and debates in the field, and highlights some of the recent changes in our conception of these issues. Certainly, there have been many changes since Gabriel Horn entered the field, and he has been instrumental in several of them. This book is a celebration of the scientific research to which he contributed so much. With the Millennium, the 'Decade of the Brain' has come to an end, but the exciting work that is going on—and of which this book is a reflection—suggests that we have entered the Century of Cognitive Neuroscience. In many respects, the study of brain and cognition is still in its infancy, and research in the new millennium will continue to cast new light on these problems, and lead us into fascinating new vistas. Gabriel Horn has often led the way. For those of us who work or have worked with him, he is a great inspiration.

It was a joy to work on this book. I am grateful to all the contributors for their willingness to write a chapter. They were all enthusiastic about contributing to a book in honor of Gabriel Horn, which made my task much easier. Robert Hinde is one of Gabriel's closest friends and colleagues. Previously, they collaborated in organizing a conference and editing a book (*Short-term Changes in Neural Activity and Behaviour*. G. Horn and R.A. Hinde, eds. Cambridge University Press, 1970), which in some way is a forerunner of the present volume. I am delighted that Robert wrote a Foreword for this book. Thanks are due to Vanessa Whitting, Martin Baum, Kate Martin, and their assistants at Oxford University Press for their help in preparing this book. I am very grateful to Gabriel Horn for being a mentor and a friend, and for the many years of fruitful and stimulating collaboration. I also thank him for writing a chapter for this volume. Finally, I want to thank my wife, Zsuzsi, for putting up with my editing efforts at odd hours, and for being who she is.

J.J.B.
Leiden
August 2000

PART ONE   MECHANISMS OF PERCEPTION AND ATTENTION

INTRODUCTION

The first section of this book is concerned with brain mechanisms of perception and attention. It will become clear that Gabriel Horn has played a pioneering role in these fields of research, e.g. concerning body-part-centered visual receptive fields (Horn and Hill, 1969), multisensory integration (Horn and Hill, 1966), attention (Horn, 1965; Horn and Wiesenfeld, 1974) and perceptual predispositions (Horn and McCabe, 1984). Pioneering work is not immediately universally accepted, and Horn's studies ar no exception. For instance, his evidence for visual receptive fields in the cortex changing with body tilt met with considerable scepticism at first. It is gratifying to see that contemporary research, some of which is presented in the present volume, has completely vindicated and extended Horn's original results (Tomko *et al.*, 1981; Jay and Sparks, 1984; Graziano *et al.*, Chapter 1).

In the opening chapter of this section, Michael Graziano, Mary Wheeler and Charles Gross give a fascinating account of recent developments in the study of 'how the primate brain encodes and remembers visuomotor space'. Traditionally, the central sulcus was thought to be the dividing line between sensory areas in the parietal cortex and the motor areas in the frontal cortex. Graziano *et al.* make it quite clear that the brain is much more complicated than that, with considerable overlap in function of various cortical regions. For instance, a large proportion of neurons in the premotor cortex are polysensory, as well as being active during motor acts. Some neurons respond to both tactile and visual stimulation. Interestingly, the visual receptive fields of these neurons are not centered on, say, retinal ganglion cells, but they are 'body part centered', i.e. a particular neuron in premotor cortex will not change its visual receptive field with movements of the eyes, but with movements of, for example, an arm. Graziano *et al.* propose that sensory–motor integration in the primate brain works though body-part-centered coordinate systems. The authors note that the concept of

body-part-centered visual receptive fields was fore-shadowed by the pioneering work of Gabriel Horn and his collaborators in the 1960s and 1970s (Horn and Hill, 1969; Horn *et al.*, 1972), who showed that the receptive fields of neurons in the striate cortex of the cat are modified by body tilt.

The theme of polysensory integration is continued in the following chapter, by Barry Stein, Mark Wallace, Terrence Stanford and John MacHaffie. These authors concentrate on the role of the superior colliculus (SC) of the cat in the integration of information from different senses, an approach that Gabriel Horn had pioneered more than 30 years earlier in the rabbit (Horn and Hill, 1966). Stein *et al.* show that there is a high degree of receptive field alignment in polysensory neurons in the SC, which they suggest is crucial for multisensory integration. The essence of multisensory integration in the SC is that changes in responsiveness of individual neurons in the SC to multiple sensory inputs are more than the sum of the changes in responsiveness to the individual stimuli. These characteristics of the system can also be measured behaviorally. Multisensory integration in the SC is critically dependent upon input from a restricted part of the cortex. Although it is tempting to suggest that this part of the cortex in the cat is functionally equivalent to the region of the primate premotor cortex discussed in the previous chapter, as yet there is insufficient evidence that this is so. In the last part of their chapter, Stein *et al.* show how in cats (unlike monkeys), there is a maturation of poly-sensory characteristics of SC neurons over the first months of life, with sometimes abrupt changes in individual neurons.

Stein *et al.* give a very good working definition of what is known as the *binding problem*: 'how is it we are able to perceive objects as unitary entities when the many features of a complex stimulus are processed separately in different populations of neurons residing in different regions of the nervous system?' (for recent reviews, see Singer, 1999 and other contributions to the September 1999 issue of *Neuron*). This binding problem is central to the following chapter by Wolf Singer. He argues that the brain can process stimulus information accurately within the millisecond range. Such amazing precision cannot rely on the activity of individual neurons, or even on the tuned responses of a 'line' of neurons, but needs a neuronal assembly, such as originally proposed by Hebb (1949). Singer goes on to argue that in a cell assembly, the significance of the responses of individual neurons becomes context dependent, 'and hence in which relationship to others a particular response occurs is of relevance for the interpretation of an assembly code'. The key to the relatedness of the responses of neurons in an assembly is in the synchronicity of individual discharges. Neurons need to be able to synchronize their discharges with a precision that is within the millisecond range. As Singer puts it, '...the nervous system binds the pattern elements that induce synchronized responses and interprets them as components of a coherent figure'. He goes on to suggest that neuronal responses can also become synchronized internally, in the absence of external stimuli. Towards the end of his chapter, Singer argues that response synchonization also plays a role in memory. Later in this book, Malcolm Brown provides a beautiful demonstration of the likely importance of synchronized firing of neurons in the perirhinal cortex of monkeys during recognition memory tests.

John Duncan gives an overview of recent developments in the behavioral and neural analysis of attention. First, he describes the most important behavioral aspects of selective attention. Two important features are competition and bias. The former indicates that, as it were, different stimuli are competing for attention, while the latter suggests that stimuli that may be equally salient may be attended to differentially, depending on their relevance for the current behavioral context. Duncan briefly discusses Bundesen's (1990) Theory of Visual Attention that provides a good model incorporating these aspects of attention. In the second half of this chapter, Duncan discusses the possible neural substrates for visual attention, on the basis of what he calls the *integrated competition hypothesis*. This hypothesis incorporates some of the principles of visual attention derived from behavioral studies, namely competition and bias. Furthermore, it is suggested that the neural substrate for visual attention is not limited to a particular brain region, but that most, if not all visually responsive regions are involved. Neurophysiological data from monkeys and

neuropsychological evidence from human patients with restricted lesions that broadly support the hypothesis are reviewed. At the same time, Duncan concedes that a lot of work is needed to reconcile the neural data with the behavioral evidence. He suggests that a neural network model might be the key to a comprehensive integration of these two domains.

In the final chapter of this section, Johnson and Bolhuis review evidence from animals and humans on the role of predispositions in perceptual development. Their early joint work on filial predispositions in the domestic chick was performed in Gabriel Horn's laboratory in Cambridge (for an earlier review, see Johnson and Bolhuis, 1991). Horn and McCabe (1984) published a re-analysis of a series of experiments involving bilateral lesions to the intermediate and medial hyperstriatum, an area of the chick forebrain that is crucial for the acquisition and retention of imprinting (for reviews, see Horn, 1985, 1998, Chapter 19). In the chick, the system underlying the filial predisposition and that underlying learning (imprinting) are neurally and behaviorally dissociable. A similar distinction can be made in face perception in neonatal human infants, as shown by, for example, the work of Johnson and his collaborators (e.g. Johnson and Morton, 1991). Given the right conditions, neonatal human infants can show a preference for face-like stimuli over non-face-like stimuli. This preference is subserved by subcortical structures, which have a developmental advantage over the neocortex. It is likely that learning the characteristics of individual faces is subserved by the cortex. Thus, there is an interesting parallel in two separate systems underlying perceptual development in chicks and human infants. The authors argue that the notion of predispositions goes beyond the simple idea that cognitive systems are somehow 'innate'. They end their chapter with a consideration of the possible function of predispositions in the development of social behavior.

REFERENCES

Bundesen, C. (1990) A theory of visual attention. *Psychological Review*, 97, 523–547.

Hebb, D.O. (1949) *The Organization of Behavior*. Wiley, New York.

Horn, G. (1965) Physiological and psychological aspects of selective perception. In: Lehrman, D.S. Hinde, R.A. and Shaw, E. (eds), *Advances in the Study of Animal Behaviour*, Vol. 1. Academic Press, New York, pp. 155–215.

Horn, G. (1985) *Memory, Imprinting, and the Brain*. Clarendon Press, Oxford.

Horn, G. (1998) Visual imprinting and the neural mechanisms of recognition memory. *Trends in Neurosciences*, 21, 300–305.

Horn, G. and Hill, R.M. (1966) Responsiveness to sensory stimulation of units in the superior colliculus and subjacent tectotegmental regions of the rabbit. *Experimental Neurology*, 14, 199–223.

Horn, G. and Hill, R.M. (1969) Modifications of receptive fields of cells in the visual cortex occurring spontaneously and associated with body tilt. *Nature*, 221, 186–188.

Horn, G. and McCabe, B.J. (1984) Predispositions and preferences. Effects on imprinting of lesions to the chick brain. *Animal Behaviour*, 32, 288–292.

Horn, G. and Wiesenfeld. Z. (1974) Attention in the cat: electrophysiological and behavioural studies. *Experimental Brain Research*, 21, 67–82.

Horn, G., Stechler, G. and Hill, R.M. (1972) Receptive fields of units in the visual cortex of the cat in the presence and absence of bodily tilt. *Experimental Brain Research*, 15, 113–132.

Jay, M.F. and Sparks, D.L. (1984) Auditory receptive fields in primate superior colliculus shift with changes in eye position. *Nature*, 309, 345–347.

Johnson, M.H. and Bolhuis, J.J. (1991) Imprinting, predispositions and filial preference in the chick. In: Andrew. R.J. (ed.), *Neural and Behavioural Plasticity*. Oxford University Press, Oxford, pp. 133–156.

Johnson, M.H. and Morton, J. (1991) *Biology and Cognitive Development: The Case of Face Recognition*. Blackwell Publishers, Oxford.

Singer, W. (1999) Neuronal synchrony, a versatile code for the definition of relations? *Neuron*, 24, 49–65.

Tomko, D.L., Barbaro, N.M. and Ali, F.N. (1981) Effect of body tilt on receptive field orientation of simple visual cortex neurons in unanaesthetized cats. *Experimental Brain Research*, 43, 309–314.

1 FROM VISION TO ACTION: HOW THE PRIMATE BRAIN ENCODES AND REMEMBERS VISUOMOTOR SPACE

Michael S.A. Graziano, Mary E. Wheeler and Charles G. Gross

INTRODUCTION

In 1870, Fritsch and Hitzig first studied primary motor cortex in the monkey brain using electrical stimulation and, in 1881, Hermann Munk used lesion methods to localize the primary visual cortex in the occipital lobe (cited in Gross, 1998). Only now, more than 100 hundred years later, has neuroscience begun to identify the neuronal pathways that connect these two areas. We are finally beginning to understand the routes through which vision is transformed into action.

Some of the hypothesized visuomotor pathways through the monkey cortex are shown in Figure 1.1 (Desimone and Ungerleider, 1989; Felleman and Van Essen, 1991; Goodale et al., 1994; Wise et al., 1997; Graziano and Gross, 1998b). Information from the eye passes through the lateral geniculate nucleus to primary visual cortex, is processed further by extrastriate visual areas, and reaches the posterior parietal cortex (shown in black in Figure 1.1B). The various posterior parietal areas are thought to encode the movement and spatial locations of objects. This set of parietal areas projects to a variety of frontal lobe areas, such as the frontal and supplementary eye fields, involved in oculomotor control, and the premotor and supplementary motor areas, involved in movements of the head and limbs. These areas, in turn, modulate the activity of motor structures such as primary motor cortex, the spinal cord and eye movement generators in the midbrain and brainstem.

The line between sensory and motor traditionally lies at the central sulcus. A major advance of the past few years, however, is the realization that the planning of movement begins in specialized subregions of the parietal lobe itself (Snyder et al., 1997), and that the processing of sensory space around the body continues into premotor cortex (Fogassi et al., 1996;

Graziano and Gross, 1998b). Indeed, there is accumulating evidence that premotor cortex may participate in a variety of complex sensory and cognitive functions that had never before been ascribed to it, such as visual attention (Graziano and Gross, 1998a) and memory of the locations of objects (Graziano et al., 1997b). Recent evidence suggests that understanding the actions of other individuals may involve using the premotor cortex to process how those actions are coordinated (Gallese and Goldman, 1998).

In this chapter, we concentrate on the visuospatial properties of premotor cortex. In the following section, we describe how single neurons in the ventral part of premotor cortex of the monkey encode the visual, tactile, auditory and even mnemonic space near the body. These neurons represent the locations of nearby objects with respect to individual body parts, in 'body-part-centered' coordinates. This spatial representation is well suited to guide movements of the head and arms toward, away from or around nearby objects. We then consider psychophysical evidence to suggest that a similar, body-part-centered encoding of space is used for the control of movement in humans. In the final section, we briefly review the growing literature on the functional imaging of premotor cortex in the human brain.

REPRESENTATION OF SPACE IN VENTRAL PREMOTOR CORTEX

The ventral premotor cortex, or area PMv, is located in the frontal lobes just posterior to the arcuate sulcus and anterior to primary motor cortex (Figure 1.1). Sensory information can reach PMv through projections from the parietal lobe (Jones and Powell, 1970; Mesulam et al., 1977; Kunzle, 1978; Matelli et al., 1986; Cavada and Goldman-Rakic, 1989), and PMv

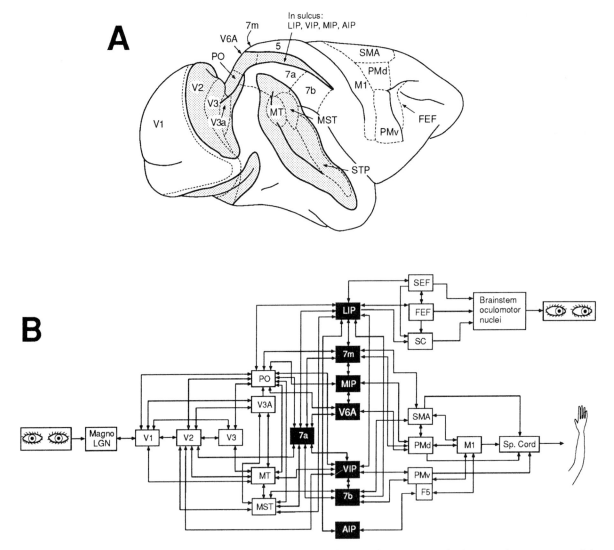

Figure 1.1. Visuomotor pathways of the monkey brain. Top: lateral view of macaque cerebral cortex showing some of the cortical areas involved in the representation of visual space and visuomotor coordination. Major posterior sulci have been 'opened up' to show the buried cortex in grey. Bottom: some of the neuronal pathways by which visual information entering the eye might guide movement of the eyes and limbs. Areas shown in black are in the posterior parietal lobe. SEF, supplementary eye fields; FEF, frontal eye fields; SC, superior colliculus; SMA, supplementary motor area; PMv, ventral premotor cortex; LIP, lateral intraparietal area; VIP, ventral intraparietal area; MIP, medial intraparietal area; AIP, anterior intraparietal area. Adapted from Graziano and Gross (1998b).

can influence movement through its projections to primary motor cortex and the spinal cord (Matsumura and Kubota, 1979; Muakkassa and Strick, 1979; Godschalk *et al.*, 1984; Leichnetz, 1986; Matelli *et al.*, 1986; Barbas and Pandya, 1987; Dum and Strick, 1991; He *et al.*, 1993). Most neurons in PMv respond to tactile stimuli, and about 40% also respond to visual stimuli (Rizzolatti *et al.*, 1981; Graziano *et al.*, 1994,

1997a; Fogassi *et al.*, 1996). These bimodal, visual–tactile neurons are especially numerous in the posterior half of PMv, termed F4; while area F5, the anterior portion of PMv that extends into the posterior bank of the arcuate sulcus, is more involved in the musculature of the fingers and the control of grasp (Gentilucci *et al.*, 1988). Recent evidence (Fogassi *et al.*, 1999) suggests that the cortical region in which bimodal, visual–tactile neurons are found may extend upward from F4 into dorsal premotor cortex (PMd; see Figure 1.1). Here we confine the discussion to the bimodal neurons found in the posterior part of PMv, because they have been studied most extensively; however, similar properties may well exist in PMd.

For the bimodal cells in PMv, the tactile receptive field is located on the face, shoulder, arm or upper torso, and the visual receptive field extends from the approximate region of the tactile receptive field into the immediately adjacent space. PMv is organized somatotopically: from dorsal to ventral, the map progresses from the arm to the face to the inside of the mouth (Graziano *et al.*, 1997a). Visual responses are not found in the mouth representation. Figure 1.2 shows the tactile receptive fields (shaded) and the associated visual receptive fields for two typical bimodal neurons related to the face (Figure 1.1A) and arm (Figure 1.1B). About 20% of the bimodal neurons continue to respond to objects in the visual receptive field even after the lights are turned out and the object is no longer visible (Graziano *et al.*, 1997b). Such neurons apparently 'remember' the locations of nearby objects. Neurons with a tactile response on the side and back of the head often respond to auditory stimuli near the head (Graziano *et al.*, 1999). Regard-

less of the intensity of the sound, if the source is more than about 0.5 m from the head, these neurons do not respond. The multimodal neurons in PMv, therefore, represent the space immediately surrounding the body through touch, audition, vision and memory.

For almost all bimodal cells with a tactile receptive field on the arm, when the arm is placed in different positions, the visual receptive field moves with the arm (Graziano *et al.*, 1994, 1997a). In contrast, when the eyes move, the visual receptive field does not move, but remains anchored to the arm (Gentilucci *et al.*, 1983; Fogassi *et al.*, 1992, 1996; Graziano *et al.*, 1994, 1997a; Graziano and Gross, 1998a). Thus these cells encode the locations of nearby visual stimuli with respect to the arm, i.e. in 'arm-centered' coordinates. Such information can be used to guide the arm toward or away from nearby objects. Some bimodal neurons have tactile receptive fields restricted to the forearm or upper arm. The adjacent visual receptive fields would be useful for guiding those portions of the arm, such as for avoiding or nudging an object or reaching around an obstacle. Other neurons have tactile receptive fields on the hand, and the associated visual receptive fields would be useful for reaching toward nearby objects. A high percentage of arm-related bimodal neurons in PMv are active during movements of the arm, and electrical stimulation of these neurons causes arm movements (Gentilucci *et al.*, 1988).

Other evidence from the monkey supports the hypothesis that reaching with the arm may be controlled in an arm-centered coordinate system. Caminiti *et al.* (1990) recorded from an area on the border of PMv, PMd and primary motor cortex, and found that each neuron responded best as the monkey reached in a particular direction, i.e. the neuron had a motor field. When the arm was moved to a different position, the motor field also moved, rotating roughly with the arm. On average, across the population of neurons, the motor fields were arm centered, moving by the same amount that the shoulder joint rotated, just as the visual receptive fields in our experiments were arm centered.

As described above, premotor cortex also contains a tactile representation of the face and a visual representation of the space near the face. For most bimodal cells with a tactile receptive field on the face, when the head is rotated, the visual receptive field moves with the head (Graziano *et al.*, 1997a). When the eyes move, the visual receptive fields do not move, but remain anchored to the head (Gentilucci *et al.*, 1983;

A   **B**

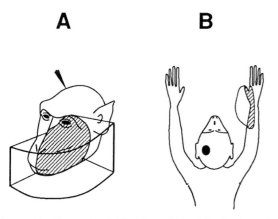

Figure 1.2. Receptive fields of two bimodal, visual–tactile neurons in PMv. (**A**) The tactile receptive field (shaded) is on the snout, mostly contralateral to the recording electrode (indicated by the arrowhead) but extending partially onto the ipsilateral side of the face. The visual receptive field (boxed) is contralateral and confined to a region of space within ~10 cm of the tactile receptive field. (**B**) The tactile receptive field for this neuron is on the hand and forearm contralateral to the recording electrode (indicated by the black dot), and the visual receptive field (outlined) surrounds the tactile receptive field. Adapted from Graziano and Gross (1998b).

Fogassi *et al.*, 1992, 1996; Graziano *et al.*, 1994, 1997a; Graziano and Gross, 1998a). These visual receptive fields, therefore, encode the locations of nearby stimuli relative to the head, in 'head-centered' coordinates, and would be useful for guiding the head toward or away from nearby stimuli, such as for biting, kissing, or flinching. More than half of these head-related bimodal neurons respond during specific voluntary movements of the head (Graziano *et al.*, 1997a).

In summary, neurons in PMv represent the spatial locations of objects within about reaching distance of the body. Any object that enters that critical region of space will activate PMv, whether the monkey senses the object through touch, vision or audition, or even if the monkey is in the dark and 'remembers' that the object is present. The representation of space in PMv is not static, unitary or Euclidian, however. Instead, it is composed of sensory receptive fields anchored to different parts of the body, moving as those body parts move, i.e. in body-part-centered coordinates. We have suggested that such body-part-centered coordinates provide a general mechanism for sensory–motor integration (Graziano *et al.*, 1994, 1997a).

OTHER BODY-PART-CENTERED COORDINATES

Visual receptive fields that do not move with the eye have been reported in a number of different brain areas and species. Such cells have been found by Schlag *et al.* (1980) in the thalamus of the cat, by Pigarev and Rodionova (1988) in parietal cortex of the cat, by Galletti *et al.* (1993) in parietal area V6A of the monkey, and by Duhamel *et al.* (1997) in the ventral intraparietal area of the monkey. Although these visual receptive fields did not move with the eye, it was not clear what part of the body or world they did move with. Therefore, the spatial coordinate systems in these brain areas remain unknown. Wiersma (1966) found visual receptive fields in the crayfish that were influenced by the otolith organs. When the animal's whole body was rotated, the visual receptive fields remained constant with respect to the gravitational vertical. Visual fields influenced by the tilt of the body were also reported in striate cortex of the cat by Gabriel Horn, to whom this book is dedicated (Horn and Hill, 1969).

The frontal eye fields, lateral intraparietal area and the intermediate and deep layers of the superior col-

liculus all guide saccadic eye movements by means of visual and auditory receptive fields that are fixed to the retina (Bruce, 1990; Sparks, 1991; Duhamel *et al.*, 1992; Stricanne *et al.*, 1996). There is evidence that even the tactile receptive fields in the superior colliculus may be anchored to the eye (Groh and Sparks, 1996), i.e. the neurons in these areas encode the location of the target with respect to the fovea, in retinocentric coordinates, even if the target is not a visual one. Such information would be useful for guiding the fovea toward the target. These areas therefore use a type of body-part-centered coordinate system, the body part in this case being the eye ball. The advantage of body-part-centered coordinates is that sensory information about the location of the target can serve as a motor error signal guiding movement toward or away from the target.

EVIDENCE OF BODY-PART-CENTERED COORDINATES IN HUMANS

Is there any evidence that humans use body-part-centered coordinate systems to guide movement? Most studies of visuomotor integration in humans have concentrated on arm movements, specifically reaching toward visual targets. As we discuss below, a number of these studies suggest that the location of the target and the path of the hand movement are encoded in hand-, arm- or shoulder-centered coordinates. Thus humans do appear to use body-part-centered coordinates to guide reaching. We would suggest that these psychophysical results reflect the presence of body-part-centered visual receptive fields in premotor cortex.

Prablanc *et al.* (1986) showed that reaching toward a small visual target is more accurate when the target is visible throughout the reach than when the target is visible only briefly at the beginning of the reach. This result indicates that the reach is not pre-programmed, but depends on the continuous adjustment of the position of the hand relative to the target, i.e. the spatial information most relevant during reaching is body part centered: the relative location of target and hand.

Soechting and Flanders (1989) asked subjects to point to remembered targets, and analyzed the pattern of errors. They found that the errors were most systematic when plotted in a coordinate system whose origin was located roughly at the shoulder. This origin was somewhat variable between tests, ranging in location from the eye to the upper arm. Our hypothesis of body-part-centered coordinate systems, however, predicts that reaching with the hand should be guided by a coordinate system whose origin is fixed to the hand, not to the shoulder. It is important to note that visual information first enters the brain in retinal, or eye-centered, coordinates, and is presumably transformed through many intermediate stages before arriving at hand- or arm-centered coordinates in premotor cortex (Graziano and Gross, 1998b). Therefore, any errors in reaching toward a target may reflect an accumulation across many different coordinate frames. The exact parameters of the reaching task may bias which processing stage and, therefore, which coordinate system contributes most to the systematic errors. Indeed, Gordon *et al.* (1994), using a similar procedure involving reaching toward remembered targets, found different results from those of Soechting and Flanders and concluded that the errors were most systematic in a hand-centered coordinate frame. More recently, McIntyre *et al.* (1998) found that the pattern of errors during reaching supported both an eye-centered and an arm-centered reference frame. Thus, these studies, in which small errors in pointing are analyzed to determine the coordinate system involved in reaching, may well be measuring a summation of many different coordinate systems that lead up to the hand- or arm-centered coordinate systems found in premotor cortex. Taken together, they suggest that visually guided reaching makes use of arm-centered coordinates at some point in the processing sequence.

Tipper *et al.* (1992) found evidence that attention to visual stimuli during a reaching task may be arm centered. In their study, subjects reached for a target while avoiding a distracting stimulus. The reaction times were longer when the distractor lay roughly between the hand and the target. The critical region of visual space, in which the distractor had maximum effect, was anchored to the hand and moved if the hand was placed in different starting locations. This result could be explained by arm-centered visual receptive fields such as those found in monkey premotor cortex.

The psychophysical studies discussed above all emphasize the control of reaching. The study by Tipper *et al.* (1992) investigates visual attention, but again in the context of visually guided reaching. There is evidence that motor planning, such as planning a reach or a saccadic eye movement to a par-

ticular location in space, may feed back on other parts of the brain and influence attention to that location in space (Rizzolatti *et al.*, 1987; Knowler *et al.*, 1994). In this view, covert motor planning is one of the many ways in which spatial attention is shifted from one location to another. If arm movements are planned in arm-centered coordinates, then it may be possible to demonstrate arm-centered spatial attention even when the subject is not explicitly performing a reaching task.

There are two studies that may show this effect of arm position on visual attention. Driver and Spence (1998) found that a touch on the hand enhanced processing of visual stimuli in the space near the hand. When the hand was placed in different locations, the enhanced region of visual space also moved, remaining anchored to the hand.

In another experiment on the relationship between arm position and visual attention, di Pellegrino *et al.* (1997) studied unilateral spatial deficits in stroke patients. In this type of patient, if a single stimulus is presented on the contralesional side, the subject can detect and report the stimulus. If two stimuli are presented simultaneously, one to each side, the patient ignores the contralesional stimulus and reports only the ipsilesional one. This phenomenon is called extinction, and is thought to be caused by an imbalance in attention in which the ipsilesional stimulus out-competes the contralesional one (see Duncan, Chapter 4). In the study by di Pellegrino *et al.* (1997), subjects were asked to detect a tactile stimulus applied to the contralesional hand. When a visual stimulus was presented near the ipsilesional hand, the subjects no longer reported the tactile stimulus, i.e. the tactile stimulus had been extinguished by the competing visual stimulus. The critical region of visual space, in which the competing stimulus was most effective, surrounded the ipsilesional hand and moved if the hand was moved.

In summary, there is accumulating evidence that the human brain uses arm-centered coordinates, both for visually guided reaching and for spatial attention in general. Other coordinate systems and other methods of spatial processing must also be used by the human brain. It is our hypothesis that arm-centered coordinates are especially relevant to the final stages of planning an arm movement under visual guidance, and that head, leg or other body-part-centered coordinate systems would be found if visually guided movements of those body parts were studied.

FUNCTIONAL IMAGING OF PREMOTOR CORTEX IN THE HUMAN BRAIN

Humans presumably have a homolog to the monkey PMv, but the exact location of the area in the human brain is not certain. Frontal lobe lesions produce spatial and visuomotor neglect, but the lesions are relatively large and sometimes include the parietal lobe (Husain and Kennard, 1996). The best evidence for the location of PMv in humans comes from functional imaging studies using positron emission tomography (PET) and functional magnetic resonance imaging (fMRI; see also Dolan, Chapter 17). As described below, many studies that involve visuomotor guidance or visuospatial judgement about objects in relation to the body activate a ventral region in human premotor cortex (Brodmann's area 6). This region is in roughly the same anatomical location as the arm representation of monkey PMv.

In one such experiment using fMRI, Vallar *et al.* (1999) studied the encoding of body-centered space. Subjects viewed a stimulus that oscillated from side to side on a screen. The subjects pressed a button each time they judged the stimulus to be aligned with their own body midline. As a control task, the subjects pressed the button each time the stimulus changed direction at the edge of its trajectory. In comparison with the control task, the spatial judgement task activated regions of the parietal lobe and also a ventral part of premotor cortex. This result matches the single neuron findings in monkeys, in that ventral premotor cortex was active during the representation of space relative to the body.

A number of imaging studies have investigated spatially guided goal-directed movement. In one study using PET (Winstein *et al.*, 1997), subjects moved a stylus rapidly between two visual targets, tapping one and then the other. This study found activation in a range of motor and premotor areas, including the PMv. Several other studies have found activation in a similar ventral part of premotor cortex during observation of objects and motor imagery of grasping and manipulating those objects (Decety *et al.*, 1994; Stephan *et al.*, 1995). Observation of tools, silent naming of tools and silent naming of a tool's use all activated PMv (Martin *et al.*, 1995, 1996; Grafton *et al.*, 1997; Grabowski *et al.*, 1998). Perhaps the subjects imagined grasping the tool as they named it.

Many studies of motor and visuomotor function do not show activation in PMv. For example, studies investigating the preparation or execution of complex finger movement sequences (Rao *et al.*, 1993; Jenkins *et al.*, 1994), motor sequence learning (Grafton *et al.*, 1995; Deiber *et al.*, 1997; Hazeltine *et al.*, 1997; Honda *et al.*, 1998), pointing (Kawashima *et al.*, 1994; Inoue *et al.*, 1998), reaching (Grafton *et al.*, 1996) and several other motor tasks (Deiber *et al.*, 1991; Van Oostende *et al.*, 1997; Grafton *et al.*, 1998; Iacoboni *et al.*, 1998) found activity in more dorsal portions of human premotor cortex and the supplementary motor area but little activity in PMv. One possible reason why these tasks did not activate PMv is that, although many of them were visually cued, few were visually guided. The visual targets were often stationary or the motor actions simple enough and repeated often enough that they did not require constant sensory guidance.

In summary, a ventral region of premotor cortex in the human brain is active in at least some tasks that require spatial and visuomotor processing, suggesting that it may have similar functions to monkey PMv.

CONCLUSIONS

To represent the space around our bodies, and to move within that space, we must put together vision, touch, audition and proprioception, and integrate them with the control of movement. Studies in monkeys and humans are beginning to clarify where and how these signals are combined in the brain. Multisensory and motor signals converge in the posterior parietal lobe. The processing of space and movement continues in premotor areas in the frontal lobe. In particular, area PMv appears to represent the space immediately surrounding the face, arms and upper torso in body-part-centered coordinates. These body-part-centered coordinates can provide a general mechanism for guiding movements of the limbs and head toward, away from or around the everyday objects that surround us.

REFERENCES

Barbas, H. and Pandya, D.N. (1987) Architecture and frontal cortical connections of the premotor cortex (area 6) in the rhesus monkey. *Journal of Comparative Neurology*, 256, 211–228.

Bruce, C.J. (1990) Integration of sensory and motor signals in primate frontal eye fields. In: Edelman, G.M. Gall, W.E. and Cowan, W.M. (eds), *From Signal to Sense: Local and Global Order in Perceptual Maps*. Wiley-Liss, New York, pp. 261–314.

Caminiti, R., Johnson, P.B. and Urbano A. (1990) Making arm movements within different parts of space: dynamic aspects in the primate motor cortex. *Journal of Neuroscience*, 10, 2039–2058.

Cavada, C. and Goldman-Rakic, P.S. (1989) Posterior parietal cortex in rhesus monkey: II: evidence for segregated corticocortical networks linking sensory and limbic areas with the frontal lobe. *Journal of Comparative Neurology*, 287, 422–445.

Decety, J., Perani, D., Jeannerod, M., Bettinardi, V., Tadary, B., Woods, R., Mazziotta, J.C. and Fazio, F. (1994) Mapping motor representations with positron emission tomography. *Nature*, 371, 600–602.

Deiber, M.P., Passingham, R.E., Colebatch, J.G., Friston, K.J., Nixon, P.D. and Frackowiak, R.S. (1991) Cortical areas and the selection of movement: a study with positron emission tomography. *Experimental Brain Research*, 84, 393–402.

Deiber, M.P., Wise, S.P., Honda, M., Catalan, M.J., Grafman, J. and Hallett, M. (1997) Frontal and parietal networks for conditional motor learning: a positron emission tomography study. *Journal of Neurophysiology*, 78, 977–991.

Desimone, R. and Ungerleider, L.G. (1989) Neural mechanisms of visual processing in monkeys. In: Boller, F. and Grafman, J. (eds), *Handbook of Neuropsychology*, Vol. 2. Elsevier, Amsterdam, pp. 267–299.

di Pellegrino, G., Ladavas, E. and Farne, A. (1997) Seeing where your hands are. *Nature*, 388, 730.

Driver, J. and Spence, C. (1998) Crossmodal attention. *Current Opinion in Neurobiology*, 8, 245–253.

Duhamel, J.R., Colby, C.L. and Goldberg, M.E. (1992) The updating of the representation of visual space in parietal cortex by intended eye movements. *Science*, 255, 90–92.

Duhamel, J., Bremmer, F., BenHamed, S. and Gref, W. (1997) Spatial invariance of visual receptive fields in parietal cortex neurons. *Nature*, 389, 845–848.

Dum, R.P. and Strick, P.L. (1991) The origin of corticospinal projections from the premotor areas in the frontal lobe. *Journal of Neuroscience*, 11, 667–689.

Felleman, D.J. and Van Essen, D.C. (1991) Distributed hierarchical processing in primate cerebral cortex. *Cerebral Cortex*, 1, 1–48.

Fogassi, L., Gallese, V., di Pellegrino, G., Fadiga, L., Gentilucci, M., Luppino, M., Pedotti, A. and Rizzolatti, G. (1992) Space coding by premotor cortex. *Experimental Brain Research*, 89, 686–690.

Fogassi, L., Gallese, V., Fadiga, L., Luppino, G., Matelli, M. and Rizzolatti, G. (1996) Coding of peripersonal space in inferior premotor cortex (area F4). *Journal of Neurophysiology*, 76, 141–157.

Fogassi, L., Raos, V., Franchi, G., Gallese, V., Luppino, G. and Matelli, M. (1999) Visual responses in the dorsal premotor area F2 of the macaque monkey. *Experimental Brain Research*, 128, 194–199.

Gallese, V. and Goldman, A. (1998) Mirror neurons and the simulation theory of mind-reading. *Trends in Cognitive Sciences*, 2, 493–501.

Galletti, C., Battaglini, P.P. and Fattori, P. (1993) Parietal neurons encoding spatial locations in craniotopic co-ordinates. *Experimental Brain Research*, 96, 221–229.

Gentilucci, M., Scandolara, C., Pigarev, I.N. and Rizzolatti, G. (1983) Visual responses in the postarcuate cortex (area 6) of the monkey that are independent of eye position. *Experimental Brain Research*, 50, 464–468.

Gentilucci, M., Fogassi, L., Luppino, G., Matelli, M., Camarda, R. and Rizzolatti, G. (1988) Functional organization of inferior area 6 in the macaque monkey. I. Somatotopy and the control of proximal movements. *Experimental Brain Research*, 71, 475–490.

Godschalk, M., Lemon, R.N., Kuypers, H.G.J.M. and Ronday, H.K. (1984) Cortical afferents and efferents of monkey postarcuate area: an anatomical and electrophysiological study. *Experimental Brain Research*, 56, 410–424.

Goodale, M.A., Meenan, J.P., Bültoff, H., Nicolle, D.A., Murphy, K.J. and Racicot, C.I. (1994) Separate neural pathways for the visual analysis of object shape in perception and prehension. *Current Biology*, 4, 604–610.

Gordon, J., Ghilardi, M.F. and Ghez, C. (1994) Accuracy of planar reaching movements. I. Independence of direction and extent variability. *Experimental Brain Research*, 99, 97–111.

Grabowski, T.J., Damasio, H. and Damasio, A.R. (1998) Premotor and prefrontal correlates of category-related lexical retrieval. *Neuroimage*, 7, 232–243.

Grafton, S.T., Hazeltine, E. and Ivry, R. (1995) Functional mapping of sequence learning in normal humans. *Journal of Cognitive Neuroscience*, 7, 497–510.

Grafton, S.T., Fagg, A.H., Woods, R.P. and Arbib, M.A. (1996) Functional anatomy of pointing and grasping in humans. *Cerebral Cortex*, 6, 226–237.

Grafton, S.T., Fadiga, L., Arbib, M.A. and Rizzolatti, G. (1997) Premotor cortex activation during observation and naming of familiar tools. *Neuroimage*, 6, 231–236.

Grafton, S.T., Fagg, A.H. and Arbib, M.A. (1998) Dorsal premotor cortex and conditional movement selection: a PET functional mapping study. *Journal of Neurophysiology*, 79, 1092–1097.

Graziano, M.S.A. and Gross, C.G. (1998a) Visual responses with and without fixation: neurons in premotor cortex encode spatial locations independently of eye position. *Experimental Brain Research*, 118, 373–380.

Graziano, M.S.A. and Gross, C.G. (1998b) Spatial maps for the control of movement. *Current Opinion in Neurobiology*, 8, 195–201.

Graziano, M.S.A., Yap, G.S. and Gross, C.G. (1994) Coding of visual space by premotor neurons. *Science*, 266, 1054–7.

Graziano, M.S.A., Hu, X.T. and Gross, C.G. (1997a) Visuospatial properties of ventral premotor cortex. *Journal of Neurophysiology*, 77, 2268–2292.

Graziano, M.S.A., Hu, X.T. and Gross, C.G. (1997b) Coding the locations of objects in the dark. *Science*, 277, 239–241.

Graziano, M.S.A., Reiss, L.A.J. and Gross, C.G. (1999) A neuronal representation of the location of nearby sounds. *Nature*, 397, 428–430.

Groh, J.M. and Sparks, D.L. (1996) Saccades to somatosensory targets. III. Eye-position-dependent somatosensory activity in primate superior colliculus. *Journal of Neurophysiology*, 75, 439–453.

Gross, C.G. (1998) *Brain, Vision, Memory: Tales in the History of Neuroscience*. MIT Press, Cambridge, Massachusetts.

Hazeltine, E., Grafton, S.T. and Ivry, R. (1997) Attention and stimulus characteristics determine the locus of motor-sequence encoding. A PET study. *Brain*, 120, 123–140.

He, S., Dum, R.P. and Strick, P.L. (1993) Topographic organization of corticospinal projections from the frontal lobe: motor areas on the lateral surface of the hemisphere. *Journal of Neuroscience*, 13, 952–980.

Honda, M., Deiber, M.P., Ibanez, V., Pascual-Leone, A., Zhuang, P. and Hallet, M. (1998) Dynamic cortical involvement in implicit and explicit motor sequence learning. A PET study. *Brain*, 121, 2159–2173.

Horn, G. and Hill, R.M. (1969) Modifications of receptive fields of cells in the visual cortex occurring spontaneously and associated with body tilt. *Nature*, 221, 186–188.

Husain, M. and Kennard, C. (1996) Visual neglect associated with frontal lobe infarction. *Journal of Neurology*, 243, 652–657.

Iacoboni, M., Woods, R.P. and Mazziotta, J.C. (1998) Bimodal (auditory and visual) left frontoparietal circuity for sensorimotor integration and sensorimotor learning. *Brain*, 121, 2135–2143.

Inoue, K., Kawashima, R., Satoh, K., Kinomura, S., Goto, R., Koyama, M., Sugiura, M., Ito, M. and Fukuda, H. (1998) Pet study of pointing with visual feedback of moving hands. *Journal of Neurophysiology*, 79, 117–125.

Jenkins, I.H., Brooks, D.J., Nixon, P.D., Frackowiak, R.S.J. and Passingham, R.E. (1994) Motor sequence learning: a study with positron emission tomography. *Journal of Neuroscience*, 14, 3775–3790.

Jones, E.G. and Powell, T.P.S. (1970) An anatomical study of converging sensory pathways within the cerebral cortex of the monkey. *Brain*, 93, 739–820.

Kawashima, R., Roland, P.E. and O'Sullivan, B.T. (1994) Fields in human motor areas involved in preparation for reaching, actual reaching, and visuo-motor learning: a positron emission tomography study. *Journal of Neuroscience*, 14, 3462–3474.

Knowler, E., Anderson, E., Dosher, B. and Blaser, E. (1995) The role of attention in the programming of saccades. *Vision Research*, 35, 1897–1916.

Kunzle, H. (1978) An autoradiographic analysis of the efferent connections from premotor and adjacent prefrontal regions (areas 6 and 8) in *Macaca fascicularis*. *Brain and Behavioral Evolution*, 15, 185–234.

Leichnetz G.R. (1986) Afferent and efferent connections of the dorsolateral precentral gyrus (area 4, hand/arm region) in the macaque monkey, with comparison to area 8. *Journal of Comparative Neurology*, 254, 460–492.

Martin, A., Haxby, J.V., Lalonde, F.M., Wiggs, C.L. and Ungerleider, L.G. (1995) Discrete cortical regions associated with knowledge of color and knowledge of action. *Science*, 270, 102–105.

Martin, A., Wiggs, C.L., Ungerleider, L.G. and Haxby, J.V. (1996) Neural correlates of category-specific knowledge. *Nature*, 379, 649–652.

Matelli, M., Camarda, R., Glickstein, M. and Rizzolatti, G. (1986) Afferent and efferent projections of the inferior area 6 in the macaque monkey. *Journal of Comparative Neurology*, 255, 281–298.

Matsumura, M. and Kubota, K. (1979) Cortical projection to hand–arm motor area from post-arcuate area in macaque monkeys: a histological study of retrograde transport of horseradish peroxidase. *Neuroscience Letters*, 11, 241–246.

McIntyre, J., Stratta, F. and Lacquaniti, F. (1998) Short-term memory for reaching to visual targets: psychophysical

evidence for body-centered reference frames. *Journal of Neuroscience*, 18, 8423–8435.

Mesulam, M.-M., Van Hoesen, G.W., Pandya, D.N. and Geschwind, N. (1977) Limbic and sensory connection of the inferior parietal lobule (area PG) in the rhesus monkey: a study with a new method for horseradish peroxidase histochemistry. *Brain Research*, 136, 393–414.

Muakkassa, K.F. and Strick, P.L (1979) Frontal lobe inputs to primate motor cortex: evidence for four somatotopically organized 'premotor' areas. *Brain Research*, 177, 176–182.

Pigarev, I.N. and Rodionova, E.I. (1988) Neurons with visual receptive fields independent of the position of the eyes in cat parietal cortex. *Sensornie Sistemi*, 2, 245–254.

Prablanc, C., Pelisson, D. and Goodale, M.A. (1986) Visual control of reaching movements without vision of the limb. I. Role of retinal feedback of target position in guiding the hand. *Experimental Brain Research*, 62, 293–302.

Rao, S.M., Binder, J.R., Bandettini, P.A., Hammeke, T.A., Yetkin, F.Z., Jesmanowicz, A. *et al.* (1993) Functional magnetic resonance imaging of complex human movements. *Neurology*, 43, 2311–2318.

Rizzolatti, G., Scandolara, C., Matelli, M. and Gentilucci, M. (1981) Afferent properties of periarcuate neurons in macaque monkeys. II. Visual responses. *Behavioural Brain Research*, 2, 147–163.

Rizzolatti, G., Riggio, L., Dascola, I. and Umilta, C. (1987) Reorienting attention across the horizontal and vertical meridians: evidence in favor of a premotor theory of attention. *Neuropsychologia*, 25, 31–40.

Schlag, J., Schlag-Rey, M., Peck, C.K. and Joseph, J.P. (1980) Visual responses of thalamic neurons depending on the direction of gaze and the position of targets in space. *Experimental Brain Research*, 40, 170–184.

Snyder, L.H., Batista, A.P. and Andersen, R.A. (1997) Coding of intention in the posterior parietal cortex. *Nature*, 386, 167–170.

Sparks, D.L. (1991) The neural encoding of the location of targets for saccadic eye movements. In: Paillard, J. (ed.), *Brain and Space*. Oxford University Press, New York, pp. 3–19.

Stephan, K.M., Fink, G.R., Passingham, R.E., Silbersweig, D., Ceballos-Baumann, A.O., Frith, C.D. and Frackowiak, R.S.J. (1995) Functional anatomy of the mental representation of upper extremity movements in healthy subjects. *Journal of Neurophysiology*, 73, 373–386.

Stricanne, B., Andersen, A. and Mazzoni, P. (1996) Eye-centered, head-centered and intermediate coding of remembered sound locations in area LIP. *Journal of Neurophysiology*, 76, 2071–2076.

Soechting, J.F. and Flanders, M. (1989) Sensorimotor representations for pointing to targets in three-dimensional space. *Journal of Neurophysiology*, 62, 582–594.

Tipper, S.P., Lortie, C. and Baylis, G.C. (1992) Selective reaching: evidence for action-centered attention. *Journal of Experimental Psychology: Human Perception and Performance*, 18, 891–905.

Vallar, G., Lobel, E., Galati, G., Berthoz, A., Pizzamiglio, L. and Bihan, D. (1999) A fronto-parietal system for computing egocentric spatial frame of reference in humans. *Experimental Brain Research*, 124, 281–286.

Van Oostende, S., Van Heck, P., Sunaert, S., Nuttin, B. and Marchal, G. (1997) fMRI studies of the supplementary motor area and the premotor cortex. *Neuroimage*, 6, 181–190.

Wiersma, C.A.G. (1966) Integration in the visual pathway of crustacea. *Symposium for the Society of Experimental Biology*, 20, 151–177.

Winstein, C.J., Grafton, S.T. and Pohl, P.S. (1997) Motor task difficulty and brain activity: investigation of goal-directed reciprocal aiming using positron emission tomography. *Journal of Neurophysiology*, 77, 1581–1594.

Wise, S.P., Boussaoud, D., Johnson, P.B. and Caminiti, R. (1997) Premotor and parietal cortex: corticocortical connectivity and combinatorial computations. *Annual Review of Neuroscience*, 20, 25–42.

2 INTEGRATING INFORMATION FROM DIFFERENT SENSES IN THE SUPERIOR COLLICULUS

Barry E. Stein, Mark T. Wallace, Terrence R. Stanford and John G. McHaffie

INTRODUCTION

It is interesting to note that many of the most timely discussions of sensory and intersensory function reiterate long-standing philosophical and biological speculations. Indeed, the often recurring arguments about whether the same stimulus produces equivalent sensory impressions in different individuals or whether the senses can provide reliable information about the world were issues that provoked enthusiastic debate during the Platonic age of ancient Greece (for a discussion, see Watson, 1968). Followers of Protagoras, known as the Sophists, argued that sensory impressions are subjective and idiosyncratic, and, as a result, real knowledge of the world is impossible. Plato, although less damning in his critique of sensory information, was still less than enamored of its veracity and dependability. Not being a proponent of the experimental method, he felt that the senses provide only shadows, or reflections, of universal truths, and that these truths are approachable only via the mind or 'soul'.

It was Plato's intellectual successor in Athens, Aristotle, whose scientific and philosophical postulates have an almost eerie modernity. He believed that while sensory information is an essential first step in the acquisition of knowledge, it first must be interpreted and placed in context by higher order processes. This sounds much like any current treatise on perception. Aristotle's views of the aggregate function of the various senses seem particularly fitting in the current context in which problems inherent in understanding intersensory processes are approached. For Aristotle was one of the first to grapple with the concept of intersensory integration. He recognized that while each of the five senses provides us with different information, we perceive a single world. His conclusion was that there must be mechanisms whereby the information derived from different sensory organs is brought together into a unified whole, a view that anticipated modern discussions of what has become known as the 'binding' problem. In other words, how is it we are able to perceive objects as unitary entities when the many features of a complex stimulus are processed separately in different populations of neurons residing in different regions of the nervous system? The problem is the same regardless of whether these different stimulus features are extracted and processed by different populations of modality-specific neurons (e.g. visual versus auditory) or by different populations of neurons within a modality (e.g. those in the visual system primarily responsive to motion, or color or form).

Although the brain obviously has little difficulty in solving this 'problem', there currently is no generally accepted unifying hypothesis that explains how it accomplishes this feat. While the purpose of the present chapter is not to discuss the binding problem *per se* (but see Treisman, 1996; Hardcastle, 1998; Singer, Chapter 3), its discussion of the convergence and integration of multiple sensory inputs is certainly germane to this problem.

THE CONVERGENCE OF MULTIPLE SENSORY INPUTS

There is a vast literature detailing the anatomical, physiological and psychophysical properties of the different senses. The greatest emphasis has been placed on vision, audition and somesthesis (including pain), in part because we depend heavily on these senses to evaluate events in the external world and in part because these modalities, and their related neural structures, are most amenable to experimental manipulation and evaluation. Because most of these inquiries have been focused on a single sensory modality, one could form the impression that the fundamental architecture of the brain restricts information processing to a sense-by-sense analysis. However, there are many areas of the brain that are 'multisensory' by virtue of the fact that they receive converging inputs from two or more senses. These areas are quite common outside the primary projection pathways and are present at all levels of the neuraxis (see also Graziano *et al.*, Chapter 1). Indeed, the ability to segregate sensory information within the primary sensory nuclei reflects a more recent evolutionary development than the pooling of information from multiple senses. For example, primordial unicellular organisms are believed to have had more than one type of sensory receptor and were, therefore, both a multisensory cell and a multisensory organism. Such an organism would be a *de facto* multisensory integrator, because all sensory inputs would contribute to the cell's membrane potential via the current fluxes they influenced. Many primitive invertebrates are also unable to sequester specific sensory signals because of the nature of their cellular contacts, and the segregation of information on a sense-by-sense basis probably did not occur in nature until the appearance of rather advanced multicellular organisms (for a review, see Stein and Meredith, 1993).

In all higher order animals, the foundation for integrating cross-modality information is provided by the anatomical convergence of inputs from multiple senses onto common neuronal pools (Figure 2.1).

Because this takes place in a variety of structures that are widely dispersed throughout the nervous system, and because these structures are involved in many different functions, multisensory integration undoubtedly has widespread influences on perception and behavior. The possibility that we may come to understand the neural principles underlying this integration was the motivation for much of the research described in this chapter.

At first inspection, it may seem counterintuitive that information from different senses is integrated commonly in the nervous system, not only because so much biological energy appears to have been devoted to evolving unique sets of peripheral receptors for each sense, but because each of the senses is so closely tied to a unique subjective impression. Although we commonly may refer to the smell of grass as green, there really is no equivalence in the different senses for the peculiar sensations they evoke. Thus, pitch is exclusive to the auditory system, tickle and itch to the somatosensory system, hue to the visual system, saltiness to the gustatory system, etc. The unique nature of these subjective impressions is underscored by the difficulty in trying to describe music to the congenitally deaf or color to the congenitally blind.

How, then, can these modality-specific impressions be maintained if the inputs from the different senses are integrated in widespread areas of the brain? The answer appears to lie in a peculiar duality that exists in the nervous systems of higher organisms. The primary projection nuclei are designed specifically for processing modality-specific information and are probably responsible for the specificity of the sub-

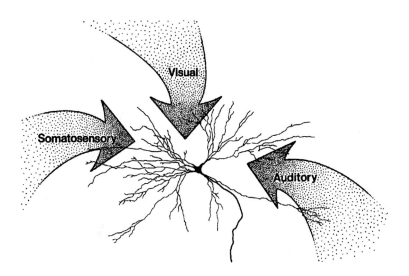

Figure 2.1. Inputs from multiple sensory modalities converge on individual neurons at many levels of the neuraxis. From Stein and Meredith (1993).

jective impressions that characterize each sense. In contrast, other regions are designed for integrating information regardless of its modality-specific source. These multisensory regions are unlikely to play a significant role in evoking the unique subjective impressions that characterize each modality, but, as noted earlier, are likely to play critical roles in assessing environmental cues and guiding reactions to them. For example, the detection and reaction to a given modality-specific stimulus is significantly enhanced in the presence of a stimulus from another sensory modality (Stein *et al.*, 1989). Thus, the latencies of eye movements to visual or auditory stimuli can be substantially longer than those for combined stimuli (Zahn *et al.*, 1978; Zambarbieri *et al.*, 1982; Lueck *et al.*, 1990; Perrott *et al.*, 1990; Lee *et al.*, 1991; Hughes *et al.*, 1994; Frens *et al.*, 1995; Corneil and Munoz, 1996; Goldring *et al.*, 1996). These cross-modal interactions have been shown to be influenced by attention (Spence and Driver, 1996).

Because it is difficult to imagine any situation in a normal environment in which cues from only one modality are present, multisensory integration is almost certainly a continuous process. Yet, it is one of which we are generally unaware. This is best illustrated when multiple sensory cues are discordant, thereby producing any one of a host of striking cross-modality illusions. One such illusion is the 'McGurk effect' (McGurk and McDonald, 1976). It is particularly popular among speech professionals because it demonstrates how important sight is in understanding speech. In an example of this illusion, when one hears the word 'bows' but sees the mouth form the word 'goes' the perception is 'doze' or 'those', a synthesis of the visual and auditory inputs. The sight of moving lips can also cause us to mislocate a sound, an effect referred to as the 'ventriloquism effect' (Howard and Templeton, 1966) for obvious reasons, and one we experience whenever we watch a movie. Even though the actors move across a very wide screen, and the sound originates from speakers fixed in space and far from their images on the screen, their voices always seem to be coming from their mouths. Cross-modality illusions can be obtained with a variety of sensory combinations, and an interesting tactile–auditory illusion called the 'parchment-skin illusion' has been reported recently by Jousmaki and Hari (1998). In this case, one's tactile perception of roughness is strongly influenced by the frequency of a sound one hears through headphones.

The list of cross-modality illusions is quite long and, although fascination with a number of them has produced a wealth of perceptual and behavioral observations (for further discussion, see Welch and Warren, 1986; Stein and Meredith, 1993), there have been relatively few corresponding neural studies. In part, this paucity of neural information was due to the inherent problems in assessing interactions among modalities and linking these observations to specific perceptual or behavioral events. In recent years, however, a midbrain structure, the superior colliculus (SC), has been used as an effective model system with which to examine these processes at the level of the individual neuron and relate these neural phenomena to overt behaviors.

THE SUPERIOR COLLICULUS (SC) AS A MODEL FOR UNDERSTANDING MULTISENSORY INTEGRATION

The SC has been a productive model for these studies because it contains a high incidence of multisensory neurons, making it possible to make numerous observations of how multisensory neurons respond to various stimulus combinations. Equally important, however, is the fact that the SC is at the interface between sensory and motor processing. This organization enables parallels to be drawn between the impact of various stimulus combinations on sensory activity and their impact on motor behaviors (i.e. orienting) mediated by the SC. Specifically, the circuitry of the SC is believed to use visual, auditory and somatosensory inputs in concert (as well as individually) to initiate coordinated movements of the eyes, ears, head and body toward the location of these stimuli (Stein *et al.*, 1989; see also Sprague and Meikle, 1965; Schneider, 1969; Casagrande *et al.*, 1972; Goodale and Murison, 1975; Sparks, 1986; Stein and Meredith, 1991, 1993).

Comparing the data obtained from the SC with multisensory integration in cortical neurons has also provided intriguing insights into the possibility that some of the same principles of integration may be used by neurons in very different circuits to influence very different perceptual and behavioral processes (e.g. see Stein and Wallace, 1996). Before discussing the specifics of SC multisensory integration, however, it is helpful first to examine briefly some of the organizational principles of the structure that are relevant to this phenomenon. Because it is the deep layers of the SC that contain its multisensory neurons (super-ficial layer neurons are purely visual), as well as the premotor circuitry through which it effects overt responses, it is this division that will be the focus of discussion. Furthermore, because most of the data regarding SC multisensory integration come from experiments in cats, unless otherwise stated, this will be the referent species.

Most deep layer SC neurons have sensory responses, but some have been found to be exclu-sively premotor, while others are both sensory and premotor. Many neurons are selective for the location of sensory stimuli and/or for the metrics (i.e. ampli-tude and direction) of a shift in gaze. This selectivity is manifested in neurons with sensory-related proper-ties by each neuron responding only to stimuli within the restricted region of space called its receptive field. Such neurons may be unimodal (responding only to visual, auditory or somatosensory stimuli and having a single receptive field) or multisensory, responding to stimuli from two or even three sensory modalities and having multiple receptive fields (one for each effective modality). Analogously, neurons with motor-related activity exhibit their selectivity via their move-ment fields; they discharge only in association with orienting movements (e.g. gaze shifts) within a particular range of amplitudes and directions.

TOPOGRAPHIC REGISTER AMONG SENSORY AND MOTOR REPRESENTATIONS

Both the sensory and motor representations in the SC are organized topographically. Accordingly, the locus of sensory-related activity shifts with the spatial location of the sensory stimulus, while the locus of motor-related activity depends on the vector (i.e. the amplitude and direction) of the desired orienting movement. At first glance, it would seem that a simple point-to-point correspondence between sen-sory and motor topographies could serve as a very efficient mechanism for translating sensory signals into appropriate motor commands. However, the problem of establishing meaningful alignment be-tween SC sensory and motor maps is not as straight-forward as one might think. The difficulty arises because each sensory system uses its own frame of reference for locating stimuli: the visual axes are referred to the retina, acoustic axes to the head (i.e. the relative position of the ears) and the location of a

tactile stimulus is referred to the body surface. Further complicating the issue is the fact that these sensory reference frames can move independently of one another, thereby eliminating the possibility of a one-to-one correspondence between a coordinate in one reference frame and that in another. Neither is there a unique relationship between the position of a stimulus in any sensory coordinate frame and the vector of a movement that would be required to orient to it. For example, the amplitude and direction of a gaze shift required to look at a stimulus on the forearm (or forepaw) depends on many factors, including the relative positions of the limb, the head and the eyes. Similarly, the gaze shift required to look toward an auditory stimulus changes as a function of the position of the eyes in the orbit.

If each sensory modality were encoded in its native reference frame (i.e. eye-centered, head-centered or body-centered), fixed registration between the indivi-dual sensory and motor topographies would not be possible. However, studies of gaze using behaving animals indicate that compensatory mechanisms attempt to maintain receptive field register and con-sistency between the loci of sensory- and motor-related activity when the eyes move within the head. These studies have shown that auditory and somato-sensory receptive fields can be remapped dynamically as a function of eye position in the orbit (Jay and Sparks, 1987a,b; Hartline *et al.*, 1995; Peck *et al.*, 1995; Groh and Sparks, 1996) and suggest that 'sensory' representations in the SC have been translated from their native reference frames to a common 'motor' coordinate frame (e.g. see Sparks and Nelson, 1987).

The translation of sensory signals into a common coordinate frame ensures registration among modality-specific sensory receptive fields and, consequently, guarantees that motor responses will be consistent across stimulus modalities. Along with its implica-tions for sensorimotor transformation, receptive field register is crucial for multisensory integration (see below). While studies in awake animals have revealed this feature of the sensory maps, details of this cross-modal receptive field register have been best studied in anesthetized cats in which the eyes, ears and body are all directed forward. This posture, which places the individual sensory coordinate frames in approxi-mate alignment, permits detailed comparisons of the modality-specific maps. The results of such studies suggest a high degree of spatial register among the maps representing visual, auditory and somato-sensory space. Visually responsive neurons with receptive fields in forward or central visual space are located in the rostral portion of the structure, along with neurons having forward or central auditory receptive fields and neurons having somatosensory receptive fields on the head and face. At progressively more caudal locations, visual and auditory receptive fields are located more peripherally in space, and somatosensory receptive fields are located more caudally on the body. In a similar manner, the superior–inferior axis of sensory space is laid out along the medial–lateral axis of the SC (Stein and Meredith, 1993). As would be expected, the topographies of the sensory representations are consistent with the topography of the motor map. For example, a visual or auditory stimulus located slightly to the left and up would produce activity in the rostro-medial aspect of the right SC, a region in which premotor activity results in a small leftward gaze shift with an upward component (for details of the SC motor topography, see Sparks, 1986). The functional details of the motor representation have been best described for eye movements and combined eye–head gaze shifts (described below) but, presumably, the same principles apply to other types of movement (e.g. ear movements) (Robinson, 1972; Roucoux and Crommelinck, 1976; Harris, 1980; Stein and Clamann, 1981; McHaffie and Stein, 1982; Sparks, 1986; McIlwain, 1991).

This topographic sensory scheme is not specific to the cat, but has also been demonstrated in monkey (Wallace *et al.*, 1996), hamster (Tiao and Blakemore, 1976; Chalupa and Rhoades, 1977; Finlay *et al.*, 1978; Stein and Dixon, 1979), mouse (Drager and Hubel, 1975; Benedetti, 1991), rat (McHaffie *et al.*, 1989), rabbit (Horn and Hill, 1966) and guinea pig (King and Palmer, 1985). It has also been found in the optic tecta (the non-mammalian homolog of the SC) of birds, reptiles, amphibians and fish (Hartline *et al.*, 1978; Stein and Gaither, 1981; Knudsen, 1982; Bullock, 1984; see also Stein and Meredith, 1993). The fact that this same organizational plan is apparent at different phyletic levels and in animals living in varying habitats suggests that it is not only an ancient one, but one that is adaptable in very different ecological situations. As might be expected, receptive field alignment shows the greatest fidelity among multisensory neurons and, as discussed below, plays a critical role in dictating the nature of multisensory interactions. Though the fidelity of cross-modality receptive field alignment is particularly striking in multisensory SC neurons (Figure 2.2), similar cross-modality receptive field register is found in individual neurons in other

multisensory structures, especially in cortex (e.g. see Bruce *et al.*, 1981; Rizzolatti *et al.*, 1981a,b; Duhamel *et al.*, 1991; Wallace *et al.*, 1992; Ramachandran *et al.*, 1993; Stein *et al.*, 1993; Fogassi *et al.*, 1996; Graziano *et al.*, 1997; see also Graziano *et al.*, Chapter 1), suggesting that its importance may transcend SC-mediated functions, and may in fact represent a universal organizational principle for multisensory structures throughout the brain.

MULTISENSORY INTEGRATION

The spatial correspondence among the multiple receptive fields of an individual multisensory neuron is important in the current context because maintaining this correspondence is critical for the integration of multisensory information (see below). At the neural level, the integration of multiple sensory inputs can result in a dramatic increase in the number of impulses evoked above that elicited by the

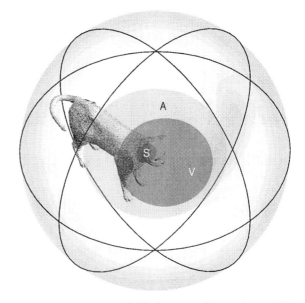

Figure 2.2. Receptive field alignment characterizes multisensory neurons. In this schematized diagram, the receptive fields of an individual SC neuron in the cat are shown. For this neuron, a somatosensory receptive field on the head (S; darkest shading) is matched with visual and auditory receptive fields in corresponding regions of extrapersonal space (V and A; lighter shading). Extrapersonal receptive fields are illustrated on an imaginary bubble, which surrounds the animal. Azimuthal, elevation and interaural axes are shown with lines.

individual stimuli (a 'response enhancement' that can exceed the sum of the two modality-specific responses), or a significant decrement below that elicited by either of the individual stimuli (a 'response depression' that sometimes eliminates responses altogether). Both response enhancement and response depression can be exhibited by the same neuron and depend on a variety of factors, one of which is the spatial relationship of the stimuli to one another and to their respective receptive fields.

Spatial influences on multisensory integration

When two different sensory stimuli originate from the same location in space, as when they arise from the same event, they fall within the respective (overlapping) receptive fields of a given multisensory neuron. Such a combination usually yields a substantially enhanced neural response (Figure 2.3). If, on the other

hand, the stimuli are spatially disparate (and unlikely to be causally related), so that one of them originates from a location outside its modality-specific receptive field, no enhancement of the response to the other stimulus occurs (Figure 2.3). Also, if that stimulus falls within the inhibitory region of its receptive field, it will depress (and may eliminate) responses to the other stimulus (Kadunce *et al.*, 1997). Note that whereas response enhancement could serve to facilitate orienting responses to a stimulus combination at a particular spatial location, response depression serves to prevent such responses to conflicting movement goals resulting from spatially disparate stimulus combinations.

Effectiveness

The effectiveness of the individual stimuli in activating a given multisensory neuron also plays an import-

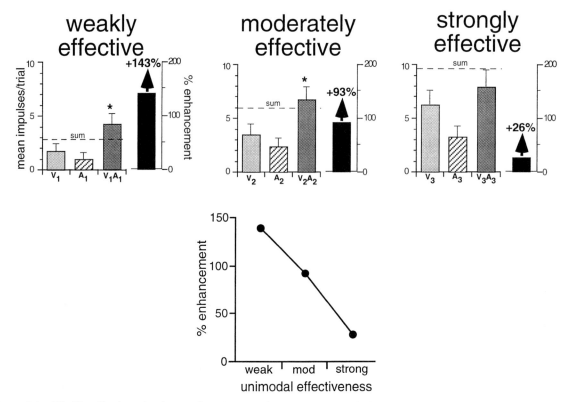

Figure 2.4. Weakly effective stimulus combinations result in proportionately larger response enhancements. In these histograms and summary bar graphs illustrating responses from a single SC neuron, the pairing of visual and auditory stimuli that are weakly effective when presented individually results in a large superadditive (i.e. greater than the sum) interaction (top left). When those stimuli are made more effective, the combined response becomes an additive interaction (top middle) and, finally, a subadditive interaction when the stimuli are made strongly effective (top right). The bottom graph plots the change in enhancement as a function of stimulus effectiveness. *P <0.05.

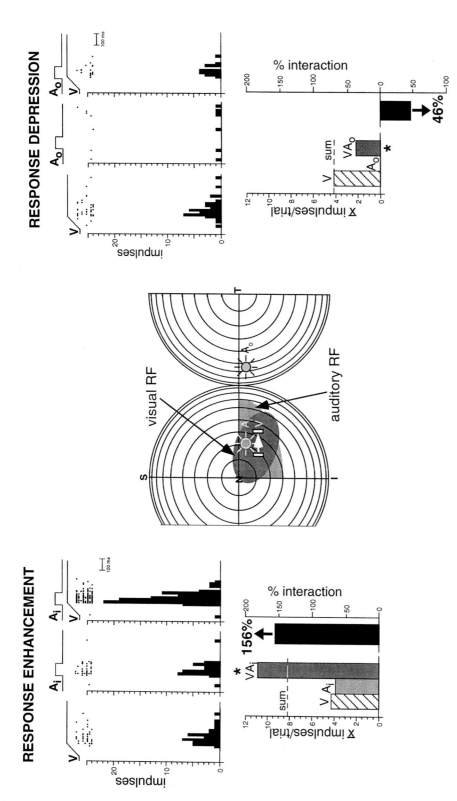

Figure 2.3. Response enhancement and response depression are often found in the same multisensory neuron and depend on the spatial relationships of the stimuli. The visual and auditory receptive fields of this representative SC neuron are shown as shaded regions plotted onto a conventional representation of visual and auditory space (center). In this representation, each concentric circle represents 10°, and the right half circle shows the caudal half of contralateral auditory space. Icons show the locations of the visual (V; moving bar of light) and auditory (A; broad band noise burst from a fixed speaker) stimuli used in the sensory tests. Rasters, histograms and summary bar graphs show that when either stimulus is presented within its receptive field (V and A_i), a modest sensory response is elicited (left). However, the combination of these stimuli results in a significant response enhancement that exceeds the sum of the two unimodal responses. In contrast, when the auditory stimulus is presented outside its receptive field (A_o), its pairing with the same visual stimulus results in a significant response depression (right). S = superior, I = inferior, N = nasal, T = temporal. *P <0.05.

ant role in determining the magnitude of the neural response produced by their combined presentation. Thus, the more effective a given modality-specific stimulus is when presented alone, the less the response to it can be enhanced by the addition of a stimulus from the second modality. However, when each modality-specific stimulus is only mimimally effective, their combination results in a response that often exceeds the response predicted by summing the two unimodal responses (i.e. a superadditive interaction). This principle, known as *inverse effectiveness*, is illustrated in Figure 2.4.

Time

The relative timing of multisensory stimuli is also an important factor in determining the magnitude of their interaction. When stimuli are widely separated in time, they are, not surprisingly, treated as independent events. Nevertheless, the temporal delay during which multisensory interactions can occur is quite long, and for some neurons can be hundreds of milliseconds (Meredith *et al.*, 1987; Wallace and Stein, 1997a). Such a broad temporal window for integration obviates the need for inputs from different modalities to arrive at the neuron at precisely the same time in

order to be integrated. This relatively broad temporal window is critical because neurons throughout the nervous system have very different response latencies to different sensory modalities. For example, auditory and somatosensory response latencies for SC neurons are of the order of 10–25 ms, while their visual response latencies range from 40 to 120 ms. However, the effect of each sensory input lasts for some time and, if during this period a sensory input from a second modality arrives, it will be integrated with that of the first.

Multisensory neurons show a good deal of variability in the optimum temporal intervals that give rise to maximal response enhancements. Some show their greatest response enhancement when the stimuli are presented simultaneously, whereas others prefer a lag between the onset of one stimulus and the onset of the other. Despite these differences in temporal tuning, most neurons show a reasonably sharp decline in their response magnitude when the stimulus onset asynchrony is 50–100 ms from the optimum, as depicted in Figure 2.5 (see also Meredith *et al.*, 1987; Wallace and Stein, 1997a). This finding suggests that such neurons are tuned to events that take place at different distances from the animal and thus respond best to stimuli that have onset asynchronies consistent with these distances.

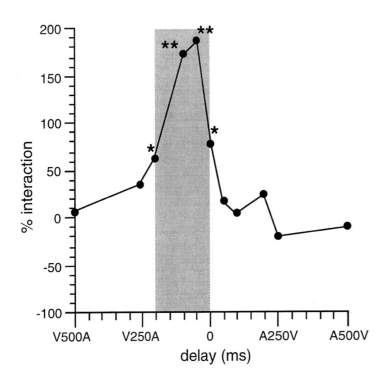

Figure 2.5. Multisensory interactions can take place within a broad temporal window. In this plot of interactive magnitude as a function of temporal interval for a single SC neuron, significant enhancements (shading) are seen for intervals ranging from when the visual stimulus precedes the auditory stimulus by 200 ms (V200A) to when the two are presented simultaneously (0). Note that for this neuron the maximal multisensory interaction was seen when the visual stimulus preceded the auditory stimulus by 50 ms. *P <0.05; **P <0.01.

SC-MEDIATED MULTISENSORY BEHAVIORS

Neurons in the SC gain direct access to regions of the brainstem and spinal cord that influence movements of the eyes, ears and head by means of a crossed descending pathway—the predorsal bundle (see Stein and Meredith, 1991). Because the vast majority of SC neurons projecting into this pathway are responsive to sensory stimuli, and most of these are multisensory (Meredith *et al.*, 1992; Wallace *et al.*, 1993), it seemed reasonable to suppose that the same conditions that enhance or degrade the activity of these neurons would enhance or degrade SC-mediated behaviors.

To examine this possibility, several cats were acclimated to a dimly illuminated apparatus in which light-emitting diodes (LEDs) and speakers were placed at 15° intervals (Figure 2.6). The animals were then trained to fixate directly ahead and to orient toward and approach any LED that was illuminated and/or any speaker from which a brief, low-intensity noise was presented (whenever the two cues were presented simultaneously during training, they were always at the same location). During testing, the simultaneous presentation of the sound and light at the same location enhanced the performance of animals more than was expected using statistical predictions based on reactions to either stimulus alone. Enhanced responding to the visual stimulus was also obtained in animals that had learned to 'ignore' the sounds during training (they were never rewarded for responding to them) and in animals that never had any experience with the sounds during training. On the other hand, when animals were trained to respond only to the visual stimulus, the presence of an auditory stimulus 60° away from the visual stimulus substantially decreased the probability of correct responses to that visual stimulus (Stein *et al.*, 1989). The results of these behavioral experiments reflected the predictions based on the physiological studies described earlier.

THE CRITICAL NATURE OF CORTICAL INFLUENCES ON SC NEURONS

One might suppose that any neuron capable of responding to multiple sensory cues would also be capable of integrating those inputs, and that the source of its various afferents would not be particularly important. The strategy adopted to examine this

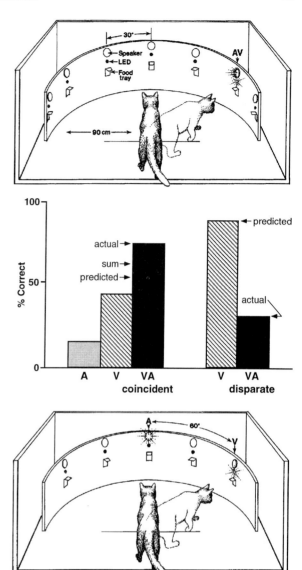

Figure 2.6. Paradigms examining multisensory orientation behaviors to spatially coincident (top) and spatially disparate (bottom) stimulus combinations. After training to a criterion level of response (see text for details), the impact of such combinations on multisensory orientation responses was examined. The center graph summarizes the data for spatially coincident (VA coincident) and spatially disparate (VA disparate) trials. Note that the percentage of actual correct responses is enhanced above both predicted and summed levels in the coincident condition, whereas such responses are depressed in the disparate condition. Adapted from Stein and Meredith (1993).

hypothesis was to deactivate selected inputs to a multisensory SC neuron temporarily and examine the resultant effects on its multisensory integration capabilities. The use of this strategy depends on the SC neuron being the site of converging inputs from different modalities (rather than simply reflecting the responses of multisensory neurons located elsewhere), and recent observations have shown that visual, auditory and somatosensory inputs converge on individual SC neurons in various combinations (Wallace *et al.*, 1993). The rationale of the strategy also assumes that the neuron receives multiple inputs from each modality (otherwise deactivating the modality's one operating input channel would simply render the neuron unresponsive to stimuli in that modality). Fortunately, inputs to SC neurons are derived from a host of both ascending and descending (corticotectal) visual, auditory and somatosensory structures (Edwards *et al.*, 1979; Huerta and Harting, 1984; Stein and Meredith, 1991). For example, a visual–somatosensory SC neuron may receive both ascending and descending visual and somatosensory inputs (Clemo and Stein, 1984; Wallace *et al.*, 1993). When we began to examine the nature of these ascending and descending inputs, we were surprised to learn that the conservative hypothesis that all inputs are equivalent, and thus capable of conferring an integrative capacity on a multisensory neuron, was incorrect.

Projections from an area of cortex, the anterior ectosylvian sulcus (AES), proved to be unexpectedly important for SC multisensory integration. The AES is divided into three separate unimodal regions: a somatosensory area, SIV (Clemo and Stein, 1982); a visual area, AEV (Mucke *et al.*, 1982; Olson and Graybiel, 1987); and an auditory area, Field AES (FAES) (Clarey and Irvine, 1986). All three of these AES subdivisions project heavily to the SC and do so in a convergent fashion (Stein *et al.*, 1983; Norita *et al.*, 1986; Meredith and Clemo, 1989; Wallace *et al.*, 1993). When these corticotectal inputs are deactivated, many multisensory SC neurons can still respond to their various modality-specific inputs (e.g. deactivating FAES does not eliminate auditory responses), but they lose their ability to integrate these inputs to produce an enhanced response (Figure 2.7). Consistent with this is the observation that in the small number of SC multisensory neurons in which integration could not be demonstrated, no AES inputs could be demonstrated (Wallace and Stein, 1994). Apparently, this cortical region plays a key role in the cross-modality

associative functions of the SC. Presumably, its influences would also be necessary to mediate multisensory orientation functions.

To examine this possibility, several cats were trained in the perimetry device described earlier, and their orientation and approach behaviors to visual and auditory stimuli were then tested in the presence and absence of AES inputs. This was accomplished

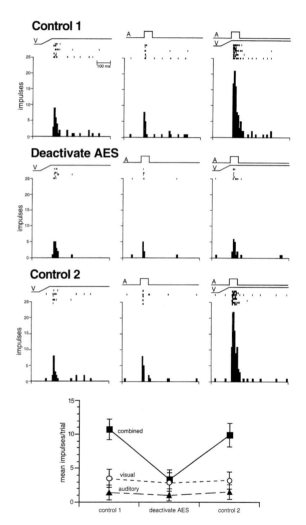

Figure 2.7. Multisensory integration in individual SC neurons is abolished by deactivation of AES cortex. Rasters and histograms at the top show the unimodal (i.e. V, A) and multisensory (i.e. VA) responses of a representative visual–auditory neuron prior to cortical deactivation (control 1), during the deactivation of AES (deactivate AES) and 8 min after the cooling was ended (control 2). Note that while unimodal responses remain during AES deactivation, the large enhancement seen in response to the stimulus combination is eliminated. The bottom graph plots the summary data for this neuron's responses for each condition.

by rendering the AES temporarily inactive by infusing it with the local anesthetic lidocaine through indwelling cannulae (Fiure. 2.8). Whereas deactivating the AES had no demonstrable effect on an animal's ability to respond correctly to a single modality-specific stimulus, it severely compromised the characteristic response enhancement to spatially coincident stimulus combinations and the response

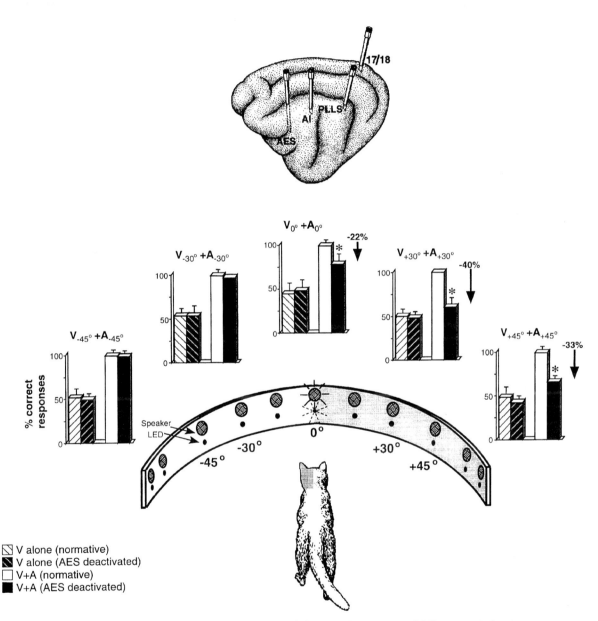

Figure 2.8. Deactivation of AES alters multisensory orientation behaviors. Deactivation of different cortical regions was accomplished by means of lidocaine injections through indwelling chronically implanted cannulae (top). Behavioral data at the bottom are shown for AES deactivation alone. Histograms illustrate this animal's behavioral responses to visual and to spatially coincident combined visual–auditory stimuli before (normative) and during AES deactivation. Data from five stimulus locations are shown. Whereas deactivation of the left AES (shading on cat) had little effect on unimodal or multisensory responses to stimuli in the ipsilateral hemifield, such deactivation significantly reduced the enhancement seen to multisensory combinations in the contralateral hemifield (shading on perimeter). *P <0.05. AI = primary auditory cortex, PLLS = posterolateral lateral suprasylvian cortex, 17/18 = primary visual cortex. Adapted from Wilkinson *et al.* (1996).

depression to spatially disparate combinations (Figure 2.8; see also Wilkinson *et al.*, 1996). These effects could not be induced by deactivating other visual or auditory cortical regions.

Together, the physiological and behavioral results indicate that a functional cortical–SC axis must be maintained in order to support the multisensory synthesis that goes on in SC neurons and is expressed in orientation and approach behaviors. More recent observations (H. Jiang, B.E. Stein and J.G. McHaffie, unpublished) have suggested that cortical areas adjacent to the AES may also participate in this circuit.

THE MATURATION OF MULTISENSORY INTEGRATION

Some argue that the brain's ability to synthesize information from different sensory modalities is likely to be innate and, therefore, present at birth (Bower, 1977; Marks, 1978; Maurer and Maurer, 1988; Turkewitz and Mellon, 1989; Meltzoff, 1990). In contrast to this 'Primitive Unity' hypothesis is the perspective that the newborn must first learn to associate among the various sensory impressions in order to relate them to one another, obviously necessitating postnatal experience with sensory cues (Von Helmholtz, 1968; Piaget, 1952). Although this conflict has centered primarily on the perceptual capabilities of human infants (e.g. see Stein *et al.*, 1999), it is just as relevant to animal models. For this reason, we began exploring the maturation of multisensory integration in SC neurons of the cat.

In altricial mammals such as the cat, the brain undergoes a great deal of postnatal maturation before it can subserve adult-like behaviors. The minimal sensory and sensorimotor capabilities of the neonatal kitten reflect an immaturity of many central nervous system structures, including the SC, and provide little hint of the impressive skills which the animal will develop later. However, from the experimental perspective, the gradual postnatal development of the cat SC provides an opportunity to use this system as a model to examine how SC neurons develop their sensory responses, and especially their striking ability to synthesize cross-modality information.

The immaturity of the newborn cat SC is evident in the paucity of its electrical activity. Few of its neurons exhibit spontaneous activity, and fewer still are responsive to sensory stimuli (see Stein *et al.*, 1973).

However, as if to prepare the animal for its most immediate postnatal task of nuzzling its mother in search of milk, at least some tactile-responsive neurons in the SC (and other somatosensory structures) become active in late fetal stages (Stein *et al.*, 1973). From a functional perspective, the structure is purely somatosensory at this time. It is not until about 5 days postnatal (dpn) that neurons responsive to auditory cues appear (though none of these are multisensory), and the first deep layer visual neurons are not present until about 3 weeks postnatal (although visual neurons in the purely visual superficial layers are active at 6–7 dpn (Stein *et al.*, 1973; Kao *et al.*, 1994; Wallace and Stein, 1997a).

The receptive fields of neonatal SC sensory neurons are extremely large, regardless of whether they are unimodal or multisensory (Figure 2.9). Visual receptive fields cover much of the contralateral visual field, and somatosensory receptive fields cover most of the contralateral body. Auditory receptive fields are completely unformed (i.e. omni-

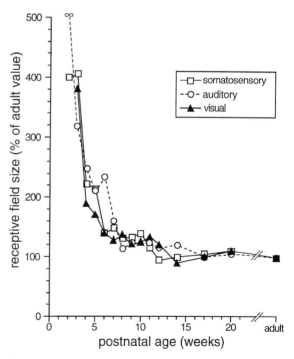

Figure 2.9. Receptive fields for each of the modalities represented in the SC decline in size during postnatal development. Following their appearance, the individual receptive fields of multisensory neurons decline precipitously in size over a 2–4 week period, which is followed by a slower decline over the ensuing 2–4 weeks. From Wallace and Stein (1997a).

directional), so that responses are evoked to stimuli anywhere in space. As postnatal maturation proceeds, there is a progressive reduction in the size of receptive fields until the characteristic adult-like alignment becomes evident (Wallace *et al.*, 1995; Wallace and Stein, 1996, 1997a,b). A similar contraction of SC receptive fields during postnatal life has been noted in monkey (Wallace *et al.*, 1995, 1997), ferret (King *et al.*, 1996), owl (Brainard and Knudsen, 1995), guinea pig (Withington-Wray *et al.*, 1990) and mouse (Benedetti, 1991).

The functional ontogeny of multisensory neurons in cat SC parallels that of their unimodal counterparts, with the first being auditory–somatosensory neurons that appear at 12 dpn. In contrast, visually responsive multisensory neurons do not appear until about 3 weeks postnatal. Achieving the adult-like number of multisensory neurons is a very gradual developmental process that is not completed until about 3 months postnatal (Figure 2.10) (Wallace and Stein, 1997a). Thus, on the basis of data from this neural model, one might conclude that there is little to support the contention that multisensory processes are innate. However, unlike the newborn cat, the rhesus monkey does have multisensory SC neurons at birth (see Wallace *et al.*, 1997), thus emphasizing the very wide variations among species in their levels of maturation at birth. Although no in-depth comparisons have been made of the maturational rate of the cat and monkey SC, it is not until the second month of postnatal life that neurons in the cat SC seem as mature as those in the newborn primate.

MATURATION OF CROSS-MODALITY RECEPTIVE FIELD SLIGNMENT AND MULTISENSORY INTEGRATION

By the end of the second month of the cat's postnatal life, visual-, auditory- and somatosensory-responsive neurons abound in the SC, and they are quite responsive to natural sensory cues. The animal is also very responsive to these cues and will rapidly orient to them, and coordinated orienting responses can be evoked readily with low-intensity electrical stimulation of the SC (Stein *et al.*, 1973, 1980; Norton, 1974; Stein, 1984; Wallace and Stein, 1997a). Furthermore, the sensory (and motor) maps have established their close topographic register, and there are many active multisensory neurons.

It might reasonably be argued that the point at which an individual SC neuron develops the ability to respond to inputs from different modalities (i.e. becomes multisensory) is the more appropriate time to test the necessity of experience for multisensory integration. Although it seemed highly likely that neurons that were already able to respond to more than one modality-specific stimulus would integrate these different inputs when they were presented together, it was surprising to note that this is not the case. In both cat (Wallace and Stein, 1997a) and monkey (Wallace *et al.*, 1995), the youngest multisensory neurons generally respond to the combination of two different sensory cues in the same way that they respond when one or the other cue is presented individually (i.e. they fail to demonstrate response

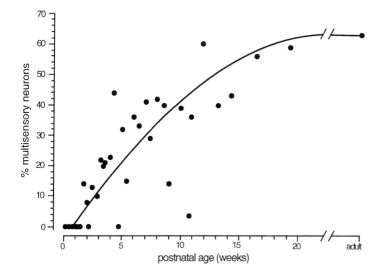

Figure 2.10. The developmental chronology of multisensory neurons in the SC. Note the gradual rise in the proportion of multisensory neurons with increasing postnatal age. Adapted from Wallace and Stein (1997a).

enhancements or depressions). The maturation of their integrative capacity was followed closely in cat, and it became evident that this capacity increases only gradually during postnatal development. Although the time frame may differ, it is expected that a similar trend will be evident in the monkey.

The observation that the multisensory properties of the SC develop only gradually in postnatal life (see Wallace and Stein, 1997a) is in contrast to expectations based on the idea of a primitive unity among the senses. Nevertheless, it remains possible that neurons with mature integrative capabilities are present in the human infant SC and/or in other more perceptually oriented structures in the nervous system. However, the sequential appearance of somatosensory, auditory and then visual responses in this structure (Stein *et al.*, 1973; Wallace and Stein, 1997a) is consistent with the idea, developed in several non-human species, that there is a developmental window during which there is a focus on developing the fundamental organization and information-processing capabilities of one sensory modality before repeating this process for another and, presumably, before dealing with the most complicated task of integrating their different signals (for a discussion of the possible adaptive significance of sequential sensory development, see Turkewitz and Kenny, 1985).

Although the maturation of the population of multi-sensory SC neurons is a gradual process, at the level of the individual neuron it seems quite abrupt (Figure 2.11). When an SC neuron is first capable of exhibiting response enhancements and depressions, it does so in the same fashion as an adult neuron. The magnitude of the changes are similar, the same spatial requirements apply, and inverse effectiveness holds. The one obvious difference between neonatal and adult multi-sensory neurons that is evident thus far is that the former have a much narrower window of time during which response enhancements can take place. The neonate seems to require near simultaneous presentation of the different sensory stimuli in order to exhibit an integrated product (Wallace and Stein, 1997b), though this issue remains to be explored further.

In light of the importance of corticotectal influences described earlier, it seemed likely that the functional onset of cortical influences on SC neurons is a critical step in developing the capacity to integrate cross-modality cues. If this input from the AES develops abruptly on individual SC neurons, it would also explain their abrupt maturation with respect to multi-sensory integration. Indeed, previous studies of the maturation of visual corticotectal influences have

shown an abrupt functional onset (see Stein and Gallagher, 1981). Thus far, the data are consistent with this idea. Neurons unable to integrate multisensory cues exhibit little evidence of AES corticotectal influences. However, once a neuron is capable of integrating cross-modality cues, its integration is lost when the AES is deactivated temporarily (unpublished observations).

CONCLUDING REMARKS

Although commonalities in the sensory maps, cross-modality receptive field register and multisensory integration have been stressed here, this should not be interpreted to indicate that there are no differences among species. The particular visual and auditory stimuli that have most ready access to these neurons will certainly differ in different animals. Substantial species differences exist in the ability to discern high-frequency sounds, different spectral compositions of light, or even to use self-generated sounds (e.g. bats, cetaceans) to evaluate the environment. Furthermore, the primacy of one modality over another will differ among species (e.g. vision is primary in primates, sound in bats, somesthesis in the blind mole) as will the relevance and presumptive effectiveness of different stimulus configurations, speeds of movement, etc. Undoubtedly, these species differences are reflected in the convergence patterns of SC neurons and response properties of individual SC multi-sensory neurons. Nevertheless, it is likely that the same principles guide the integration of these multiple sensory cues.

Similarly, multisensory neurons abound in many areas of the brain other than the SC. Thus far, when the same tests of multisensory integration described above have been conducted in cortical multisensory neurons, similar results have been obtained (see Wallace *et al.*, 1992; Ramachandran *et al.*, 1993), suggesting that a core of common multisensory principles exists at different levels of the brain. Presumably, this ensures that there is a coordination of multisensory enhancement or depression in the multiple areas involved in each of the components of an integrated behavior.

ACKNOWLEDGEMENTS

We thank Nancy London for editorial assistance. The research described here was supported by NIH grants EY06562 and NS22543.

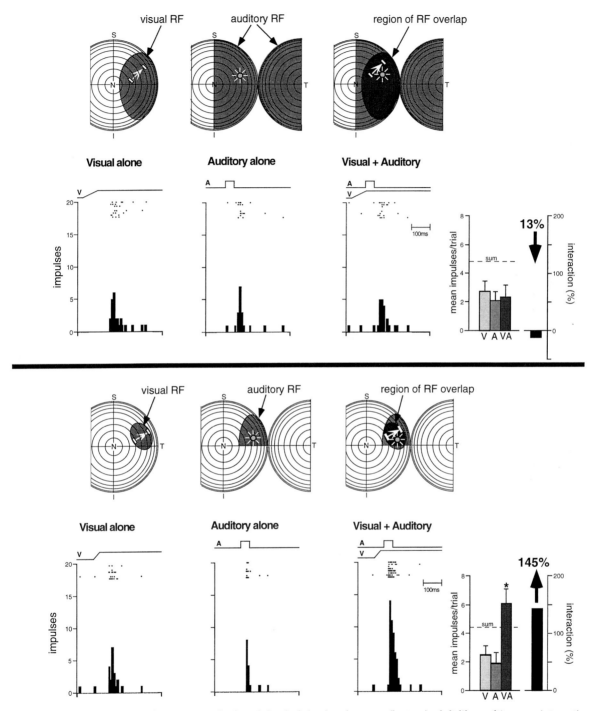

Figure 2.11. In the same animal, neurons can be found that lack (top) and possess (bottom) adult-like multisensory integration. The conventions for representing receptive fields and neuronal responses are the same as in Figure 2.3. Data are taken from a pair of neurons in the same electrode penetration that were separated by only 150 μm. In the top figure, note the large receptive fields and the lack of enhancement in response to the stimulus combination. In the bottom figure, note the adult-like receptive fields and the enhanced response to the stimulus combination. From Wallace and Stein (1997a).

REFERENCES

Benedetti, F. (1991) The postnatal emergence of a functional somatosensory representation in the superior colliculus of the mouse. *Developmental Brain Research*, 60, 51–58.

Bower, T.G.R. (1977) *A Primer of Infant Development.* W.H. Freeman, San Francisco.

Brainard, M.S. and Knudsen, E.I. (1995) Dynamics of visually guided auditory plasticity in the optic tectum of the barn owl. *Journal of Neurophysiology*, 73, 595–614.

Bruce, C., Desimone, R. and Gross, C.G. (1981) Visual properties of neurons in a polysensory area in superior temporal sulcus of the macaque. *Journal of Neurophysiology*, 46, 369–384.

Bullock, T.H. (1984) Physiology of the tectum mesencephali in elasmobranchs. In: Vanegas, H. (ed.), *Comparative Neurology of the Optic Tectum.* Plenum Press, New York, pp. 47–68.

Calvert, G.A., Brammer, M.J. and Iversen, S.D. (1998) Crossmodal identification. *Trends in Cognitive Sciences*, 2, 247–253.

Casagrande, V.A., Harting, J.K., Hall, W.C. and Diamond, I.T. (1972) Superior colliculus of the tree shrew: a structural and functional subdivision into superficial and deep layers. *Science*, 177, 444–447.

Chalupa, L.M. and Rhoades, R.W. (1977) Responses of visual, somatosensory, and auditory neurones in the golden hamster's superior colliculus. *Journal of Physiology (London)*, 207, 595–626.

Clarey, J.C. and Irvine, D.R.F. (1986) Auditory response properties of neurons in the anterior ectosylvian sulcus of the cat. *Brain Research*, 386, 12–19.

Clemo, H.R. and Stein, B.E. (1982) Somatosensory cortex: a new somatotopic representation. *Brain Research*, 235, 162–168.

Clemo, H.R. and Stein, B.E. (1984) Topographic organization of somatosensory corticotectal influences in cat. *Journal of Neurophysiology*, 51, 843–858.

Corneil, B.D. and Munoz, D.P. (1996) The influence of auditory and visual distractors on human orienting gaze shifts. *Journal of Neuroscience*, 16, 8193–81207.

Drager, U.C. and Hubel, D.H. (1975) Responses to visual stimulation and relationship between visual, auditory and somatosensory inputs in mouse superior colliculus. *Journal of Neurophysiology*, 38, 690–713.

Duhamel, J.-R., Colby, C.L. and Goldberg, M.E. (1991) Congruent representations of visual and somatosensory space in single neurons of monkey ventral intraparietal cortex (area VIP). In: Paillard, J. (ed.), *Brain and Space.* Oxford University Press, New York, pp. 223–236.

Edwards, S.B., Ginsburgh, C.L., Henkel, C.K. and Stein, B.E. (1979) Sources of subcortical projections to the superior colliculus in the cat. *Journal of Comparative Neurology*, 184, 309–330.

Finlay, B.L., Schneps, S.E., Wilson, K.G. and Schneider, G.E. (1978) Topography of visual and somatosensory projections to the superior colliculus of the golden hamster. *Brain Research*, 142, 223–235.

Fogassi, L., Gallese, V., Fadiga, L., Luppino, G., Matelli, M. and Rizzolatti, G. (1996) Coding of peripersonal space in inferior premotor cortex (area F4). *Journal of Neurophysiology*, 76, 141–157.

Frens, M.A. and Van Opstal, A.J. (1995) A quantitative study of auditory-evoked saccadic eye movements in two dimensions. *Experimental Brain Research*, 107, 103–117.

Goldring, J.E., Dorris, M.C., Corneil, B.D., Ballantyne, P.A. and Munoz, D.P. (1996) Combined eye–head gaze shifts to visual and auditory targets in humans. *Experimental Brain Research*, 111, 68–78.

Goodale, M.A. and Murison, R.C.C. (1975) The effects of lesions of the superior colliculus on locomotor orientation and the orienting reflex in the rat. *Brain Research*, 88, 243–261.

Graziano, M.S., Hu, T. and Gross, C.G. (1997) Visuospatial properties of ventral premotor cortex. *Journal of Neurophysiology*, 77, 2268–2292.

Groh, J.M. and Sparks, D.L. (1996) Saccades to somatosensory targets. III. Eye-position-dependent somatosensory activity in primate superior colliculus. *Journal of Neurophysiology*, 75, 439–453.

Hardcastle, V.G. (1998) The binding problem. In: Bechtel, W. and Graham, G. (eds), *A Companion to Cognitive Science.* Blackwell, Malden, Massachusetts, pp. 555–565.

Harris, L.R. (1980) The superior colliculus and movements of the head and eyes in cats. *Journal of Physiology*, 300, 367–391.

Hartline, P.H., Kass, L. and Loop, M.S. (1978) Merging of modalities in the optic tectum: infrared and visual integration in rattlesnakes. *Science*, 199, 1225–1229.

Hartline, P.H., Pandey Vimal, R.L., King, A.J., Kurylo, D.D. and Northmore, D.P.M. (1995) Effects of eye position on auditory localization and neural representation of space in superior colliculus of cats. *Experimental Brain Research*, 104, 402–408.

Horn, G. and Hill, R.M. (1966) Responsiveness to sensory stimulation of units in the superior colliculus and subjacent tectotegmental regions of the rabbit. *Experimental Neurology*, 14, 199–223.

Howard, I.P. and Templeton, W.B. (1966) *Human Spatial Orientation.* Wiley, London.

Huerta, M.F. and Harting, J.K. (1984) The mammalian superior colliculus. Studies of its morphology and connections. In: Vanegas, H. (ed.), *Comparative Neurology of the Optic Tectum.* Plenum, New York, pp. 687–773.

Hughes, H.C., Reuter-Lorenz, P.A., Nozawa, G. and Fendrich, R. (1994) Visual–auditory interactions in sensorimotor processing: saccades versus manual responses. *Journal of Experimental Psychology: Human Perception and Performance*, 20, 131–153.

Jay, M.F. and Sparks, D.L. (1987a) Sensorimotor integration in the primate superior colliculus. I. Motor convergence. *Journal of Neurophysiology*, 57, 22–34.

Jay, M.F. and Sparks, D.L. (1987b) Sensorimotor integration in the primate superior colliculus. II. Coordinates of auditory signals. *Journal of Neurophysiology*, 57, 35–55.

Jousmaki, V. and Hari, R. (1998) Parchment-skin illusion: sound-biased touch. *Current Biology*, 8, R190.

Kadunce, D.C., Vaughan, J.W., Wallace, M.T., Benedek, G. and Stein, B.E. (1997) Mechanisms of within- and crossmodality suppression in the superior colliculus. *Journal of Neurophysiology*, 78, 2834–2847.

Kao, C.Q., McHaffie, J.G., Meredith, M.A. and Stein, B.E. (1994) Functional development of a central visual map in cat. *Journal of Neurophysiology*, 72, 266–272.

King, A.J. and Palmer, A.R. (1985) Integration of visual and auditory information in bimodal neurones in the guinea-pig superior colliculus. *Experimental Brain Research*, 60, 492–500.

King, A.J., Schnupp, J.W.H., Carlile, S., Smith, A.L. and Thompson, I.D. (1996) The development of topographically-aligned maps of visual and auditory space in the superior colliculus. *Progress in Brain Research*, 112, 335–350.

Knudsen, E.I. (1982) Auditory and visual maps of space in the optic tectum of the owl. *Journal of Neuroscience*, 2, 1177–1194.

Lee, C., Chung, S., Kim, J. and Park, J. (1991) Auditory facilitation of visually guided saccades. *Society for Neuroscience Abstracts*, 17, 862.

Lueck, C.J., Crawford, T.J., Savage,C.J. and Kennard, C. (1990) Auditory–visual interaction in the generation of saccades in man. *Experimental Brain Research*, 82, 149–157.

Marks, L.E. (1978) *The Unity of the Senses: Interrelations Among the Modalities*. Academic Press, New York.

Maurer, D. and Maurer, C. (1988) *The World of the Newborn*. Basic Books, New York.

McGurk, H. and MacDonald, J. (1976) Hearing lips and seeing voices. *Nature*, 264, 746–748.

McHaffie, J.G. and Stein, B.E. (1982) Eye movements evoked by electrical stimulation in the superior colliculus of rats and hamsters. *Brain Research*, 247, 243–253.

McHaffie, J.G., Kao, C.-Q. and Stein, B.E. (1989) Nociceptive neurons in the rat superior colliculus: response properties, topography, and functional implications. *Journal of Neurophysiology*, 62, 510–525.

McIlwain, J.T. (1991) Distributed spatial coding in the superior colliculus—a review. *Visual Neuroscience*, 6, 3–14.

Meltzoff, A.N. (1990) Towards a developmental cognitive science: the implications of cross-modal matching and imitation for the development of representation and memory in infants. *Annals of the New York Academy of Sciences*, 608, 1–37.

Meredith, M.A. and Clemo, H.R. (1989) Auditory cortical projection from the anterior ectosylvian sulcus (Field AES) to the superior colliculus in the cat: an anatomical and electrophysiological study. *Journal of Comparative Neurology*, 289, 687–707.

Meredith, M.A., Nemitz, J.W. and Stein, B.E. (1987) Determinants of multisensory integration in superior colliculus neurons: I. Temporal factors. *Journal of Neuroscience*, 10, 3215–3229.

Meredith, M.A., Wallace, M.T. and Stein, B.E. (1992) Visual, auditory and somatosensory convergence in output neurons of the cat superior colliculus: multisensory properties of the tecto-reticulo-spinal projection. *Experimental Brain Research*, 88, 181–186.

Mucke, L., Norita, M., Benedek, G. and Creutzfeldt, O. (1982) Physiologic and anatomic investigation of a visual cortical area situated in the ventral bank of the anterior ectosylvian sulcus of the cat. *Experimental Brain Research*, 46, 1–11.

Norita, M., Mucke, L., Benedek, G., Albowitz, B., Katoh, Y. and Creutzfeldt, O.D. (1986) Connections of the anterior ectosylvian visual area (AEV). *Experimental Brain Research*, 62, 225–240.

Norton, T.T. (1974) Receptive-field properties of superior colliculus cells and development of visual behavior in kittens. *Journal of Neurophysiology*, 37, 674–690.

Olson, C.R. and Graybiel, A.M. (1987) Ectosylvian visual area of the cat: location, retinotopic organization, and connections. *Journal of Comparative Neurology*, 261, 277–294.

Peck, C.K., Baro, J.A. and Warder, S.M. (1995) Effects of eye position on saccadic eye movements and on the neuronal responses to auditory and visual stimuli in cat superior colliculus. *Experimental Brain Research*, 103, 227–242.

Perrott, D.R., Saberi, K., Brown, K. and Strybel, T.Z. (1990) Auditory psychomotor coordination and visual search performance. *Perception and Psychophysics*, 48, 214–226.

Piaget, J. (1952) *The Origins of Intelligence in Children*. International Universities Press, New York.

Ramachandran, R., Wallace, M.T. and Stein, B.E. (1993) Distribution and properties of multisensory neurons in rat cerebral cortex. *Society for Neuroscience Abstracts*, 19, 1447.

Rizzolatti, G., Scandolara, C., Matelli, M. and Gentilucci, M. (1981a) Afferent properties of periarcuate neurons in macaque monkeys. I. Somatosensory responses. *Behavioural Brain Research*, 2, 125–146.

Rizzolatti, G., Scandolara, C., Matelli, M. and Gentilucci, M. (1981b) Afferent properties of periarcuate neurons in macaque monkeys. II. Visual responses. *Behavioural Brain Research* 2, 147–163.

Robinson, D.A. (1972) Eye movements evoked by collicular stimulation in the alert monkey. *Vision Research*, 12, 1796–1808.

Roucoux, A. and Crommelinck, M. (1976) Eye movements evoked by superior colliculus stimulation in the adult cat. *Brain Research*, 106, 349–363.

Schneider, G.E. (1969) Two visual systems: brain mechanisms for localization and discrimination are dissociated by tectal and cortical lesions. *Science*, 163, 895–902.

Sparks, D.L. (1986) Translation of sensory signals into commands for control of saccadic eye movements: role of the primate superior colliculus. *Physiological Reviews*, 66, 118–171.

Sparks, D.L. and Nelson, J.S. (1987) Sensory and motor maps in the mammalian superior colliculus. *Trends in Neurosciences*, 10, 312–317.

Spence, C. and Driver, J. (1996) Audiovisual links in endogenous covert spatial attention. *Journal of Experimental Psychology: Human Perception and Performance*, 22, 1005–1030.

Sprague, J.M. and Meikle, T.H., Jr (1965) The role of the superior colliculus in visually guided behavior. *Experimental Neurology*, 11, 115–146.

Stein, B.E. (1984) Development of the superior colliculus. *Annual Review of Neuroscience*, 7, 95–125.

Stein, B.E. and Clamann, H.P. (1981) Control of pinna movements and sensorimotor register in cat superior colliculus. *Brain Behavior and Evolution*, 19, 180–192.

Stein, B.E. and Dixon, J.P. (1979) Properties of superior colliculus neurons in the golden hamster. *Journal of Comparative Neurology*, 183, 269–284.

Stein, B.E. and Gaither, N.S. (1981) Sensory representation in reptilian optic tectum: some comparisons with mammals. *Journal of Comparative Neurology*, 202, 69–87.

Stein, B.E. and Gallagher, H.L. (1981) Maturation of cortical control over superior colliculus cells in cat. *Brain Research*, 223, 429–435.

Stein, B.E. and Meredith, M.A. (1991) Functional organization of the superior colliculus. In: Leventhal, A.G. (ed.), *The Neural Basis of Visual Function*. Macmillan, Hampshire, UK, pp. 85–110.

Stein, B.E. and Meredith, M.A. (1993) *The Merging of the Senses*. MIT Press, Cambridge, Massachusetts.

Stein, B.E. and Wallace, M.T. (1996) Comparisons of cross-modality integration in midbrain and cortex. *Progress in Brain Research*, 112, 289–299.

Stein, B.E., Labos, E. and Kruger, L. (1973) Sequence of changes in properties of neurons of superior colliculus of the kitten during maturation. *Journal of Neurophysiology*, 36, 667–679.

Stein, B.E., Clamann, H.P. and Goldberg, S.J. (1980) Superior colliculus: control of eye movements in neonatal kittens. *Science*, 210, 78–80.

Stein, B.E., Spencer, R.F. and Edwards, S.B. (1983) Cortico-tectal and corticothalamic efferent projections of SIV somatosensory cortex in cat. *Journal of Neurophysiology*, 50, 896–909.

Stein, B.E., Meredith, M.A., Honeycutt, W.S. and McDade, L. (1989) Behavioral indices of multisensory integration: orientation of visual cues is affected by auditory stimuli. *Journal of Cognitive Neuroscience*, 1, 12–24.

Stein, B.E., Meredith, M.A. and Wallace, M.T. (1993) The visually-responsive neuron and beyond: multisensory integration in cat and monkey. *Progress in Brain Research*, 95, 79–90.

Stein, B.E., Wallace, M.T. and Stanford, T.R. (1999) Merging sensory signals in the brain: the development of multisensory integration in the superior colliculus. In: Gazzaniga, M.S. (ed.), *The New Cognitive Neurosciences*. MIT Press, Cambridge, Massachusetts, pp. 55–71.

Tiao, Y.-C. and Blakemore, C. (1976) Functional organization in the superior colliculus of the golden hamster. *Journal of Comparative Neurology*, 168, 483–504.

Treisman, A. (1996) The binding problem. *Current Opinion in Neurobiology*, 6, 171–178.

Turkewitz, G. and Kenny, P.A. (1985) The role of developmental limitations of sensory input on sensory/perceptual organization. *Journal of Developmental and Behavioral Pediatrics*, 6, 302–306.

Turkewitz, G. and Mellon, R.C. (1989) Dynamic organization of intersensory function. *Canadian Journal of Psychology*, 43, 286–307.

Von Helmholtz, H. (1968) The origin of the correct interpretation of our sensory impressions. In: Warren, R.M. and Warren, R.P. (eds), *Helmholtz on Perception: Its Physiology and Development*. Wiley, New York, pp. 247–266.

Wallace, M.T. and Stein, B.E. (1994) Cross-modal synthesis depends on input from cortex. *Journal of Neurophysiology*, 71, 429–432.

Wallace, M.T. and Stein, B.E. (1996) Development of auditory responsiveness, topography, and functional convergence with visual inputs in cat superior colliculus (SC). *Society for Neuroscience Abstracts*, 22, 636.

Wallace, M.T. and Stein, B.E. (1997a) Development of multisensory neurons and multisensory integration in cat superior colliculus. *Journal of Neuroscience*, 17, 2429–2444.

Wallace, M.T. and Stein, B.E. (1997b) Development of somatosensory responses, topography, and interactions with other sensory modalities in cat superior colliculus (SC). *Society for Neuroscience Abstracts*, 23, 1541.

Wallace, M.T., Meredith, M.A. and Stein, B.E. (1992) Integration of multiple sensory modalities in cat cortex. *Experimental Brain Research*, 91, 484–488.

Wallace, M.T., Meredith, M.A. and Stein, B.E. (1993) Converging influences from visual, auditory, and somatosensory cortices onto output neurons of the superior colliculus. *Journal of Neurophysiology*, 69, 1797–1809.

Wallace, M.T., McHaffie, J.G. and Stein, B.E. (1995) Sensory response properties in the superior colliculus (SC) of the newborn rhesus monkey. *Society for Neuroscience Abstracts*, 21, 655.

Wallace, M.T., Wilkinson, L.K. and Stein, B.E. (1996) Representation and integration of multiple sensory inputs in primate superior colliculus. *Journal of Neurophysiology*, 76, 1246–1266.

Wallace, M.T., McHaffie, J.G. and Stein, B.E. (1997) Visual response properties and visuotopic representation in the newborn monkey superior colliculus. *Journal of Neurophysiology*, 78, 2732–2741.

Watson, R.I. (1968) *The Great Psychologists: From Aristotle to Freud*. 2nd edn. Lippincott, New York.

Welch, R.B. and Warren, D.H. (1986) Intersensory interactions. In: Boff, K.R., Kaufman, L. and Thomas, J.P. (eds), *Handbook of Perception and Human Performance: I. Sensory Processes and Perception*. Wiley, New York, pp. 1–36.

Wilkinson, L.K., Meredith, M.A. and Stein, B.E. (1996) The role of anterior ectosylvian cortex in cross-modality orientation and approach behavior. *Experimental Brain Research*, 112, 1–10.

Withington-Wray, D.J., Binns, K.E. and Keating, M.J. (1990) The developmental emergence of a map of auditory space in the superior colliculus of the guinea pig. *Developmental Brain Research*, 51, 225–236.

Zahn, J.R., Abel, L.A. and Dell'Osso, L.F. (1978) Audio-ocular response characteristics. *Sensory Processes*, 2, 32–37.

Zambarbieri, D., Schmid, R., Magenes, G. and Prablanc, C. (1982) Saccadic responses evoked by presentation of visual and auditory targets. *Experimental Brain Research*, 47, 417–427.

3   RESPONSE SYNCHRONIZATION, A NEURONAL CODE FOR RELATEDNESS

Wolf Singer

INTRODUCTION

In order to arrive at a precise description of perceptual objects, usually a large number of both temporal and non-temporal variables need to be encoded and evaluated jointly. Because the coding capacity of individual cells is limited—the only variable for the encoding of information is the temporal pattern of action potential sequences—there is a need for parallel processing. When searching for effective coding mechanisms, it is helpful to consider the performance limits in the various coding dimensions. Particularly crucial is temporal resolution because low temporal resolution would rule out a number of coding strategies. I begin, therefore, with a review of data that permit inferences on the temporal precision of neuronal signaling and on processing speed.

PRECISION

There is increasing evidence that neuronal networks can encode, transmit and evaluate the temporal structure of stimuli with astounding precision. The highest degree of temporal resolution is probably reached in the specialized circuits of the auditory system that exploit latency differences for the location and identification of objects. Here, coincidence detection is achieved with a precision in the submillisecond range (Carr, 1993). Although signal transduction in the retina is slower than in the ear, the visual system, too, is capable of resolving temporal patterns with a precision in the millisecond range. Thus, timing differences in the millisecond range are readily exploited for perceptual grouping (Leonards *et al.*, 1996; Alais *et al.*, 1998; Leonards and Singer, 1998; Usher and Donelly, 1998; but see Kiper *et al.*, 1996). The visual system

binds simultaneously appearing pattern elements and segregates them from elements presented with temporal offset, whereby offset, intervals of less than 10 ms are sufficient for perceptual grouping (Leonards *et al.*, 1996). Interestingly, the perceptibility of temporal variables can dissociate from their effect on cognitive processes. Two tones are perceived as individual events only if segregated by tens of milliseconds (e.g. Joliot *et al.*, 1994), while much shorter offset times can be exploited for sound localization. Likewise, flicker is perceivable only up to interflash intervals of 20–30 ms, and the ability to judge the temporal order of two successively presented stimuli is limited to similar intervals. This is in sharp contrast to the system's ability to exploit offset intervals below 10 ms for perceptual grouping.

These psychophysical studies suggest several important conclusions. First, information about the temporal variables of stimuli can be encoded and transmitted over several processing stages with a precision in the millisecond range, in specialized systems even in the submillisecond range. Second, there is a mechanism which is capable of evaluating the temporal co-variation of responses, i.e. the degree of their synchronicity, with a resolution that is far beyond the temporal resolution of conscious perception. Third, the mechanism that exploits temporal co-variation of responses for perceptual grouping interprets simultaneous, i.e. synchronized, responses as related and segregates them from responses that follow a different time course.

Electrophysiological evidence confirms the ability of neuronal networks to transmit temporally modulated responses with a precision in the millisecond range over several processing stages. In the auditory cortex of owl monkeys, species-specific calls evoke responses whose temporal modulation is so precise that both intratrial variability across neurons and intertrial variability for responses to the same call remain in the range of a few milliseconds (deCharms and Merzenich, 1996). The visual system appears to operate with comparable precision: first, cortical responses to flicker are so well locked to the stimuli that cross-correlation functions between simultaneously recorded responses of different neurons are indistinguishable from correlations computed between responses to subsequent stimuli (Rager and Singer, 1998). Secondly, cross-correlations between simultaneously recorded responses of retinal ganglion cells, relay neurons in the lateral geniculate and cortical cells show that the oscillatory patterning of retinal responses is transmitted reliably to the cortex (Castelo-Branco *et al.*, 1998). Given the high frequency of the retinal oscillations (up to 100 Hz), this implies that the timing of discharges can be transmitted over several synaptic stages with a resolution in the millisecond range, at least when the discharges in parallel channels are synchronized precisely. This temporal fidelity of synaptic transmission is not confined to primary sensory pathways but also holds for intracortical interactions. Cortical neurons can engage in oscillatory firing patterns in the γ-frequency range and synchronize their responses with millisecond precision over surprisingly large distances, indicating that cortical networks can also handle temporally structured activity with low temporal dispersion (Engel *et al.*, 1992, 1997; Singer and Gray, 1995; König *et al.*, 1996; for the monkey, see also Buracas *et al.*, 1998).

At first sight, this evidence for the ability of neuronal networks to handle temporal patterns with remarkable precision appears to be incompatible with the relatively long time constants of synaptic transmission and integration. It is commonly held that these are in the range of tens of milliseconds and thus an order of magnitude longer than the resolvable temporal intervals. However, simulation studies indicate that such precision is readily obtained with neurons that operate with conventional time constants if one allows for population coding in reciprocally coupled parallel channels (Diesmann *et al.*, 1996). In this case, neurons at the same processing level synchronize their discharges, and these highly coherent pulse packets are then conveyed with minimal dispersion across several synaptic stages as postulated for synfire chains (Abeles, 1991).

PROCESSING SPEED

The same apparent incompatibility that one suspects between the slow time constants of neurons and the temporal precision of processing exists between the low discharge rate of cortical neurons and the high speed of processing. Estimates based on reaction times, evoked potentials and latencies of single-cell responses suggest that recognition of patterns of average complexity can occur within less than 100 ms. This leaves only a few tens of milliseconds per processing stage to perform the computations necessary for the selection and grouping of responses (Rolls and Tovee, 1994; Thorpe *et al.*, 1996). A cortical neuron can, on average, emit maximally 3–4 spikes within the interval of interest if one assumes a Poissonian distribution of interspike intervals. If one allows for bursting, the modulation depth can be increased by a few more spikes; but since these discharges cannot be distributed arbitrarily over the relevant temporal window if stimulus timing is also to be encoded, the dynamic range for the transmission of rate coded information is very narrow. Because the nervous system cannot afford to average across successive stimuli as neurophysiologists do, the only option is population coding and joint evaluation of the responses of a large number of neurons responding to the same stimulus (see, for example, Shadlen and Newsome, 1998).

RATE CODING VERSUS TEMPORAL CODING

There has been considerable disagreement on the question of whether neurons in the central nervous system encode information solely by varying their discharge rate (Shadlen and Newsome, 1994, 1998) or whether additional information is contained in the precise temporal relationships between the discharges in a population of neurons (Softky and Koch, 1993; Softky, 1995; König *et al.*, 1996; Buracas *et al.*, 1998; Stevens and Zador, 1998). The arguments presented above suggest that this may be an ill-posed question and that both coding regimes co-exist. If a population of neurons is to signal the onset of a stimulus or fluctuations of its energy with a precision in the millisecond range, it can only do so if the amplitude of the population response increases and decreases with similar time constants, i.e. within milliseconds. Furthermore, the temporal pattern of the population output must reflect the pattern of the input signals with a precision and resolution in the millisecond range. Thus, if signals are to be transmitted with high temporal precision, it is important when exactly and in which temporal relationship the units constituting a population emit their action potentials. This, however, violates a basic criterion advocated as constitutive for rate codes. Concepts on rate coding are based on the assumption that the precise timing of spikes in a discharge sequence is irrelevant and that the only parameter that is of importance is the frequency of spikes. However, what is important in a population code is the number (frequency) of spikes in a time slice *across* the population, and this number can be changed either by modulating discharge frequency of individual cells or by changing the relative timing of spikes in parallel channels without altering the discharge rate. The reason why pure rate codes have been considered sufficient is probably that most investigations have concentrated on the processing of non-temporal features that are encoded in the amplitude of sustained responses of individual neurons. As long as only this variable is studied, the precise temporal relationships among the spikes in the input connections indeed is not important. However, when relationships need to be defined between signals in parallel channels or when precise timing information needs to be transmitted, precise temporal relationships among discharges in parallel channels are important and carry information. The latter follows from the fact that the amplitude and the temporal patterning of the output of a population can be changed radically by scrambling the relative timing of the input spikes without changing the average discharge rate of the inputs to the population—the average being defined over intervals long enough to define a rate.

The arguments presented so far suggest the following conclusions. (i) Neuronal networks of the mammalian brain including the neocortex can handle timing information with a resolution in the millisecond range. (ii) Neuronal computations of average complexity are executed within a few tens of milliseconds per processing stage. (iii) Because of these temporal constraints, individual neurons can contribute only a few spikes to each computational step. (iv) Hence, information about both temporal and nontemporal stimulus features has to be conveyed by population coding. (v) For the definition of these population codes, precise timing relationships among the discharges of the participating neurons are crucial because variations of these relationships change the information conveyed by the population, even if these variations do not affect the average firing rate. If these conclusions are valid, the precise timing relationships

among the discharges of neuronal populations carry information and hence can be exploited for coding, and in particular for the definition of relationships. In the next section, it will be shown that there is a recurring need to define relationships among simultaneously active neurons at all levels of sensory processing where population codes are used, and the proposal is put forward that these relationships are defined by internal temporal patterning of discharges.

A NEED FOR RELATIONAL CODES

A major problem with which representational systems are confronted is the combinatorial complexity of the relationships that need to be analyzed and represented. In the context of cognitive functions, combinatorial problems arise from the fact that each perceptual object is defined by a unique constellation of features. Although the variety of basic feature dimensions that nervous systems exploit to classify perceptual objects is limited, the diversity of possible constellations is, for all practical purposes, virtually unlimited. Thus, cognitive systems have to explore a huge combinatorial space when searching for the consistent relationships among features that define a perceptual object. Combinatorial problems of a similar nature have to be solved for the programing and execution of movements. Although the elementary components of motor acts—the movements of individual muscle fibers—are limited in number, the diversity of movements that can be composed by combining the elementary components in ever changing constellations is again virtually infinite.

In order to evaluate relationships, activity conveyed in parallel channels has to be compared. In the primary visual cortex of mammals, for example, relationships among the responses of co-linearly aligned retinal ganglion cells are evaluated by making the output of these ganglion cells converge onto individual cortical neurons (Hubel and Wiesel, 1962; Reid and Alonso, 1995). In this way, the feature 'orientation' is extracted and represented. This strategy of evaluating and representing relationships by selective combination of feed-forward connections is iterated in prestriate cortical areas and leads to neurons that encode increasingly complex relationships among elementary features (Tanaka *et al.*, 1991). Representing features and their constellations by the tuned responses of individual cells (labeled line coding) is rapid and reliable because it can be realized by simple feed-forward processing. However, if used as the only representational mechanism, it requires too many neurons (Sejnowski, 1986; Engel *et al.*, 1992). This is true not only for the representation of complex perceptual objects but also for the encoding of elementary features such as the precise orientation of a contour. Given the high resolution with which contours of a particular orientation and location can be distinguished, one would require an astronomical number of neurons if location and orientation of contours were encoded in a one-to-one relationship by sharply tuned neurons.

A complementary strategy is needed, therefore, that permits utilization of the same set of neurons for the representation of different features at low levels, and of perceptual objects at high levels of processing. As proposed by Hebb (1949) and subsequently elaborated by numerous authors, this can be achieved with assembly coding (Braitenberg, 1978; Edelman, 1987; Palm, 1990; Gerstein and Gochin, 1992). In this case, particular features and relationships among features are signaled by the coordinated activity of an *ensemble* of cells. A neuron tuned to a particular feature can then contribute to the representation of all objects containing this feature by joining different assemblies. The requirements for the generation of assembly codes are that: (i) feature-selective neurons are associated in variable constellations into different assemblies; (ii) grouping occurs in a context-dependent way; and (iii) the joint responses of cells constituting an assembly are labeled so that they can be distinguished by subsequent processing stages as components of one coherent representation and do not get confounded with simultaneous responses of other cells that signal unrelated contents. Thus, there is a fundamental difference between labeled line codes and assembly codes: in the former, the semantic content of a response is defined solely by the invariant position of a neuron in the network. In an assembly code, additional relational information is contained in the specific combination of dynamically grouped responses. The meaning of individual responses becomes context dependent and hence in which relationship to others a particular response occurs is of relevance for the interpretation of an assembly code.

Numerous theoretical studies have addressed the question of how assemblies can self-organize on the basis of cooperative interactions within associative neuronal networks (for reviews, see Hebb, 1949; Braitenberg, 1978; Edelman, 1987; Palm, 1990; Gerstein

and Gochin, 1992) and have provided solutions compatible with the functional architecture of the cerebral cortex (for a review, see Singer, 1995). The most critical question is, however, how responses of cells that have been grouped into an assembly can be tagged as related. An unambiguous signature of relatedness is absolutely crucial for assembly codes because the meaning of responses changes with the context in which they are interpreted. Hence, false conjunctions are deleterious. Unfortunately, the risk of false conjunctions is constitutive in assembly coding for the following reason: assembly codes only economize on neuron numbers if the same cells can be bound into different assemblies at different times. Since complex scenes usually consist of spatially overlapping and contiguous contours, there will often be situations when the same group of neurons ought to be recruited simultaneously into different assemblies. If two contours are close or overlapping, there will always be a set of cells that respond to both contours even if these differ in certain features and ought to be processed separately. Segregating the respective populations spatially is no solution. This scenario would be equivalent to labeled line coding—except that now each 'line' would consist of an autonomous group of dozens of broadly tuned cells. It would require more neurons than would implementing sharply tuned cells right away. In addition, as a matter of principle, populations or assemblies that share common neurons but describe different features or objects cannot overlap in time. They have to be generated successively in order to avoid their merging. Processing speed is thus critically limited by the rate at which populations or assemblies can be formed and dissolved. At peripheral levels of processing where perceptual grouping has to be achieved for many, often spatially contiguous features, the alternation rate between populations or assemblies coding for different features or conjunctions of features has to be considerably faster than the rate at which different objects can be perceived and represented. The reason is that the results of the various grouping operations need to be interpreted jointly by higher processing stages in order to evaluate relationships of higher order. Hence, the multiplexed results of low-level grouping must alternate quickly enough to permit their association at higher processing stages even though they are transmitted as a sequence.

What is needed then is a mechanism that permits association of distributed responses on a time scale that is fast enough to be compatible with the known processing speed. Hence, at a particular processing stage, grouping of responses needs to be accomplished within a few tens of milliseconds.

As proposed by Hebb (1949), the simplest way to define an assembly is to increase conjointly the discharge rate of cells that have become grouped into an assembly. This selectively increases the salience of the grouped responses and thereby ensures further joint processing of the selected responses. However, if the lifetime of such assemblies has to be kept in the range of tens of milliseconds or less, the same strategy needs to be applied as for the precise signaling of temporal stimulus features. The discharges of the selected cells need to co-vary on a time scale that is considerably shorter than the interval needed to compute the rate of a cell, i.e. responses need to be selected and bound together by synchronizing their discharges with a precision in the millisecond range. Thus, it is again of importance when exactly the cells grouped into an assembly emit their spikes rather than how many spikes they produce on average. Synchronicity of individual discharges becomes the tag for the relatedness of responses, and this tag is as efficient as coherent rate increases because synchronization also jointly increases the salience of the grouped responses. Moreover, synchronization of discharges defines relationships with much higher temporal precision than coherent rate increases. Thus, defining relationships by synchronization permits rapid regrouping of responses by shifting of spike timing without changing the average rate of the respective responses. Hence, grouping through synchronization can be, but need not be, accomplished without concomitant rate changes, and this provides the option to use modifications of average rates in parallel for other functions.

SYNCHRONIZATION BY STIMULUS LOCKING AND INTERNAL INTERACTIONS

In sensory systems, and in particular in the auditory and somatosensory system, precise synchronization of discharges typically results from the locking of responses to temporally structured stimuli. As discussed above, this externally induced synchronicity of discharges is used as a signature of relatedness; the nervous system binds the pattern elements that induce synchronized responses and interprets them as components of a coherent figure, and it does so with a temporal resolution below 10 ms.

The notion that precise temporal contiguity of discharges serves as a fundamental cue of relatedness can also be deduced from the nature of learning rules. The most critical parameter in use-dependent synaptic modifications is timing. Whether a synapse undergoes long-term potentiation (LTP) or long-term depression (LTD) depends on the relative timing between the incoming excitatory postsynaptic potential (EPSP) and the outgoing spike, whereby offsets of a few milliseconds are critical (Gerstner *et al.*, 1996; Markram *et al.*, 1997; for a discussion of LTP, see Winder and Kandel, Chapter 10). Since spike generation usually requires cooperativity among numerous excitatory inputs, synapses of synchronously active inputs tend to get strengthened while synapses that are active with temporal offset relative to the spike-generating inputs tend to weaken. The result is a selective association of synchronously active input connections.

Thus, there is both psychophysical and electrophysical evidence that synchronized discharges such as those that result from temporally contiguous stimuli are bound perceptually, and eventually lead to long-lasting association of synchronously active neurons due to synaptic modifications.

The question remains then of how the nervous system achieves grouping and binding of responses to stimuli that lack a distinct temporal structure and evoke sustained responses that provide no temporal grouping cues. Does it use an entirely different strategy, in which case different learning rules would also have to be implemented, or is there a way to use the synchronization of responses as a signature of relatedness also for non-temporal stimulus properties?

Following the discoveries (i) that the responses of cortical neurons to visual stimuli often exhibit an oscillatory patterning which is not stimulus locked (Gray and Singer, 1987); (ii) that these temporally structured discharges can become synchronized for neurons distributed both within (Gray and Singer, 1987, 1989) and across cortical areas (Gray *et al.*, 1989; Engel *et al.*, 1991a,b,c); and (iii) that synchronization probability reflects common Gestaltcriteria of perceptual grouping (Gray *et al.*, 1989; Engel *et al.*, 1992; Kreiter and Singer, 1992, 1996; Freiwald *et al.*, 1995), we have proposed that the cerebral cortex imposes a temporal microstructure on otherwise sustained responses and uses this temporal patterning to express through synchronization the degree of relatedness of the responses (for a review, see Singer, 1999). This temporal patterning and synchronization can be achieved in two ways. First, additional spikes can be inserted in the respective window, in which case one could observe an increase in the average rate of the individual neurons. Secondly, spikes that would have occurred anyway could be shifted so as to occur within the critical window, in which case one would have no rate change. In both cases, when summed across the population, one measures increased spike density within the interval where discharges are synchronized. However, because the time of occurrence of internally generated synchronized events is not locked to any external event, the synchronized epochs cannot be detected in averaged response histograms taken from individual cells. The only way to detect internally generated synchrony is to record simultaneously from more than one unit and to perform correlation analysis (e.g. Gray *et al.*, 1989) or spike counts across parallel channels (e.g. Riehle *et al.*, 1997).

Based on the hypothesis that synchronization serves as a binding mechanism (von der Malsburg, 1985), we postulated and subsequently obtained evidence that synchronization probability reflects common Gestaltcriteria for perceptual grouping. Responses to contours that share groupable features become synchronized, while responses to contours that are commonly perceived as unrelated are not synchronized (Gray *et al.*, 1989; Engel *et al.*, 1991b,c; Kreiter and Singer, 1992, 1996; Freiwald *et al.*, 1995). Since then, a large number of studies have been performed to investigate the occurrence and the mechanisms of internally generated temporal response patterns and their synchronization. These studies will not be discussed here since they are covered in several recent reviews (Singer and Gray, 1995; Singer *et al.*, 1997). The main outcome of these studies was that internal synchronization of responses is a frequent phenomenon in many cerebral structures. These temporal patterns often have an oscillatory component which is best revealed by jointly recording the activity of several adjacent cells. The reason why population responses reveal oscillations better than single-cell discharges are twofold. First, individual cells tend to skip oscillation cycles in an irregular manner and, second, oscillatory epochs are usually short and oscillation frequencies variable. This means that the periodicity of oscillatory population responses often is not apparent in the firing patterns of individual cells, even if their discharges are phase locked precisely to the oscillatory activity of the population.

Evidence is also increasing that the responses of neurons can become *synchronized* by internal mechanisms independently of the temporal structure of stimuli. These synchronization phenomena often occur in conjunction with an oscillatory patterning of responses, but they are also seen in the absence of oscillations (for a review, see Singer, 1993; Singer and Gray, 1995; Singer *et al.*, 1997).

If this internally generated synchronization were to serve as a signature of relatedness, as is the case for stimulus-locked synchronization of responses, it needs to fulfill several requirements. (i) Its precision should be in the millisecond range to permit multiplexing of different assemblies at a rate fast enough to be compatible with known processing speed. (ii) For the same reason, it must be possible to synchronize responses within a few tens of milliseconds. (iii) One should find evidence that synchronized activity is more effective than non-synchronized activity in driving cells in target structures because precise synchronization can only serve as a tag of relatedness if it effectively enhances the salience of the synchronized responses. (iv) There should be a close correlation between the occurrence of these precise and rapidly changing synchronization patterns on the one hand and perceptual or motor processes on the other. Ideally, one should be able to predict behavior from the occurrence of specific synchronization patterns.

SPEED

The postulate that internally generated synchronization must be established very rapidly (within maximally a few tens of milliseconds) has received theoretical and experimental support only recently. Simulations with spiking neurons revealed that networks of appropriately coupled units can undergo very rapid transitions from uncorrelated to synchronized states (Bauer and Pawelzik, 1993; Deppisch *et al.*, 1993; Gerstner and van Hemmen, 1993; van Vreeswijk *et al.*, 1994; Hopfield and Hertz, 1995; Gerstner, 1996). Rapid transitions from independent to synchronized firing are also observed in natural networks. In visual centers, it is not uncommon for neurons to engage in synchronous activity, often with additional oscillatory patterning, at the very same time that they increase their discharge rate in response to the light stimulus (Gray *et al.*, 1992; Neuenschwander and Singer, 1996; Castelo-Branco *et al.*, 1998).

Recently, combined *in vitro* and *in vivo* experiments have suggested a new synchronization mechanism that operates extremely quickly and permits a rapid read out of the grouping criteria that reside in the functional architecture of cortical connections (Volgushev *et al.*, 1997). This mechanism exploits two properties, first, the ability of oscillating cells to delay their output relative to incoming EPSPs and, secondly, the oscillatory-patterning of ongoing cortical activity.

When the membrane potential of a cell undergoes an oscillatory modulation, EPSPs with an *N*-methyl-D-aspartate (NMDA) receptor-mediated component evoke spikes not necessarily at the time of their occurrence but only when the cell reaches the peak of the next depolarizing cycle. The reason for this is that the depolarization removes the magnesium ion that blocks the NMDA receptor at resting potential, so that receptors still occupied by glutamate are reactivated. Thus, in cells with an oscillating membrane potential, responses can become considerably delayed, whereby the maximal possible delay interval depends on the oscillation frequency and can amount to almost the duration of one cycle. With such a mechanism, responses to temporally dispersed EPSPs can become synchronized within less than an oscillation cycle.

This option appears to be exploited for the synchronization of responses to stimuli that possess groupable features. Response latencies of cortical neurons fluctuate in the range of about 20 ms for identical, repeatedly presented stimuli. The new finding is that these fluctuations of response latency are often correlated across cortical columns (Fries *et al.*, 1997b). In this case, synchronization of the early response phase is better than expected from mere stimulus locking. This rapid synchronization of the very first spikes of a response is due to ongoing, oscillatory fluctuations of the cells' membrane potential. These oscillations delay or advance responses to light stimuli depending on the timing of the stimulus relative to the phase of the ongoing oscillation, leading to synchronization of onset latencies in cells located in coherently oscillating columns. In this case, then, synchronization is achieved by latency adjustment, using the delay mechanism identified in the *in vitro* experiments. Irrespective of when the EPSP is generated relative to the phase of the oscillation cycle, the first discharge is likely to occur shortly after the peak of the respective next depolarizing cycle.

In case the ongoing fluctuations of cortical activity are not random and not simply noise but—as suggested by a different approach by Arieli *et al.* (1996)—exhibit specific spatiotemporal patterns, the latency adjustments could be exploited for rapid per-ceptual grouping. The only additional requirement is that the grouping criteria which reside in the functional architecture of the intracortical association connections are translated into specific spatiotemporal patterns of membrane potential fluctuations. Columns encoding groupable features should oscillate in phase. Anatomical evidence indicates that the cortico-cortical association connections preferentially link columns coding for related features that tend to be grouped perceptually (Gilbert and Wiesel, 1989; Ts'o and Gilbert, 1988; Malach *et al.*, 1993; Schmidt *et al.*, 1997), and physiological data suggest that these cortico-cortical connections contribute to the synchronization of spatially segregated groups of neurons (Engel *et al.*, 1991a; Löwel and Singer, 1992; König *et al.*, 1993). It appears likely then that the functional architecture of these association connections is translated continuously into coordinated fluctuations of neuronal excitability which reflect dynamically the system's 'knowledge' of grouping rules. Inevitably, the pattern of these fluctuations is also modified by top-down influences from higher cortical areas and by immediately preceding changes of sensory input. Both effects would be equivalent to the function commonly attributed to attentional mechanisms, the selection and binding of expected events, as a consequence either of bottom-up priming or of intentional top-down selection (see also Duncan, Chapter 4). The observed fluctuations could thus be equivalent to the system's updated expectancy that is determined by the fixed, locally installed grouping rules, by top-down influences and preceding sensory input that influences subsequent selection, grouping and binding of actual input patterns. Seen in this context, ongoing activity assumes the function of a predictor against which incoming activity is matched. One of the effects of matching these predictions with incoming signals is a rapid temporal regrouping of output activity (see Figure 3.1).

ATTENTION-GATED BINDING BY RATE CHANGES

Another strategy to express expectancies and to bias grouping of incoming signals is of course to increase tonically the excitability of selected groups of neurons. This would lead to sustained enhancement of discharge rates in selected transmission channels and hence to a sustained increase in the salience of the selected responses. Such prolonged modifications of

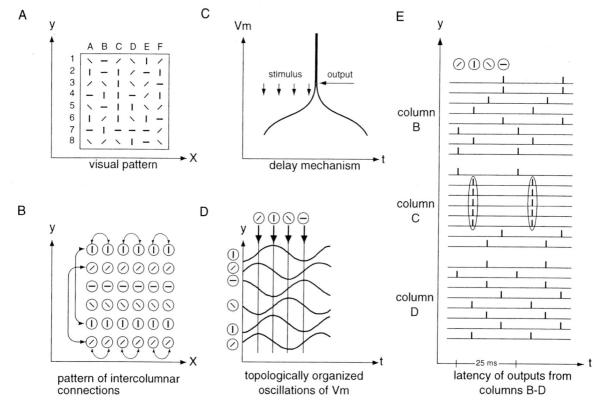

Figure 3.1. A putative mechanism for the rapid conversion of perceptual grouping rules into a temporal code. (**A**) Due to the grouping criterion of co-linearity, the vertical bars in column C and the horizontal bars in row 7 are bound together and are perceived as the letter L. (**B**) In agreement with anatomy, it is assumed that cortical columns preferring similar orientations are coupled preferentially. (**C**) Schematic representation of the mechanism that delays the output of a cell with oscillating membrane potential until the depolarizing peak of the respective next oscillation cycle is reached (horizontal arrow) irrespective of when the EPSPs are generated (vertical arrows). (**D**) Due to preferential coupling, cells preferring the same orientation are assumed to exhibit coherent oscillations of their membrane potential, but oscillations of cells with different preferences are assumed to be phase shifted. Thus, cells sharing the same preferences will emit synchronized responses and cells with differing preferences will emit temporally offset responses. (**E**) Latency distribution of discharges of cells responding to pattern elements in columns B, C and D of (A). Latencies correspond to the phase-shifted oscillations of cells preferring different orientations as depicted in (D). Note that the cells responding to the co-linear bars in column C (A) discharge synchronously, which allows for rapid binding of the respective responses.

the discharge rate occur in association with shifts in selective attention (Luck *et al.*, 1997). However, if the expected or selected content is encoded in the format of assemblies, the same superposition problems arise as for rate-defined assembly codes. It is not possible to express different expectancies simultaneously if the expected contents are represented by cell populations that overlap and share a subset of units. Again, rapid multiplexing of different expectancies within the same population of cells would be a solution. As discussed above, this can be achieved by shortening the time constants of the coherent excitability fluctuations, or, in other terms, by increasing the frequency

of the fluctuations. Evidence is available from experiments in cats (Bouyer *et al.*, 1981; Roelfsema *et al.*, 1996), monkeys (Bressler *et al.*, 1993; Sanes and Donoghue, 1993; Munk *et al.*, 1996; Murthy and Fetz, 1996a,b; De Oliveira *et al.*, 1997; Donoghue *et al.*, 1998) and humans (Sheer, 1984; Tallon-Baudry *et al.*, 1996, 1997, 1998) that highly synchronized oscillatory fluctuations of cortical activity in the β- and γ-frequency range occur over the involved cortical areas during the preparatory phase of cognitive or sensori-motor performance. This contingency suggests the possibility that the generation of temporally patterned excitability fluctuations prior to the appearance of expected stimuli is the expression of attentional mechanisms. These highly coherent temporal patterns become more prominent once stimuli have appeared and actual processing is resumed, but they collapse immediately once a solution is found and a response executed (see, for example, Roelfsema *et al.*, 1996). This tight correlation between the internal generation of synchronous high-frequency oscillatory fluctuations of cortical activity and distinct phases of cognitive and motor behavior is compatible with the view that these coherent fluctuations are related both to the expression of expectancies and to the subsequent generation of representations.

What, then, could be the function of the frequently observed, attention-dependent sustained changes of response amplitude? As discussed above for feedforward processing, response selection and grouping through synchronization does not exclude transportation of additional information by shifting the average level of activity with a time course that is much slower than that of the high-frequency fluctuations. In top-down processing, such tonic modulations could be used to stabilize representations once they have been disambiguated and hence become eligible as objects of attention (Roelfsema *et al.*, 1998). It should be noted, however, that selection and stabilization of assemblies by attention can only take place once grouping is accomplished, because grouping precedes identification and identification is a prerequisite for the organization of object-centered attention. Also, only one object can be selected at any given moment in time if the assemblies representing different objects overlap. Thus, when object-centered attention is expressed by sustained rate increases, assemblies can only be selected at a rate corresponding to the time course of the tonic rate increases because of the superposition problems discussed above. Since attentional states are apparently associated not only with sustained rate increases but also with enhanced oscillatory patterning and synchronization of responses in the γ-frequency range, the possibility should be considered that attentional mechanisms operate at two complementary levels: first, by enhancing the efficacy of the interactions which lead to oscillatory patterning and synchronization of responses, they could contribute to the generation of multiple expectancies that are interleaved temporally and alternate on a rapid time scale. This top-down effect could facilitate the disambiguation of population responses through temporal grouping and thereby accelerate the formation of 'expected' assemblies. Secondly, by tonically

increasing the excitability of successfully grouped neurons, attentional mechanisms could prolong the duration of the multiplexing process and thereby contribute to the stabilization of the selected assemblies over perceptually relevant time scales. If in this case oscillations and synchrony disappear, it would indicate that only a single assembly is selected or a set of assemblies that do not overlap. If the enhanced responses are still oscillatory and synchronized, it would indicate that multiplexing is still required because the selected assemblies share common neurons. In both cases, the observed rate increase would partly be a reflection of the fact that a given neuron contributes spikes more often and over a longer period of time either to a single, tonically sustained assembly or to a sequence of different, rapidly alternating assemblies.

RELATIONSHIPS BETWEEN RESPONSE SYNCHRONIZATION, COGNITION AND MOTOR PERFORMANCE

One line of support for a functional role for the oscillatory patterning of responses in the β- and γ-frequency range and for precise synchronization comes from the finding that these phenomena are particularly well expressed when the brain is in an activated state, i.e. when the electroencephalogram (EEG) is desynchronized and exhibits high power in the β- and γ-frequency range (Munk *et al.*, 1996; Herculano *et al.*, 1999). Such EEG patterns are characteristic for the aroused, attentive as well as for the dreaming brain and thus for states in which sensory representations can be activated. Conversely, both the oscillatory patterning of responses in the γ-frequency range and the precise synchronization disappear when anesthesia is deepened and, or if, the animal is in slow wave sleep and the EEG exhibits prominent delta activity. In this case, synchronization collapses long before the amplitudes of neuronal responses become attenuated (unpublished observations).

Direct relationships between response synchronization and perception have been found in cats who suffered from strabismic amblyopia, a developmental impairment of vision associated with suppression of the amblyopic eye, reduced visual acuity and disturbed perceptual grouping (crowding) in this eye. Quite unexpectedly, the responses of individual neurons in the primary visual cortex fail to reflect these deficits (for references, see Roelfsema *et al.*,

1994). The only significant correlate of amblyopia was the drastically reduced ability of neurons driven by the amblyopic eye to synchronize their responses (Roelfsema *et al.*, 1994), and this accounts well for the perceptual deficits: impaired synchronization reduces the salience of responses and therefore can explain the suppression of signals from the amblyopic eye. Moreover, deficiencies in the synchronizing mechanism are bound to impair the disambiguation of population codes, and this can account for the reduced visual acuity and the crowding phenomenon.

Another close correlation between response synchronization and perception has been found in experiments on binocular rivalry that again were performed in strabismic animals (Fries *et al.*, 1997a). Due to experience-dependent modifications of processing circuitry (Löwel and Singer, 1992), perception in non-amblyopic strabismic subjects always alternates between the two eyes. We have exploited this phenomenon of rivalry to investigate how neuronal responses that are selected and perceived differ from those that are suppressed and excluded from supporting perception (Figure 3.2). The outcome of these experiments was surprising because the responses of neurons in areas 17 and 18 were not attenuated during epochs during which they were excluded from controlling eye movements and supporting perception. A close and highly significant correlation existed, however, between changes in the strength of response synchronization and the outcome of rivalry. Cells mediating responses of the eye that won in interocular competition increased the synchronicity of their responses upon presentation of the rival stimulus to the other, losing eye, while the reverse was true for cells driven by the eye that became suppressed. Thus, selection of responses for further processing appeared to be achieved by modulating the degree of synchronization rather than the amplitude of responses.

These results are direct support for the hypothesis that precise temporal relationships between the discharges of spatially distributed neurons are important in cortical processing and that synchronization may be exploited to increase jointly the salience of the responses selected for further processing. The important point here is that this selection apparently is achieved without enhancing the average discharge rate of the selected responses or inhibiting the non-selected responses.

Recent studies on the effects of synchronization on synaptic transmission and integration demonstrate

that precisely synchronized inputs are indeed more efficient in driving target cells in visual pathways (see, for example, Alonso *et al.*, 1996; Usrey *et al.*, 1998). The same holds for the cooperativity among cortical neurons and their effect on subcortical target structures. Brecht *et al.* (1998) recently have studied cortico-tectal interactions by recording simultaneously from several areas of the visual cortex (A17, A18 and suprasylvian areas) and superficial layers of the superior colliculus. They found that responses of tectal cells become synchronized to responses of cortical cells if the respective cell groups are activated by the same contour, suggesting synchronization of tectal responses by cortico-tectal projections. Of particular importance in the present context is that this synchronizing effect was enhanced strongly when the responses of cortical cells were themselves well synchronized among each other, irrespective of whether the considered cortical cells were located within a single cortical area or were distributed across different areas. This indicates that cortical cells are more effective in driving common tectal target cells when their responses are synchronized than when they fire independently. Again, these changes in coupling cannot be explained by rate changes. When neurons synchronize their responses, this is usually not associated with an increase in discharge rate; rather, the average discharge rate remains either unchanged or decreases (Herculano *et al.*, 1999).

Taken together, these results support the notion that neuronal networks are capable of evaluating the temporal relationships among the discharges of neuronal populations with a precision in the millisecond range and that they exploit this ability to define relationships among distributed responses with high temporal resolution. Such a relationship-defining mechanism seems indispensable whenever contents are encoded by populations or ensembles of neurons because these require flexible and rapid binding of distributed responses into functionally coherent representations. It appears, then, as if the cerebral cortex applied two complementary coding strategies: first, an explicit representation of features and their conjunctions in the tuned responses of individual neurons, and, secondly, an implicit representation of features and their conjunctions in dynamically associated populations (ensembles) of neurons, each of which is tuned to only a subcomponent of the represented content. The first strategy seems to be applied for the representation of a limited set of features and combinations of features and is with all likelihood reserved for items that occur very frequently and/or are of particular behavioral importance, such as, for example, faces and their expression. The second strategy seems to be reserved for the representation of all those items for which an explicit representation cannot be realized, either because the explicit representation by sharply tuned neurons would require too many neurons or because the contents to be represented are too infrequent to warrant the implementation of specialized neurons. Also, the second strategy seems to be the only way to represent novel contents as there cannot be specialized neurons for them at

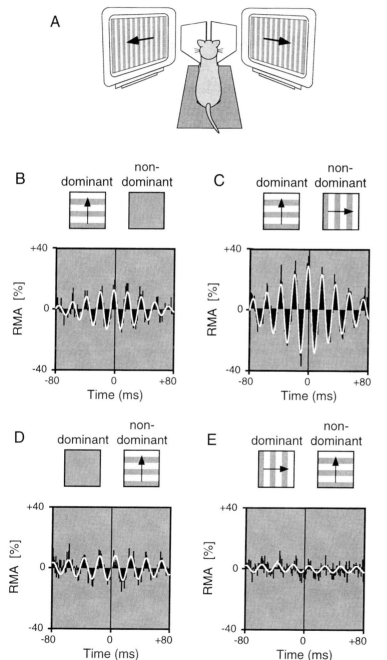

Figure 3.2. Neuronal synchronization under conditions of binocular rivalry. (**A**) Using two mirrors, different patterns were presented to the two eyes of strabismic cats. (**B–E**) Normalized cross-correlograms for two pairs of recording sites activated by the eye that won (**B** and **C**) and lost (**D** and **E**) in interocular competition, respectively. Insets above the correlograms indicate stimulation conditions. Under monocular stimulation (B), cells driven by the winning eye show a significant correlation which is enhanced after introduction of the rival stimulus to the other eye (C). The reverse is the case for cells driven by the loosing eye (compare conditions D and E). The white continuous line superimposed on the correlograms represents a damped cosine function fitted to the data. RMA, relative modulation amplitude of the center peak in the correlogram, computed as the ratio of peak amplitude over offset of correlogram modulation. This measure reflects the strength of synchrony. Modified from Fries *et al.* (1997a).

first encounter. However, if novel items acquire high behavioral significance, as is the case for stimuli used in experiments with trained monkeys, it appears as if these would then become represented explicitly by specialized neurons. In conclusion, then, labeled line and assembly coding are by no means incompatible. Rather, the two strategies ideally complement each other and it should be interesting to examine how implicit assembly codes can be converted into explicit labeled line codes by learning.

REFERENCES

Abeles, M. (1991) *Corticonics*. Cambridge University Press, Cambridge.

Alais, D., Blake, R. and Lee, S.-H. (1998) Visual features that vary together over time group together over space. *Nature Neuroscience*, 1, 160–164.

Alonso, J.-M., Usrey, W.M. and Reid, R.C. (1996) Precisely correlated firing in cells of the lateral geniculate nucleus. *Nature*, 383, 815–819.

Arieli, A., Sterkin, A., Grinvald, A. and Aertsen, A. (1996) Dynamics of ongoing activity: explanation of the large variability in evoked cortical responses. *Science*, 273, 1868–1871.

Bauer, H.-U. and Pawelzik, K. (1993) Alternating oscillatory and stochastic dynamics in a model for a neuronal assembly. *Physica D*, 69, 380–393.

Bouyer, J.J., Montaron, M.F. and Rougeul, A. (1981) Fast fronto-parietal rhythms during combined focused attentive behaviour and immobility in cat: cortical and thalamic localizations. *Electroencephalography and Clinical Neurophysiology*, 51, 244–252.

Braitenberg, V. (1978) Cell assemblies in the cerebral cortex. In: Heim, R. and Palm, G. (eds), *Architectonics of the Cerebral Cortex. Lecture Notes in Biomathematics 21, Theoretical Approaches in Complex Systems*. Springer-Verlag, Berlin, pp. 171–188.

Brecht, M., Singer, W. and Engel, A.K. (1998) Correlation analysis of corticotectal interactions in the cat visual system. *Journal of Neurophysiology*, 79, 2394–2407.

Bressler, S.L., Coppola, R. and Nakamura, R. (1993) Episodic multi-regional binding at multiple frequencies during visual task performance by the macaque monkey. *Nature*, 366, 153–156.

Buracas, G., Zador, A., Deweese, M. and Albright, T. (1998) Efficient discrimination of temporal patterns by motion-sensitive neurons in primate visual cortex. *Neuron*, 20, 959–969.

Carr, C.E. (1993) Processing of temporal information in the brain. *Annual Review of Neuroscience*, 16, 223–243.

Castelo-Branco, M., Neuenschwander, S. and Singer, W. (1998) Synchronization of visual responses between the cortex, lateral geniculate nucleus, and retina in the anesthetized cat. *Journal of Neuroscience*, 18, 6395–6410.

DeCharms, R.C. and Merzenich, M.M. (1996) Primary cortical representation of sounds by the coordination of action-potential timing. *Nature*, 381, 610–613.

Deppisch, J., Bauer, H.-U., Schillen, T.B., König, P., Pawelzik, K. and Geisel, T. (1993) Alternating oscillatory and stochastic states in a network of spiking neurons. *Network*, 4, 243–257.

De Oliveira, S.C., Thiele, A. and Hoffmann, K.P. (1997) Synchronization of neuronal activity during stimulus expectation in a direction discrimination task. *Journal of Neuroscience*, 17, 9248–9260.

Diesmann, M., Gewaltig, M.-O. and Aertsen, A. (1996) Characterization of synfire activity by propagating 'pulse packets'. In: Bower, J. (ed.), *Computational Neuroscience Trends in Research*. Academic Press, San Diego, pp. 59–64.

Donoghue, J.P., Sanes, J.N., Hatsopoulos, N.G. and Gaál, G. (1998) Neural discharge and local field potential oscillations in primate motor cortex during voluntary movements. *Journal of Neurophysiology*, 79, 159–173.

Edelman, G.M. (1987) *Neural Darwinism: The Theory of Neuronal Group Selection*. Basic Books, New York.

Engel, A.K., König, P., Kreiter, A.K. and Singer, W. (1991a) Interhemispheric synchronization of oscillatory neuronal responses in cat visual cortex. *Science*, 252, 1177–1179.

Engel, A.K., König, P. and Singer, W. (1991b) Direct physiological evidence for scene segmentation by temporal coding. *Proceedings of the National Academy of Sciences of the United States of America*, 88, 9136–9140.

Engel, A.K., Kreiter, A.K., König, P. and Singer, W. (1991c) Synchronization of oscillatory neuronal responses between striate and extrastriate visual cortical areas of the cat. *Proceedings of the National Academy of Sciences of the United States of America*, 88, 6048–6052.

Engel, A.K., König, P., Kreiter, A.K., Schillen, T.B. and Singer, W. (1992) Temporal coding in the visual cortex: new vistas on integration in the nervous system. *Trends in Neurosciences*, 15, 218–226.

Engel, A.K., Roelfsema, P.R., Fries, P., Brecht, M. and Singer, W. (1997) Role of the temporal domain for response selection and perceptual binding. *Cerebral Cortex*, 7, 571–582.

Freiwald, W.A., Kreiter, A.K. and Singer, W. (1995) Stimulus dependent intercolumnar synchronization of single unit responses in cat area 17. *NeuroReport*, 6, 2348–2352.

Fries, P., Roelfsema, P.R., Engel, A.K., König, P. and Singer, W. (1997a) Synchronization of oscillatory responses in visual cortex correlates with perception in interocular rivalry. *Proceedings of the National Academy of Sciences of the United States of America*, 94, 12699–12704.

Fries, P., Roelfsema, P.R., Singer, W. and Engel, A.K. (1997b) Correlated variations of response latencies due to synchronous subthreshold membrane potential fluctuations in cat striate cortex. *Society for Neuroscience Abstracts*, 23, 499.

Gerstein, G.L. and Gochin, P.M. (1992) Neuronal population coding and the elephant. In: Aertsen, A. and Braitenberg, V. (eds), *Information Processing in the Cortex, Experiments and Theory*. Springer-Verlag, Berlin, pp. 139–173.

Gerstner, W. (1996) Rapid phase locking in systems of pulse-coupled oscillators with delays. *Physical Review Letters*, 76, 1755–1758.

Gerstner, W. and Van Hemmen, J.L. (1993) Coherence and incoherence in a globally coupled ensemble of pulse-emitting units. *Physical Review Letters*, 7, 312–315.

Gerstner, W., Kempter, R., van Hemmen, J.L. and Wagner, H. (1996) A neuronal learning rule for sub-millisecond temporal coding. *Nature*, 383, 76–78.

Gilbert, C.D. and Wiesel, T.N. (1989) Columnar specificity of intrinsic horizontal and cortico-cortical connections in cat visual cortex. *Journal of Neuroscience*, 9, 2432–2442.

Gray, C.M. and Singer, W. (1987) Stimulus-specific neuronal oscillations in the cat visual cortex: a cortical functional unit. *Society for Neuroscience Abstracts*, 13, 404.3.

Gray, C.M. and Singer, W. (1989) Stimulus-specific neuronal oscillations in orientation columns of cat visual cortex. *Proceedings of the National Academy of Sciences of the United States of America*, 86, 1698–1702.

Gray, C.M., König, P., Engel, A.K. and Singer, W. (1989) Oscillatory responses in cat visual cortex exhibit inter-columnar synchronization which reflects global stimulus properties. *Nature*, 338, 334–337.

Gray, C.M., Engel, A.K., König, P. and Singer, W. (1992) Synchronization of oscillatory neuronal responses in cat striate cortex—temporal properties. *Visual Neuroscience*, **8**, 337–347.

Hebb, D.O. (1949) *The Organization of Behavior: A Neuropsychological Theory*. Wiley, New York.

Herculano, S., Munk, M.H.J., Neuenschwander, S. and Singer, W. (1999) Precisely synchronized oscillatory firing patterns require cortical activation. *Journal of Neuroscience*, 19, 3992–4010.

Hopfield, J.J. and Hertz, A.V.M. (1995) Rapid local synchronization of action potentials: toward computation with coupled integrate-and-fire neurons. *Proceedings of the National Academy of Sciences of the United States of America*, 92, 6655–6662.

Hubel, D.H. and Wiesel, T.N. (1962) Receptive fields, binocular interaction and functional architecture in the cat's visual cortex. *Journal of Physiology (London)*, 160, 106–154.

Joliot, M., Ribary, U. and Llinás, R. (1994) Human oscillatory brain activity near 40 Hz coexists with cognitive temporal binding. *Proceedings of the National Academy of Sciences of the United States of America*, 91, 11748–11751.

Kiper, D.C., Gegenfurtner, K.R. and Movshon, J.A. (1996) Cortical oscillatory responses do not affect visual segmentation. *Vision Research*, 36, 539–544.

König, P., Engel, A.K., Löwel, S. and Singer, W. (1993) Squint affects synchronization of oscillatory responses in cat visual cortex. *European Journal of Neuroscience*, 5, 501–508.

König, P., Engel, A.K. and Singer, W. (1996) Integrator or coincidence detector? The role of the cortical neuron revisited. *Trends in Neurosciences*, 19, 130–137.

Kreiter, A.K. and Singer, W. (1992) Oscillatory neuronal responses in the visual cortex of the awake macaque monkey. *European Journal of Neuroscience*, 4, 369–375.

Kreiter, A.K. and Singer, W. (1996) Stimulus-dependent synchronization of neuronal responses in the visual cortex of the awake macaque monkey. *Journal of Neuroscience*, 16, 2381–2396.

Leonards, U. and Singer, W. (1998) Two segmentation mechanisms with differential sensitivity for colour and luminance contrast. *Vision Research*, 38, 101–109.

Leonards, U., Singer, W. and Fahle, M. (1996) The influence of temporal phase differences on texture segmentation. *Vision Research*, 36, 2689–2697.

Löwel, S. and Singer, W. (1992) Selection of intrinsic horizontal connections in the visual cortex by correlated neuronal activity. *Science*, 255, 209–212.

Luck, S.J., Chelazzi, L., Hillyard, S.A. and Desimone, R. (1997) Neural mechanisms of spatial selective attention in areas V1, V2, and V4 of macaque visual cortex. *Journal of Neurophysiology*, 77, 24–42.

Malach, R., Amir, Y., Harel, M. and Grinvald, A. (1993) Relationship between intrinsic connections and functional architecture revealed by optical imaging and *in vivo* targeted biocytin injections in primate striate cortex. *Proceedings of the National Academy of Sciences of the United States of America*, 90, 10469–10473.

Markram, H., Lübke, J., Frotscher, M. and Sakmann, B. (1997) Regulation of synaptic efficacy by coincidence of postsynaptic Aps and EPSPs. *Science*, 275, 213–215.

Munk, M.H.J., Roelfsema, P.R., König, P., Engel, A.K. and Singer, W. (1996) Role of reticular activation in the modulation of intracortical synchronization. *Science*, 272, 271–274.

Murthy, V.N. and Fetz, E.E. (1996a) Oscillatory activity in sensorimotor cortex of awake monkeys: synchronization of local field potentials and relation to behavior. *Journal of Neurophysiology*, **76**, 3949–3967.

Murthy, V.N. and Fetz, E.E. (1996b) Synchronization of neurons during local field potential oscillations in sensorimotor cortex of awake monkeys. *Journal of Neurophysiology*, 76, 3968–3982.

Neuenschwander, S. and Singer, W. (1996) Long-range synchronization of oscillatory light responses in the cat retina and lateral geniculate nucleus. *Nature*, 379, 728–733.

Palm, G., (1990) Cell assemblies as a guideline for brain research. *Concepts in Neuroscience*, 1, 133–147.

Rager, G. and Singer, W. (1998) The response of cat visual cortex to flicker stimuli of variable frequency. *European Journal of Neuroscience*, 10, 1856–1877.

Reid, R.C. and Alonso, J.M. (1995) Specificity of monosynaptic connections from thalamus to visual cortex. *Nature*, 378, 281–284.

Riehle, A., Grün, S., Diesmann, M. and Aertsen, A. (1997) Spike synchronization and rate modulation differentially involved in motor cortical function. *Science*, 278, 1950–1953.

Roelfsema, P.R., König, P., Engel, A.K., Sireteanu, R. and Singer, W. (1994) Reduced synchronization in the visual cortex of cats with strabismic amblyopia. *European Journal of Neuroscience*, 6, 1645–1655.

Roelfsema, P.R., Engel, A.K., König, P. and Singer, W. (1996) The role of neuronal synchronization in response selection: a biologically plausible theory of structured representations in the visual cortex. *Journal of Cognitive Neuroscience*, 8, 603–625.

Roelfsema, P.R., Lamme, V.A.F. and Spekreijse, H. (1998) Object-based attention in the primary visual cortex of the macaque monkey. *Nature*, 395, 376–381.

Rolls, D.T. and Tovee, M.J. (1994) Processing speed in the cerebral cortex and the neurophysiology of visual masking. *Proceedings of the Royal Society of London B*, 257, 9–15.

Sanes, J.N. and Donoghue, J.P. (1993) Oscillations in local field potentials of the primate motor cortex during voluntary movement. *Proceedings of the National Academy of Sciences of the United States of America*, 90, 4470–4474.

Schmidt, K.E., Goebel, R., Löwel, S. and Singer, W. (1997) The perceptual grouping criterion of colinearity is reflected by anisotropies of connections in the primary visual cortex. *European Journal of Neuroscience*, 9, 1083–1089.

Sejnowski, T.R. (1986) Open questions about computation in cerebral cortex. In: McClelland, J.L. and Rumelhart, D.E. (eds), *Parallel Distributed Processing*, Vol. 2. MIT Press, Cambridge, Massachusetts, pp. 372–389.

Shadlen, M.N. and Newsome, W.T. (1994) Noise, neural codes and cortical organization. *Current Opinion in Neurobiology*, 4, 569–579.

Shadlen, M.N. and Newsome, W.T. (1998) The variable discharge of cortical neurons: implications for connectivity, computation, and information coding. *Journal of Neuroscience*, 18, 3870–3896.

Sheer, D.E. (1984) Focused arousal, 40 Hz EEG, and dysfunction. In: Elbert, T., Rockstroh, B., Lutzenberger, W. and Birbaumer, N. (eds), *Self-regulation of the Brain and Behavior*. Springer Verlag, Berlin, pp. 66–84.

Singer, W. (1993) Synchronization of cortical activity and its putative role in information processing and learning. *Annual Review of Physiology*, 55, 349–374.

Singer, W. (1995) Development and plasticity of cortical processing architectures. *Science*, 270, 758–764.

Singer, W. (1999) Neuronal synchrony, a versatile code for the definition of relations? *Neuron*, 24, 49–65

Singer, W. and Gray, C.M. (1995) Visual feature integration and the temporal correlation hypothesis. *Annual Review of Neuroscience*, 18, 555–586.

Singer, W., Engel, A.K., Kreiter, A.K., Munk, M.H.J., Neuenschwander, S. and Roelfsema, P.R. (1997) Neuronal assemblies: necessity, signature and detectability. *Trends in Cognitive Sciences*, 1, 252–261.

Softky, W.R. (1995) Simple codes versus efficient codes. *Current Opinion in Neurobiology*, 5, 239–247.

Softky, W.R. and Koch, C. (1993) The highly irregular firing of cortical cells is inconsistent with temporal integration of random EPSPs. *Journal of Neuroscience*, 13, 334–350.

Stevens, C.F. and Zador, A.M. (1998) Input synchrony and the irregular firing of cortical neurons. *Nature Neuroscience*, 1, 210–217.

Tallon-Baudry, C., Bertrand, O., Delpuech, C. and Pernier, J. (1996) Stimulus specificity of phase-locked and non-phase-locked 40Hz visual responses in human. *Journal of Neuroscience*, 16, 4240–4249.

Tallon-Baudry, C., Bertrand, O., Delpuech, C. and Pernier, J. (1997) Oscillatory γ-band (30–70Hz) activity induced by a visual search task in humans. *Journal of Neuroscience*, 17, 722–734.

Tallon-Baudry, C., Bertrand, O., Peronnet, F. and Pernier J. (1998) Induced γ-band activity during the delay of a visual short-term memory task in humans. *Journal of Neuroscience*, 18, 4244–4254.

Tanaka, K., Saito, H., Fukada, Y. and Moriya, M. (1991) Coding visual images of objects in the inferotemporal cortex of the macaque monkey. *Journal of Neurophysiology*, 66, 170–189.

Thorpe, S., Fize, D. and Marlot, C. (1996) Speed of processing in the human visual system. *Nature*, 38, 520–522.

Ts'o, D.Y. and Gilbert, C.D. (1988) The organization of chromatic and spatial interactions in the primate striate cortex. *Journal of Neuroscience*, 8, 1712–1727.

Usher, M. and Donnelly, N. (1998) Visual synchrony affects binding and segmentation in perception. *Nature*, 394, 179–182.

Usrey, W.M., Reppas, J.B. and Reid, R.C. (1998) Paired-spike interactions and synaptic efficacy of retinal inputs to the thalamus. *Nature*, 395, 384–387.

Van Vreeswijk, D., Abbott, L.F. and Ermentrout, G.B. (1994) When inhibition not excitation synchronizes neural firing. *Journal of Computational Neuroscience*, 1, 313–321.

Volgushev, M., Voronin, L.L., Chistiakova, M. and Singer, W. (1997) Relations between long-term synaptic modifications and paired-pulse interactions in the rat neocortex. *European Journal of Neuroscience*, 9, 1656–1665

von der Malsburg, C. (1985) Nervous structures with dynamical links. *Berichte der Bunsengesellschaft für Physikalische Chemie*, 89, 703–710.

4 VISUAL ATTENTION IN MIND AND BRAIN

John Duncan

INTRODUCTION

In this chapter, I address the problem of selective attention, in particular the direction of attention to one object rather than another in our cluttered, complex visual world. In cognitive psychology, based largely on studies of human behavior and performance, attention has been a central topic at least since the publication of Broadbent's *Perception and Communication* in 1958. In the subsequent 40 years, a large body of experimental and theoretical work has established basic properties of attentional function at this behavioral level. More recently, the expansion of cognitive neuroscience has led to increasing attempts to understand the implementation of attentional functions at the neurophysiological level. Indeed, through a combination of well-defined behavioral questions and firm basis in known sensorimotor physiology, the problem of attention is establishing itself as one of the higher mental functions especially well suited to the converging methods of the cognitive neuroscience approach.

It is clear from everyday experience that objects in the visual world in a sense *compete* for our attention. Thus devoting attention to one thing implies withdrawing it from others, leaving us with a detailed awareness of some objects but little if any awareness of others. By and large, furthermore, our attention tends to be focused on objects of relevance to current behavior. Thus competition is *biased* by the context of current tasks or concerns, relevant objects competing strongly while irrelevant—though perhaps equally salient—objects are ignored. In this chapter, I consider attention from the perspective of these two problems, competition and bias.

In part, no doubt, the selection of relevant information from a visual scene is accomplished by eye movements. Certainly we tend to fixate objects of current concern, giving them the advantage of foveal representation on the retina. At the same time, it is an everyday experience that we can attend selectively away from the point of fixation, showing that additional, internal mechanisms supplement the selection of relevant information by gaze direction. Indeed it is easy to see why this should be the case: since attended objects come in all shapes and sizes, it will not generally be possible to select them simply by favoring input at the fovea. In this chapter, in any case, the focus is not on the control of eye movements, but on those internal selection mechanisms differentiating 'attended' from 'unattended' inputs.

The chapter has two main sections. The first deals with general principles of attentional function established in behavioral studies. Such principles may be regarded as *constraints* shaping theory at the behavioral level, and indeed, I show how they are aptly captured by a specific quantitative account, Bundesen's (1990) Theory of Visual Attention or TVA. The second section turns to the issue of neural implementation, reviewing electrophysiological and neuropsychological studies in human and monkey.

BEHAVIORAL STUDIES

Competition

A simple example (Duncan, 1993b) illustrates the problem of competition. In this experiment, each stimulus display (Figure 4.1A) consisted of two grating patches, one unpredictably positioned to the left or right of fixation (the *horizontal* stimulus), the other above or below (the *vertical* stimulus). Each possible stimulus position was marked by a frame of four dots (Figure 4.1), and a central dot marked the

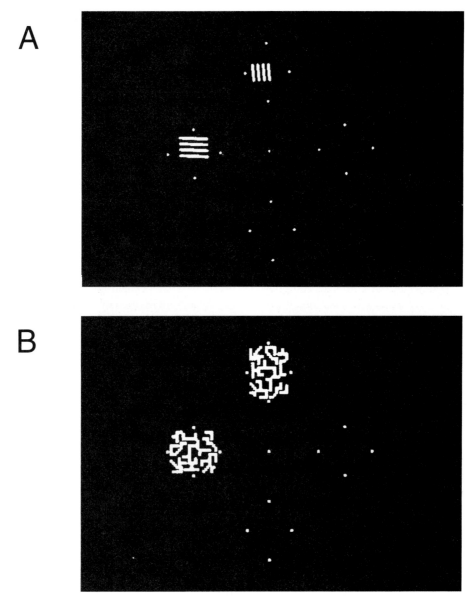

Figure 4.1. Example stimuli from Duncan (1993b). (**A**) Gratings; (**B**) masks.

point of fixation. Stimuli were exposed briefly (100–150 ms), and followed immediately by a masking display (Figure 4.1B) used to restrict any remaining visual impression of the gratings after their offset.

In one *focused attention* condition, the subject was required to identify just the length of the horizontal grating. There were two alternative lengths for this stimulus, and the subject simply indicated after each exposure which length he or she thought had been presented. Central fixation was maintained throughout; to encourage this, the subject did not know in advance of the display whether the critical stimulus would be presented to the left or right, and displays themselves were too brief to permit directed eye movements after display onset. In this condition, with only one relevant object in the display, the proportion of correct responses was 0.94. A second focused attention condition required the subject to identify just the length of the vertical stimulus; here the proportion correct was 0.80. The critical comparison is with the third condition, *divided attention*. In this case, the subject was required to identify the lengths of both stimuli. This time, accordingly, two separate reports were made at the end of each trial, one for the horizontal and another for the vertical. Now, with two relevant objects competing for attention, proportion correct dropped to 0.80 for the horizontal stimulus and 0.66 for the vertical.

In the general version of this experiment, two visual stimuli are presented. For the most part, I will concentrate on experiments with brief stimuli—typically exposed for less than 200 ms—which cannot be identified perfectly. In focused attention control conditions, the subject is asked to identify some property of just one stimulus. In the divided attention condition, properties of both stimuli must be identified simultaneously. As in the above example, a variety of means are used to ensure constant eye position across conditions. Typically, nevertheless, there is decreased accuracy in the divided attention condition. Subjectively, diverting attention to one stimulus makes the other harder to see. This decrease of accuracy when two stimuli must be processed—the *divided attention decrement*—provides the behavioral measure of attentional competition.

Many variations of this simple experiment are possible. Subjects can be asked to identify different attributes of the presented stimuli, from simple features such as color, motion or line orientation, to more complex properties such as shape or identity. Discriminations can be relatively easy or relatively difficult. There can be variation in spatial and temporal relationships between attended stimuli. In the following sections, I review some of the basic principles established by experiments of this sort.

Ubiquity of attentional competition

Many theories have proposed that attentional competition should be seen only for certain kinds of visual judgement. An early view, for example, was that competition reflected limited capacity for processing complex stimulus attributes such as the shape and meaning of a word (see, for example, Broadbent, 1958; Neisser, 1967). In contrast, unlimited capacity was proposed for simultaneous processing of simpler features such as color and size, implying that for these there should be no divided attention decrement. At least in its early versions, the influential feature integration theory of Treisman and Gelade (1980) made a

similar suggestion: attentional competition was relevant only to the processing of complex combinations of visual features, not elementary features themselves.

As outlined above, however, the simple competition experiment suggests no distinctions of this sort. Certainly there is a divided attention decrement for the identification of complex shapes and feature conjunctions (Broadbent, 1958; Treisman and Schmidt, 1982). Very similar decrements, however, attach to the processing of many elementary visual features, including size, line orientation, spatial frequency, color, brightness, texture, motion and spatial location (Duncan, 1984, 1993a,b; Duncan and Nimmo-Smith, 1996; see also, for example, Lindsay *et al.*, 1967; Wing and Allport, 1972; Long, 1975). With only a few possible exceptions (Braun and Sagi, 1991; Bonnel *et al.*, 1992), decrement is almost universal in experiments of this sort.

This ubiquity of attentional competition corresponds well with everyday experience. When we are fully absorbed in attention to one object, very little is known of others; indeed we may be unaware even of the existence of other salient events in the environment (Rock *et al.*, 1992), let alone their detailed properties. In this respect, competition is a central aspect of awareness and use of any aspect of visual information.

Object-based competition

What factor sets the limit to simultaneous processing of multiple inputs? Is it the number of discriminations to be made, or the total information processed (Broadbent, 1958)? Is it the spatial area over which attention must be distributed? In fact, the key consideration appears to be the *number of objects* to be attended (Neisser, 1967; Duncan, 1984).

Consider a display containing two objects, e.g. grating patches like those shown in Figure 4.1, this time varying in both size and exact location within their surrounding frame of dots (Duncan, 1993a). One may now require 'divided attention' in several different ways. First, as we have already considered, one may ask the subject to identify *the same* property of each object, i.e. both sizes or both locations. Secondly, one may ask for identification of *different properties* of the two objects, e.g. size of one and location of the other. Since different visual features are processed to some extent in different, specialized regions of the primate brain (see later), it is interesting to ask what happens when these different systems are asked to work concurrently on different objects in the scene. In fact, divided attention decrements are very similar in the same- and different-property cases (Duncan, 1993a,b). Thirdly, one may ask for identification of *both properties* of both objects. Though the amount of information to be processed has now increased, this has no effect on performance: Accuracy is just as high as it is when only one property of each object must be identified (Duncan, 1993b). Fourthly, one may ask for identification of *both properties of a single object*, e.g. both size and location of the horizontal stimulus. Now the results are very different: all divided attention decrement is eliminated. In other words, when a subject must identify two properties of the same object, each property is identified exactly as well as it is in a control condition requiring identification of this property on its own (Duncan, 1984, 1993a,b; Duncan and Nimmo-Smith, 1996).

For the display of Figure 4.1, the spatial distribution of information is very different in one- and two-object cases. Visual attention often has been likened to a mental spotlight facilitating perception in a selected region of space (Eriksen and Hoffman, 1973; Posner *et al.*, 1980); according to such a model, the one-object case would be easy because both relevant visual features were present in the same location, allowing the spotlight to encompass both simultaneously. In fact, however, divided attention decrements are much the same in the two-object case, whether objects are spatially separate as in Figure 4.1, or overlapping at the fixation point (Duncan, 1984; Vecera and Farah, 1994).

Perhaps the clearest separation of object- and space-based effects can be made with transparent motion displays (Valdes-Sosa *et al.*, 1998b). If two completely overlapping patterns of random dots rotate in opposite directions, one set rotating clockwise and the other set anticlockwise, they are perceived as two separate sheets, presented at exactly the same spatial location but moving in opposite directions. Now suppose that subjects must identify either two properties of a single sheet, or one property of each. Again, there is a divided attention decrement only in the two-object case (Valdes-Sosa *et al.*, 1998b).

Together, these experiments show that the key factor in attentional competition is neither the nature nor number of discriminations to be made, nor simply the spatial layout of relevant information (though spatial factors can be important in more complex displays; see, for example, Hoffman and Nelson, 1981; Lavie and Driver, 1996). Rather it is *the number of objects* to be attended at one time.

Parallel processing extended in time

Since the early 1960s (e.g. Estes and Taylor, 1966), two classes of models have been applied to attentional phenomena. According to high-speed serial models, competition arises because some stage of visual processing can deal with only one input at a time. To process an array of multiple objects, this serial process moves rapidly from one to another. A typical rate hypothesized in such models is 50 ms/item, accounting for the manifest ability to complete processing of a multiple-element array in just a few hundred milliseconds (e.g. Estes and Taylor, 1966; Treisman and Gelade, 1980). Competition according to these models is viewed as competitive access to the serial stage; if this stage is dealing with one input, others must wait until it is finished. The alternative is limited-capacity parallel processing (e.g. Atkinson *et al.*, 1969). Here multiple attended items can be processed simultaneously, each for a much longer period of time. Competition now is viewed as reduced speed or accuracy of processing any one item as the number of simultaneously processed items increases.

By varying the interval between one attended input and another, we can obtain a direct measurement of the time course of attentional competition. An experiment by Duncan *et al.* (1994) provides an illustration. Stimuli are illustrated in Figure 4.2A. On each trial, two alphanumeric characters were presented, a number 2 or 5, appearing in a horizontal position (left or right of fixation, cf. Figure 4.1), and a letter T or L, appearing in a vertical position (above or below). Characters were presented only for a period of 45–60 ms, calibrated to bring performance below 100% correct, and followed by a masking pattern of random contours. The two stimuli, number and letter, were presented in random order, with an interval (stimulus onset asynchrony or SOA) of 0–900 ms between their onsets.

In one focused attention condition, as before, subjects were asked just to pay attention to the number, i.e. to the horizontal positions, and to identify it as 2 or 5. Responses were unspeeded, and made at the end of the whole stimulus sequence. In a second focused attention condition, subjects identified just the letter occurring in a vertical position. Mean accuracy in these focused attention conditions is shown by the upper function in Figure 4.2B. In this figure, data for the *first* character presented on each trial are plotted at negative SOAs, while data for the *second* character are plotted at positive SOAs. For example, results at SOA

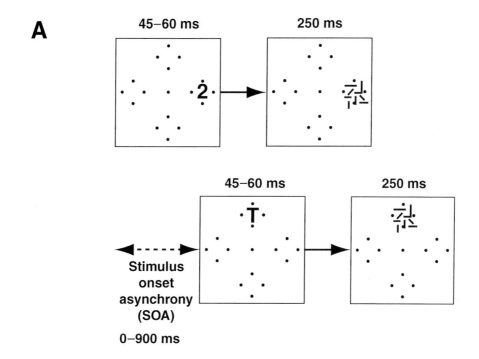

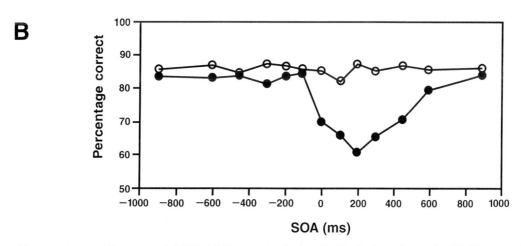

Figure 4.2. The experiment of Duncan *et al.* (1994). (**A**) Events of a single trial. The horizontal stimulus (digit) appeared randomly to the left or right of fixation, followed immediately by a mask in the same location. The vertical stimulus (letter) appeared randomly above or below fixation, also followed immediately by a mask. The order of horizontal and vertical stimuli was random, the second following the first by a delay of 0–900 ms (onset to onset). (**B**) Mean percent correct identification in focused attention (○) and divided attention (●).

= –300 show mean accuracy for an attended number when it preceded an unattended letter by 300 ms, and for an attended letter when it preceded an unattended number by 300 ms. The results showed that, in these focused attention conditions, performance was unaffected by SOA: the accuracy of identifying a single attended character was independent of temporal separation from a preceding or following unattended item.

In the divided attention condition, both characters were to be identified on each trial. Again, responses were unspeeded, and given at the end of the stimulus sequence. The results (Figure 4.2B, lower function) were very different from those of the control conditions. Again the first item presented on each trial was identified well, independently of temporal separation (Figure 4.2B, negative SOAs). At separations up to around 500 ms, however, the second item suffered substantial interference. A separation of 900 ms was needed before accuracy returned to control levels. Other experiments have shown very much the same with two inputs presented successively at fixation (e.g. Broadbent and Broadbent, 1987; Raymond *et al.*, 1992). The results show that, even with very brief visual inputs, the time course of attentional competition is at least several hundred milliseconds; two attended inputs must be separated by half a second or more before competition is eliminated.

Such results are quite incompatible with conventional serial models. According to such models, interference between one item and the next should be eliminated by a separation of the order of 50 ms, allowing the serial process to be finished with the first item by the time it should begin on the second. Instead, the results suggest competition over a much longer time course, in line with the proposal of extended, parallel but limited-capacity processing.

Results like these make another useful point. Evidently, in the experiments we are considering, we are dealing with competition in stimulus *input* rather than response *output*. Two targets can be reported well as long as they are not *presented* close together in time (Duncan, 1980).

Bias

We turn now from competition to bias, i.e. selective processing of those inputs most relevant to current behavior. As in the focused attention conditions of the above experiments, some parts of the input are defined as *targets* to be identified, while others are defined as *non-targets* to be ignored. Our topic in this section is how competition can be biased such that targets are processed while non-targets are not.

A good example is the *partial report* experiment (e.g. Sperling, 1960; von Wright, 1970; Bundesen *et al.*, 1985). An array of several objects (e.g. filled and outline letters; see Figure 4.3) is presented briefly. Some rule (e.g. 'report only the filled letters') defines some objects as targets to be identified and reported, others as non-targets to be ignored. Again responses are unspeeded and the measure is the accuracy of target identification. In this experiment, we can manipulate both the number of targets (Figure 4.3A versus B) and the number of non-targets (Figure 4.3A versus C) in the array. Evidently each target will be identified less well as the number of targets increases, reflecting attentional competition in the standard way (X identified less well in Figure 4.3B than in A). However, what will happen with non-targets? If the task context is effective in producing the desired competitive bias, targets will compete strongly to be processed, while non-targets will compete weakly if at all. In the extreme case, performance would be unaffected by the number of non-targets in the display; target identification would be just as good whether non-targets were present or absent (report of X as good in Figure 4.3C as in A). At the opposite extreme, there could be no effective bias. In this case, non-targets would compete as strongly as targets; adding non-targets to the array would have just as harmful an effect as adding targets (report of X as bad in Figure 4.3C as in B). Thus the experiment provides a scale for measurement of bias under a range of visual and task conditions.

Many visual features can bias competition

In the above example, target selection is based on a filled–outline distinction. Many variants of the partial report experiment are possible, however, including selection by location (e.g. reporting just items from one row of a display), by a variety of simple object features such as color, brightness or size (e.g. reporting just red items, just dim items or just small items), or even by more complex categorizations (e.g. reporting letters while ignoring numbers). In all these cases, there is evidence for some effective bias; adding non-targets to the display is less harmful than adding targets (e.g. Sperling, 1960; von Wright, 1970; Duncan, 1983; Bundesen *et al.*, 1985).

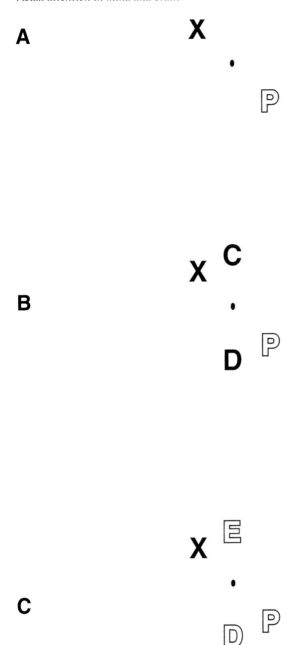

Figure 4.3. Example stimuli for partial report. The task is to identify just the filled letters, with a variable number of targets (**A** versus **B**) and non-targets (**A** versus **C**).

Flexibility is a key requirement for attentional control: in principle, any kind of object, at any level of scale, can be the most relevant to current concerns. In correspondence with this requirement, the data

indeed suggest that many different selection rules can be used to produce preferential target processing.

Efficiency of selection is continuously variable
Though some degree of selective target processing is seen in many different contexts, partial report experiments of the sort described above show that the *degree* of bias varies widely from one context to another (Bundesen *et al.*, 1985; Shibuya, 1993). Some selection rules, e.g. selection based on a large difference in color, are more effective than others, e.g. selection based on alphanumeric category (Bundesen *et al.*, 1985). Indeed, cases can be found with no apparent selectivity at all (Duncan, 1987).

In fact, most work examining the efficiency of selection has used a variant of partial report, the visual search task (Neisser, 1963). In this variant, a single target is present in an array of multiple non-targets; the time to find the target is plotted as a function of the number of presented non-targets, usually with unlimited exposure duration. In the easiest cases, this function is flat: adding non-targets to the array is without effect, corresponding to the most efficient cases of partial report. In harder cases, the slope increases up to 100 ms or more per added non-target (Duncan, 1987). For the visual search task, it is impossible to know what slope value would correspond to zero selectivity—equal processing of targets and non-targets—because the case of processing N non-targets is not compared with the corresponding case of processing N targets. Still, the method provides a convenient way to compare selectivity in different task contexts (see, for example, Treisman and Gelade, 1980; Treisman and Gormican, 1988).

Not surprisingly, the single main factor determining the slope of the search function is the similarity between targets and non-targets. Whatever the visual feature distinguishing these two, increasing the similarity of targets and non-targets increases search slope (Treisman and Gormican, 1988; Duncan and Humphreys, 1989). A second major factor is similarity of the non-targets themselves; a target stands out well, for example, against a background of identical non-targets (Farmer and Taylor, 1980; Duncan and Humphreys, 1989). A *search surface* (Duncan and Humphreys, 1989) summarizing the joint effects of these two variables is shown in Figure 4.4; using this surface, it is easy to design search tasks of any arbitrary level of difficulty, whatever the visual feature (color, motion, shape, etc.) or combination of features

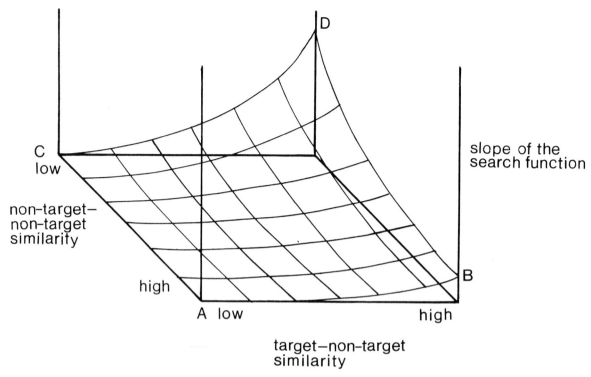

Figure 4.4. Search surface illustrating variable search efficiency (slope) as a joint function of target–non-target and non-target–non-target similarity. Reproduced with permission from Duncan and Humphreys (1989).

(e.g. conjunctions of color and shape) used to distinguish targets from non-targets.

Controlling competitive bias with information that cannot itself be reported

Consider a partial report experiment in which the task is to identify only red letters. As we have seen, targets may compete strongly to be processed, so that performance is very sensitive to the number of targets in the display, while non-targets compete weakly, so that the number of non-targets is rather unimportant.

In this case, a plausible explanation might be that color can be processed with little attentional competition, while letter identity cannot (Broadbent, 1971). Color is processed first, serving to reject non-targets. Only targets require competitive processing of shape.

This line of reasoning fails, however, when exactly the same information serves both to distinguish targets from non-targets, and to support target reports. A good example is the task of reporting digits and ignoring letters. Very probably, a character must be identified before it can be classified as a digit or a

letter, yet still it can be found that performance is sensitive mainly to the number of targets (digits), non-targets having modest (Duncan, 1983) or negligible (Duncan, 1980) competitive impact. Simpler distinctions between targets and non-targets (e.g. detecting tilted lines among verticals) can be used to make the same point (Duncan, 1985).

How can it be that non-targets in such a task can be rejected with little competitive impact, while targets must compete to be identified or reported explicitly? The data suggest that, at the time of input, the same visual information is used in two rather different processing phases, with different properties. In the first phase, information is used to set competitive strengths high for targets and low for non-targets. Though in one sense one may say that targets are already 'identified' in this phase, such identification is not yet sufficient to support explicit report or control of behavior. Subjectively, it seems that the target has not yet reached awareness. For that, the further, competitive processing phase is needed, guided by the first phase so that now targets are processed preferentially (Duncan, 1980). Subjectively, attention is drawn to targets in the display, with little awareness of non-targets.

The essential distinction between processing of targets and non-targets casts light on a point raised earlier. As we have seen, it has been suggested often that simple visual features such as color can be processed without attentional competition. Generally, however, such proposals have been based on the results of visual search studies, i.e. on processing of multiple non-targets. When subjects must identify explicitly the colors of two separate targets, color, like any other visual feature, shows clear competitive effects (Duncan and Nimmo-Smith, 1996). Again the results imply a two-phase architecture, the first phase setting competitive strengths, the second enabling explicit behavior.

Bundesen's (1990) Theory of Visual Attention (TVA)

Together, the principles outlined in the previous sections provide constraints helping to shape an appropriate attentional theory. In this section, I give a brief outline of one theory, Bundesen's TVA (1990), that combines these principles in the context of a specific quantitative form.

A fundamental idea in TVA is that objects in a visual display *race* to be identified. When an identification is made, it is placed into a limited-capacity visual short-term memory (VSTM), and is then available for report and the control of explicit behavior. Biased competition is introduced by modulating the speed of processing for each object in the race.

Exponential processing dynamics

Consider first the identification of a single object presented in an otherwise empty field. According to TVA, the probability of identifying this object increases exponentially as a function of time. Indeed, exponential functions provide good fits to data measuring the probability of correct identification as a function of exposure duration (interval between stimulus onset and onset of a subsequent masking pattern) (see Bundesen, 1998a).

Competition through modulation of rate

When several objects are processed together, competition is reflected in a reduced processing rate for each one. Specifically, the rate parameter of an exponential function indicates how quickly identification takes place. In Figure 4.5, for example, the function relating probability of identification to processing time is shown separately for three different rate parameters. In TVA, it is these rate parameters that decrease when objects compete to be processed.

Evidently, TVA implements competition by limited-capacity parallel processing. Furthermore, it models identification of all visual features—that an object is the color red, the letter E, positioned in a certain location—in the same way, so that all categorizations are subject to competitive modulation.

Bias by attentional weighting

How strongly is processing rate reduced in a multiple-object display? According to TVA, each object *i* is given an *attentional weight* w_i. For each object, the basic processing rate, i.e the rate obtained when this object is processed alone, is multiplied by the ratio of its own attentional weight divided by the sum of weights for all objects in the display. Thus objects with high weights (relative to others in the display) are processed relatively well, and, at the same time, they produce strong interference with processing of other objects (adding substantially to the denominator of each weight ratio). Objects with low weights are processed poorly, and produce only weak interference (adding little to the denominator of each weight ratio).

An object's weight ratio modulates the processing of all that object's features. Thus TVA implements object-based competition; the key consideration is the relative weighting of different objects in a display, not which features of those objects are to be processed.

Weight setting by match to a target category

How are attentional weights set? In a first stage of processing, every object in the input is matched against a set of *pertinent* target categories defining the relevant inputs for this task. For example, pertinent categories might be 'objects in a certain row' (selection by location), 'red objects' (selection by feature) or 'letters' (selection by category). To the extent that any object is similar to one of the target categories, its attentional weight is increased.

Thus TVA implements flexible selection rules by allowing task-dependent definition of target pertinence. The quantitative implementation of matching between input objects and target categories leads naturally to variable efficiency of attentional

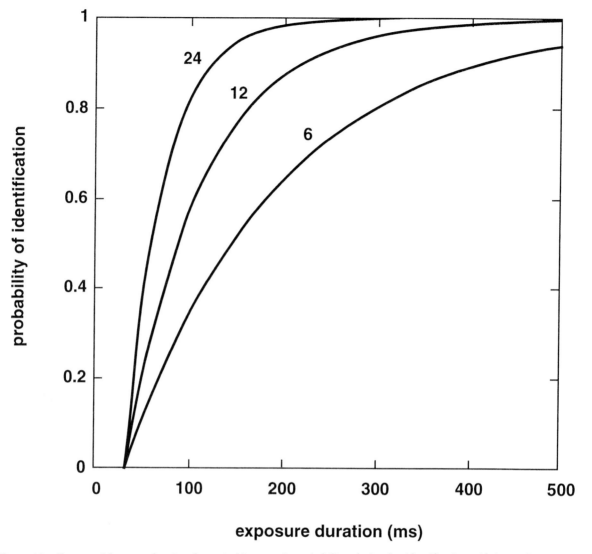

Figure 4.5. Exponential curves showing the typical increase in probability of stimulus identification with increasing exposure duration. The parameter is the exponential rate constant. As shown, a minimum exposure of the order of 30 ms is usually required before processing begins.

weighting: when non-target objects are very unlike the target category, they receive low weights and contribute little to attentional competition; when they are closely similar to targets, they receive high weights and compete strongly. TVA also implements the two phases of visual processing discussed above; though attentional weights are set early on, explicit reports and behavior can only be based on categorizations subsequently entered into VSTM.

Beyond its agreement with important qualitative principles, the quantitative form of TVA—its expo-nential processing dynamics, competition through modulation of processing rate, weight setting by match to target categories—allows detailed, quantitative fits to data from many different kinds of experiment, including measurements of both accuracy and speed as a function of numbers of targets and non-targets in partial report, visual search and many other tasks (Bundesen, 1990, 1998a,b). As one would hope, parameters of the theory respond appropriately to experimental manipulations targeting one or another aspect of attentional function; for example, altering the selection rule in partial report affects only the relative weights of targets and non-targets, leaving basic processing rates, short-term memory capacity, etc. unaffected (Bundesen *et al.*, 1985; see also Shibuya, 1993). Without doubt, the theory has some restrictions of scope; at the same time, it aptly captures a great deal of what we currently know about attentional functions at the level of behavioral measurements.

Open questions

Of course, very many questions remain open at the behavioral level. We may take just one as an example. What is the relationship between competitive phenomena in vision and the more general issue of performance decrements in dual tasks? Our everyday experience of limited attentional capacity is not restricted to visual perception; much more generally, absorption in one line of thought or action implies withdrawal from others. One common view is that many separate reasons exist for 'limited capacity' or interference between concurrent activities (e.g. Allport, 1980). For example, similar tasks (e.g. two verbal or two spatial tasks) will sometimes interfere more strongly than dissimilar tasks (one verbal and one spatial), implying conflict in material-specific processing systems (e.g. Baddeley, 1986). Indeed, some experiments suggest little interference between the identification of concurrent visual and auditory inputs (Treisman and Davies, 1973; Duncan *et al.*, 1997b), implying that competition in strictly visual experiments is largely modality specific. At the same time, there are cases of very substantial interference between speeded response to an auditory input and concurrent unspeeded identification of a brief visual input (Jolicoeur, 1999). Though this chapter emphasizes competition within vision, this is evidently only one example of a much broader set of competitive phenomena in cognition in general.

NEURAL IMPLEMENTATION

Many brain systems are active concurrently in response to visual input. These include the many cortical 'visual areas' in the posterior part of the brain, specialized for different aspects of visual processing and in part for processing separate visual attributes such as color, motion, location and shape (Desimone and Ungerleider, 1989). Visually driven activity is also seen, however, in a variety of more motor and sensorimotor regions such as premotor cortex and the frontal eye fields, and throughout a broad area of prefrontal cortex (e.g. Rainer *et al.*, 1998). Among others, visually responsive subcortical structures include the superior colliculus, involved in control of eye movements, and a number of different thalamic nuclei. In the second part of this chapter, I turn to the neural implementation of attentional functions in the context of this widely distributed network of visually responsive brain systems.

Without doubt, we are not yet in a position to make a detailed mapping between principles established in behavioral studies and neurophysiological mechanisms. At the same time, the discussion may be guided by the outline of a scheme for object-based attentional competition, and for how such competition may be biased by current behavioral context (Desimone and Duncan, 1995; Duncan, 1996; Duncan *et al.*, 1997a). The scheme rests on three proposals. First, we suggest that processing is competitive in many and perhaps most visually responsive brain systems. Increased response to one object is associated with decreased response to others, for example because responses to different objects are mutually inhibitory. Such competition, we suggest, is the neural equivalent of attentional competition at the behavioral level. Secondly, we suggest that behaviorally relevant objects are given a competitive advantage by pre-activation or priming of corresponding neural populations (Walley and Weiden, 1973; Harter and Aine, 1984). When the task requires attention to red objects, for example, neurons responding to red are primed in color-selective parts of the network. Such priming implements bias of attentional competition by behavioral context. Thirdly, competition is *integrated* between one brain system and another; as an object gains dominance in any one part of the network, it tends also to take control of the remainder. As a whole, the network tends to settle into a state in which the same object is dominant throughout, making its different properties concurrently available for control of behavior. Together, this set of proposals may be termed the *integrated competition hypothesis* (Duncan, 1996). The following sections review the physiological and neuropsychological evidence bearing on this general view.

Physiological studies

Competition and non-target suppression in the extrastriate cortex

The first relevant results come from single-cell recording studies of attentional competition in the visual cortex of the behaving monkey. A useful illustration is a recent study of responses in infero-temporal (IT) cortex during a simple form of visual search (Chelazzi *et al.*, 1998; see also Chelazzi *et al.*, 1993). Receiving projections from earlier regions of extrastriate cortex, IT is a high-level visual area involved in the final stages of object recognition (Desimone and Ungerleider, 1989). Cells in IT have large, bilateral receptive fields generally including the fovea; they are typically selective for complex object features such as combinations of color and shape.

The stimuli for our experiment were complex, multicolored pictures presented on a computer monitor. For any given cell, the experiment began by selecting three stimuli: one, the good stimulus, selected to produce a strong positive response from the cell; a second, the poor stimulus, selected to produce little or no response; and a third, the neutral stimulus, selected with no specific response requirement. In the experiment proper, we were interested in the cell's response to arrays consisting of (i) the good stimulus alone, (ii) the poor stimulus alone and (iii) the good and poor stimulus together; use of the neutral stimulus will be explained below.

Following stimulus selection, responses were recorded during several hundred trials of search. Each trial began with onset of a fixation point in the center of the screen. Once fixation was achieved, a first stimulus, the cue, was presented, also at screen center. This cue could be any one of the three stimuli selected for the experiment. At this point, the monkey simply had to hold fixation, remembering the cue as his *target* for the current trial. Following a brief delay (typically 1500 ms), a search array of one or two (different) stimuli was presented. For the data to be described here, the array was presented in the visual field contralateral to the recording site, within the receptive field of the recorded cell. On half of the trials, the previously specified target was present in the array, in an unpredictable location. It appeared either alone (one-stimulus arrays) or accompanied by a non-target (two-stimulus arrays). On remaining trials, the target was absent, the array consisting of one or two non-targets. The monkey's task was to make an immediate saccade to the target if present, otherwise to hold fixation for a further period.

Responses to several possible arrays are shown in Figure 4.6. These are average responses from 58 individually recorded cells, with zero on the time axis indicating array onset. Responses to one- and two-stimulus non-target arrays are shown in Figure 4.6A,

and responses to corresponding target arrays in Figure 4.6B.

Consider first the non-target arrays (Figure 4.6A). The strongest response occurred to the good stimulus presented on its own. The poor stimulus on its own produced little or no response. The key results concern response to the two-stimulus array consisting of good and poor stimuli together. (On these trials, the specified target was the third, neutral stimulus.) Though the good stimulus was present in the receptive field, responses to this stimulus were weakened by the additional presence of the poor stimulus. Such data strongly imply some form of competition or interference between concurrent stimuli in the array.

The target array data (Figure 4.6B) are perhaps even more informative. Responses to single good or poor stimuli were much the same whether these appeared as targets (Figure 4.6B) or non-targets (Figure 4.6A). The data suggest that, in the absence of competing array elements, the IT response is influenced little by behavioral context. When both good and poor stimuli were present in the array, however, responses depended strongly on which of these was the target. Following an initial on-discharge, response to the good stimulus in the array was sustained when this stimulus was the target. In this case, indeed, responses approached those given to the good stimulus presented on its own. Following a similar on-discharge, however, responses to the good stimulus were later suppressed if this stimulus was the non-target and the accompanying poor stimulus was the target. Indeed, when the poor stimulus was the target, responses again approached those given to this poor stimulus on its own.

Such results are exactly what one would expect from a process of biased competition. When two stimuli are presented together, they compete for representation in IT. If both are non-targets, such competition is equally balanced, producing intermediate results. If one is a target, however, it dominates the competition; responses to this stimulus are maintained while responses to non-targets are suppressed. The overall result is that, by the time the animal makes its eye movement, only cells responsive to the current target are strongly active in IT.

The key result in this experiment is the differential response to the two-stimulus array, depending on whether the good stimulus is target (attended) or non-target (ignored). Viewed either as relative enhancement of target responses or relative suppression of non-target responses, such a differential response has

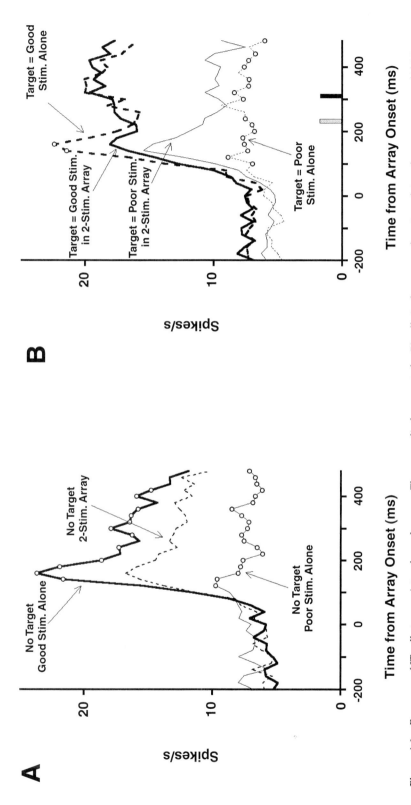

Figure 4.6. Response of IT cells to a variety of search arrays. The mean discharge rate for 58 cells is shown as a function of time from array onset. (**A**) Non-target arrays. (**B**) Target arrays, with bars on the abscissa showing mean saccadic latency for one-stimulus (dotted) and two-stimulus (filled) arrays. For the data presented here, arrays consisted of the good stimulus alone, the poor stimulus alone or both together (2-Stim.). Reproduced with permission from Chelazzi *et al.* (1998).

been observed throughout much of the monkey visual system, including posterior parietal cortex (Bushnell *et al.*, 1981), concerned in particular with spatial and visuomotor processing, the motion-sensitive areas MT and MST (Treue and Maunsell, 1996), the extrastriate regions V2 and V4 (Moran and Desimone, 1985; Motter, 1994; Luck *et al.*, 1997) and, more recently, primary visual cortex or V1 itself (Roelfsema *et al.*, 1998; see also Motter, 1993). Much the same undoubtedly can be observed in frontal and motor regions too (e.g. Schall *et al.*, 1995; Rainer *et al.*, 1998). Measurements of human brain activity using event-related brain potentials (ERPs; Van Voorhis and Hillyard, 1977), positron emission tomography (PET; Heinze *et al.*, 1994) and functional magnetic resonance imaging (fMRI; Martínez *et al.*, 1999) show a similar widespread suppression of responses to ignored or non-target objects. ERP studies have excellent temporal resolution; they show that the earliest cortical response, presumably arising in V1, is similar for attended and unattended inputs (Martínez *et al.*, 1999). Even in V1, however, responses to unattended inputs may be suppressed late in their time course (Roelfsema *et al.*, 1998; Martínez *et al.*, 1999).

As in behavioral studies, an important property of target enhancement and/or non-target suppression is that it reflects the structure of the selected target object, not just an attended region of space. In a transparent motion display, for example, the ERP generated by an event on the unattended dot field is suppressed substantially while, over exactly the same spatial region, there is good response to the attended field (Valdes-Sosa *et al.*, 1998a). In monkey V1, if the animal is set to attend to one irregularly curved line while ignoring another, cells responding to different segments along the attended line are enhanced simultaneously, even though attended and unattended lines may cross (Roelfsema *et al.*, 1998).

Together, the results reviewed in this section support the first major proposal of the integrated competition hypothesis. As reflected in suppression of responses to unattended or non-target stimuli, there is widespread, object-based competition throughout much of the sensorimotor network.

Priming of target-selective neurons
In many regions of the brain, single-cell recording has shown selective activity in *delays* preceding an anticipated stimulus or movement. Such delay activity is seen in motor and premotor cortex preceding an arm

movement (e.g. Godschalk *et al.*, 1985), in prefrontal and parietal cortex preceding eye movements (e.g. Gnadt and Andersen, 1988; Funahashi *et al.*, 1989), in inferotemporal cortex during matching of successive stimuli (e.g. Fuster *et al.*, 1985) and so on. According to the integrated competition hypothesis, such delay activity should be used to produce a competitive advantage for targets. When a given type of stimulus is defined as relevant to the current task, neurons responsive to that stimulus should be pre-activated or primed.

Again the data of Chelazzi *et al.* (1998) provide an illustration. During the interval following the cue, the screen was empty except for the central fixation point. In IT, however, neural activity reflected cue identity. In the majority of cells, there was a sustained increase in firing rate for those trials on which the cue was this cell's good stimulus. In a control experiment, such selective delay activity was eliminated when it was unnecessary for the monkey to remember the cue, simply maintaining fixation until a reward was given. For IT as a whole, the data imply that, in the interval preceding the search array, there was enhanced activity in those cells responsive to the current target. Very similar results have been described recently for shape-selective cells in area LIP of the parietal cortex (Sereno and Maunsell, 1998).

More broadly, the specialization of different extrastriate regions implies that very different regions should show priming activity in different task contexts. An instruction to attend to objects with a certain shape, location or movement should produce priming activity in areas where shape, location or movement respectively are coded. In the Chelazzi *et al.* (1998) experiment, behavioral relevance was defined by the *identity* of the target stimulus. Correspondingly, priming activity was seen in IT, whose neurons are selective for object identity. In spatial selection tasks, the monkey is cued instead to attend to whatever stimulus appears in a given *location*. Location information is weak in IT, since receptive fields are large; it is much better in earlier visual areas, where receptive fields are much smaller. Correspondingly, neurons in both V2 and V4 show increased activity when a monkey is cued to attend to a location within their receptive field (Luck *et al.*, 1997).

Though the above experiments concern extrastriate cortex, selective delay activity related to forthcoming targets can be at least as conspicuous in other regions of the brain. In both spatial and non-spatial selection tasks, such activity is particularly robust in prefrontal cortex (e.g. Fuster *et al.*, 1985; Funahashi *et al.*, 1989; Miller *et al.*, 1996). Very plausibly, the frontal lobe is one source of the signals establishing an appropriate competitive bias in posterior visual areas (Desimone and Duncan, 1995).

In some experiments, there has been little evidence of selective extrastriate delay activity (McAdams and Maunsell, 1999), and undoubtedly more work is needed to establish exactly when such activity is seen. Meanwhile, however, the results give preliminary support to this second aspect of the integrated competition hypothesis: when a certain type of stimulus is defined as relevant to the current task, neurons responsive to that stimulus can be pre-activated throughout widespread regions of visually responsive cortex.

Lesion studies

Extinction: imbalanced competition between left and right
The other major findings bearing upon the integrated competition hypothesis come from lesion studies. Of particular relevance is the phenomenon of *extinction* (Bender, 1952). Since the brain's representation of space is predominantly crossed, it is typical that lesions on one side of the brain will impair sensory and motor operations on the opposite side of space. In extinction, such impairments are exaggerated when the input or movement on the contralesional side is accompanied by a simultaneous input or movement on the ipsilesional or less affected side. In the most extreme cases, ipsilesional inputs may extinguish all awareness of concurrent contralesional events. This phenomenon rather directly suggests imbalanced competition between events on the two sides (Posner *et al.*, 1984; Kinsbourne, 1987).

Commonly, extinction has been associated with a broader set of phenomena termed *unilateral neglect* (Bisiach and Vallar, 1988; see Weiskrantz, Chapter 18). Clinically, patients with neglect may fail to eat food on one side of the plate, veer to one side while walking, omit one side of a drawing or fail to read words on one side of a page. Since these broader spatial deficits are associated most commonly with right parietal lesions, it has often been proposed that this region is involved specifically in attentional control. According to the integrated competition hypothesis, on the other hand, extinction should be a rather common consequence of lesions weakening the representation of one side of space. Since competition is widespread throughout the sensorimotor network, many different lesions should be associated with com-

petitive imbalance. In line with this prediction, it does appear that extinction itself is associated with a much wider variety of lesions than the full-blown neglect syndrome, including in monkeys the superior colliculus, the lateral nucleus of the pulvinar and extrastriate area V4 (Desimone *et al.*, 1990a,b), and in humans a wide variety of subcortical and cortical structures (Vallar *et al.*, 1994). In somesthesis, indeed, extinction can even be associated with lesions of the peripheral nervous system, a touch on the affected part of the body passing undetected when it is accompanied by a simultaneous touch elsewhere (Bender, 1952).

Illustrative data from a partial report task are shown in Figure 4.7 (Duncan, 1996; for a fuller account, see Duncan *et al.*, 1999). In this experiment, patients reported only letters in a specified color, red or green, in different trial blocks. Targets in each hemifield were presented either alone, or accompanied by a non-target (other color), or a second target, in the opposite hemifield. In Figure 4.7A are shown data for a patient with a right parietal lesion. Targets on either side were identified well when they were presented alone. A right-sided target was still identified well when a letter was also present on the left; adding an item on the right, however, substantially reduced accuracy on the left, especially when this additional right-sided item was itself a target. These results, typical of extinction, are exactly those one would expect if competitive weights were determined jointly by task instruction and lesion location, with higher weights for targets than for non-targets, and higher weights for ipsilesional than for contralesional items.

Similar results for quite a different lesion are shown in Figure 4.7B. For this patient, the lesion was in the occipitotemporal cortex of the left hemisphere, producing a conventional picture of reading deficit and right upper field loss. The extinction pattern, however, was equally evident here, a contralesional (now right-sided) target suffering especially severely from a competing ipsilesional (left-sided) item.

At first sight, it is tempting to see extinction as a simple spatial phenomenon, reflecting biased competition between left and right sides. Based on what we have said about normal behavior, however, we might expect such competition also to be modulated by non-spatial aspects of object structure. Indeed, extinction is weakened when array elements to the left and right appear to be parts of a single object, e.g. an arrow with its shaft on one side and its head on the other (Ward *et al.*, 1994). Even when objects on the two sides are clearly distinct, non-spatial factors contribute to

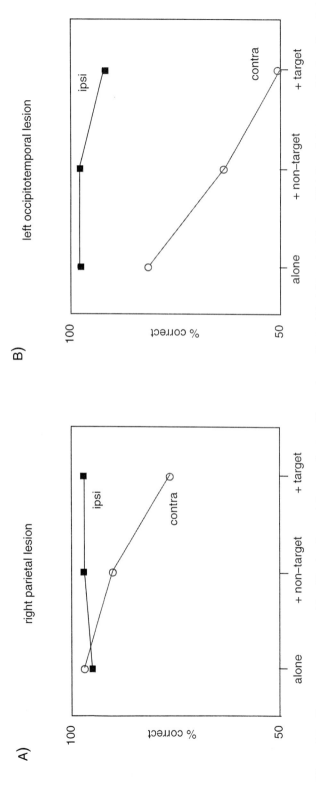

Figure 4.7. Percent correct target identification in partial report for two illustrative patients: (**A**) right parietal lesion; (**B**) left occipitotemporal lesion. Targets in ipsilesional (ipsi) and contralesional (contra) visual fields were presented alone (left point), or accompanied by either a non-target (middle point), or a second target (right point), in the opposite hemifield. Reproduced with permission from Duncan (1996).

the overall pattern of competitive dominance. In an experiment by Ward and Goodrich (1996), for example, separate line drawings were presented to the left and right. Though the task was simply to detect whether anything was present on the left and/or right sides, a nonsense shape on the contralesional side was much more likely to be extinguished than a drawing of a familiar shape. Another point of contact with normal studies is that extinction occurs over a time course of several hundred of milliseconds. Though the effect is strongest with simultaneous stimulation, some extinction of a brief contralesional stimulus can remain even when the ipsilesional event follows 500–1000 ms later (di Pellegrino *et al.*, 1997).

Extinction, in sum, may be seen as an imbalance in the normal process of attentional competition, produced by any lesion selectively weakening one part of the input. In line with the integrated competition hypothesis, the results show that such a competitive imbalance can be produced by lesions in many different parts of the nervous system.

Spatial integration

A further important result from lesion studies concerns integration between different parts of the sensorimotor network. According to the integrated competition hypothesis, different sensorimotor systems have a strong tendency to cohere, so that a dominant object in one tends also to take control of others. This property is essential if a local bias in one part of the network, for example a bias to prefer stimuli with a certain motion, is to translate into global selection of a whole object description, with all of its different properties and implications for action. Indeed, studies of spatial bias after brain lesions suggest exactly this sort of coherence.

One striking example is feedback from motor to visual bias. Robertson and North (1994), for example, showed that right-sided bias in a reading task can be reduced substantially by asking the patient to make occasional, irrelevant movements of the left hand. Similarly, rightward visual bias can be diminished by vestibular stimulation inducing leftward orienting (Rubens, 1985), or by left-sided stimulation on the body (Vallar *et al.*, 1995). Though these procedures doubtless have their initial effects on very different lateralized systems, the end result in all cases is a generalized attentional shift.

Indeed, this tendency to cross-modal spatial integration is also evident in studies of normal subjects. For example, listening to a speaker on the left is facili-

tated by turning the eyes, head or even trunk in that direction (Morais, 1975), while ignoring a vibration on one hand is helped by turning the eyes away (Driver and Grossenbacher, 1996). Broadly speaking, any spatial bias has a tendency to generalize, encouraging multiple sensorimotor systems to converge to work on the same, selected region of input.

Open questions

Useful though it may be in general outline, it is evident that the integrated competition hypothesis leaves many problems outstanding. For example, though some computational accounts of integration have been proposed (e.g. Phaf *et al.*, 1990), we know little of how such integration is actually achieved at the neural level. Even more importantly, the neurophysiological data already show evident exceptions to a generalized integration process.

Again the study of Chelazzi *et al.* (1998) can be used as an illustration. Earlier, we considered displays in which competing stimuli were presented together in one visual field, the field contralateral to the recording site. Bearing in mind that IT cells have large, bilateral receptive fields, however, we can also ask what happens with one stimulus in each field. In this case, results were very different: the responses of each cell were dominated, not by the attended stimulus, but by the stimulus in the contralateral field. With one stimulus in each field, in other words, different stimuli were dominant simultaneously in different hemispheres; at the behavioral level, in contrast, there is no suggestion that targets in opposite hemifields can be processed together without mutual competition. The puzzle becomes even more striking in earlier visual areas, where receptive fields are smaller. In both V4 (Moran and Desimone, 1985) and MT/MST (Treue and Maunsell, 1996), competition is most strongly evident when two stimuli lie within a single cell's receptive field. Again this implies that stimuli spaced far apart are processed simultaneously in separate parts of the extrastriate network (separate regions of the same visual area); but again, competition is clear in behavior. For the future, a key question is exactly how these neural data map onto unified competition at the behavioral level.

CONCLUSIONS

Broadly speaking, the neural data we have considered are consistent with the behavioral principles reviewed in the first section of this chapter, and with the outlines of TVA. Indeed, the integrated competition hypothesis is motivated directly by the ideas of temporally extended, object-based competition, and by a requirement for flexible, context-based bias.

At the same time, it remains the case that current neurophysiological data make little contact with much of what we know at the behavioral level. The good quantitative fit of TVA to behavioral data implies that, at the neural level, we should be seeking an account that generates similar basic equations: exponential processing dynamics, competition by modulation of processing rate and variably efficient weight setting. The bridge needed here is perhaps a neural network model which, facing one way, can be linked directly to the physiological data but, facing the other, can generate quantitative behavior as prescribed by TVA.

As one example, we reviewed behavioral data implying two rather separate phases of visual processing, the first phase setting attentional weights, the second, competitive phase generating explicit stimulus identification. Neurophysiological data indeed suggest that all objects in a visual display produce an initial activation of visually responsive cortex, followed by a later phase of competitive interaction (Figure 4.6). However, can such data—and the idea of competitive bias by advance priming—lead to a quantitative account of the form implied by behavioral work?

Already, however, the approach we have taken suggests an interesting perspective on the relationship between behavioral and neural levels. Perhaps the most conventional assumption is that functional entities defined at the behavioral level, i.e. competition, selection and attention, map onto anatomical entities at the neural level, such that a particular cognitive function is undertaken by a particular neural system. According to the integrated competition hypothesis, however, there is no localized system responsible for visual attention: even the components of this function, such as competition and priming, have no distinct localization. Instead of being the province of a particular part of the sensorimotor network, attention is seen as a *state* of the network as a whole; an object is 'attended' as multiple brain systems converge to work on its multiple properties and implications for behavior.

REFERENCES

Allport, D.A. (1980) Attention and performance. In: Claxton G. (ed.), *Cognitive Psychology: New Directions*. Routledge and Kegan Paul, London, pp. 112–153.

Atkinson, R.C., Holmgren, J.E. and Juola, J.F. (1969) Processing time as influenced by the number of elements in a visual display. *Perception and Psychophysics*, 6, 321–326.

Baddeley, A.D. (1986) *Working Memory*. Oxford University Press, Oxford.

Bender, M.B. (1952) *Disorders in Perception*. Charles C. Thomas, Springfield, Illinois.

Bisiach, E. and Vallar, G. (1988) Hemineglect in humans. In: Boller, F. and Grafman, J. (eds), *Handbook of Neuropsychology*, Vol. 1. Elsevier, Amsterdam, pp. 195–222.

Bonnel, A.-M., Stein, J.-F. and Bertucci, P. (1992) Does attention modulate the perception of luminance changes? *Quarterly Journal of Experimental Psychology*, 44A, 601–626.

Braun, D. and Sagi, D. (1991) Texture-based tasks are little affected by second tasks requiring peripheral or central attentive fixation. *Perception*, 20, 483–500.

Broadbent, D.E. (1958) *Perception and Communication*. Pergamon Press, London.

Broadbent, D.E. (1971) *Decision and Stress*. Academic Press, London.

Broadbent, D.E. and Broadbent, M.H.P. (1987) From detection to identification: response to multiple targets in rapid serial visual presentation. *Perception and Psychophysics*, 42, 105–113.

Bundesen, C. (1990) A theory of visual attention. *Psychological Review*, 97, 523–547.

Bundesen, C. (1998a) A computational theory of visual attention. *Philosophical Transactions of the Royal Society of London, Series B*, 353, 1271–1281.

Bundesen, C. (1998b) Visual selective attention: outlines of a choice model, a race model and a computational theory. *Visual Cognition*, 5, 287–309.

Bundesen, C., Shibuya, H. and Larsen, A. (1985) Visual selection from multielement displays: a model for partial report. In: Posner, M.I. and Marin, O.S.M. (eds), *Attention and Performance XI*. Erlbaum, Hillsdale, New Jersey, pp. 631–649.

Bushnell, M.C., Goldberg, M.E. and Robinson, D.L. (1981) Behavioral enhancement of visual responses in monkey cerebral cortex. I. Modulation in posterior parietal cortex related to selective visual attention. *Journal of Neurophysiology*, 46, 755–772.

Chelazzi, L., Miller, E.K., Duncan, J. and Desimone, R. (1993) A neural basis for visual search in inferior temporal cortex. *Nature*, 363, 345–347

Chelazzi, L., Duncan, J., Miller, E.K. and Desimone, R. (1998) Responses of neurons in inferior temporal cortex during memory-guided visual search. *Journal of Neurophysiology*, 80, 2918–2940.

Desimone, R. and Duncan, J. (1995) Neural mechanisms of selective visual attention. *Annual Review of Neuroscience*, 18, 193–222.

Desimone, R. and Ungerleider, L.G. (1989) Neural mechanisms of visual processing in monkeys. In: Boller, F. and Grafman, J. (eds), *Handbook of Neuropsychology*, Vol. 2. Elsevier, Amsterdam, pp. 267–299.

Desimone, R., Li, L., Lehky, S., Ungerleider, L. and Mishkin, M. (1990a) Effects of V4 lesions on visual discrimination performance and on responses of neurons in inferior temporal cortex. *Society for Neuroscience Abstracts*, 16, 621.

Desimone, R., Wessinger, M., Thomas, L. and Schneider, W. (1990b) Attentional control of visual perception: cortical and subcortical mechanisms. *Cold Spring Harbor Symposia on Quantitative Biology*, 55, 963–971.

di Pellegrino, G., Basso, G. and Frassinetti, F. (1997) Spatial extinction on double asynchronous stimulation. *Neuropsychologia*, 35, 1215–1223.

Driver, J. and Grossenbacher, P.G. (1996) Multimodal spatial constraints on tactile selective attention. In: Inui T. and McClelland, J.L. (eds), *Attention and Performance XVI*. MIT Press, Cambridge, Massachusetts, pp. 209–235.

Duncan, J. (1980) The locus of interference in the perception of simultaneous stimuli. *Psychological Review*, 87, 272–300.

Duncan, J. (1983) Perceptual selection based on alphanumeric class: evidence from partial reports. *Perception and Psychophysics*, 33, 533–547.

Duncan, J. (1984) Selective attention and the organization of visual information. *Journal of Experimental Psychology: General*, 113, 501–517.

Duncan, J. (1985) Visual search and visual attention. In: Posner, M.I. and Marin, O.S.M. (eds), *Attention and Performance XI*. Erlbaum, Hillsdale, New Jersey, pp. 85–104.

Duncan, J. (1987) Attention and reading: wholes and parts in shape recognition. In: Coltheart M. (ed.), *Attention and Performance XII*. Erlbaum, Hillsdale, New Jersey, pp. 39–61.

Duncan, J. (1993a) Coordination of what and where in visual attention. *Perception*, 22, 1261–1270.

Duncan, J. (1993b) Similarity between concurrent visual discriminations: dimensions and objects. *Perception and Psychophysics*, 54, 425–430.

Duncan, J. (1996) Cooperating brain systems in selective perception and action. In: Inui T. and McClelland, J.L. (eds), *Attention and Performance XVI*. MIT Press, Cambridge, Massachusetts, pp. 549–578.

Duncan, J. and Humphreys, G. (1989) Visual search and stimulus similarity. *Psychological Review*, 96, 433–458.

Duncan, J. and Nimmo-Smith, M.I. (1996) Objects and attributes in divided attention: surface and boundary systems. *Perception and Psychophysics*, 58, 1076–1084.

Duncan, J., Ward, R. and Shapiro, K. (1994) Direct measurement of attentional dwell time in human vision. *Nature*, 369, 313–315.

Duncan, J., Humphreys, G. and Ward, R. (1997a) Competitive brain activity in visual attention. *Current Opinion in Neurobiology*, 7, 255–261.

Duncan, J., Martens, S. and Ward, R. (1997b) Restricted attentional capacity within but not between sensory modalities. *Nature*, 387, 808–810.

Duncan, J., Bundesen, C., Olson, A., Humphreys, G., Chavda, S. and Shibuya, H. (1999) Systematic analysis of deficits in visual attention. *Journal of Experimental Psychology: General*, 128, 450–478.

Eriksen, C.W. and Hoffman, J.E. (1973) The extent of processing of noise elements during selective encoding from visual displays. *Perception and Psychophysics*, 14, 155–160.

Estes, W.K. and Taylor, H.A. (1966) Visual detection in relation to display size and redundancy of critical elements. *Perception and Psychophysics*, 1, 9–16.

Farmer, E.W. and Taylor, R.M. (1980) Visual search through color displays: effects of target–background similarity and background uniformity. *Perception and Psychophysics*, 27, 267–272.

Funahashi, S., Bruce, C.J. and Goldman-Rakic, P.S. (1989) Mnemonic coding of visual space in the monkey's dorsolateral prefrontal cortex. *Journal of Neurophysiology*, 61, 331–349.

Fuster, J.M., Bauer, R.H. and Jervey, J.P. (1985) Functional interactions between inferotemporal and prefrontal cortex in a cognitive task. *Brain Research*, 330, 299–307.

Gnadt, J.W. and Andersen, R.A. (1988) Memory related motor planning activity in posterior parietal cortex of macaque. *Experimental Brain Research*, 70, 216–220.

Godschalk, M., Lemon, R.N., Kuypers, H.G.J.M. and Van der Steen, J. (1985) The involvement of monkey premotor cortex neurones in preparation of visually cued arm movements. *Behavioural Brain Research*, 18, 143–157.

Harter, M.R. and Aine, C.J. (1984) Brain mechanisms of visual selective attention. In: Parasuraman, R. and Davies, D.R. (eds), *Varieties of Attention*. Academic Press, Orlando, Florida, pp. 293–321.

Heinze, H.J., Mangun, G.R., Burchert, W., Hinrichs, H., Scholz, M., Münte, T.F., Gös, A., Scherg, M., Johannes, S., Hundeshagen, H., Gazzaniga, M.S. and Hillyard, S.A. (1994) Combined spatial and temporal imaging of brain activity during visual selective attention in humans. *Nature*, 372, 543–546.

Hoffman, J.E. and Nelson, B. (1981) Spatial selectivity in visual search. *Perception and Psychophysics*, 30, 283–290.

Jolicoeur, P. (1999) Restricted attentional capacity between sensory modalities. *Psychonomic Bulletin and Review*, 6, 87–92.

Kinsbourne, M. (1987) Mechanisms of unilateral neglect. In: Jeannerod, M. (ed.), *Neurophysiological and Neuropsychological Aspects of Neglect*. North-Holland Publishers, Amsterdam, pp. 69–86.

Lavie, N. and Driver, J. (1996) On the spatial extent of attention in object-based visual selection. *Perception and Psychophysics*, 58, 1238–1251.

Lindsay, P.H., Taylor, M.M. and Forbes, S.M. (1968) Attention and multi-dimensional discrimination. *Perception and Psychophysics*, 4, 113–117.

Long, J. (1975) Reduced efficiency and capacity limitation in multidimension signal recognition. *Quarterly Journal of Experimental Psychology*, 27, 599–614.

Luck, S.J., Chelazzi, L., Hillyard, S.A. and Desimone, R. (1997) Mechanisms of spatial selective attention in areas V1, V2 and V4 of macaque visual cortex. *Journal of Neurophysiology*, 77, 24–42.

Martínez, A., Anllo-Vento, L., Sereno, M.I., Frank, L.R., Buxton, R.B., Dubowitz, D.J., Wong, E.C., Hinrichs, H., Heinze, H.J. and Hillyard, S.A. (1999) Involvement of striate and extrastriate visual cortical areas in spatial-selective attention: combined evidence from fMRI and event-related potentials. *Nature Neuroscience*, 2, 364–369.

McAdams, C.J. and Maunsell, J.H.R. (1999) Effects of attention on the orientation tuning functions of single neurons in macaque area V4. *Journal of Neuroscience*, 19, 431–441.

Miller, E.K., Erickson, C.A. and Desimone, R. (1996) Neural mechanisms of visual working memory in prefrontal cortex of the macaque. *Journal of Neuroscience*, 16, 5154–5167.

Morais, J. (1978) Spatial constraints on attention to speech. In: Requin, J. (ed.), *Attention and Performance VII*. Erlbaum, Hillsdale, New Jersey, pp. 245–260.

Moran, J. and Desimone, R. (1985) Selective attention gates visual processing in the extrastriate cortex. *Science*, 229, 782–784.

Motter, B.C. (1993) Focal attention produces spatially selective processing in visual cortical areas V1, V2 and V4 in the presence of competing stimuli. *Journal of Neurophysiology*, 70, 909–919.

Motter, B.C. (1994) Neural correlates of attentive selection for color or luminance in extrastriate area V4. *Journal of Neuroscience*, 14, 2178–2189.

Neisser, U. (1963) Decision-time without reaction-time: experiments in visual scanning. *American Journal of Psychology*, 76, 376–385.

Neisser, U. (1967) *Cognitive Psychology*. Appleton-Century-Crofts, New York.

Phaf, R.H., van der Heijden, A.H.C. and Hudson, P.T.W. (1990) SLAM: a connectionist model for attention in visual selection tasks. *Cognitive Psychology*, 22, 273–341.

Posner, M.I., Snyder, C.R.R. and Davidson, B.J. (1980) Attention and the detection of signals. *Journal of Experimental Psychology: General*, 109, 160–174.

Posner, M.I., Walker, J.A., Friedrich, F. and Rafal, R.D. (1984) Effects of parietal injury on covert orienting of attention. *Journal of Neuroscience*, 4, 1863–1874.

Rainer, G., Asaad, W.F. and Miller, E.K. (1998) Selective representation of relevant information by neurons in the primate prefrontal cortex. *Nature*, 393, 577–579.

Raymond, J.E., Shapiro, K.L. and Arnell, K.M. (1992) Temporary suppression of visual processing in an RSVP task: an attentional blink? *Journal of Experimental Psychology: Human Perception and Performance*, 18, 849–860.

Robertson, I.H. and North, N.T. (1994) One hand is better than two: motor extinction of left hand advantage in unilateral neglect. *Neuropsychologia*, 32, 1–11.

Rock, I., Linnett, C.M., Grant, P. and Mack, A. (1992) Perception without attention: results of a new method. *Cognitive Psychology*, 24, 502–534.

Roelfsema, P.R., Lamme, V.A.F. and Spekreijse, H. (1998) Object-based attention in the primary visual cortex of the macaque monkey. *Nature*, 395, 376–381.

Rubens, A.B. (1985) Caloric stimulation and unilateral visual neglect. *Neurology*, 35, 1019–1024.

Schall, J.D., Hanes, D.P., Thompson, K.G. and King, D.J. (1995) Saccade target selection in frontal eye field of macaque. 1. Visual and premovement activation. *Journal of Neuroscience*, 15, 6905–6918.

Sereno, A.B. and Maunsell, J.H.R. (1998) Shape selectivity in primate lateral intraparietal cortex. *Nature*, 395, 500–503.

Shibuya, H. (1993) Efficiency of visual selection in duplex and conjunction conditions in partial report. *Perception and Psychophysics*, 54, 716–732.

Sperling, G. (1960) The information available in brief visual presentations. *Psychological Monographs*, 74 (11, Whole No. 498).

Treisman, A.M. and Davies, A. (1973) Divided attention to ear and eye. In: Kornblum, S. (ed.), *Attention and Performance IV*. Academic Press, London, pp. 101–117.

Treisman, A.M. and Gelade, G. (1980) A feature integration theory of attention. *Cognitive Psychology*, 12, 97–136.

Treisman, A.M. and Gormican, S. (1988) Feature analysis in early vision: evidence from search asymmetries. *Psychological Review*, 95, 15–48.

Treisman, A.M. and Schmidt, H. (1982) Illusory conjunctions in the perception of objects. *Cognitive Psychology*, 14, 107–141.

Treue, S. and Maunsell, J.H.R. (1996) Attentional modulation of visual motion processing in cortical areas MT and MST. *Nature*, 382, 539–541.

Valdes-Sosa, M., Bobes, M.A., Rodriguez, V. and Pinilla, T. (1998a) Switching attention without shifting the spotlight: object-based attentional modulation of brain potentials. *Journal of Cognitive Neuroscience*, 10, 137–151.

Valdes-Sosa, M., Cobo, A. and Pinilla, T. (1998b) Transparent motion and object-based attention. *Cognition*, 66, B13–B23.

Vallar, G., Rusconi, M.L., Bignamini, L., Geminiani, G. and Perani, D. (1994) Anatomical correlates of visual and tactile extinction in humans: a clinical CT scan study. *Journal of Neurology, Neurosurgery, and Psychiatry*, 57, 464–470.

Vallar, G., Rusconi, M.L., Barozzi, S., Bernardini, B., Ovadia, D., Papagno, C. and Cesarani, A. (1995) Improvement of left visuo-spatial hemineglect by left-sided transcutaneous electrical stimulation. *Neuropsychologia*, 33, 73–82.

Van Voorhis, S. and Hillyard, S.A. (1977) Visual evoked potentials and selective attention to points in space. *Perception and Psychophysics*, 22, 54–62.

Vecera, S.P. and Farah, M.J. (1994) Does visual attention select objects or locations? *Journal of Experimental Psychology: General*, 123, 146–160.

von Wright, J.M. (1970) On selection in visual immediate memory. In: Sanders, A.F. (ed.), *Attention and Performance III*. North-Holland Publishers, Amsterdam, pp. 280–292.

Walley, R.E. and Weiden, T.D. (1973) Lateral inhibition and cognitive masking: a neuropsychological theory of attention. *Psychological Review*, 80, 284–302.

Ward, R. and Goodrich, S.J. (1996) Differences between objects and non-objects in visual extinction: a competition for attention. *Psychological Science*, 3, 177–180.

Ward, R., Goodrich, S.J. and Driver, J. (1994) Grouping reduces visual extinction: neuropsychological evidence for weight linkage in visual selection. *Visual Cognition*, 1, 101–129.

Wing, A. and Allport, D.A. (1972) Multidimensional encoding of visual form. *Perception and Psychophysics*, 12, 474–476.

5 PREDISPOSITIONS IN PERCEPTUAL AND COGNITIVE DEVELOPMENT

Mark H. Johnson and Johan J. Bolhuis

INTRODUCTION

Two opposing views traditionally have dominated the study of brain and behavioral development. From one perspective, the newborn's brain has been characterized as a *tabula rasa* upon which experience writes new information. From the other viewpoint, the brain of the newborn is seen as being composed of 'innate domain-specific modules' through which information about the environment is processed in a manner much the same as that in the mature animal. Horn (1985, 1992), among others, has advanced a middle ground position in which the brain comes equipped with 'predispositions' (Horn and McCabe, 1984; Horn, 1985; Johnson and Morton, 1991) or 'prefunctional perceptual mechanisms' (Hogan, 1988). It has become increasingly apparent that such predispositions exert a powerful influence on the subsequent perceptual and cognitive development of animals and man (for reviews, see, for example, Horn, 1985; Johnson and Bolhuis, 1991; Bolhuis, 1996). In this chapter, we will review some of the evidence for predispositions in the cognitive development of animals and humans. We will emphasize that the concept of 'predispositions' is quite different from the arcane notion that perceptual mechanisms or cognitive systems are somehow 'innate' (cf. Bolhuis, 1999a, in press). In particular, we will focus in detail on two related examples of predispositions, early filial preferences in the chick and face preferences in the human newborn. We will use the examples to examine in more detail two basic questions about predispositions: (i) what are the mechanisms underlying predispositions? and (ii) what are the functions of predispositions?

PREDISPOSITIONS AND PERCEPTUAL PREFERENCES IN ANIMALS

Predispositions play an important role in a number of animal developmental paradigms. They have been found to be involved in bird song learning (Marler, 1991) and the development of auditory preferences in ducklings (Gottlieb, 1980). Further, there is an important influence of predispositions in the perception of faces in neonatal human infants (Johnson and Morton, 1991; de Haan and Halit, in press) and in the development of filial preferences in chicks (Johnson *et al.*, 1985; Johnson and Bolhuis, 1991; Bolhuis, 1996). In the study of the development of filial preferences in chicks, we have used the term filial predispositions (Bolhuis, 1996). These were defined as perceptual preferences that develop in young animals without specific experience with the particular stimuli involved (e.g. Bolhuis and Honey, 1998; Bolhuis, 1999a).

A predisposition for species-specific sounds has been demonstrated in song learning in certain avian species (Marler, 1987, 1991). Songbird species need to learn their song from a tutor male (Marler, 1976; DeVoogd, 1994). Under certain circumstances, young males of some species can learn their songs, or at least part of their songs, from tape recordings of tutor songs. When fledgling male song sparrows (*Melospiza melodia*) and swamp sparrows (*Melospiza georgiana*) were exposed to taped songs that consisted of equal numbers of songs of both species, they preferentially learnt the songs of their own species. Males of both species are able to sing the songs of the other species. Thus it appears that perceptual predispositions are involved in what Marler (1991) called 'the sensitization of young sparrows to conspecific song' (p. 200).

In an extensive series of experiments, Gottlieb (e.g. 1971, 1980, 1982) investigated the mechanisms underlying the preferences that young ducklings of a number of species show for the maternal call of their own species over that of other species. Gottlieb (1971) found that differential behavior towards the species-specific call could already be observed in an early embryonic stage, before the animal started to vocalize itself. However, a post-hatching preference for the conspecific maternal call was only found when the animals received exposure to embryonic contact-contentment calls, played back at the right speed (Gottlieb, 1980) and with a natural variation (Gottlieb, 1982), within a certain period in development (Gottlieb, 1985). Thus, the expression of a species-specific predisposition in ducklings is dependent on particular experience earlier in development (see below, and Gottlieb, 1980; Bolhuis, 1996).

A filial predisposition in the domestic chick

The development of filial behavior in the chick involves two systems that are neurally and behaviorally dissociable (Horn, 1985, 1998; Johnson and Bolhuis, 1991; Johnson and Morton, 1991; Bolhuis, 1996; Bolhuis and Honey, 1998). Filial imprinting is the process through which social preferences of young animals (mainly precocial birds) become restricted to a particular stimulus as a result of exposure to that stimulus (for a review, see Bolhuis, 1991; see also Bateson, Chapter 15; Horn, Chapter 19). Horn and his collaborators found that in domestic chicks, a restricted region of the forebrain (the intermediate and medial hyperstriatum ventrale or IMHV) is crucially involved in imprinting (for reviews, see Horn, 1985, 1998; see also Horn, Chapter 19). Neural evidence that distinguished two different systems came

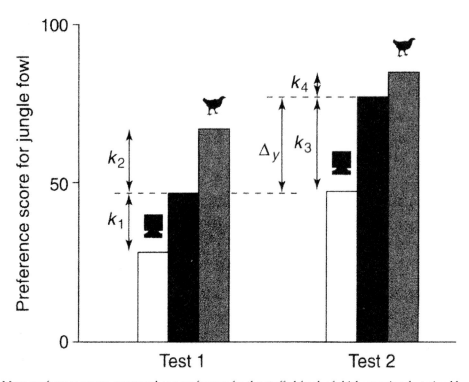

Figure 5.1. Mean preference scores, expressed as a preference for the stuffed fowl, of chicks previously trained by exposure to a rotating stuffed jungle fowl, a rotating red box, or exposed to white light (black bars). Preference scores are defined as activity when attempting to approach the stuffed jungle fowl divided by total approach activity during the test. Preferences were measured in a simultaneous test either 2 h (Test 1) or 24 h (Test 2) after the end of training. k_1–k_4 represent the differences between the preferences of the trained chicks and the controls; Δ_y represents the difference in preference between the control chicks at Test 2 and at Test 1. See text for further explanation. From Horn (1985), by permission of Oxford University Press, after Johnson *et al.* (1985).

from a study (Horn and McCabe, 1984) showing that the effects of bilateral lesions to the IMHV were much greater in chicks that were trained by exposing them to a rotating red box than in chicks that received imprinting training with a rotating stuffed jungle fowl (*Gallus gallus spadiceus*). Behavioral evidence for the existence of a predisposition was provided by a study in which day-old dark-reared chicks received imprinting training by exposing them to either a rotating red box or a rotating stuffed jungle fowl hen (Johnson *et al.*, 1985; see Figure 5.1). Chicks in a control group were exposed to white overhead light for the same amount of time. The approach preferences of the chicks were measured in a subsequent test where the two training stimuli were presented simultaneously. Preferences were tested at either 2 h (Test 1) or 24 h (Test 2) after the end of training. At Test 1, the chicks preferred the object to which they had been exposed previously. At Test 2, there was a significantly greater preference for the fowl in both experimental groups as well as in the light-exposed control group. Thus, the preference for the jungle fowl increased from the 2 h to the 24 h test, and did so regardless of the stimulus with which the chicks had been trained.

These results suggested to us that the preferences of trained chicks are influenced by at least two different systems. On the one hand, there is an effect of experience with particular stimuli (reflected in the differences k_1–k_4 in Figure 5.1), i.e. filial imprinting takes place. On the other hand, there is an emerging predisposition to approach stimuli resembling conspecifics (reflected in Figure 5.1 as Δ_y for the control group). The results in Figure 5.1 suggest that training with a particular stimulus is not necessary for the predisposition to emerge. In subsequent studies, it was found that visual experience was not necessary to 'trigger' or induce (Gottlieb, 1976; Bolhuis, 1996) the predisposition. The predisposition can emerge in dark-reared chicks, provided that they receive a certain amount of non-specific stimulation within a certain period in development (Johnson *et al.*, 1989).

Stimulus selection in filial predispositions

The stimulus characteristics that are important for the filial predisposition to be expressed were investigated in chicks that had developed the predisposition, in tests involving an intact stuffed jungle fowl versus a series of increasingly degraded versions of a stuffed jungle fowl (Johnson and Horn, 1988). The degraded versions ranged from one where different parts of the stuffed fowl (wings, head, torso or legs) were reassembled in an unnatural way, to one in which the pelt of a jungle fowl had been cut into small pieces that were stuck onto a rotating box. The intact model was preferred only when the degraded object possessed no distinguishable jungle fowl features. In addition, chicks did not prefer an intact jungle fowl model over an alternative object that contained only the head and neck of a stuffed fowl. Thus, the head and neck region contains stimuli that are relevant for the predisposition. In subsequent experiments, it was found that the chicks did not prefer a stuffed jungle fowl hen over a stuffed Gadwall duck (*Anas strepera*) or even a stuffed pole cat (*Mustela putorius*). Thus, the predisposition is not species or even class specific. Subsequent studies showed that eyes are an important stimulus, but that other aspects of the stimulus are also sufficient for the expression of a predisposition (Bolhuis, 1996).

Filial predispositions and early learning

It is important to distinguish between a concept of predispositions as a filter or 'template' (Marler, 1976), restricting the information that the animal can store in memory, or, alternatively, an interpretation of predispositions as acting independently of the effects of learning during development. In order to investigate this issue, Bolhuis *et al.* (1989) allowed dark-reared chicks to develop the predisposition. The chicks were then trained by exposing them to a rotating red or blue box. In subsequent preference tests, it was found that these chicks, after the predisposition had developed, were still capable of learning the characteristics of these conspicuous objects. These results suggest that, rather than the predisposition constraining the information that can be stored, the two mechanisms interact at the behavioral level, i.e. the activated predisposition will bias the chick's approach response to certain stimuli, and the animal may learn the characteristics of those stimuli; but the chick is still capable of learning the characteristics of other objects.

Neural mechanisms underlying filial predispositions

Although lesion studies led to the original discovery in the chick of the emerging predisposition (Horn and McCabe, 1984), little is known about the underlying neural and physiological mechanisms. Johnson and Horn (1986) found that the development of the predisposition was not affected by early bilateral lesions to the IMHV. Thus, it is likely that the neural substrate involved in the predisposition is located outside the IMHV. However, recent electrophysiological findings (Brown and Horn, 1994; see also Horn, Chapter 19) suggest that this neural substrate may influence neuronal activity in the IMHV. Brown and Horn (1994) trained dark-reared chicks by exposing them to a rotating red box or a rotating blue cylinder. One day after the end of imprinting training, recordings were made from groups of neurons in the left IMHV. There was an effect of training on the response to presentation of a stuffed jungle fowl. A significantly higher proportion of responses to the fowl were excitatory in trained chicks (68%), irrespective of the training object, than in dark-reared chicks (7%). Thus, imprinting training altered the responsiveness of neurons in IMHV to an unfamiliar stimulus that is important for a filial predisposition. Further research is needed to elucidate the nature of these effects.

Johnson *et al.* (1989) showed that there is a sensitive period (between ~14 and 42 h after hatching) during which non-specific stimulation can induce the filial predisposition in domestic chicks (cf. Bolhuis *et al.*, 1989; Bolhuis and Horn, 1997). Davies *et al.* (1992) found that injections of the catecholaminergic neurotoxin DSP4 delayed the onset of the sensitive period for the induction of the predisposition in dark-reared chicks. Unlike vehicle-injected controls, DSP4-treated chicks did not show a significant preference for the jungle fowl over the red box when they had been placed in the wheels at 24 or 36 h after hatching. However, DSP4-treated chicks showed a significant preference for the fowl when they had been placed in the wheels at 42 or 48 h after hatching, i.e. at times when this wheel placement did not induce a significant preference in the controls. A similar delay in the onset of the sensitive period is achieved after early equithesin anesthesia (Bolhuis and Horn, 1997). After the preference tests, Davies *et al.* (1992) determined the levels of dopamine and noradrenaline in forebrain samples containing predominantly IMHV. In control chicks, there was a significant negative correlation between forebrain dopamine concentration and preference score for the fowl; no such correlation was found for noradrenaline. As the authors note, if dopamine is involved in the expression of the predisposition, it likely to involve brain regions outside the IMHV, as lesions to this structure do not affect the predisposition (Johnson and Horn, 1986).

It is not known whether catecholamines are involved in the *induction* of the predisposition. It has been suggested that androgens may have such a role (Bolhuis *et al.*, 1985, 1986; Horn, 1985). Bolhuis *et al.* (1986) reported that in chicks trained by exposure to a stuffed jungle fowl, there was a significant positive correlation between plasma levels of testosterone and preference score for the stuffed fowl. No such relationship was found in chicks trained by exposure to a rotating red box. Further, subcutaneous injections of a long-lasting testosterone ester shortly after hatching significantly increased the mean preference score of chicks trained on a stuffed fowl, not that of red box-trained chicks. These findings suggest that the preference for the stuffed fowl is limited by the concentration of androgens in the plasma, and they led to the suggestion (Bolhuis *et al.*, 1985; Horn, 1985) that testosterone may be involved in the development of the predisposition. Horn (1985) suggested that increased levels of testosterone or other hormones could render the systems involved in the predisposition operational (for further discussion, see Bolhuis, 1996).

PREDISPOSITIONS AND PERCEPTUAL PREFERENCES IN HUMAN INFANTS

In many respects, conducting behavioral experiments in human infants shares features in common with animal studies, since the testing methods used have to elicit non-verbal responses. These methods also have to engage the natural behavior and interests of the infant in order for a reasonable amount of data to be collected. It is no surprise, therefore, that some of the early pioneers in infancy research were animal researchers who adapted their existing methods. For example, in the early, 1960s, Robert Fantz developed a preferential looking time paradigm for testing infants which was taken directly from his earlier work with domestic chicks (Fantz, 1964). Preferential looking, and related paradigms such as habituation–dishabituation, remains in widespread use in infant laboratories today. While there are similarities in some of the behavioral paradigms used, obviously the more direct neural interventions possible with animals cannot be applied to infants. However, in this section, we will describe new non-invasive functional imaging methods that allow us to begin to ask questions about the neural basis of perceptual development in human infants.

A continuing debate with regard to the abilities of infants over the first few months of life concerns whether the visual and auditory preferences they demonstrate are best accounted for by the increasing capacities of the central nervous system, or whether we need only suppose growth in peripheral receptors such as the retina. Until recently, the psychobiological approach to infancy was associated commonly with the assumption that development in peripheral receptors and the earliest stages of sensory processing were sufficient to account for most transitions in the behavior of infants. In contrast, psychologists and ethologists with less interest in the neural basis of behavior were generally more inclined to focus on the importance of central 'cognitive' mechanisms in accounting for developmental changes over the first few months of life. However, the emergence of cognitive neuroscience approaches to aspects of cognition such as face recognition (Perrett *et al.*, 1985) and visual attention (Posner and Petersen, 1990) in adults has stimulated work on the neural basis of cognition during early infancy (de Schonen and Mathivet, 1990; Johnson, 1997; Nelson and Bloom, 1997). In this section, we focus on the example of face processing in human infants, and in particular on the properties and probable neural basis of these abilities. However, first let us consider the issue of central versus peripheral limitations on infant perception in a little more detail.

This debate perhaps has raged most fiercely with regard to the visual capacities and preferences of the human newborn, since the immaturity of the eye is clearly a limiting factor on early visual capacities. A number of models in which infants' preferences are predicted by hypothesized limitations on the contrast sensitivity function due to peripheral receptors have been proposed (Stevens, 1992). In one version of this approach (Banks and Shannon, 1993), 'ideal observers' were constructed from an analysis of the morphology of neonatal photoreceptors and optics, and compared with those from adults. This allowed estimates of the contribution of optical and receptoral immaturity, as opposed to neural immaturity, to deficits in infant spatial and chromatic vision. Observed differences in spatial and chromatic vision between adults and infants turn out to be significantly greater than predicted from the ideal observer analysis, indicating that central nervous system immaturity is a contributing factor in the neonate's visual perception. This, and other evidence from the development of visual orienting (see Johnson, 1990), leads to the conclusion that at least some of the changes in behavior observed in infancy may be attributed to development in brain regions such as the cerebral cortex, rather than merely reflecting sensory limitations. In what follows, we examine these issues with regard to the particular domain of face recognition.

Neurodevelopmental mechanisms of face perception

Psychophysical studies of human infant vision have suggested that the amount of information obtainable from a face in early infancy is very limited. For example, some authors (e.g. Souther and Banks, 1979) have argued that a 1-month-old infant may be able to discern only the grossest features of the face: the outer contour defined by the hairline, and vague darker areas in the region of the eyes and mouth. A related claim about the visual capacities of infants over the first 2 months of life is that they attend to the boundaries of stimuli in preference to the interior, the so-called 'externality effect' (Johnson, 1990). This factor, taken together with the supposed limitations in sensitivity mentioned previously, leads to the expectation of poor face recognition abilities in infants under 2 months of age.

While the prevailing view, and until recently most of the evidence, supported the contention that it is not until about 2 or 3 months of age that infants learn about the arrangement of features that compose a face (for reviews, see Maurer, 1985; Nelson and Ludemann, 1989), one study suggested that newborn infants as young as 10 min old will track (by means of head and eye movements) a face-like pattern further than various 'scrambled' face patterns (Goren *et al.*, 1975). Due to the importance of this study, and its being somewhat controversial for methodological reasons, Johnson and colleagues (Johnson *et al.*, 1991) attempted to replicate it with several changes to improve the methodology.

As in the original study, newborn infants (within the first hour of life) were required to track different patterned stimuli. This procedure differs markedly from that employed by most other investigators. Rather than the infant viewing one or more stimuli in static locations and measuring the length of time spent looking at the stimuli, in the Goren *et al.* tracking procedure the dependent measure is how far the infant will turn its head and/or eyes in order to keep a moving stimulus in view. The stimulus is moved slowly away from the midline and the angle at which

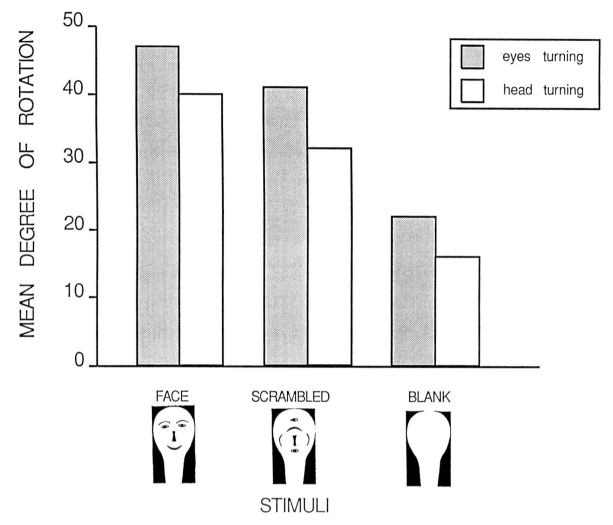

Figure 5.2. The mean extent of head and eye turning to follow the slowly moving stimuli indicated. The face stimulus was tracked significantly further than either of the other two by both head- and eye-turning measures. Data from Johnson *et al.* (1991, Experiment 1).

the infant disengages its eyes from the stimulus is recorded. Our sample consisted of normal, healthy, newborns who were tested within the first hour after birth. The stimuli employed were three head-shaped, head-sized, two-dimensional white forms with black features of a human face, similar to those used by Goren and colleagues (see Figure 5.2).

The mean head- and eye-turning responses to the three stimuli are shown in Figure 5.2. The extent of the eye turns to the *face* were significantly greater than those to the *scrambled face*, which, in turn, were greater than those to the *blank* stimulus. The same differences were found by measuring the extent of head turning.

The results obtained in this experiment clearly replicated the findings of Goren and her colleagues: neonates tracked a face-like pattern further than a 'scrambled' face pattern. Clearly, there are a number of differences between the face stimulus and other patterns that could have given rise to this differential responding. For example, given that newborn infants may not be able to resolve the details that constitute a facial feature, it may be that they are simply responding to the three high-contrast areas or blobs that correspond to the correct spatial arrangement of eyes and mouth in a face. In order to investigate this issue, and in an attempt to replicate once again the original

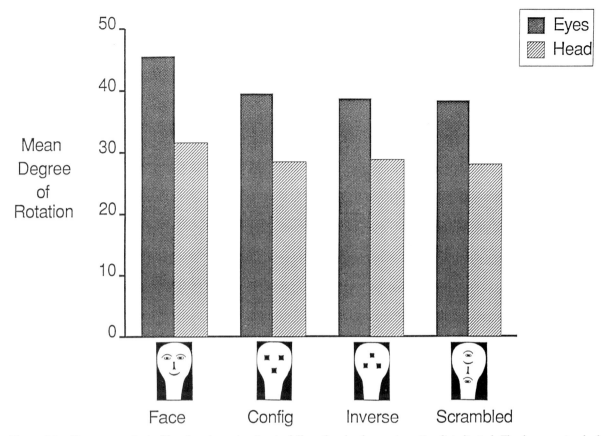

Figure 5.3. The mean extent of head and eye turning to follow the slowly moving stimuli indicated. The face was tracked significantly further than all of the other stimuli except 'config.' by the eye movement measure. Data from Johnson *et al.* (1991, Experiment 2).

finding (in a different hospital and geographical location), a second experiment with the stimulus set shown in Figure 5.3 was conducted.

Once again, the subjects were normal newborns, this time with a mean age at start of testing of 43 min. The results from the eye movement analysis revealed a significant preference for the face pattern over all of the stimuli except the one possessing the configuration of elements of a face (see Figure 5.2). While the findings of Goren *et al.* were replicated for a third time with this measure (see also Maurer and Young, 1983), whether newborns will track a face further by head turning remains an open question since no significant differences were found with this measure in this experiment (or that of Maurer and Young, 1983).

The results of this and several other experiments (for reviews, see Johnson and Morton, 1991; Morton and Johnson, 1991) indicated that there is no consistent difference between the detailed schematic face

and the face-like three blobs. While the information necessary to elicit the preferential tracking may be not specific to the details of face features, the evidence obtained so far suggests that it may be specific to the arrangement of elements that compose a face. More recently, the finding that newborns are biased to orient toward simple face-like patterns has been replicated using different procedures, but always ones in which infants orient more frequently to face patterns outside the foveal field (Valenza *et al.*, 1996; Simion *et al.*, 1998; Macchi Cassia *et al.*, in press).

Theories of infants' face recognition have followed roughly the same divide as was discussed earlier; some researchers have argued for the importance of sensory limitations in determining the preference for faces in young infants (the sensory hypothesis) while others have argued for the importance of central factors (configural hypothesis). The fundamental assumption of sensory hypotheses is that certain classes of stimuli are preferred by young infants as a result of the general properties of the early stages of visual processing. By this view, any preference for face-like patterns over other stimuli is simply due to their general psychophysical properties matching those of the developing visual system. In contrast, the configural view holds that no single psychophysical dimension can account for infants' responses to faces. Rather, the infant's nervous system, like that of some other species (Horn, 1985), contains some rudimentary configural information relevant to the detection of conspecifics.

A large number of stimulus variables have been proposed as determining infants' preferences for looking at stimuli, such as contour density, size, brightness, complexity and number of elements. However, perhaps the most successful predictor of infants' preferences over the first few months of life is the linear systems model (LSM) devised by Banks and colleagues (e.g. Banks and Salapatek, 1981; Banks and Ginsburg, 1985). This model, a form of the sensory hypothesis, predicts infants' preferences according to the amplitude spectrum of the stimulus filtered through the contrast sensitivity function for that age group (for details, see Stevens, 1992). The phase information (loosely corresponding to the structural pattern) is specifically unimportant in determining preference according to this model. Kleiner (1987) argued that the LSM could account for face preferences in newborn infants on the basis of an ingenious experiment in which she crossed the phase and amplitude of a face stimulus and a lattice pattern. Consistent with the predictions of the LSM (that face preference is determined by amplitude spectra alone), infants showed a preference for the amplitude spectra of a face over that of the lattice, and no preference between the lattice and the crossed stimulus with the phase of the face. This pattern of results indicates that the phase of the face alone is not influencing preference. However, Kleiner's experiment also produced an important and strong result not predicted by the LSM: the schematic face (phase and amplitude of a face) was very strongly preferred over the crossed stimulus with only the amplitude of the face (and the phase of the lattice). As stated earlier, the LSM explicitly claims that phase information is unimportant to preference. However, the results of Kleiner's study indicate that face phase information is crucially important when combined with the appropriate amplitude. In other words, decomposing a face stimulus into phase and amplitude spectra may not be of

utility for predicting preferences for this class of stimulus. Rather, some form of configural description involving the inter-relationship between elements may be of more value.

The debate between structure and sensory theorists with regard to infant face recognition continues (for arguments in support of the 'structure' hypothesis, see Morton *et al.*, 1990; Morton and Johnson, 1991; Morton, 1993; and in support of the 'sensory' hypothesis, see Kleiner and Banks, 1987; Kleiner, 1990, 1993; Slater, 1993). Leaving aside the details of this ongoing debate, the following facts are clear.

(i)   The extent to which face stimuli are tracked by newborns relative to most other stimuli cannot be accounted for by the LSM (and several variants thereof) alone (Johnson and Morton, 1991; Valenza *et al.*, 1996). Face stimuli are always tracked further than is predicted purely on the basis of their amplitude spectra.

(ii) The LSM is fairly successful at predicting preferences between scrambled and non-face stimuli in tracking and preferential looking experiments, a least until 3 or 4 months of age.

(iii) Checkerboards designed to be at the optimal spatial frequency for newborn infants can be tracked further than the face pattern (Morton, *et al.*, 1990; Johnson and Morton, 1991), implying that spatial frequency contributes to some extent to infant preferences, even when the stimuli are faces. However, on other occasions, simple face patterns are even preferred to optimal spatial frequency patterns (Valenza *et al.*, 1996).

(iv) Stimuli which are equated for amplitude spectra will be optimal for determining the nature and extent of configural information about faces. For example, in some experiments, upright face patterns are preferred over identical but inverted patterns (Valenza *et al.*, 1996).

The above considerations suggest partially independent effects of faces and spatial frequency in determining newborn visual preferences, and that no unidimensional psychophysical variable can explain the newborn's preferential orienting to faces. Clearly, convoluted psychophysical descriptions which involve multiple independent factors can be generated to produce rudimentary face detectors (see Johnson and Morton, 1991), but these are arbitrary redescriptions of configural information.

At this point then, we can conclude that human infants have at least some predispositions that go beyond simple sensory or receptor biases. One view of what causes such predispositions in the human infant is that there are 'innate cortical modules' for abilities such as face processing (Rodman *et al.*, 1993; Farah, in press), i.e. there is an area of cerebral cortex pre-wired through genetic and molecular mechanisms for the purpose of processing information about faces. Roughly speaking, the evidence for this view is that (i) newborns show a face-specific predisposition and (ii) neuroimaging and neuropsychological studies of adults have revealed that certain cortical areas are involved specifically in face processing. It is but a short step from this to assume that the newborn preference is supported by the same neural circuits involved in adult face processing. However, two lines of evidence make us sceptical about this view. We start with the first line of evidence which indicates that the newborn predisposition does not depend on the same cortical areas as are important in adults. The second line of evidence shows that there are dynamic changes in the cortical processing of faces over the first year of life.

Johnson and Morton (Johnson and Morton, 1991; Morton and Johnson, 1991) hypothesized that the predisposition to orient to face-like patterns observed in the newborn is not subserved by the same cortical pathways as are involved in face processing in adults on the following grounds. Indirect sources of evidence support the hypothesis that the preferential orienting to faces found in newborn infants is largely (but probably not exclusively) mediated by subcortical neural circuitry. Two of these considerations are (i) its developmental time course and (ii) the testing methods required to elicit the behavior.

Evidence from a variety of sources indicates that visual orienting and attention in the newborn infant are largely, though not exclusively, supported by subcortical structures such as the superior colliculus and the pulvinar, and that it is not until after 1 month of age that cortical pathways come to dominate subcortical circuits (see Johnson, 1990). To investigate the developmental time course of the preferential tracking of faces, three age groups of infants were studied, 5, 10 and 19 weeks, in a similar paradigm to that used with neonatal infants (Johnson, *et al.*, 1991, Expt. 3). Analysis of variance revealed no significant effects in the older age groups, but the face was tracked significantly further than all the other stimuli in the 5-week-old infants. Because the older infants failed to show preferential tracking of the face, we divided the 5-week-old sample into two, with the younger group

having an age range of 22–30 days, and the older group a range of 34–43 days. This post-hoc analysis revealed that most of the group effect was due to the younger infants: only in this group was the face tracked significantly further. This result indicates that the preferential tracking of faces may decline between 4 and 6 weeks after birth. The time course of this response is similar to that of other newborn responses thought to be mediated by subcortical circuits, for example the imitation of facial gestures (Maratsos, 1982; Vinter, 1986) or pre-reaching (von Hofsten, 1984). It has been suggested that the disappearance of these early reflex-like behaviors in the second month of life is due to inhibition by developing cortical circuits (see, for example, Muir *et al.*, 1989). This would also seem to be a plausible explanation for the decline observed in the tracking of faces. Thus, not only is it unlikely that the newborns have adequate cortical functioning to support the preferential tracking of faces, but this behavior declines at the same age as other behaviors thought to be mediated subcortically.

Why should the tracking task be so sensitive to newborns' preferences, whereas standard testing procedures with static stimuli are relatively ineffective? One reason is that the temporal visual field feeds more directly into the subcortical (collicular) pathway, whereas the nasal field is thought to feed more into the cortical visual pathway. In a tracking task such as that described with newborns, the stimulus is moving continually out of the central visual field and into the temporal field of one or the other eye. It has been suggested that it is this movement into the temporal field that initiates a saccade to re-foveate the stimulus in newborns (for details, see Bronson, 1974; Johnson, 1990). Unless specific situations are set up, this temporal field-driven orienting will not always occur with static presentations of stimuli, explaining why face preferences are rarely elicited clearly in other types of newborn testing procedures. Thus, the tracking task may tap effectively into the capacities of the subcortical oculomotor pathway.

To these two lines of evidence originally cited by Johnson and Morton (1991), we can now add two more. The first of these concerns the prediction that the predisposition should be evident in the temporal visual field, but not in the nasal field. As mentioned earlier, this is because the temporal field is thought to feed more heavily into the collicular (subcortical) pathway (Rafal *et al.*, 1991; but see Williams *et al.*, 1995). To test this prediction, Simion *et al.* (1998) patched one eye of their infant subjects and displayed face-like or control patterns in either the temporal or nasal field of the open eye. They observed that, in accordance with the prediction, there was preferential orienting to the face-like pattern only in the temporal field and not in the nasal field. Interestingly, a recent study by Johnson *et al.* (2000) provided evidence that spatial frequency preferences may be dominated more by nasal visual field input. Thus, with binocular full field viewing in behavioral testing paradigms, nasal and temporal field preference systems may compete for expression in behavior.

Finally, Mancini and colleagues (2000) tested the hypothesis more directly by examining face preferences in infants who unfortunately had suffered perinatal damage to parts of the cerebral cortex. While these infants showed a variety of deficits in more complex aspects of face processing, even those with widespread damage to visual cortical regions showed the bias to orient to simple face-like patterns. Thus, in the cases studied so far, damage to visual cortical areas does not appear to impair the predisposition. When taken together, these various strands of evidence are consistent with the view that the predisposition evident in newborns has a different neural basis from the more complex aspects of face processing studied in adults.

We now turn to a second line of evidence concerning the development of the cortical basis of face processing observed in adults. There is evidence that there are dynamic changes in the cortical processing of faces over the first year after birth. These data are important because they are inconsistent with the view that pre-wired dedicated circuits for face processing are activated early in life. Rather, it is more consistent with an 'interactive specialization framework' (Johnson, 2000) in which several interacting factors give rise to patterns of cortical specialization for function.

There is now a considerable body of evidence from neuroimaging and neuropsychological studies on adults identifying particular cortical pathways activated during face processing. One such area studied is the fusiform face area (FFA), a region of ventral temporal cortex that lies anterior to V4 (Halgren *et al.*, 1997). In a series of studies, it has been shown that this cortical area is more active while viewing faces than while viewing objects (Sergent *et al.*, 1992; Kanwisher *et al.*, 1997), hands (Kanwisher *et al.*, 1997), scrambled faces (Puce *et al.*, 1995) or textures (Malach *et al.*, 1995; Puce *et al.*, 1996), and while matching faces than while matching locations (Courtney *et al.*, 1997),

houses (Wojciulik *et al.*, 1998) or hands (Kanwisher *et al.*, 1997). These results support the view that the activation of the FFA in response to faces cannot be accounted for by visual complexity, stimulus meaningfulness or simple perceptual properties of faces. If adults are, in addition, required to remember facial identity, activation in these ventral occipito-temporal areas is correlated negatively with delay, suggesting that these regions are more involved in the initial encoding of faces and less in retaining memories of them (Haxby *et al.*, 1995; Courtney *et al.*, 1996, 1997).

Turning to scalp-recorded electrophysiological responses (ERPs), Bentin *et al.* (1996) identified a component of the ERP which occurs around 170 ms after the presentation of a face, and which is localizable in some subjects to parts of the inferior temporal cortex. In many, but not all, adults the specificity of this region for face processing tends to be lateralized, with the right side being more face specific than the left. This finding confirms reports with other brain imaging methods (Kanwisher *et al.*, 1997). Using a high-density ERP recording system, de Haan *et al.* (1998) replicated Bentin's finding with adults, and gave the same task to 6-month-old infants. High-density ERP recordings are possible in infants through the use of the Geodesic sensor net (Tucker, 1993) which is easily installed and comfortable to wear (see Figure 5.4).

The results for infants were both similar to and different from those obtained with adults. The results were similar in that there was a face-selective effect observed in the ERP. However, the results were different in a number of ways that suggest that infants at this age are still only partially specialized for face processing (for more details, see de Haan and Halit, in press; Johnson and de Haan, in press). For brevity, we illustrate just two of these differences here, the first of which concerns the differential responses observed when processing human and monkey faces. In this experiment, infant and adult subjects viewed upright and inverted monkey faces. We used monkey faces because they are different from, yet closely related to, human faces, and thus likely to be good stimuli for assessing the extent to which cortical processing of faces becomes specialized for our own species. We used inverted faces as control stimuli since they have the same basic visual properties as upright faces yet are known not to engage face-specific mechanisms.

As in previous studies, adults showed clear modulation of the N170 over posterior temporal sites

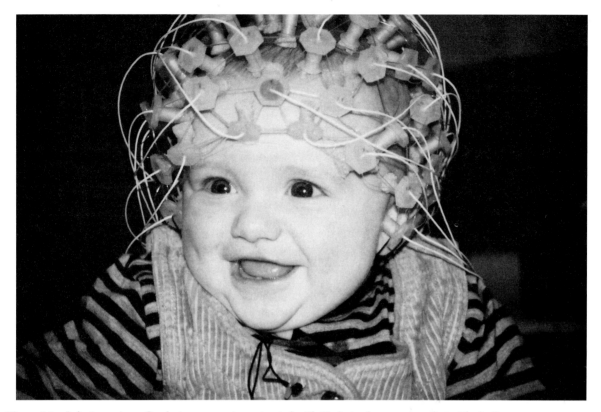

Figure 5.4. Infant wearing a Geodesic sensor net constructed with 62 electrodes sewn together with elastic.

according to the nature of the stimulus. The upright human face elicited a different response from the other three stimuli, indicating different processing of this stimulus. In contrast, the infants showed a similar evoked pattern for the upright monkey face as for the upright human face, suggesting that their face-processing pathways are not yet species specific: unlike in adults, a monkey face will engage these pathways as well as a human face.

A second way in which the cortical processing of faces in infants may differ from that observed in adults concerns lateralization. While, as discussed above, most normal adults show clearer evidence for face-specific processing on the right than on the left, most infants show a more bilateral pattern, suggesting that there is a process of increasing localization during postnatal life.

In conclusion, the in-depth investigation of a predisposition in the human infant has revealed it to be more than just a bias in sensory receptors or in the earliest stages of visual processing. However, we have argued that neither is it due to cortical circuitry

specifically pre-specified for that function. Rather, the predisposition appears to be the product of a bias in subcortical structures, perhaps in interaction with some partially active cortical structures. The pulvinar is one subcortical nucleus that has been suggested as possibly being critically involved (Johnson, 1997), but further research is required.

DISCUSSION

In this chapter, we have focused on two questions concerning predispositions and perceptual development: first, what are the mechanisms underlying perceptual predispositions; secondly, what are the functions of predispositions, in particular, how important are predispositions to the emergence of natural social behavior? In this discussion, we take a broader perspective, which includes both animal and human development, to these questions. First, we briefly consider interpretations of predispositions as being 'innate'.

Predispositions are not 'innate'

It is now common parlance in the study of animal behavior that it is meaningless to label a certain behavior pattern as 'innate' (Lehrman, 1970). Nevertheless, the assumption that predispositions are in some way 'innate' is still lurking in the minds of some authors. Bateson (1999) pointed out that there are at least seven different meanings of the word 'innate', namely 'present at birth; being a behavioral difference caused by a genetic difference; adapted over the course of evolution; unchanging throughout development; shared by all members of a species; present before the behavior serves any function; and not learned'. We will not repeat the arguments against the use of the concept of 'innate' in behavior research (Lehrman, 1970; cf. Bolhuis, 1999b); we will merely summarize the evidence, mainly from work on animals, that illustrates the inadequacy of applying the concept to predispositions.

Predispositions are not static phenomena, but they have a developmental dynamism that is the result of a continuous interaction between the individual and its internal and external environment. As we have seen, both auditory predispositions in ducklings (Gottlieb, 1980, 1982, 1985) and visual predispositions in domestic chicks (Horn, 1985; Johnson and Bolhuis, 1991) only develop after appropriate (but often non-specific) external experience. In the case of ducklings, the auditory experience had to be of a certain nature and with a particular variation in order to maintain certain predispositions. Both auditory and visual predispositions were dependent on the inducing or maintaining experience being delivered within a sensitive period. Furthermore, this sensitive period itself is not a static phenomenon, but can be delayed by certain manipulations of the animal's internal environment. All these results show that predispositions are the result of a complex interaction between the individual and its environment, very much in the way that Lehrman (1970) envisaged the developmental dynamic.

Mechanisms underlying predispositions

As we have illustrated, the mechanisms of predispositions can be studied through both neural and behavioral experimentation. Usually, the most effective strategy has been to combine neural and behavioral approaches into a single integrated program of research. The first conclusion which can be reached is

that both for human infants and for chicks, visual predispositions to orient to conspecifics appear to be more than just sensory biases. For example, even when we examined some sophisticated psychophysical theories of infant visual preferences, predictions seem to break down when faces are involved, with faces always eliciting more looking than predicted purely on the basis of their psychophysical properties. We are not denying that there are sensory biases that influence preference behavior in young vertebrates; indeed, they are clearly established. However, there also appear to be preferences based on inputs which are defined by more than a single psychophysical dimension, and these preferences can interact with sensory biases to influence behavior.

One obvious candidate mechanism for such predispositions is that they are supported by the same neural mechanisms as those that mediate processing of that class of stimulus in adults. For example, the tendency of newborn humans to orient to faces could be supported by the same ventral cortical visual pathway structures that mediate face processing in adults, or the specific predisposition in chicks could be mediated by the IMHV. In at least these cases, however, evidence indicates that these specific predispositions are supported by other parts of the brain. Thus, while these predispositions are the result of more than biases in early sensory processing, they do not appear to engage the same neural mechanisms as are involved in adults.

The function of predispositions

Given that the predisposition for faces we have discussed is not controlled by the same ventral pathway circuits as those in adults, what is its purpose? Why did evolution select for a behavior which is not related directly to an adult ability (cf. Oppenheim, 1981; Bolhuis, 1999b)? We suggest, by analogy with the two-process model of filial imprinting in chicks, that the human infant predisposition serves to bias the input to plastic neural circuits. In the human, these would be structures and pathways along the ventral cortical stream of visual processing. A lot of exposure to faces over the first days, weeks and months of life would contribute to selecting and tuning the appropriate circuits for face processing in adults.

The fact that these predispositions are not mediated by the same structures as in adults raises a question as to their purpose. Why would evolution select for such predispositions? For both the chick and the human newborn, we have argued (Johnson and Bolhuis, 1991; Johnson and Morton, 1991; Bolhuis, 1996) have argued that a primary purpose for the predispositions is to ensure the appropriate input for subsequent specialization and learning. In the case of human infants, we presented evidence that the specialization of the ventral visual pathway for face processing is a gradual process that takes some months. This observation is consistent with the view that for such specialization to develop appropriately requires exposure to faces. In the case of chicks, attending to adult conspecifics ensures that learning involving the IMHV (imprinting) is centered on an appropriate stimulus. In the case of humans, attending and responding to faces may also be of immediate adaptive value by ensuring that parents are engaged and bonded to their offspring. We suspect that simpler biases, such as those for certain spatial frequencies of pattern in human infants, serve no particular adaptive purpose, and merely reflect properties of the maturing nervous system.

Predispositions and social behavior

Virtually all of the specific predispositions we have reviewed in this chapter have relevance to social behavior. We postulate that there is a specific reason for this; namely that the newly born or hatched animal is bombarded with a variety of conspicuous moving objects, and it is vital for it to discriminate and attend preferentially to those which will be of greatest relevance to its subsequent survival. There is continuing debate about this issue among those studying human cognitive development. While the traditional view has been that infants gradually learn about the significance of social stimuli over the first few months of life, others have suggested recently that infants initially interpret the behavior of all moving stimuli as social (i.e. as 'agents' capable of having intentions) (e.g. Csibra and Gergely, 1998). While future research on this topic is required, it may be that such predispositions provide the essential foundations for building a social brain.

ACKNOWLEDGEMENTS

This chapter is dedicated to our mentor Gabriel Horn. We are grateful to him for his guidance and support, for his friendship and for fruitful scientific collaboration throughout the years that we worked in his laboratory and beyond. M.J. acknowledges financial support from MRC Programme grant G97 15587, EU Biomed grant BMH4-CT97-2032 and Birkbeck College.

REFERENCES

Banks, M.S. and Ginsburg, A.P. (1985) Early visual preferences: a review and new theoretical treatment. In: Reese, H.W. (ed.), *Advances in Child Development and Behavior*. Academic Press, New York, pp. 207–246.

Banks, M.S. and Salapatek, P. (1981) Infant pattern vision: a new approach based on the contrast sensitivity function. *Journal of Experimental Child Psychology*, 31, 1–45.

Banks, M.S. and Shannon, E. (1993) Spatial and chromatic visual efficiency in human neonates. In: Granrud, C.E. (ed.), *Visual Perception and Cognition in Infancy*. Erlbaum, Hillsdale, New Jersey, pp. 1–46.

Bateson, P. (1999) Foreword. In: Bolhuis, J.J. and Hogan, J.A. (eds), *The Development of Animal Behavior. A Reader*. Blackwell Publishers, Oxford, pp. ix–xi.

Bentin, S., Allison, T., Puce, A., Perez, E. and McCarthy, G. (1996) Electrophysiological studies of face perception in humans. *Journal of Cognitive Neuroscience*, 8, 551–565.

Bolhuis J.J. (1991) Mechanisms of avian imprinting: a review. *Biological Reviews*, 66, 303–345.

Bolhuis J.J. (1996) Development of perceptual mechanisms in birds: predispositions and imprinting. In: Moss, C.F. and Shettleworth, S.J. (eds), *Neuroethological Studies of Cognitive and Perceptual Processes*. Westview Press, Boulder, Colorado, pp. 158–184.

Bolhuis, J.J. (1999a) Early learning and the development of filial preferences in the chick. *Behavioural Brain Research*, 98, 245–252.

Bolhuis, J.J. (1999b) The development of animal behavior. From Lorenz to neural nets. *Naturwissenschaften*, 86, 101–111.

Bolhuis, J.J. (in press) Biological approaches to the study of perceptual and cognitive development. In: Kalverboer, A.F. and Gramsbergen, A. (eds), *Brain and Behaviour in Human Development: A Sourcebook*. Kluwer Academic Publishers, Dordrecht, in press.

Bolhuis, J.J. and Honey, R.C. (1994) Within-event learning during filial imprinting. *Journal of Experimental Psychology: Animal Behavior Processes*, 20, 240–248.

Bolhuis J.J. and Honey R.C. (1998) Imprinting, learning and development: from behaviour to brain and back. *Trends in Neurosciences*, 21, 306–311.

Bolhuis, J.J. and Horn, G. (1997) Delayed induction of a filial predisposition in the chick after anaesthesia. *Physiology & Behavior*, 62, 1235–1239.

Bolhuis, J.J., Johnson, M.H. and Horn, G. (1985) Effects of early experience on the development of filial preferences in the domestic chick. *Developmental Psychobiology*, 18, 299–308.

Bolhuis, J.J., McCabe, B.J. and Horn, G. (1986) Androgens and imprinting. Differential effects of testosterone on filial preferences in the domestic chick. *Behavioral Neuroscience*, 100, 51–56.

Bolhuis, J.J., Johnson, M.H. and Horn, G. (1989) Interacting mechanisms during the formation of filial preferences: the development of a predisposition does not prevent learning. *Journal of Experimental Psychology: Animal Behavior Processes*, 15, 376–382.

Bronson, G.W. (1974) The postnatal growth of visual capacity. *Child Development*, 45, 873–890.

Brown, M.W. and Horn, G. (1994) Learning-related alterations in the visual responsiveness of neurons in a memory system of the chick brain. *European Journal of Neuroscience*, 6, 1479–1490.

Courtney, S.M., Ungerleider, L.G., Keil, K. and Haxby, J.V. (1996) Object and spatial visual working memory activate separate systems in human cortex. *Cerebral Cortex*, 6, 39–49.

Courtney, S.M., Ungerleider, L.G., Keil, K. and Haxby, J.V. (1997) Transient and sustained activity in a distributed neural system for human working memory. *Nature*, 386, 608–611.

Csibra, G. and Gergely, G. (1998) The teleological origins of mentalistic action explanations: a developmental hypothesis. *Developmental Science*, 1, 255–259.

Davies, D.C., Johnson, M.H. and Horn, G. (1992) The effect of the neurotoxin DSP4 on the development of a predisposition in the domestic chick. *Developmental Psychobiology*, 25, 251–259.

de Haan, M. and Halit, H. (in press) The development and neural basis of face recognition during infancy. In: Kalverboer, A.F. and Gramsbergen, A. (eds), *Brain and Behaviour in Human Development: A Sourcebook*. Kluwer Academic Publishers, Dordrecht, in press.

de Haan, M., Oliver, A. and Johnson, M.H. (1998) Electrophysiological correlates of face processing by adults and 6-month-old infants. *Journal of Cognitive Neuroscience, Annual Meeting Supplement*, 36.

de Schonen, S. and Mathivet, E. (1990) Hemispheric asymmetry and interhemispheric communication of face processing in infancy. *Child Development*, 61, 1192–1205.

DeVoogd, T.J. (1994) The neural basis for the acquisition and production of bird song. In: Hogan, J.A. and Bolhuis, J.J. (eds), *Causal Mechanisms of Behavioural Development*. Cambridge University Press, Cambridge, pp. 49–81.

Fantz, R.L. (1964) Visual experience in infants: decreased attention to familiar patterns relative to novel ones. *Science*, 46, 668–670.

Farah, M.J. (in press) Early commitment of neural substrates for race recognition. *Cognitive Neuropsychology*, in press.

Goren, C.C., Sarty, M. and Wu, P.Y.K. (1975) Visual following and pattern discrimination of face-like stimuli by newborn infants. *Pediatrics*, 56, 544–549.

Gottlieb, G. (1971) *Development of Species Identification in Birds*. University of Chicago Press, Chicago.

Gottlieb, G. (1976) The roles of experience in the development of behavior and the nervous system. In: Gottlieb, G. (ed.), *Neural and Behavioral Specificity: Studies in the Development of Behavior and the Nervous System*. Academic Press, New York, pp. 237–280.

Gottlieb, G. (1980) Development of species identification in ducklings: VI. Specific embryonic experience required to maintain species-typical perception in Peking ducklings. *Journal of Comparative and Physiological Psychology*, 94, 579–587.

Gottlieb, G. (1982) Development of species identification in ducklings: IX. The necessity of experiencing normal variations in embryonic auditory stimulation. *Developmental Psychobiology*, 15, 507–517.

Gottlieb, G. (1985) Development of species identification in ducklings: XI. Embryonic critical period for species-typical perception in the hatchling. *Animal Behaviour*, 33, 225–233.

Halgren, E., Dale, A.M., Sereno, M.K., Tootell, R.B.H., Marinkovic, K. and Rosen, B.R. (1997) Location of fMRI responses to faces anterior to retinotopic cortex. *Neuroimage*, 5, S150.

Haxby, J.V., Ungerleider, L.G., Horwitx, B., Rapoport, S.I. and Grady, C.L. (1995) Hemispheric differences in neural systems for face working memory: a PET-rCBF study. *Human Brain Mapping*, 3, 68–82.

Hogan, J.A. (1988) Cause and function in the development of behavior systems. In: Blass, E.M. (ed.), *Handbook of Behavioral Neurobiology*, Vol. 9. Plenum Press, New York, pp. 63–106.

Horn, G. (1985) *Memory, Imprinting, and the Brain*. Clarendon Press, Oxford.

Horn, G. (1992) Brain mechanisms of memory and predispositions: interactive studies of cerebral function and behaviour. In: Johnson, M.H. (ed.), *Brain Development and Cognition: A Reader*. Blackwell, Oxford, pp. 485–513.

Horn, G. (1998) Visual imprinting and the neural mechanisms of recognition memory. *Trends in Neurosciences*, 21, 300–305.

Horn, G. and McCabe, B.J. (1984) Predispositions and preferences. Effects on imprinting of lesions to the chick brain. *Animal Behaviour*, 32, 288–292.

Johnson, M.H. (1990) Cortical maturation and the development of visual attention in early infancy. *Journal of Cognitive Neuroscience*, 2, 81–95.

Johnson, M.H. (1997) *Developmental Cognitive Neuroscience: An Introduction*. Blackwell, Oxford.

Johnson, M.H. (2000) Functional brain development in infants: elements of an interactive specialization framework. *Child Development*, 71, 75–81.

Johnson, M.H. and Bolhuis, J.J. (1991) Imprinting, predispositions and filial preference in the chick. In: Andrew R.J. (ed.), *Neural and Behavioural Plasticity*. Oxford University Press, Oxford, pp. 133–156.

Johnson, M.H. and de Haan, M. (in press) Developing cortical specialization for visual–cognitive function: the case of face recognition. In: McClelland, J.L. and Siegler, R.S. (eds), *Mechanisms of Cognitive Development: Behavioral & Neural Perspectives*. Lawrence Erlbaum Associates, Hillsdale, New Jersey, in press.

Johnson, M.H. and Horn, G. (1986) Is a restricted brain region of domestic chicks involved in the recognition of individual conspecifics? *Behavioural Brain Research*, 20, 109–110.

Johnson, M.H. and Horn, G. (1988) Development of filial preferences in dark-reared chicks. *Animal Behaviour*, 36, 675–683.

Johnson, M.H. and Morton, J. (1991) *Biology and Cognitive Development: The Case of Face Recognition*. Blackwell, Oxford.

Johnson, M.H., Bolhuis, J.J. and Horn, G. (1985) Interaction between acquired preferences and developing predispositions during imprinting. *Animal Behaviour*, 33, 1000–1006.

Johnson, M.H., Davies, D.C. and Horn, G. (1989) A sensitive period for the development of a predisposition in dark-reared chicks. *Animal Behaviour*, 37, 1044–1046.

Johnson, M.H., Dziurawiec, S., Ellis, H.D. and Morton, J. (1991) Newborns' preferential tracking of face-like stimuli and its subsequent decline. *Cognition*, 40, 1–19.

Johnson, M.H., Farroni, T., Brockbank, M. and Simion, F. (in press) Preferential orienting to faces in four month olds: analysis of temporal–nasal visual field differences. *Developmental Science*, in press.

Kanwisher, N., McDermott, J. and Chun, M.M. (1997) The fusiform face area: a module in human extrastriate cortex specialized for face perception. *Journal of Neuroscience*, 17, 4302–4311.

Kleiner, K.A. (1987) Amplitude and phase spectra as indices of infant's pattern preferences. *Infant Behavior and Development*, 10, 49–59.

Kleiner, K.A. (1990) Models of neonates' preferences for face-like patterns: a response to Morton, Johnson and Maurer. *Infant Behavior and Development*, 13, 105–108.

Kleiner, K.A. (1993) Specific vs non-specific face recognition device. In: de Boysson-Bardies, B., de Schonen, S., Jusczyk, P., MacNeilage, P. and Morton, J. (eds), *Developmental Neurocognition: Speech and Face Processing in the First Year of Life*. Kluwer Academic Publishers, Dordrecht, pp. 103–108.

Kleiner, K.A. and Banks, M.S. (1987) Stimulus energy does not account for 2-month old preferences. *Journal of Experimental Psychology: Human Perception and Performance*, 13, 594–600.

Lehrman, D.S. (1970) Semantic and conceptual issues in the nature–nurture problem. In: Aronson, L.R., Tobach, E., Lehrman, D.S. and Rosenblatt, J.S. (eds), *Development and Evolution of Behavior*. Freeman, San Francisco, pp. 17–52.

Macchi Cassia, V., Simion, F. and Umilta, C. (in press) Face preference at birth: the role of an orienting mechanism. *Developmental Science*, in press.

Malach, R., Reppas, J.B., Benson, R.R., Kwong, K.K., Jiang, H., Kennedy, W.A., Ledden, P.J., Brady, T.J., Rosen, B.R. and Tootell, R.B. (1995) Object-related activity revealed by functional magnetic resonance imaging in human occipital cortex. *Proceedings of the National Academy of Sciences of the United States of America*, 92, 8135–8139.

Mancini, J., Casse-Perrot, C., Giusiano, B., Girard, N., Camps, R., Deruelle, C. and de Schonen, S. (2000) Face processing development after a perinatal unilateral brain lesion. *Child Development*, in press.

Maratsos, O. (1982) Trends in the development of early imitation in infancy. In: Bever, T.G. (ed.), *Regressions in Development: Basic Phenomena and Theories*. Lawrence Erlbaum, Hillsdale, New Jersey, pp. 81–101.

Marler, P. (1976) Sensory templates in species-specific behavior. In: Fentress, J. (ed.), *Simpler Networks and Behavior*. Sinauer, Sunderland, Massachusetts, pp. 314–329.

Marler, P. (1987) Sensitive periods and the roles of specific and general sensory stimulation in birdsong learning. In: *Imprinting and Cortical Plasticity. Comparative Aspects of Sensitive Periods*. Rauschecker, J.P. and Marler, P. (eds), John Wiley & Sons, New York, pp. 99–135.

Marler, P. (1991) Song-learning behavior: the interface with neuroethology. *Trends in Neurosciences*, 14 199–206.

Maurer, D. (1985) Infants perception of faceness. In: Field, T.N. and Fox, N. (eds), *Social Perception in Infants*. Ablex, New Jersey, pp. 73–100.

Maurer, D. and Young, R.E. (1983) Newborns' following of natural and distorted arrangements of facial features. *Infant Behavior and Development*, 6, 127–131.

Morton, J. (1993) Mechanisms in infant face processing. In: *Developmental Neurocognition: Speech and Face Processing in the First Year of Life*. de Boysson-Bardies, B., de Schonen, S., Jusczyk, P., MacNeilage, P. and Morton, J. (eds), Kluwer Academic Publishers, Dordrecht, pp. 93–102.

Morton, J. and Johnson, M.H. (1991) CONSPEC and CONLERN: a two-process theory of infant face recognition. *Psychological Review*, 98, 164–181.

Morton, J., Johnson, M.H. and Maurer, D. (1990) On the reasons for newborns' responses to faces. *Infant Behavior and Development*, 13, 99–103.

Muir, D.W., Clifton, R.K. and Clarkson, M.G. (1989) The development of a human auditory localization response: a U-shaped function. *Canadian Journal of Psychology*, 43 199–216.

Nelson, C.A. and Bloom, F.E. (1997) Child development and neuroscience. *Child Development*, 68, 970–987.

Nelson, C.A. and Ludemann, P.M. (1989) Past, current and future trends in infant face perception research. *Canadian Journal of Psychology*, 43, 183–198.

Oppenheim, R.W. (1981) Ontogenetic adaptations and retrogressive processes in the development of the nervous system and behaviour: a neuroembryological perspective. In: Connolly, K.J. and Prechtl, H.F.R. (eds), *Maturation and Development: Biological and Psychological Perspective*. Lippincott, Philadelphia, pp. 73–109.

Perrett, D.I., Mistlin, A.J., Potter, D.D., Smith, P.A.J., Head, A.S., Chitty, A.J., Broennimann, R., Milner, A.D. and Jeeves, M. (1985) Functional organisation of visual neurones processing face identify. In: Ellis, H.D., Jeeves, M.A., Newcombe, F. and Young, A. (eds), *Aspects of Face Processing*. Martinus Nijhoff, Dordrecht, pp.

Posner, M.I. and Petersen, S.E. (1990) The attention system of the human brain. *Annual Review of Neuroscience*, 13, 25–42.

Puce, A., Allison, T., Gore, J.C. and McCarthy, G. (1995) Face-sensitive regions in human extrastriate cortex studied by functional MRI. *Journal of Neurophysiology*, 74, 1192–1199.

Puce, A., Allison, T., Asgari, M., Gore, J.C. and McCarthy, G. (1996) Differential sensitivity of human visual cortex to faces, letterstrings, and textures: a fMRI study. *Journal of Neuroscience*, 16, 5205–5215.

Rafal, R., Henik, A. and Smith, J. (1991) Extrageniculate contributions to reflex visual orienting in normal humans—a temporal hemifield advantage. *Journal of Cognitive Neuroscience*, 10, 358–364.

Rodman, H.R., Scalaidhe, S.P. and Gross, C.G. (1993) Response properties of neurons in temporal cortical visual areas of infant monkeys. *Journal of Neurophysiology*, 70, 1115–1136.

Sergent, J., Ohta, S. and McDonald, B. (1992) Functional neuroanatomy of face and object processing. A positron emission tomography study. *Brain*, 115, 15–36.

Simion, F., Valenza, E., Umilta, C. and Dalla Barba, B. (1998) Preferential orienting to faces in newborns: a temporal–

nasal asymmetry. *Journal of Experimental Psychology: Human Perception and Performance*, 24, 1399–1405.

Slater, A.M. (1993) Visual perceptual abilities at birth: implications for face perception. In: *Developmental Neurocognition: Speech and Face Processing in the First Year of Life*. de Boysson-Bardies, B., de Schonen, S., Jusczyk, P., MacNeilage, P. and Morton, J. (eds), Kluwer Academic Publishers, Dordrecht, pp. 125–134.

Souther, A. and Banks, M. (1979) The human face: a view from the infant's eye. In: *Society for Research in Child Development*, San Francisco.

Stevens, B.R. (1992) Uses of linear systems models of infant pattern vision. *Advances in Infancy Research*, 7, 1–38.

Tucker, D. (1993) Spatial sampling of head electrical fields: the geodesic sensor net. *Electroencephalography and Clinical Neurophysiology*, 87, 154–163.

Valenza, E., Simion, F., Macchi Cassia, V. and Umilta, C. (1996) Face preference at birth. *Journal of Experimental Psychology: Human Perception and Performance*, 22, 892–903.

Van Kampen, H.S. and Bolhuis, J.J. (1991) Auditory learning and filial imprinting in the chick. *Behaviour*, 117, 303–319.

Vinter, A. (1986) The role of movement in eliciting early imitations. *Child Development*, 57, 66–71.

von Hofsten, C. (1984) Developmental changes in the organisation of prereaching movements. *Developmental Psychology*, 20, 378–388.

Williams, C., Azzopardi, P. and Cowey, A. (1995) Nasal and temporal retinal ganglion-cells projecting to the midbrain—implications for blindsight. *Neuroscience*, 65, 577–586.

Wojciulik, E., Kanwisher, N. and Driver, J. (1998) Covert visual attention modulates face-specific activity in the human fusiform gyrus: fMRI study. *Journal of Neurophysiology*, 79, 1574–1578.

PART TWO   LEARNING AND MEMORY: MOLECULES, CELLS AND CIRCUITS

INTRODUCTION

In Part two, a number of leading paradigms are reviewed that investigate the brain mechanisms of learning and memory at the level of molecules, neurons and neuronal circuits. It will become clear that some of the chapters in this section of the book could quite easily have been included in Part Three ('Cognitive systems in animals and humans'), simply because several paradigms concerned with learning and memory operate at different levels of analysis. For example, the chapters by Smulders and DeVoogd and by Brown are concerned with the cognitive systems of spatial learning in birds and mammalian recognition memory, respectively, which would have justified inclusion in Part Three. However, within their respective paradigms, they concentrate on mechanisms at the cellular and circuit level, which was the reason for placing them in the current section.

Two important questions in the search for the neural substrates of learning and memory can be summarized as: what is happening, and where? The second of these questions can be rephrased as: is the neural substrate for information storage localized in the brain? Some authors have argued that such a localization of function is essential for a successful analysis of the neural mechanisms of learning and memory (e.g. Horn, 1985, 1998, Chapter 19; Thompson and Krupa, 1994, King and Thompson, Chapter 12). Gabriel Horn and his collaborators have been pioneers in attempting to localize the neural substrate of memory (Horn, 1985, Chapter 19). The argument is that, in order to be able to analyze the neuronal correlates of learning and memory, you have to know where in the brain to look for these correlates. A well-known attempt at localization of function was that of Karl Lashley who was 'in search of the engram' (Lashley, 1950), the engram being the 'mark' or 'trace' left in the brain by the learning experience. Lashley conducted an extensive series of experiments involving lesions to and incisions of areas of the cortex of rats, testing the effects of these manipulations in maze tasks. His main conclusion was that the effects of his lesions were not related to their location, but to their extent. Lashley famously concluded that 'I sometimes feel, in reviewing the evidence on the localization of the memory trace, that the necessary conclusion is that learning just is not possible' (Lashley, 1950, pp. 477–478). Subsequent attempts to localize brain regions where memory is stored have been more successful, mainly because they have employed a number of different neurobiological techniques, most of which were not available in Lashley's days.

The second important question—what is happening in the brain during learning and memory?—has been answered in a number of ways, some of which are discussed in Chapter 9 of the present volume. Most investigaters agree that learning and memory involves changes in the connections between neurons (e.g. Cajal, 1911; Hebb, 1949). Cajal (1911) distinguished between Tanzi's (1893) suggestion that information storage involves changes in the effectiveness of existing connections, a view later shared by Hebb (1949), and his own view that new connections were being formed between neurons. Hebb (1949) essentially suggested that information storage involved an increase in the area of contact between the pre- and postsynaptic neuron. Horn (1998) recently discussed these and some more recent suggestions concerning mechanisms for an increase in neuronal connectivity, including an increase in the number of receptors in the postsynaptic membrane (Horn, 1962) and an increase in neurotransmitter release (Kosower, 1972).

A closely related issue concerning the 'what' question is that of *how* the putative plastic changes in neural connectivity come about. The most commonly cited suggestion was made by Donald Hebb over half a century ago, as epitomized in his famous statement:

'When an axon of cell A is near enough to excite a cell B and repeatedly or persistently takes part in firing it, some growth process or metabolic change takes place in one or both cells such that A's efficiency, as one of the cells firing B, is increased' (Hebb, 1949, p. 62).

In contemporary terms, this means that neural plasticity involves changes in neuronal connectivity as a result of simultaneous pre- and postsynaptic activity. Hebb's ideas have had an enormous influence on the study of the neural mechanisms of learning and memory (cf. Horn, 1985; Dudai, 1989; Morris, 1989), and they continue to do so, as exemplified by many chapters in the present volume. The simple elegance of his idea has stimulated theoretical approaches ever since the publication of his book (Hebb, 1949), and many attempts have been made to translate Hebb's proposals into specific synaptic mechanisms. Hebb's suggestions have also been an important driving force for the study of long-term potentiation (LTP) as a model for the neural plasticity underlying learning and memory (see below, and Dudai and Morris, Chapter 9; Winder and Kandel, Chapter 10).

Broadly speaking, the study of the neural mechanisms of learning and memory has been approached from two different angles (Dudai, 1989; Bolhuis, 1994), both of which are represented in this book. An important general approach is to study the neural changes that occur during or after a learning experience. Examples of this approach are olfactory learning (Chapter 6) and imprinting (Chapter 19). Presuppositions about the nature of the neural changes are usually quite general, it merely being presumed that information storage in the brain is reflected in changes in neuronal connectivity. At the other end of the scientific spectrum are approaches that make specific assumptions as to the substrates or mechanisms involved in learning and memory. For instance, the profound effects of lesions to the temporal lobe (including the hippocampus) on human memory (Scoville and Milner, 1957) have sparked off a huge research effort, which is also reflected in the present volume (Chapters 8–11, 16–18; see also, for example, Squire and Zola-Morgan, 1991). Another example of this approach is the presumed importance of LTP as a mechanism that may be similar to (or the same as) the neural mechanisms underlying learning and memory (Chapters 9 and 10). In practice, these two general approaches are often combined (cf. Horn, 1985; Dudai, 1989), and surely such a synthetic approach is the way forward.

In Chapter 6, Peter Brennan and Barry Keverne review the neural mechanisms of olfactory learning in mice and sheep. Their own work on olfactory recognition memory involved in a pregnancy block in female mice is a fascinating example of how far we have come in search of the engram (Lashley, 1950). In female mice, mating leads to a memory for the smell of the male: exposure to an alien male leads to a pregnancy block. The neural substrate for this olfactory memory is localized in the accessory olfactory bulb (AOB). Briefly, the memory is represented as increased feedback inhibition of a subpopulation of neurons in the AOB. This feedback involves increased neurotransmitter release and an enlargement of postsynaptic densities at dendro-dendritic synapses in this subpopulation of neurons. Similar neural events occur in the main olfactory bulb (MOB) during the olfactory learning that is involved in ewes' recognition of their young, and during olfactory learning in young rodents. Brennan and Keverne discuss different characteristics of olfactory learning, and conclude that the underlying neural mechanisms are similar across a range of vertebrate species, as well as mollusks and insects.

David Clayton in Chapter 7 reviews the latest developments in the study of the neural mechanisms of bird song learning. Songbirds need to learn their song from an adult tutor when they are young. Until recently, it was thought that bird song was subserved by two forebrain circuits connecting a number of 'song control nuclei'. These suggestions were based mainly on lesion studies and electrophysiology (Nottebohm, 1991; De Voogd, 1994). Recently, however, introduction of the immediate early gene (IEG) technique has radically changed the field. IEGs are activated very soon after a stimulus impinges upon the cell. The protein products of IEGs return to the cell nucleus to influence the expression of late response genes. Expression of IEGs can be used as a marker for neuronal activation (Hunt *et al.*, 1987; Sagar *et al.*, 1988; Dragunow and Faull, 1989), by analyzing the expression of mRNA for the proteins, or the protein products themselves. These analytical techniques are now widely used tools in cognitive neuroscience, as can also be seen in several chapters in the present volume (Brennan and Keverne, Chapter 6; Clayton, Chapter 7; Brown, Chapter 11; Horn, Chapter 19; cf. McCabe and Horn, 1994). Clayton and his colleagues found that exposure of an adult zebra finch to an unfamiliar song leads to IEG expression in brain regions other than the conventional 'song control nuclei', notably the caudal parts of the neostriatum (NCM) and the hyperstriatum ventrale (CMHV). Clayton suggests that different parts of the songbird brain are involved in motor control, perception and template matching of song. As yet, we do not know where in the brain the information about the tutor song is stored, but recent evidence (Jin and Clayton, 1997; Bolhuis *et al.*, 2000) suggests that the NCM (and possibly the CMHV) is a likely site of storage.

Just as in the study of bird song, the neural analysis of food storing in birds often employs what I will call a 'neuroecological' approach to the study of the neural mechanisms of learning and memory. Tom Smulders and Timothy DeVoogd review some recent developments in the search for the neural mechanisms of avian food storing in Chapter 8. In a neuroecological approach, a functional or evolutionary principle is used for a comparative analysis of brain mechanisms of behavior (for some recent examples, see Balda *et al.*, 1998; Shettleworth, 1998). For instance, by comparing the brains of a food-storing bird species with those of a closely related species that does not store food, it is hoped that the neural substrate for the memory of stored food items will be revealed (cf. Krebs *et al.*, 1989). This approach has yielded important information regarding the evolution of brain and behavior. Smulders and DeVoogd argue that the avian hippocampal formation (HF) is analogous to the mammalian hippocampus. They go on to review research that suggests a role for the HF in spatial memory. These results are very interesting, but at the same time they illustrate some potential dangers of a neuroecological approach, i.e. there are numerous behavioral differences between food-storing and non-food-storing species besides the presence or absence of food storing. For instance, food storers are likely to spend more time navigating through the environment than non-storers, and the differences in HF morphology may be related to differences in these activities rather than to differences in food storing. Furthermore, the authors show that in a laboratory setting, neural differences between storers and non-storers are not always apparent, nor do these neural differences always correlate with behavioral differences. These discrepancies suggest that a neuroecological approach should always be combined with an experimental approach.

In a thought-provoking chapter, Yadin Dudai and Richard Morris provide a critical review of our current knowledge of what they term 'consolidation' (Chapter 9)—the 'what' question that I discussed above. In this context, consolidation refers to the processes occurring at the level of the neuron and the synapse during and after memory formation or its neural models. Many of their examples concern artificially induced neural plasticity, such as hippocampal LTP (Bliss and Lømo, 1973), a phenomenon

that is also discussed in some detail in the following chapter by Winder and Kandel. LTP involves long-term changes in synaptic efficacy as a result of brief high-frequency stimulation of presynaptic, afferent fibers. Interestingly, LTP induction is dependent on simultaneous depolarization of the postsynaptic cell and activation of postsynaptic receptors by presynaptic inputs. Thus, LTP appears to fit the Hebbian scheme of neuronal plasticity rather nicely, which is one reason for its popularity as a model for memory. In fact, at some stage, some journals seemed to find the subtleties of LTP more interesting than real memory itself. The use of LTP as a model for learning and memory has not been without its critics, however (e.g. Horn and McCabe, 1990). Previous efforts to investigate explicitly the relationship between LTP and memory had been pharmacological, where the NMDA receptor, which is crucial for the induction of LTP, was blocked (e.g. Morris *et al.*, 1986). Recent evidence shows that the induction of LTP in rats can be blocked completely pharmacologically, without an effect on spatial learning (Bolhuis and Reid, 1992; Bannerman *et al.*, 1995; Saucier and Cain, 1995). These findings cast doubt on the relationship between LTP and learning and memory; at the very least, they suggest that this relationship is more complex than was thought previously.

Chapter 10, by Danny Winder and Eric Kandel, is a review of recent genetic approaches to the study of learning and memory. With modern genetic techniques, individual genes can be 'knocked out' or, alternatively, overexpressed, and the effects of these manipulations on behavior or on properties of neurons can be measured. The authors' work is directed particularly at the phenomenon of LTP (Bliss and Lømo, 1973) which, as I discussed earlier, is often seen as a model for the synaptic plasticity that may underlie learning and memory. Winder and Kandel discuss genetic approaches to LTP, where the genes coding for individual proteins that are thought to play a role in some stage of LTP can be deleted or overexpressed. The authors do not ignore the pitfalls of the genetic approach. For instance, until recently, when a gene was knocked out, it was knocked out in every cell in the body, throughout the life of the individual—a complexity which leads to obvious difficulties in the interpretation of its behavioral effects. Furthermore, it is important to realize that there is not a one-to-one relationship between a gene and behavior. The problems of the interpretation of the genetic approach have been discussed in detail by Good (1996),

Keverne (1997) and Nelson and Young (1998). Winder and Kandel go on to discuss 'second generation' genetic techniques, where there is a much higher degree of spatial and temporal specificity of the genetic manipulation, for instance where in some lines of mice a gene knockout (and its effects on LTP) was found to be limited to the CA1 region of the hippocampus. It is hoped that these more sophisticated genetic techniques, together with contemporary pharmacological approaches, can shed more light on the mechanisms underlying LTP, and also of those underlying memory.

In the last chapter of this section, Malcolm Brown discusses the neural substrates of recognition memory. Later in this book, Buckley and Gaffan (Chapter 16) describe how the search for an animal model of human amnesia, after focusing on the hippocampus for decades, switched its attention to extrahippocampal neocortical structures. In fact, some time before lesion studies diverted attention to extrahippocampal structures, the evidence was already staring us in the face, coming from Brown *et al.*'s electrophysiological studies. As early as 1987, Brown and his collaborators reported that neurons in extrahippocampal temporal cortex seemed to be more important for recognition memory than neurons in the hippocampus proper (Brown *et al.*, 1987). Ironically, some researchers only seem to be convinced by lesion evidence, the very technique that had led them astray for so long! Brown *et al.* have found that neurons in the perirhinal cortex of both rats and monkeys are sensitive to the familiarity and recency of visual stimuli. In addition, a system involving the hippocampus proper is thought to be important for recognition involving the recollection of associations and the spatial context of events.

REFERENCES

Balda, R.P., Pepperberg, I.M. and Kamil, A.C. (eds) (1998) *Animal Cognition in Nature*. Academic Press, San Diego.

Bannerman, D.M., Good, M.A., Butcher, S.P., Ramsay, M. and Morris, R.G.M. (1995) Distinct components of spatial learning revealed by prior training and NMDA receptor blockade. *Nature*, 378, 182–186.

Bliss, T.V.P. and Lømo, T. (1973) Long-lasting potentiation of synaptic transmission in the dentate area of the anaesthetised rabbit following stimulation of the perforant path. *Journal of Physiology*, 232, 331–356.

Bolhuis J.J. (1994) Neurobiological analyses of behavioural mechanisms in development. In: Hogan, J.A. and Bolhuis, J.J. (eds), *Causal Mechanisms of Behavioural Development*. Cambridge University Press, Cambridge, pp. 16–46.

Bolhuis, J.J. and Reid, I.C. (1992) Effects of intraventricular infusion of the *N*-methyl-D-aspartate (NMDA) receptor antagonist AP5 on spatial memory of rats in a radial arm maze. *Behavioural Brain Research*, 47, 151–157.

Bolhuis, J.J, Zijlstra, G.G.O., Den Boer-Visser, A.M. and Van der Zee, E.A. (2000) Localized neuronal activation in the zebra finch brain is related to the strength of song learning. *Proceedings of the National Academy of Sciences of the United States of America*, 97, 2282–2285.

Brown, M.W., Wilson, F.A.W. and Riches, I.P. (1987) Neuronal evidence that inferotemporal cortex is more important than hippocampus in certain processes underlying recognition memory. *Brain Research*, 409, 158–162.

Cajal, S.R. (1911) *Histologie du Système Nerveux de l'Homme et des Vertébrés*. Maloine, Paris.

DeVoogd, T.J. (1994) The neural basis for the acquisition and production of bird song. In: Hogan, J.A. and Bolhuis, J.J. (eds), *Causal Mechanisms of Behavioural Development*. Cambridge University Press, Cambridge, pp. 49–81.

Dragunow, M. and Faull, R. (1989) The use of c-*fos* as a metabolic marker in neuronal pathway tracing. *Journal of Neuroscience Methods*, 29, 261–265.

Dudai, Y. (1989) *The Neurobiology of Memory*. Oxford University Press, Oxford.

Good, M. (1996) Targeted deletion of neuronal nitric oxide: a step closer to understanding its functional significance? *Trends in Neurosciences*, 19, 83–84.

Hebb, D.O. (1949) *The Organization of Behavior*. John Wiley & Sons, New York.

Horn, G. (1962) Some neural correlates of perception. In: Carthy, J.D. and Duddington, C.L. (eds), *Viewpoints in Biology*. Butterworth, London, pp. 242–285.

Horn, G. (1985) *Memory, Imprinting, and the Brain*. Clarendon Press, Oxford.

Horn, G. (1998) Visual imprinting and the neural mechanisms of recognition memory. *Trends in Neurosciences*, 21, 300–305.

Horn, G., Bradley, P. and McCabe, B.J. (1985) Changes in the structure of synapses associated with learning. *Journal of Neuroscience*, 5, 3161–3168.

Horn, G. and McCabe, B.J. (1990) Learning by seeing: *N*-methyl-D-aspartate receptors and recognition memory. In: Ben-Ari, Y. (ed.), *Excitatory Amino Acids and Neuronal Plasticity*. Plenum Press, New York, pp. 187–196.

Hunt, S.P., Pini, A. and Evans, G. (1987) Induction of c-*fos* like protein in spinal cord neurons following sensory stimulation. *Nature*, 328, 632–634.

Keverne, E.B. (1997) An evaluation of what the mouse knockout experiments are telling us about mammalian behaviour. *BioEssays* 19, 1091–1098.

Kosower, E.M. (1972) A molecular basis for learning and memory. *Proceedings of the National Academy of Sciences of the United States of America*, 69, 3292–3296.

Krebs, J.R., Sherry, D.F., Healy, S.D., Perry, V.H. and Vaccarino, A.L. (1989) Hippocampal specialization of food-storing birds. *Proceedings of the National Academy of Sciences of the United States of America*, 86, 1388–1392.

Lashley, K.S. (1950) In search of the engram. *Symposia of the Society for Experimental Biology*, 4, 454–482.

McCabe, B.J. and Horn, G. (1994) Learning-related changes in Fos-like immunoreactivity in the chick forebrain after imprinting. *Proceedings of the National Academy of Sciences of the United States of America*, 91, 11417–11421.

Morris, R.G.M. (1989) Does synaptic plasticity play a role in learning and memory? In: Morris, R.G.M. (ed.), *Parallel Distributed Processing: Implications for Psychology and Neurobiology*. Oxford University Press, pp. 248–285.

Morris, R.G.M., Anderson, E., Lynch, G.S. and Baudry, M. (1986) Selective impairment of learning and blockade of long-term potentiation by an *N*-methyl-D-aspartate receptor antagonist. *Nature*, 319, 774–776.

Nelson, R.J. and Young, K.A. (1998) Behavior in mice with targeted disruption of single genes. *Neuroscience and Biobehavioral Reviews*, 22, 453–462.

Nottebohm, F. (1991) Reassessing the mechanisms and origins of vocal learning in birds. *Trends in Neurosciences*, 14, 206–211.

Sagar, S.M., Sharp, F.R. and Curran, T., (1988) Expression of c-*fos* protein in brain: metabolic mapping at the cellular level. *Science*, 240, 1328–1331.

Saucier, D. and Cain, D.P. (1995) Spatial learning without NMDA receptor-dependent long-term potentiation. *Nature*, 378, 186–189.

Scoville, W.B. and Milner, B. (1957) Loss of recent memory after bilateral hippocampal lesions. *Journal of Neurology, Neurosurgery and Psychiatry*, 20, 11–21.

Shettleworth, S.J. (1998) *Cognition, Evolution, and Behavior*. Oxford University Press, Oxford.

Squire, L.R. and Zola-Morgan, S. (1991) The medial temporal lobe memory system. *Science*, 253, 1380–1386.

Tanzi, E. (1993) I fatti e le induzioni nell' odierna istologia del systema nervoso. *Riv. Sper. Freniat. Med. Leg. Alien. Ment.*, 19, 419–472.

Thompson, R.F. and Krupa, D.J. (1994). Organization of memory traces in the mammalian brain. *Annual Review of Neuroscience*, 17, 519–549.

6 NEURAL MECHANISMS OF OLFACTORY RECOGNITION MEMORY

Peter A. Brennan and Eric B. Keverne

INTRODUCTION

In the context of learning and memory, it is of some benefit if the exceedingly complex mammalian nervous system can be reduced to some component part that provides insights into the way in which macroscopic neural assemblies function. This viewpoint has developed from the writings of Hebb (1949), in *The Organization of Behavior,* and Shimbel (1950) who were among the first to describe how some features of learning could be imitated by a simple system of neurons linked by synapses that were assumed to change their properties as a result of activity.

In more recent years, various mathematical models have been derived which describe the modification of assemblies of neuron-like units and which have properties that mimic biological memory systems (Hopfield, 1984; see also Bateson, Chapter 15). Such neural models have to be based on the details of biological systems that have been shaped by evolution. Therefore, an understanding of a simple memory system that has developed across a variety of mammalian species and a wide range of contexts could provide insights into the units from which more complex nervous systems are constructed. This does not mean to imply that reducing cortical structures to functional units provides a complete picture. Nevertheless, if neural mechanisms for memory can be served by some basic structure, then such is the nature of conservation in evolution that it is likely that variations on this arrangement will be repeated elsewhere in the brain.

A memory system that has played an important part in the organization of mammalian behavior is that of the olfactory system. Olfactory learning is important in the recognition of kin, mates and offspring, as well as which foods to eat and which territories to avoid. Extensive studies on the olfactory bulb have found that this simple tri-laminar structure is capable of long-term synaptic changes which underlie the learning of such biologically significant odors. A common feature in these examples of olfactory learning is that they occur during a sensitive period, triggered by somatosensory cues such as coitus (Keverne and de la Riva, 1982), parturition (Keverne *et al.,* 1983) or maternal grooming, and are mediated by noradrenaline (NA) release in the olfactory bulb (Gervais *et al.,* 1988; Sullivan *et al.,* 1989).

PHEROMONAL LEARNING IN MICE

The ability of a female mouse to recognize the pheromones of the male with which she has mated is one of the simplest, and most extensively studied examples of olfactory learning (Brennan *et al.,* 1990; Brennan and Keverne, 1997). Memory formation is contingent on the vagino-cervical stimulation occurring during mating and is formed during a sensitive period lasting a few hours immediately after mating (Rosser and Keverne, 1985). It is specific for the pheromones to which the female has been exposed at mating and lasts for at least 30 days (Kaba *et al.,* 1988). If the female is exposed subsequently to a strange male's pheromones, pregnancy fails, but this does not occur when she is exposed to the pheromones of the mating male. This recognition of the mating male is therefore vital to prevent the abortion of the developing embryos, which is the normal result of exposure to male pheromones during the pre-implantation period (Bruce, 1961).

Mouse pheromones and their influence on reproduction

The pheromonal signals in mouse urine are complex and not very well understood. Various small, volatile molecules are found at high concentrations in male mouse urine, are produced in a testosterone-dependent fashion and have been claimed to possess pheromonal activity, e.g. brevicomins, dihydrothiazoles, farnesones and heptanones (Novotny *et al.,* 1990) However, there is insufficient interindividual variation of these compounds to convey the individuality of the pheromonal signal that can be discriminated in the pregnancy block effect. More likely

candidates to convey the individuality of the signal are the major urinary proteins (MUPs). These are produced by a large gene family with many allelic variants (Clark *et al.,* 1985), and the total urinary pool of MUPs is highly polymorphic (Clissold and Bishop, 1982) and likely to differ among individual, wild animals. Their expression is androgen dependent, and adult males produce large quantities (5–20 mg)

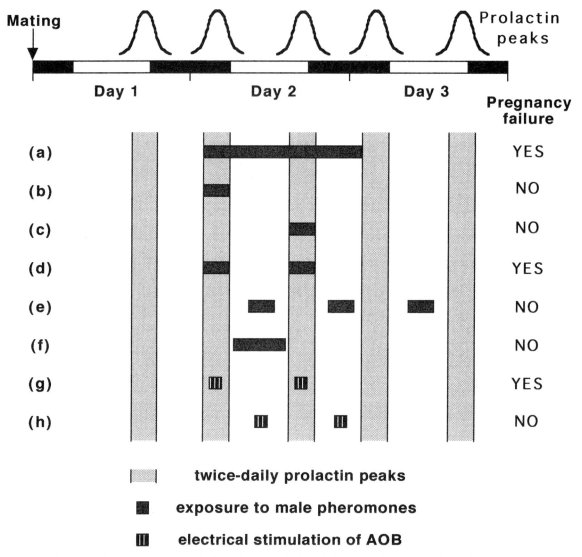

Figure 6.1. Susceptibility to pregnancy block depends on the timing of pheromonal exposure. The timing of the semi-circadian prolactin peaks initiated by mating is shown diagramatically in relation to the light/dark cycle at the top of the figure. The timing of pheromonal exposure or accessory olfactory bulb (AOB) stimulation (horizontal bars) to the prolactin peaks (vertical bars) is shown below, along with their effects on pregnancy failure. Exposure to strange male pheromones, or electrical stimulation of the AOB, during the two prolactin peaks on day 2 are effective in blocking pregnancy (a, d and g). Exposure during only one of the peaks, or exposure or stimulation between the peaks is ineffective (b, c, e, f and h).

daily. Moreover, MUPs have been reported to have a direct pheromonal effect to accelerate puberty in pre-pubertal females (Mucignat-Caretta *et al.*, 1995). Interestingly, MUPs belong to the lipocalin family of ligand-binding proteins and bind many of the small volatile molecules found in mouse urine such as brevicomins and thiazoles (Bocskei *et al.*, 1992). This raises the possibility that the complex of MUP plus bound ligand may interact with the pheromonal receptor, in a similar manner to the presentation of antigens to the T cells in the immune system.

The role of MUPs in pheromonal communication in mice is consistent with the finding of pheromonal activity in the protein fraction of male mouse urine (Marchlewska-Koj, 1981), and explains why these pheromonal effects, such as pregnancy block, are mediated via the vomeronasal system. Unlike the main olfactory system that primarily responds to volatile, airborne molecules, the vomeronasal system responds to non-volatile molecules that gain access to the nasal cavity during licking and nuzzling of urine marks. Access of pheromones to the vomeronasal organ, which is a blind-ended tubular structure in the nasal septum, requires an active pumping mechanism (Meredith and O'Connell, 1979). Lesions to the vome-ronasal organ or to the accessory olfactory bulb (AOB) of female mice prevent male pheromones from induc-ing estrus, accelerating puberty onset and blocking pregnancy (Keverne, 1983).

The block to pregnancy occurs pre-implantation, the primary endocrine change being a fall in serum pro-lactin (Reynolds and Keverne, 1979; Ryan and Schwartz, 1980; Keverne and de la Riva, 1982; Marchelwska-Koj, 1983). Evidence for this comes from experiments which show that restricted periods of exposure of female mice to male pheromones, coinci-dent with the prolactin surges following mating, block pregnancy (Figure 6.1), and do so by stimulating hypo-thalamic dopamine release, thereby inhibiting prolactin production from the anterior pituitary (Rosser *et al.*, 1989). Similarly, electrical stimulation of the mouse AOB, when coincident with prolactin surges, also blocks pregnancy (Li *et al.*, 1994). As prolactin is luteotrophic in mice, this withdrawal of luteotrophic support leads to the failure of the corpora lutea and a fall in progesterone levels, thus preventing implanta-tion and initiating a return to estrus.

The neural pathway to the tuberoinfundibular dopaminergic (TIDA) neurons in the arcuate nucleus of the hypothalamus (Figure 6.2) has been identified by electrophysiological stimulation of the AOB (Li

et al., 1989). It involves excitatory connections in the cortico-medial amygdala (Li *et al.*, 1990) and the medial preoptic area of the hypothalamus (Li *et al.*, 1992). Hence, unlike the main olfactory system, which projects extensively throughout the brain, especially to cortical areas, the vomeronasal system has a restricted subneocortical projection. This relatively direct projection to hypothalamic areas mediates pheromonal effects on endocrine state and behavior. The question arises as to whether the neural changes underlying the memory for the mating male's pheromones are confined to one locus or distributed throughout this pathway. Any permanent lesion to the pathway would disrupt the neuroendocrine output that is required to assess whether memory for-mation has occurred. Therefore, to address this ques-tion, we transiently disabled each site along the neural pathway, using local infusions of the anesthetic lignocaine, during the sensitive period for memory formation (Kaba *et al.*, 1989). When lignocaine was infused into the medial amygdala, at the second relay, formation of pheromonal memory proceeded as normal, whereas memory formation was disrupted when lignocaine was infused in the first relay in the pathway, in the AOB. Taken together with the neces-sary control procedures, these experiments imply that the AOB itself is the site for the neural changes that underpin pheromonal recognition.

Neural mechanisms for memory formation in the AOB

The synaptic circuitry of the AOB is comparatively simple (Figure 6.3), and is very similar to that of the main olfactory bulb (MOB), containing three main cell types (Mori, 1987). Mitral cells contact afferents from the vomeronasal nerve in glomeruli and project to the cortical and medial amygdala, forming the excitatory pathway for pheromonal signals. The mitral cells form reciprocal dendro-dendritic synapses with inhibitory interneurons at two levels. Periglomerular cells provide feedback inhibition at the glomerular level, controlling the input to the mitral cells. Granule cells, on the other hand, are the main class of interneuron in the AOB and regulate mitral cell output by providing feedback inhibition on their primary and secondary dendritic tree. Granule cell dendritic spines are depo-larized by excitatory glutamatergic input from mitral cells, and in turn provide feedback inhibition to the mitral cells via GABA release at the same spines (Figure 6.4A).

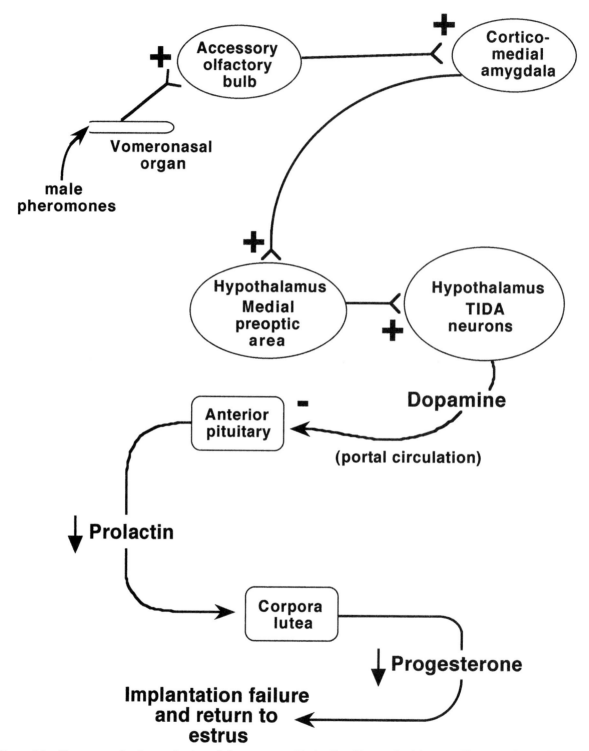

Figure 6.2. The neuroendocrine mechanism of the pregnancy block effect (Bruce effect) in mice. Pheromonal stimulation of receptors in the vomeronasal organ initiates a neuroendocrine reflex resulting in the release of dopamine by the tuberoinfundibular dopaminergic neurons in the hypothalamus. This suppresses prolactin secretion from the anterior pituitary, and the consequent removal of luteotrophic support results in a fall in progesterone levels and a return to estrus.

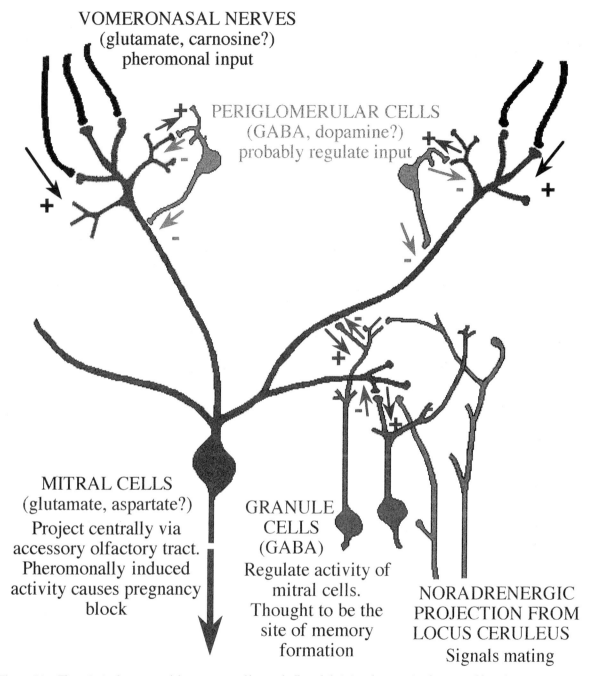

Figure 6.3.　The principal neurons of the accessory olfactory bulb and their involvement in pheromonal learning.

The AOB receives direct pheromonal input from the vomeronasal receptor neurons, but how is the occurrence of mating signaled? In a similar fashion to the MOB, the AOB receives a rich noradrenergic projection from the locus ceruleus, mainly targeted at the granule cell and external plexiform layers. Micro-dialysis studies have confirmed that NA levels in the AOB are elevated for at least 4 h following mating as a result of somatosensory stimulation during coitus (Brennan *et al.*, 1995). Moreover, specific neurotoxic

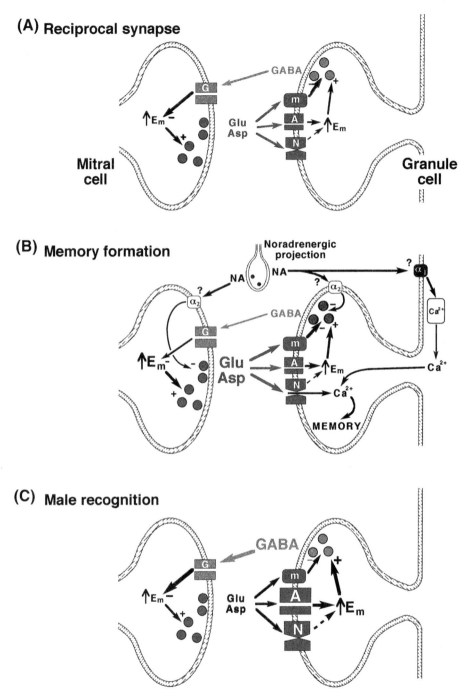

Figure 6.4. (**A**) Reciprocal synapses mediate feedback inhibition to mitral cells. Glutamate and/or aspartate released from mitral cells depolarize granule cell spines via AMPA (A) and NMDA (N) receptors. This depolarization stimulates GABA release, which inhibits mitral cell spines via $GABA_A$ receptors (G). Self-inhibition of mitral cells is regulated by $mGluR_2$ receptors (m) that locally inhibit GABA release from stimulated granule cell spines. (**B**) The association of pheromonal input to mitral cells with elevated noradrenaline (NA) leads to memory formation. The role of NA in this process is not clear but could involve an α_2-mediated disinhibition of mitral cells or an α_1-mediated release of Ca^{2+} from intracellular stores. (**C**) Memory formation is hypothesized to result in a long-lasting increase in sensitivity of the granule cell AMPA and/or NMDA receptors. This will increase the gain of the self-inhibition of mitral cells responding to the learned pheromonal signal, preventing the signal from being transmitted centrally to induce pregnancy block.

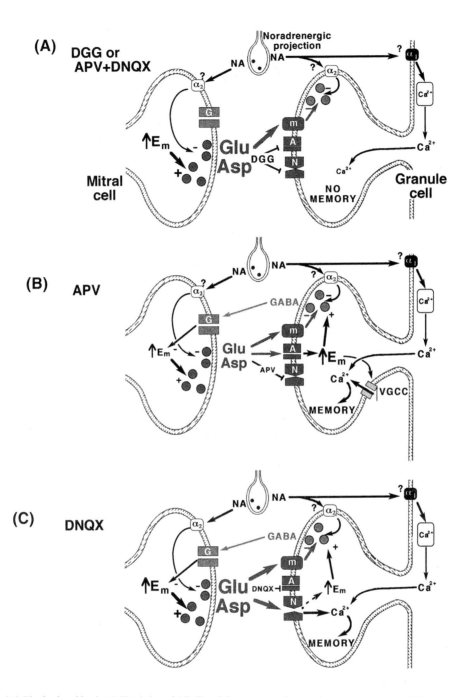

Figure 6.5. (**A**) Blockade of both AMPA (A) and NMDA (N) receptors during the sensitive period following mating prevents memory formation. This is despite the substantial disinhibition of mitral cells. (**B**) If only the NMDA receptors are blocked with APV, the mitral cells are again disinhibited. However, memory formation can still occur, probably due to the activation of voltage-dependent Ca^{2+} channels resulting from the excessive depolarization of granule cell spines mediated by AMPA receptors. (**C**) Disinhibition of mitral cells also occurs when the AMPA receptors are blocked with DNQX. In this case, memory formation probably proceeds via the activation of NMDA receptors.

lesions to the noradrenergic bulbar innervation result in a failure of memory formation, and the mated female loses her pregnancy when exposed to the familiar male (Rosser and Keverne, 1985). In the MOB, NA has been shown to decrease the release of both glutamate from mitral cells and γ-aminobutyric acid (GABA) from granule cells by a presynaptic α_2 mechanism, resulting in a disinhibition of the mitral cells (Trombley and Shepherd, 1992). A similar mechanism may be involved in learning the pheromonal signal by the AOB, as this can be prevented by local infusions of the α-noradrenergic antagonist phentolamine during the sensitive period for memory formation (Kaba and Keverne, 1988). Accordingly, NA is thought to disinhibit those mitral cells that are active as a result of pheromonal input, greatly increasing the excitation of their associated granule cells, leading to memory formation (Kaba and Nakanishi, 1995). Such a sustained excitation of mitral cells can be mimicked without mating, by local infusions of the $GABA_A$ receptor antagonist bicuculline, which blocks the feedback inhibition from granule cells. However, such infusions disinhibit mitral cells throughout the AOB regardless of their pheromonal input, leading to the formation of a non-specific memory so that no male pheromones are able to block pregnancy, even though mating has not occurred (Kaba *et al.*, 1989).

Inhibition of ionotropic glutamate receptors reduces the excitation of the inhibitory interneurons causing disinhibition of mitral cells in the AOB. However, this has different consequences for memory formation (Figure 6.5). If both NMDA and α-amino-3-hydroxy-5-methyl-4-isoxazole proprionic acid (AMPA)/kainate receptors are blocked during the sensitive period, by local infusions of a non-selective antagonist such as γ-D-glutamylglycine (DGG), memory formation is prevented, despite causing disinhibition of the mitral cells (Brennan and Keverne, 1989). In contrast, selective antagonism of either *N*-methyl-D-aspartate (NMDA) or AMPA/kainate receptors alone, using 2-amino-5-phosphonovaleric acid (APV) or 6,7-dinitroquinoxaline-2,3-dione (DNQX), respectively, fails to prevent memory formation (Brennan, 1994). This finding can be explained by the tightness of the coupling of excitation and inhibition at the reciprocal synapses. Any disruption of the excitation of granule cells causes a disinhibition of the mitral cells and intense stimulation of granule cells via the non-blocked ionotropic receptor subtype. This might raise Ca^{2+} levels in the granule cell spines and trigger memory formation in an unphysiological manner. Indeed, local infusions of

DNQX into the AOB actually form a non-specific memory, without mating having occurred, in a similar manner to bicuculline infusions (Brennan, 1994). This drug-induced memory formation does not occur with infusions of APV, suggesting that transmission via the NMDA receptor pathway is more effective in inducing memory formation than the AMPA/kainate pathway. Nevertheless, the dissociation of the different effects of bicuculline, DGG, APV and DNQX on memory formation from their common effect of disinhibiting mitral cells provides further support for the locus of induction of the memory formation being at the granule cell spines in the AOB.

In addition to ionotropic glutamate receptors, metabotropic receptors are also found on the granule cell spines and are involved in memory formation (Hayashi *et al.*, 1993; Kaba *et al.*, 1994). Infusion of the specific $mGluR_2$ agonist DCG IV in the presence of male pheromones results in memory formation specifically to those pheromones (Figure 6.6). Whereas the GABA antagonist bicuculline causes a widespread disinhibition of all mitral cells, the metabotropic glutamate agonist DCG IV facilitates the action of only those mitral cells that respond to male odor. This is because the $mGluR_2$ receptor presynaptically inhibits the release of GABA from granule cells and therefore decreases the inhibitory gain of the reciprocal synapses of mitral cells receiving pheromonal input. In this respect, it acts in a similar manner to NA and may contribute to its memory-promoting effect in the natural situation.

Hypothesis for pheromonal learning in the AOB

Despite the relative simplicity of the neural interactions in the AOB, they are sufficient to account for the formation of a pheromonal memory that is able to distinguish individuals (Brennan *et al.*, 1990). The association of elevated NA levels in the AOB at mating with the activity of those mitral cells receiving pheromonal input is hypothesized to cause a long-lasting increase in gain of their reciprocal synapses with the inhibitory granule interneurons (Figure 6.4C). This increase in inhibitory control of mitral cells can account for the memory by selectively disrupting the mating male's pheromonal signal at the level of the AOB, preventing it from being transmitted centrally to induce pregnancy block. Pheromones of a strange male will activate a different but overlapping population of mitral cells. Of these, the subpopulation of mitral cells that had not been modified by learning

(A) Bicuculline

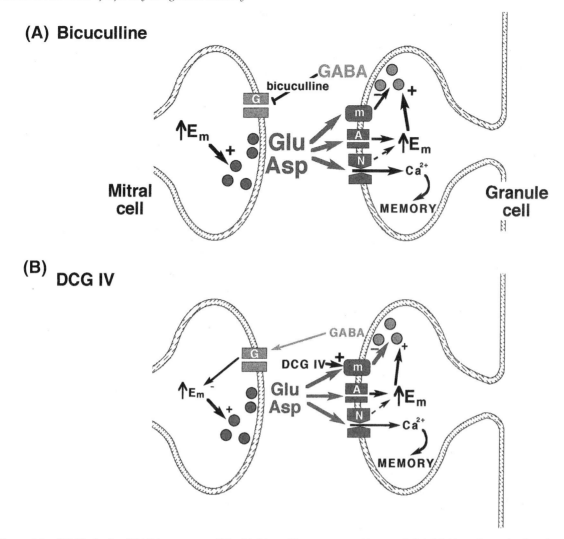

Figure 6.6. (**A**) Blockade of GABA$_A$ receptors (G) with bicuculline causes a widespread disinhibition of mitral cells. This over-stimulation of AMPA (A) and NMDA (N) receptors on the granule cell spines leads to a non-specific 'memory' formation without mating having occurred. (**B**) DCG IV is an agonist at mGluR$_2$ receptors (m) and disinhibits mitral cells by decreasing the inhibitory gain of the reciprocal synapse. However, this disinhibiton is specific to those mitral cells receiving pheromonal input, and thus a specific memory is formed without mating having occurred.

would transmit the pheromonal signal centrally and activate the neuroendocrine mechanism of pregnancy block.

Given the negative feedback occurring at the reciprocal synapses, this is unlikely to involve a complete inhibition of activity of those mitral cells responding to the learned pheromones. Instead, mathematical modeling of the system has emphasized that the frequency of mitral cell bursting would be expected to change following learning (Taylor and Keverne, 1991). Since neuroendocrine neurons fre-

quency are coded, then a change in burst firing frequency of mitral cells could interfere with the efficacy of the pheromonal signal in producing the neuroendocrine response leading to pregnancy block. According to this theory, it is not merely the pattern of active mitral cells that is being recognized at the AOB, but whether a signal is passed on to the central areas in a form to which they can respond.

It is established that the locus for induction of the changes underlying pheromonal learning is the granule cell spines of the reciprocal synapses.

Moreover, memory formation is associated with an increased length of the postsynaptic densities on granule cells that receive glutamatergic input from mitral cells (Matsuoka *et al.*, 1997), which will result in increased feedback inhibition to the mitral cells. Further evidence in support of the hypothesis that pheromonal learning involves an increased inhibitory gain of the reciprocal synapses comes from neurochemical investigations of the AOB using *in vivo* microdialysis (Brennan *et al.*, 1995). Two days following mating, a glutamate challenge to the AOB results in significantly more GABA release in mated than non-mated females. Moreover, the more natural situation of exposure to bedding from the mating male results in a significant decrease in the ratio of excitatory to inhibitory neurotransmitters in females that had mated, compared with females that had received the same amount of exposure to the bedding without mating.

Memory formation requires calmodulin-dependent processes in the AOB (Nakazawa *et al.*, 1995). Therefore, in common with other examples of synaptic plasticity, the level of Ca^{2+} within the spine is likely to be the important trigger for the long-term enhancement of the excitatory neurotransmission from the mitral to the granule cells. Ionotropic glutamatergic transmission will elevate Ca^{2+} in the granule cells either directly via NMDA receptors or indirectly via voltage-gated Ca^{2+} channels. However, the role of NA in this process is uncertain, and most theories are based on the actions of NA on cultured MOB neurons (Trombley, 1994). Kaba and Nakanishi (1995) have proposed that NA acts by disinhibiting mitral cells that are receiving pheromonal input. In conjunction with the $mGluR_2$-mediated disinhibition, this will increase the activation of NMDA and AMPA/kainate receptors sufficiently to raise Ca^{2+} levels and trigger long-term enhancement. However, there is also the possibility that NA could elevate Ca^{2+} levels directly in granule cells, via a pathway involving stimulation of α_1 noradrenergic receptors and the inositol trisphosphate (IP_3)-mediated release of Ca^{2+} from intracellular stores (Tani *et al.*, 1992).

Surprisingly, there is an indication from the microdialysis experiments that exposure to male bedding without mating has the long-term effect of increasing the levels of glutamate and aspartate released in the AOB, in response to subsequent exposure to that bedding (Brennan *et al.*, 1995). This appears to be an opposite effect to the neurochemical changes following memory formation, and can be explained by a decrease in the inhibitory gain of the reciprocal synapses, which would be expected to facilitate the transmission of the pheromonal signal. This is consistent with the priming effect of prior exposure to male pheromones on their ability to accelerate puberty in prepubertal female mice (Carreta *et al.*, 1995). At hippocampal synapses, low-frequency stimulation causes a small rise in Ca^{2+} below the threshold required to induce long-term potentiation, but above that required for long-term depression (Cummings *et al.*, 1996). A similar mechanism could explain the decreased inhibitory gain of the reciprocal synapses that appears to occur in the AOB following exposure to male pheromones without mating. In this case, pheromonal stimulation of mitral cells in the absence of NA might result in a smaller rise of Ca^{2+} in granule cell spines, leading to a long-lasting decrease in inhibitory gain of the reciprocal synapse.

OLFACTORY LEARNING IN THE MAIN OLFACTORY BULB

Lamb recognition in sheep

A similar process of olfactory learning occurs in the very different behavioral context of a ewe's recognition of her newborn lamb (Kendrick, 1994). Sheep are gregarious animals, and being seasonal breeders there are large numbers of newborns present at the same time. After parturition, the ewe rapidly forms the ability to recognize her own lamb and will reject suckling attempts from alien lambs (Poindron and Lévy, 1990). This rejection of alien lambs is important to restrict maternal investment to the ewe's own offspring and is mediated primarily by olfactory cues from their wool and skin. If the olfactory bulbs are removed, or the olfactory epithelium lesioned with $ZnSO_4$, a ewe will accept any lamb. In contrast, maternal behavior is not disrupted by section of the vomeronasal nerve, indicating that the olfactory cues are mediated solely via the main olfactory system (Lévy *et al.*, 1995b).

The sensitive period for learning the newborn lamb's odors lasts for around 2–4 h after parturition, during which the ewe will accept any lamb. After this time, ewes become highly selective, recognizing and accepting only their own lamb (Lévy *et al.*, 1991). Both the sensitive period for odor learning and the maternal behavior are dependent on the hormonal environment, but are triggered by the mechanical stimulation of the vagina and cervix occurring during parturition (Keverne *et al.*, 1983). Thus, a ewe can be induced to accept an alien lamb following manual vagino-cervical stimulation well outside the normal sensitive period (Kendrick and Keverne, 1991). Like the phero-monal learning in mice following mating, this vagino-cervical stimulation at parturition results in NA release in the olfactory bulb, which is essential for the selective recognition to occur (Lévy *et al.*, 1993). The first maternal experience has long-term consequences, as the sensitive period is much shorter for subsequent births, with the rapid development of selective recog-nition for the ewe's own offspring (Keverne *et al.*, 1993).

The development of selective lamb recognition is associated with substantial changes in the responses of neurons in the MOB (Kendrick *et al.*, 1992). Before parturition, most mitral cells recorded from a defined area of the MOB responded preferentially to the odors of food and none responded preferentially to lamb odors. Following parturition, a dramatic shift in the response preferences of mitral cells from the same region of the MOB had occurred (Figure 6.7). Now the majority of cells that showed a preferential response, did so to lamb odors, with some showing a preferen-tial response to the odors of the ewe's own lamb, and a much smaller proportion responded preferentially to food odors. These electrophysiological changes are accompanied by neurochemical changes that have been studied using *in vivo* microdialysis (Kendrick *et al.*, 1992). Prior to birth, lamb odors produced no detectable change in the release of any bulbar neuro-transmitters. After parturition, when ewes had estab-lished a selective bond with their lamb, the odor of this lamb, but not that of a strange lamb, induced a significant increase in the release of both the excita-tory amino acid glutamate, and the inhibitory trans-mitter GABA (Figue 6.7). Although both glutamate and GABA release increased in the MOB following parturition, the ratio of glutamate to GABA was significantly lower in response to the odor of the ewe's own lamb compared with that of an alien lamb. Basal release of GABA and glutamate were also significantly higher in the period after birth and, again, GABA release was significantly greater than that of glutamate.

As glutamate and GABA are the main transmitters released by mitral and granule cells, respectively, at their reciprocal synapses, the increased levels of both transmitters probably reflect an overall increase in mitral cell activity. However, in addition to this, the decreased ratio of glutamate to GABA suggests that glutamate has become more potent at eliciting GABA release, i.e. the inhibitory gain of a population of the reciprocal synapses has increased. This would change the firing frequency of those neurons that are coding for the lamb odor, and thereby alter the patterning of oscillations in the bulbar assembly with respect to these odors. This proposed mechanism has been sub-stantiated by the electrophysiological recordings during lamb recognition when more units respond to lamb odors, and some units do indeed differentiate between own and alien lambs with increased firing frequency (Kendrick *et al.*, 1992).

Olfactory learning in rodents

Olfactory learning has also been studied extensively in neonatal rats, during the postnatal period of rapid development of the olfactory system (Wilson and Sullivan, 1994). In these young animals, there appears to be a developmentally determined sensitive period, during which learning of nest odors is enhanced, perhaps analogously to visual imprinting in other species (Bolhuis, 1991). During the sensitive period, tactile stimulation mimicking maternal grooming is able to act as an unconditioned stimulus and lead to approach behavior to the conditioned odor. In com-mon with the examples of pheromonal learning in mice, and lamb recognition in sheep, NA levels are increased in the MOB of neonatal rats following tactile stimulation, and noradrenergic transmission in the MOB is necessary for odor conditioning to occur (Sullivan *et al.*, 1989). Olfactory learning in this dif-ferent species and developmental stage is also asso-ciated with substantial changes in the morphology and electrophysiology of the MOB. Following condi-tioning, Wilson *et al.* (1987) have found an increased suppression of mitral cell responses, to the condi-tioned odor compared with a novel odor, in the region of the MOB that responds to the odor. Again, these results suggest that inhibitory control of mitral cells is increased in the olfactory bulb following learning.

The fact that similar neural changes occur in the olfactory bulb across different species and different behavioral contexts suggests that these changes might be a general feature of olfactory learning. However, all of the examples that have been discussed are in some way specialized. For instance, olfactory condi-tioning in neonatal rats only occurs during a develop-mentally determined sensitive period, which may not be typical of learning in the adult animal. Similarly,

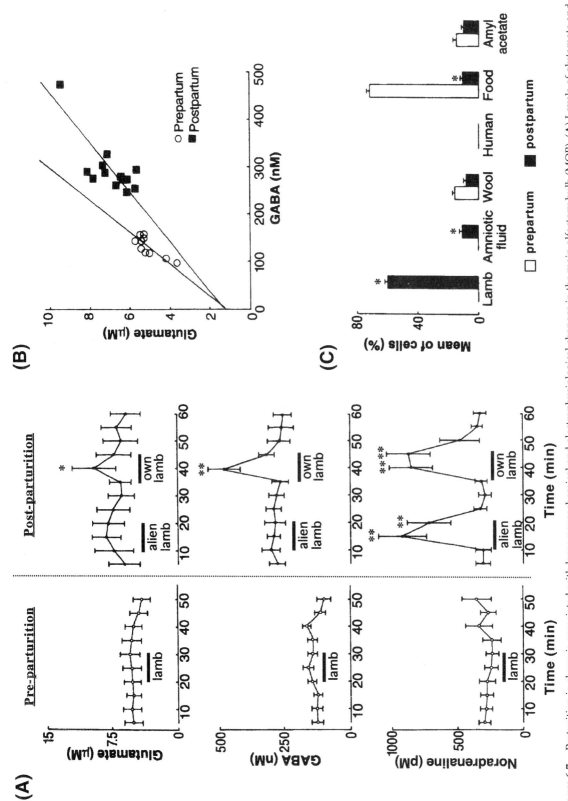

Figure 6.7. Parturition in sheep is associated with large neurochemical and electrophysiological changes in the main olfactory bulb (MOB). (A) Levels of glutamate and GABA recovered from the MOB by microdialysis are increased after parturition, specifically in response to odors from the ewe's own lamb. The noradrenaline response to lamb odors is also increased after parturition, although it does not distinguish between own and alien lambs. (B) The ratio of glutamate to GABA release in the MOB is decreased in response to the odor of the ewe's own lamb following parturition. This implies that the inhibitory control of mitral cells increased following learning. (C) The percentage of mitral cells that changed their single unit activity in response to lamb odors is increased following parturition, whereas the percentage of cells responding to food odors is decreased.

the examples of olfactory learning described in mice and sheep occur following a 'life event', requiring a major change in olfactory processing to accommodate new behavioral or neuroendocrine priorities. However, similar neurochemical changes have also been found in a simple olfactory conditioning procedure in adult mice, which is likely to be representative of less specialized odor learning. In an *in vivo* microdialysis study, Brennan *et al.* (1998) found that exposure to the conditioned odor resulted in significant increases in the levels of glutamate and GABA, indicating that the general level of activity of mitral cells in the MOB had increased. However, there was a decrease in the ratio of the excitatory to inhibitory neurotransmitters in the MOB in response to the conditioned but not the non-conditioned odor, similar to that occurring during lamb recognition. Thus, changes in the inhibitory control of mitral cells do appear to be a general feature of the neural changes in the olfactory bulb associated with odor learning. An understanding of the importance of these changes requires a fuller consideration of network interactions and their role in processing olfactory information at the bulbar level.

SPATIAL ASPECTS OF INHIBITORY INTERACTIONS

The morphology of mitral cells in the vertebrate MOB, with their extensive secondary dendritic tree in a plane tangential to the mitral cell layer, is highly suited for mediating lateral interactions with neighboring mitral cells over large areas of the bulb. These secondary dendrites ramify extensively in the external plexiform layer where they make predominantly reciprocal dendrodendritic synapses at spines on granule cell dendrites (Mori *et al.*, 1983). The activation of $mGluR_2$ receptors on the granule cell side of reciprocal synapses inhibits GABA release at those synaptic spines receiving mitral cell input (Bischofberger and Schild, 1996). This reduces localized self-inhibition mediated by the reciprocal synapses without diminishing lateral inhibition onto neighboring mitral cells that are less active. Evidence for such lateral inhibition playing an important role in olfactory processing comes from electrophysiological studies in the rabbit MOB. Mori and co-workers (Yokoi *et al.*, 1995) have found mitral cells in the dorsomedial part of the bulb that are excited by a small range of monomolecular odorants with similar chemical structures but inhibited by molecules with a

slightly different structure. For example, mitral cells in this region of the MOB may be excited during exposure to aliphatic aldehydes with chain lengths of six, seven and eight carbon atoms, but inhibited by chain lengths of five and nine.

It is therefore possible that the increased inhibitory control of mitral cells following learning may reflect changes in lateral inhibitory interactions that define the population of mitral cells responding to that odor. There is some evidence for this from electroencephalogram (EEG) recordings from the surface of the rabbit MOB. By recording the odor response from an array of 64 electrodes on the lateral side of the olfactory bulb, Freeman and co-workers have been able to show that the waveform of the response is the same across the array of electrodes but varies in amplitude. This allows the 'global' response of the MOB to an odor to be plotted as an iso-amplitude contour map across the bulbar surface. During learning, the map changes, but once an odor has become associated specifically with a behavioral response the pattern is invariant for succeeding odor presentations (Freeman and Schneider, 1982). If the reward contingencies are changed, however, the contour map also changes and, furthermore, this subtly modifies the patterns that have been established to other, previously learned odors. This demonstrates that the response of the olfactory bulb is not determined solely by glomerular input but is dependent on the lateral interactions across mitral cells. Moreover, these lateral connections are modified by odor learning, leading to the generation of a new odor response pattern from the bulb that is specific for the learned odor.

TEMPORAL ASPECTS OF INHIBITORY INTERACTIONS

The tight coupling of feedback inhibition at the reciprocal synapses can also have self-inhibitory effects that will change the temporal pattern of mitral cell activity. The importance of inhibitory interactions in temporal processing is emphasized by the presence of oscillating neural activity in the early stages of the olfactory system across animal phyla, from mollusks to vertebrates. It is also reflected in common features of the neural circuits used for the processing of odor information (Hildebrand and Shepherd, 1997), notably the presence of olfactory glomeruli and the interaction of projection neurons with local inhibitory interneurons. Indeed, reciprocal synapses are present in the olfactory structures of mammals, amphibians, reptiles, fish, insects and mollusks. This is an extremely tightly coupled version of the inhibitory feedback that occurs in other parts of the nervous system via separate synapses between excitatory and inhibitory interneurons. In many areas of the brain, the large numbers of inhibitory interneurons are thought to act as a 'clock' signal, for example synchronizing activity among neurons across large areas of cerebral cortex (Buzsáki and Chrobak, 1995). This synchronization can be revealed by cross-correlation studies of neural activity, but it is also often evident as oscillations of local field potentials resulting from the synchronized activity of neurons across large areas. Such oscillations of local field potential are a common feature of olfactory systems and have been found across the procerebral lobe of mollusks (Delaney *et al.*, 1994), the mushroom bodies of insects (Laurent and Davidowitz, 1994) and at the surface of the olfactory bulb in rabbits and rodents (Freeman and Schneider, 1982).

A distinctive feature of the odor response in mollusks is the collapse in the phase gradient that normally exists along the procerebral lobe, synchronizing the oscillations across the proximal–distal extent of the lobe (Delaney *et al.*, 1994). Moreover, the frequency of this oscillation can be increased by various neuromodulators such as dopamine as well as the intercellular messenger nitric oxide, suggesting that the oscillatory properties might be an important feature of olfactory processing. The frequency also varies in response to exposure to learned odors that have been associated with positive or negative reinforcement (Gervais *et al.*, 1996), although it is not known whether information about an odor is conveyed by the frequency of the oscillation *per se*.

The importance of oscillatory activity in odor representation is much better understood in insects. Giles Laurent's group has investigated the origin of oscillations of the local field potential (LFP) recorded from the calyx of the mushroom body of locusts in response to odor stimulation (Laurent, 1996). These LFP oscillations are not due to the response properties of the intrinsic neurons, but rather to the synchronized activity in large numbers of antennal lobe projection neurons (PNs) providing input to the mushroom body (Figure 6.8). This has been demonstrated by recording intracellular responses of antennal lobe PNs whilst simultaneously recording the local field potential from the mushroom body (Laurent and Davidowitz, 1994). Projection neurons

typically respond with different spike patterns to a range of odorants. These spike trains frequently have a complex temporal structure involving periods of excitation and inhibition during the odor presentation. Even when a PN is inhibited during the odor response, the continuing LFP oscillation in the mushroom body shows that other PNs are still responding to the odor. Furthermore, a PN's firing may be synchronized with the LFP (and, therefore, other PNs) during only part of the overall odor response. This leads to the conclusion that the population of PNs that have synchronous firing form an ensemble, but the ensemble that represents an odor is not static but dynamic, with individual PNs continually dropping out and being added to it during the odor response. Obviously, the synchronicity of PN firing is vital in this theory for defining the neuronal ensemble. This is supported by the high degree of sensitivity of the Kenyon cells in the mushroom body to the synchronicity of their input from the antennal lobe PNs.

An essential question is whether the synchronicity of firing of the antennal lobe PNs is an epiphenomenon, or whether it plays a vital role in olfactory information processing. The synchronous firing of PNs is governed by their interaction with GABAergic inhibitory interneurons in the antennal lobe (Laurent and Davidowitz, 1994). Fortunately, it has been found that picrotoxin application to the antennal lobe is able to destroy the synchronization of PNs (and, therefore, abolish LFP oscillations in the mushroom bodies) without affecting their individual firing patterns or their response specificity (MacLeod and Laurent, 1996). Thus the significance of the synchronization for olfactory processing has been tested.

Although the information contained in the spike train of individual PNs is unaffected by picrotoxin, desynchronization of the PNs has significant effects on the odor information represented by cells in the β lobes of the mushroom bodies (MacLeod *et al.*, 1998). These β-lobe neurons receive input from the Kenyon cells, which themselves receive input from antennal lobe PNs in the calyx of the mushroom bodies (Figure 6.8). Under normal conditions, β-lobe neurons have a specific response to odorants that differentiates even those that are closely related, such as a series of aliphatic alcohols. Following picrotoxin application to the antennal lobe, the distinctiveness of the responses of β-lobe neurons to similar odorants is lost. Moreover, β-lobe neurons now respond to odors that normally would not elicit a response. Thus although the spike trains of individual PNs are not significantly

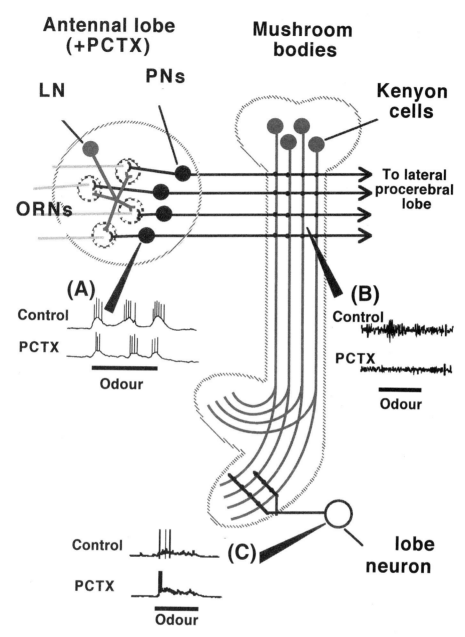

Figure 6.8. A highly simplified representation of the relationship between the antennal lobe and mushroom body in insects. Olfactory receptor neurons (ORNs) from the antennae terminate on projection neurons (PNs) in the antennal lobe. In turn, the PNs synapse on Kenyon cells in the mushroom bodies, which are highly sensitive to the synchronicity of PN activity. Local GABAergic interneurons (LNs) in the antennal lobe normally synchronize the activity of PNs during the odor response, and this synchronization can be prevented experimentally by local administration of picrotoxin (PCTX) to the antennal lobes. (**A**) The temporal structure of an individual PN's response to an odor is relatively unaffected by desynchronization. (**B**) The synchronization of PNs is normally evident in the oscillations of the local field potential recorded from the calyx of the mushroom bodies. These oscillations are abolished by the application of PCTX to the antennal lobe, demonstrating that the responses of individual PNs have been desynchronized. (**C**) Desynchronization of the antennal lobe PNs reduces the specificity of the response to an odor recorded from β-lobe neurons, which receive input from the Kenyon cells.

affected by picrotoxin, the desynchronization of their activity impairs the response specificity of more central neurons in the β-lobes. The behavioral significance of such a desynchronization has been investigated using odor conditioning of proboscis extension in the honeybee. Administration of picrotoxin to the antennal lobe during odor conditioning impairs the bees' subsequent ability to discriminate between similar, but not dissimilar odorants (Stopfer *et al.*, 1997). Thus the synchronization of PN activity by the GABAergic neurons in the antennal lobe appears to provide an extra dimension of neural space in which similar odorants can be represented and therefore discriminated more readily.

Oscillations are also found in the vertebrate olfactory system in the EEG recorded from the surface of the olfactory bulb (Freeman and Skarda, 1985; Freeman, 1991). There is a large-amplitude, low-frequency oscillation that follows the respiratory cycle but, on top of this, toward the end of inspiration, a high-frequency burst in the gamma range (30–80 Hz) occurs in response to an odor. This is due predominantly to the synchronous activity of granule cell interneurons, which are by far the most numerous neurons in the MOB. It is unlikely that the oscillatory waveform is conveying odor-specific information as it differs among each inspiratory burst for the same odor. The waveform of each oscillatory burst is the same across the extent of the MOB, but differs in amplitude, as mentioned previously. This suggests that the waveform is produced by the highly synchronized activity of granule cell interneurons, which would tend to synchronize mitral cell activity across large extents of the MOB. Thus changes in the gain of the reciprocal synapses between mitral and granule cells, following odor learning, would change the synchronization of mitral cell responses, in addition to affecting their lateral interactions. A new spatiotemporal response may thereby be generated that would specify the learned odor.

The role of the olfactory bulb is probably best appreciated by considering the example of lamb odor recognition in sheep. The complex odor of a lamb consists of a large number of components, and most of these components will be common to different lambs. For certain odors, such as food odors, generalization of the behavioral response to similar odors is appropriate as they have the same meaning to the animal. However, generalization of response is very undesirable for a ewe faced with the attentions of her own and alien lambs. Not only must the ewe's olfactory

system be able to distinguish own from alien, but they have to be linked to very different behavioral outputs. The role of the olfactory bulb is not merely to integrate the different components of a complex odor into a single representation. In addition, the olfactory bulb must change that representation during odor learning, distinguishing it from the representations of similar odors that have a different meaning for the animal and that have to be linked reliably to different behavioral outcomes by central brain areas. The olfactory bulb may be thought of as a self-organizing system that generates a spatiotemporal pattern of activity that defines meaningful odors, differentiated from those patterns of activity that characterize similar odors that are linked up to different behavioral outputs.

LONG- AND SHORT-TERM MEMORY

In addition to long-term olfactory memories, synaptic events in the olfactory bulb can also sustain short-term odor memories. While the former invariably depend on noradrenergic mechanisms, the latter are influenced by cholinergic mechanisms. Using a delayed matching-to-sample task based on olfactory cues (Ravel *et al.*, 1992), it was found that localized infusions of the muscarinic antagonist, scopolamine, impaired short-term olfactory memory. Using a 4 s delay between target odor and choice test, performance of treated rats remained unchanged, but with a 30 s delay, rats performed at random (Ravel *et al.*, 1994). It was concluded that the blocking of acetylcholine action in the olfactory bulb, contingent on odor learning, blocked odor memory storage. This is a very interesting finding since cholinergic neurons are important for the generation of theta rhythm in the hippocampus and, during exploratory sniffing both the olfactory bulb and hippocampus are dominated by theta activity (Macrides *et al.*, 1982). Furthermore, the theta rhythms in the olfactory bulb and hippocampus are often phase-locked for several seconds. Therefore, blockade of cholinergic activity in the olfactory bulb may impair short-term memory by disturbing a subset of a larger neural assembly involving not only the olfactory bulb but also the hippocampus and probably piriform cortex, especially if synchronization of oscillatory activity across neural populations is integral to learning.

The olfactory bulb is also involved in consolidation processes associated with long-term odor memory.

One of the problems associated with studies involving odor learning is control over delivery of the sensory cue. To some extent this problem can be overcome by generating odor hallucinations by direct electrical stimulation of the olfactory bulb. Rats are able to discriminate spatially distinct 'odor messages' from an array of electrodes implanted in the olfactory bulb. By infusing the local anesthetic xylocaine into the region of the stimulating electrode for 1 h following training, acquisition of the task was obtained, but retention over a 5-day period was severely impaired (Mouly *et al.*, 1993). It was concluded that for a critical period of about 1 h, changes are occurring in the olfactory bulb that are important for consolidation of long-term retention of learned olfactory cues.

Even longer term changes in the olfactory bulb have been observed which facilitate olfactory learning. A ewe's ability to recognize her lamb depends upon synaptic changes in the olfactory bulb, which are established at the first birth but facilitate the recognition process on subsequent births (Keverne *et al.*, 1993). The release of intrinsic neurotransmitters (dopamine, GABA and glutamate), as well as modulatory neurotransmitters (acetylcholine and NA) and peptides (oxytocin and vasopressin) in the olfactory bulb, has been found to differ depending on whether or not the ewe has had maternal experience (Lévy *et al.*, 1993, 1995a). The changes in underlying neural circuitry which determine these differences were shown to be established within 6 h of a ewe's first birth experience, and are probably involved in shortening the time taken to develop a selective response at subsequent births.

The first birth experience initially involves changes at the glomerular, input level, involving decreases in dopamine levels, and subsequently at deeper levels of the olfactory bulb over time. Since dopamine release in the glomerular layer presynaptically inhibits input from the olfactory nerves via a D_2 receptor, this initial decrease in dopamine would tend specifically to increase glomerular input for the own lamb odor. Normally inhibition is required to shut down noise from the diffuse odorant receptor projections, but relaxing this inhibition at the glomerular layer would enable an enormous gain in the sensitivity to component molecules that constitute the complex lamb odor. This modification of the system results in more mitral cells becoming responsive to lamb odors, as is indeed shown by electrophysiological recording, without compromising glomerular function in those modules not committed to lamb odor.

It is clear that the olfactory bulb not only acts as an interface between the olfactory receptors and the brain but also participates directly in the process of olfactory learning. The self-organizing capacity of the bulb, with its highly plastic reciprocal synapses between mitral and granule neurons, serves as a repository of past odorant associations. Even an incomplete odor message to the glomeruli recruits the rest of the bulbar network to generate the output that characterizes that odor. Of course, these changes only represent the first stage of processing underlying odor learning and recognition. How the rest of the brain links this to past odor associations and behavioral outputs is clearly important. There are extensive reciprocal interconnections between olfactory areas of the brain. There is also evidence for a spread of oscillatory activity back and forth among brain areas before, during and after odor responses, over a range of frequencies (Kay *et al.*, 1996). Thus it is likely that bulbar neurons participate in a dynamic association with neurons in the other brain areas, forming massive, but transient, functionally coherent assemblies.

REFERENCES

Bischofberger, J. and Schild, D. (1996) Glutamate and *N*-acetylaspartylglutamate block HVA calcium currents in frog olfactory bulb interneurons via an mGluR2/3-like receptor. *Journal of Neurophysiology*, 76, 2089–2092.

Bocskei, Z., Groom, C.R., Flower, D.R., Wright, C.E., Phillips, S.E.V., Cavaggioni, A. *et al.* (1992) Pheromone binding to two rodent urinary proteins revealed by X-ray crystallography. *Nature*, 360, 186–188.

Bolhuis, J.J. (1991) Mechanisms of avian imprinting: a review. *Biological Reviews*, 66, 303–345.

Brennan, P.A. (1994) The effects of local inhibition of *N*-methyl-D-aspartate and AMPA/kainate receptors in the accessory olfactory bulb on the formation of an olfactory memory in mice. *Neuroscience*, 60, 701–708.

Brennan, P.A. and Keverne, E.B. (1989) Impairment of olfactory memory by local infusions of non-selective excitatory amino acid receptor antagonists into the accessory olfactory bulb. *Neuroscience*, 33, 463–468.

Brennan, P.A. and Keverne, E.B. (1997) Neural mechanisms of mammalian olfactory learning. *Progress in Neurobiology*, 51, 457–481.

Brennan, P., Kaba, H. and Keverne, E.B. (1990) Olfactory recognition: a simple memory system. *Science*, 250, 1223–1226.

Brennan, P.A., Kendrick, K.M. and Keverne, E.B. (1995) Neurotransmitter release in the accessory olfactory bulb during and after the formation of an olfactory memory in mice. *Neuroscience*, 69, 1075–1086.

Brennan, P.A., Schellinck, H.M., de la Riva, C., Kendrick, K.M. and Keverne, E.B. (1998) Changes in neurotransmitter release in the main olfactory bulb following an olfactory conditioning procedure in mice. *Neuroscience*, 87, 583–590.

Bruce, H.M. (1961) Time relations in the pregnancy-block induced in mice by strange males. *Journal of Reproduction and Fertility*, 2, 138–142.

Buzsáki, G. and Chrobak, J.J. (1995) Temporal structure in spatially organized neuronal ensembles: a role for interneuronal networks. *Current Opinion in Neurobiology*, 5, 504–510.

Carreta, C.M., Carreta, A. and Cavaggioni, A. (1995) Pheromonally accelerated puberty is enhanced by previous experience of the same stimulus. *Physiology and Behavior*, 57, 901–903.

Clark, A.J., Chave, C.A., Ma, X. and Bishop, J.O. (1985) Analysis of mouse major urinary protein genes: variation between the exonic sequences of group 1 genes and a comparison with an active gene out with group 1 both suggest that gene conversion has occurred between MUP genes. *EMBO Journal*, 4, 3167–3171.

Clissold, P.M. and Bishop, J.O. (1982) Variation in MUP genes and MUP gene products within and between inbred lines. *Gene*, 18, 211–220.

Cummings, J.A., Mulkey, R.M., Nicoll, R.A. and Malenka, R.C. (1996) Ca^{2+} signalling requirements for long-term depression in the hippocampus. *Neuron*, 16, 825–833.

Delaney, K.R., Gelperin, A., Fee, M.S., Flores, J.A., Gervais, R., Tank, D.W. *et al.* (1994) Waves and stimulus-modulated dynamics in an oscillating olfactory network. *Proceedings of the National Academy of Sciences of the United States of America*, 91, 669–673.

Freeman, W.J. (1991) The physiology of perception. *Scientific American*, February, 34–41.

Freeman, W.J. and Schneider, W. (1982) Changes in spatial patterns of rabbit olfactory EEG with conditioning to odors. *Psychophysiology*, 19, 44–56.

Freeman, W.J. and Skarda, C.A. (1985) Spatial EEG patterns, non-linear dynamics and perception: the neo-Sherringtonian view. *Brain Research Reviews*, 10, 147–175.

Gervais, R., Holley, A. and Keverne, E.B. (1988) The importance of central noradrenergic influences on the olfactory bulb in the processing of learned olfactory cues. *Chemical Senses*, 13, 3–12.

Gervais, R., Kleinfeld, D., Delany, K.R. and Gelperin, A. (1996) Central and reflex neuronal responses elicited by odor in a terrestrial mollusk. *Journal of Neurophysiology*, 76, 1327–1339.

Hayashi, Y., Momiyama, A., Takahashi, T., Ohishi, H., Ogawa, M.R., Shigemoto, R. *et al.* (1993) Role of a metabotropic glutamate receptor in synaptic modulation in the accessory olfactory bulb. *Nature*, 366, 687–690.

Hebb, D.O. (1949) *Organization of Behavior*. John Wiley & Sons, New York.

Hildebrand, J.G. and Shepherd, G.M. (1997) Mechanisms of olfactory discrimination: converging evidence for common principles across phyla. *Annual Review of Neuroscience*, 20, 595–631.

Hopfield, J.J. (1984) Neurons with graded response have collective computational properties like those of 2-state neurons. *Proceedings of the National Academy of Sciences of the United States of America*, 81, 3088–3092.

Kaba, H. and Keverne, E.B. (1988) The effect of microinfusions of drugs into the accessory olfactory bulb on the olfactory block to pregnancy. *Neuroscience*, 25, 1007–1011.

Kaba, H. and Nakanishi, S. (1995) Synaptic mechanisms of olfactory recognition memory. *Reviews in the Neurosciences*, 6, 125–141.

Kaba, H., Rosser, A.E. and Keverne, E.B. (1988) Hormonal enhancement of neurogenesis and its relationship to the duration of olfactory memory. *Neuroscience*, 24, 93–98.

Kaba, H., Rosser, A. and Keverne, E.B. (1989) Neural basis of olfactory memory in the context of pregnancy block. *Neuroscience*, 32, 657–662.

Kaba, H., Hayashi, Y., Higuchi, T. and Nakanishi, S. (1994) Induction of an olfactory memory by the activation of a metabotropic glutamate receptor. *Science*, 265, 262–264.

Kay, L.M., Lancaster, L.R. and Freeman, W.J. (1996) Reafference and attractors in the olfactory system during odor recognition. *International Journal of Neural Systems*, 7, 489–495.

Kendrick, K.M. (1994) Neurobiological correlates of visual and olfactory recognition in sheep. *Behavioural Processes*, 33, 89–112.

Kendrick, K.M. and Keverne, E.B. (1991) Importance of vaginocervical stimulation for the formation of maternal bonding in primiparous and multiparous parturient ewes. *Physiology and Behavior*, 50, 595–600.

Kendrick, K.M., Levy, F. and Keverne, E.B. (1992) Changes in sensory processing of olfactory signals induced by birth in sheep. *Science*, 256, 833–836.

Keverne, E.B. (1983) The accessory olfactory system and its role in pheromonally mediated changes in prolactin. In: Breipohl, W. (ed.), *Olfaction and Endocrine Regulation*. IRL Press, Oxford, pp. 127–140.

Keverne, E.B. and de la Riva, C. (1982) Pheromones in mice: reciprocal interaction between the nose and brain. *Nature*, 296, 148–150.

Keverne, E.B., Lévy, F., Poindron, P. and Lindsay, D.R. (1983) Vaginal stimulation: an important determinant of maternal bonding in sheep. *Science*, 219, 81–83.

Keverne, E.B., Lévy, F., Guevara-Guzman, R. and Kendrick, K.M. (1993) Influence of birth and maternal experience on olfactory bulb neurotransmitter release. *Neuroscience*, 56, 557–565.

Laurent, G. (1996) Dynamical representation of odors by oscillating and evolving neural assemblies. *Trends in Neuroscience*, 19, 489–496.

Laurent, G. and Davidowitz, H. (1994) Encoding of olfactory information with oscillating neural assemblies. *Science*, 265, 1872–1875.

Lévy, F., Gervais, R., Kindermann, U., Litterio, M., Poindron, P. and Porter, R. (1991) Effects of early post-partum separation on maintenance of maternal responsiveness and selectivity in parturient ewes. *Applied Animal Behaviour Science*, 31, 101–110.

Lévy, F., Guevara, G.R., Hinton, M.R., Kendrick, K.M. and Keverne, E.B. (1993) Effects of parturition and maternal experience on noradrenaline and acetylcholine release in the olfactory bulb of sheep. *Behavioral Neuroscience*, 107, 662–668.

Lévy, F., Kendrick, K.M., Goode, J.A., Guevara-Guzman, R. and Keverne, E.B. (1995a) Oxytocin and vasopressin release in the olfactory bulb of parurient ewes: changes with maternal experience and effects of acetylcholine, γ-aminobutyric acid, glutamate and noradrenaline release. *Brain Research*, 669, 197–206.

Lévy, F., Locatelli, A., Piketty, V., Tillet, Y. and Poindron, P. (1995b) Involvement of the main but not the accessory olfactory system in maternal behaviour of primiparous and multiparous ewes. *Physiology and Behavior*, 57, 97–104.

Li, C.S., Kaba, H., Saito, H. and Seto, K. (1989) Excitatory influence of the accessory olfactory bulb on tuberoinfundibular arcuate neurons of female mice and its modulation by oestrogen. *Neuroscience*, 29, 201–208.

Li, C.S., Kaba, H., Saito, H. and Seto, K. (1990) Neural mechanisms underlying the action of primer pheromones in mice. *Neuroscience*, 36, 773–778.

Li, C.S., Kaba, H., Saito, H. and Seto, K. (1992) Cholecystokinin: critical role in mediating olfactory influences on reproduction. *Neuroscience*, 48, 707–713.

Li, C.S., Kaba, H. and Seto, K. (1994) Effective induction of pregnancy block by electrical stimulation of the mouse accessory olfactory bulb coincident with prolactin surges. *Neuroscience Letters*, 176, 5–8.

MacLeod, K. and Laurent, G. (1996) Distinct mechanisms for synchronization and temporal patterning of odor-encoding neural assemblies. *Science*, 274, 976–979.

MacLeod, K., Bäcker, A. and Laurent, G. (1998) Who reads temporal information contained across synchronized and oscillatory spike trains? *Nature*, 395, 693–698.

Macrides, F., Eichenbaum, H.B. and Forbes, W.B. (1982) Temporal relationships between sniffing and the limbic rhythm during odor discrimination and reversal learning. *Journal of Neuroscience*, 2, 1705–1717.

Marchlewska-Koj, A. (1981) Pregnancy block elicited by male urinary peptides in mice. *Journal of Reproduction and Fertility*, 61, 221–224.

Marchelwska-Koj, A. (1983) Pregnancy blocking by pheromones. In: Vandenbergh, J.G. (ed.), *Pheromones and Reproduction in Mammals*. Academic Press, New York, pp. 113–174.

Matsuoka, M., Kaba, H., Mori, Y. and Ichikawa, M. (1997) Synaptic plasticity in olfactory memory formation in female mice. *Neuroreport*, 8, 2501–2504.

Meredith, M. and O'Connell, R.J. (1979) Efferent control of stimulus access to the hamster vomeronasal organ. *Journal of Physiology*, 286, 301–316.

Mori, K. (1987) Membrane and synaptic properties of identified neurons in the olfactory bulb. *Progress in Neurobiology*, 29, 275–320.

Mori, K., Kishi, K. and Ojima, H. (1983) Distribution of dendrites of mitral, displaced mitral, tufted, and granule cells in the rabbit olfactory bulb. *Journal of Comparative Neurology*, 219, 339–335.

Mouly, A.M., Kindermann, U., Gervais, R. and Holley, A. (1993) Involvement of the olfactory bulb in consolidation processes associated with long-term memory in rats. *Behavioral Neuroscience*, 107, 451–475.

Mucignat-Caretta, C., Caretta, A. and Cavaggioni, A. (1995) Acceleration of puberty onset in female mice by male urinary proteins. *Journal of Physiology*, 486, 517–522.

Nakazawa, H., Kaba, H., Higuchi, T. and Inoue, S. (1995) The importance of calmodulin in the accessory olfactory bulb in the formation of an olfactory memory in mice. *Neuroscience*, 69, 585–589.

Novotny, M., Jemiolo, B. and Harvey, S. (1990) Chemistry of rodent pheromones: molecular insights into chemical signalling in mammals. In: Macdonald, D., Muller-Schwarze, W.D. and Natynczuk, S.E. (eds), *Chemical Signals in Vertebrates 5*. Oxford University Press, New York, pp. 1–22.

Poindron, P. and Lévy, F. (1990) Physiological, sensory, and experiental determinants of maternal behavior in sheep. In: Krasnegor, N.A. and Bridges, R.S. (eds), *Mammalian Parenting*. Oxford University Press, Oxford, pp. 133–156.

Ravel, N., Vigouroux, M., Elaagouby, A. and Gervais, R. (1992) Scopolamine impairs delayed matching in an olfactory task in rats. *Psychopharmacology*, 109, 439–443.

Ravel, N., Elaagouby, A. and Gervais, R. (1994) Scopolamine injection into the olfactory bulb impairs short-term olfactory memory in rats. *Behavioral Neuroscience*, 2, 317–324.

Reynolds, J. and Keverne, E.B. (1979) The accessory olfactory system and its role in the pheromonally mediated suppression of oestrus in grouped mice. *Journal of Reproduction and Fertility*, 57, 31–55.

Rosser, A. and Keverne, E.B. (1985) The importance of central noradrenergic neurones in the formulation of an olfactory memory in the prevention of pregnancy block. *Neuroscience*, 15, 1141–1147.

Rosser, A.E., Remfry, C.J. and Keverne, E.B. (1989) Restricted exposure of mice to primer pheromones coincident with prolactin surges blocks pregnancy by changing hypothalamic dopamine release. *Journal of Reproduction and Fertility*, 87, 553–559.

Ryan, K.D. and Schwartz, N.B. (1980) Changes in serum hormone levels associated with male-induced ovulation in group housed female mice. *Endocrinology*, 105, 959–966.

Shimbel, A. (1950) Contributions to the mathematical biophysics of the central nervous system with special reference to learning. *Bulletin of Mathematical Biophysics*, 12, 241–275.

Stopfer, M., Bhagavan, S., Smith, B.H. and Laurent, G. (1997) Impaired odour discrimination on desynchronization of odour-encoding neural assemblies. *Nature*, 390, 70–74.

Sullivan, R.M., Wilson, D.A. and Leon, M. (1989) Norepinephrine and learning-induced plasticity in infant rat olfactory system. *Journal of Neuroscience*, 9, 3998–4006.

Tani, A., Yoshihara, Y. and Mori, K. (1992) Increase in cytoplasmic free Ca^{2+} elicited by noradrenalin and seratonin in cultured local interneurons of the mouse olfactory bulb. *Neuroscience*, 49, 193–199.

Taylor, J.G. and Keverne, E.B. (1991) Accessory olfactory learning. *Biological Cybernetics*, 64, 301–306.

Trombley, P.Q. (1994) Noradrenergic modulation of synaptic transmission between olfactory bulb neurons in culture: implications to olfactory learning. *Brain Research Bulletin*, 35, 473–484.

Trombley, P.Q. and Shepherd, G.M. (1992) Noradrenergic inhibition of synaptic transmission between mitral and granule cells in mammalian olfactory bulb cultures. *Journal of Neuroscience*, 12, 3985–3991.

Wilson, D.A. and Sullivan, R.M. (1994) Neurobiology of associative learning in the neonate: early olfactory learning. *Behavioral and Neural Biology*, 61, 1–18.

Wilson, D.A., Sullivan, R.M. and Leon, M. (1987) Single-unit analysis of postnatal olfactory learning: modified olfactory bulb output response patterns to learned attractive odors. *Journal of Neuroscience*, 7, 3154–3162.

Yokoi, I., Mori, K. and Nakanishi, S. (1995) Refinement of odor molecules tuning by dendrodendritic synaptic inhibition in the olfactory bulb. *Proceedings of the National Academy of Sciences of the United States of America*, 92, 3371–3375.

7 THE NEURAL BASIS OF AVIAN SONG LEARNING AND PERCEPTION

David F. Clayton

INTRODUCTION

Songbirds have well-appreciated abilities to produce distinctive, often complex vocalizations. Songbird species (oscines of the order Passeriformes) number in the thousands, and comprise roughly half of all avian species. Each species produces a song with certain recognizable, species-specific characteristics. Yet individual birds of the same species may develop songs that differ significantly, and these differences may be used by conspecifics to discriminate among individuals, for example during mate selection and territorial defense (Catchpole, 1982; Kroodsma and Byers, 1991; Wiley *et al.*, 1991; Beecher *et al.*, 1996; Nowicki *et al.*, 1998). Although both males and females listen to and respond to songs, in many species the actual production of song is limited to males, who typically learn their individual song patterns by copying an older tutor (e.g. Thorpe, 1958; Konishi, 1965; Nottebohm, 1968; Immelmann, 1969; Marler and Peters, 1977; Marler and Waser, 1977; Marler, 1997).

Song learning has much appeal as a model of integrative neural function (for a comprehensive set of detailed reviews, see Brenowitz *et al.*, 1997). Song learning is a completely natural behavior that may be studied either in the field or in a laboratory setting (laboratory studies have tended to focus on the canary and the zebra finch, two species that breed readily in captivity). The information learned (sensory and motor representations of song patterns) is sufficiently complex to involve the higher centers of the telencephalon, yet song patterns can also quite easily be recorded, played back, broken down into pieces, quantified, rearranged and presented as controlled stimuli. The learning process is subject to a number of identifiable constraints, including the age of the bird, its early social experience, its gender and breeding status, and its history of exposure to other songs. Study of mechanisms underlying these constraints may provide insight into the processes that constrain learning and neural plasticity in other systems and organisms as well.

The purpose of this chapter is, first, to outline what has been learned about the basic neural circuit elements that underlie the ability of a young male songbird to copy the song of a tutor. Current evidence suggests that song learning may involve an integration of activity in three discrete subsystems, responsible respectively for vocal motor control, auditory representations and sensorimotor feedback or template matching. A second purpose of this chapter is to review insights that have come from the relatively recent application of methods for studying gene expression in this system. Singing and hearing song both induce dynamic changes in gene activity, in different parts of the song system. These observations suggest a novel role for the genome as an agent of functional integration in the nervous system, helping to direct or constrain the storage of new information to appropriate neural circuits and developmental or behavioral contexts.

SONG COPYING

A young male songbird typically develops his song in part by copying the song of one or more tutors. In many species, this process occurs only once during a restricted period in juvenile development. With sexual maturity, the song 'crystallizes' and is retained with little change throughout the rest of the bird's life (Price, 1979; Marler and Peters, 1987). Behavioral dissection of song copying in various species has led to the idea that the learning process actually involves two phases (see Figure 7.1): a 'sensitive period' during which an initial auditory memory of the model song pattern is acquired by listening to the tutor (typically the bird's father), and a 'sensorimotor' period during which the bird attempts to replicate the model song on its own through a process of trial-and-error (Marler, 1997). These two periods may be separated in time by months (as in the case of the swamp sparrow, Figure 7.1A) or they may overlap substantially (as in the zebra finch, Figure 7.1B).

How is the brain of the songbird organized to perceive, remember and reproduce a complex vocal performance? What allows—and constrains—the behavioral plasticity implicit in song learning ability? From a functional or neural-engineering perspective, at least three neural processing elements are needed

to explain the basic process of song copying. Although many details remain to be worked out, these functional elements have now been localized to discrete circuits in the songbird brain:

1. A system to control the musculature responsible for the bird's own song production, and for storing specific motor memories.
2. A system for analyzing complex auditory signals and storing representations of specific song auditory patterns (such as the sound of a tutor's song).

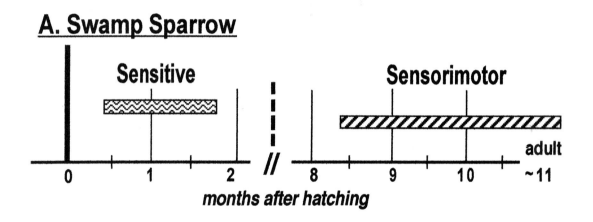

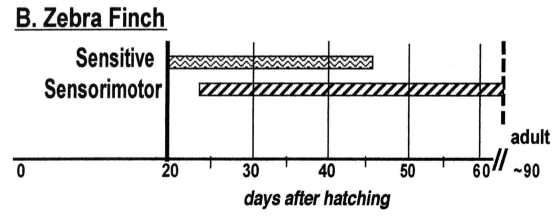

Figure 7.1.   Phases of song learning in two species. Juvenile song learning in considered to involve two processes: a sensitive phase (formation of an auditory memory of a tutor's song) and a sensorimotor phase (rehearsal of the bird's own vocal performance to match the remembered tutor song). (**A**) In the swamp sparrow, these two phases are discrete and well defined by a separation of several months (Marler and Peters, 1982). (**B**) In the zebra finch, song rehearsal can begin even before the final song model has been acquired (Immelmann, 1969).

3. A mechanism by which information in the second system influences the functional development or plasticity of the first, for example by selectively stabilizing only those motor patterns that give recognized auditory results.

SYSTEM 1: VOCAL MOTOR CONTROL

Wide appreciation of songbirds as a specific model for study of brain organization and neural mechanism began with a series of observations made in the mid-1970s in which song production by adult male canaries was the behavioral focus. Initially, brain lesions were defined that resulted in highly specific perturbations of singing behavior. Study of these lesions led to recognition of a set of large and discrete but interconnected nuclei within the telencephalon, each easily recognized within Nissl-stained brain sections (Nottebohm *et al.*, 1976). These nuclei were observed to be greatly reduced in size or even absent in females in species in which only the male sings (Nottebohm and Arnold, 1976), yet are of comparable size in males and females in duetting species (Brenowitz *et al.*, 1985; Brenowitz, 1997). Found only in oscine songbirds (Kroodsma and Konishi, 1991; Gahr *et al.*, 1993; Brenowitz, 1997), the 'song control nuclei' are believed to represent specializations that evolved in the context of more ancient and universal pathways for motor control, auditory processing and sensorimotor integration (Brenowitz, 1991).

The four major telencephalic nuclei are known best by acronyms:

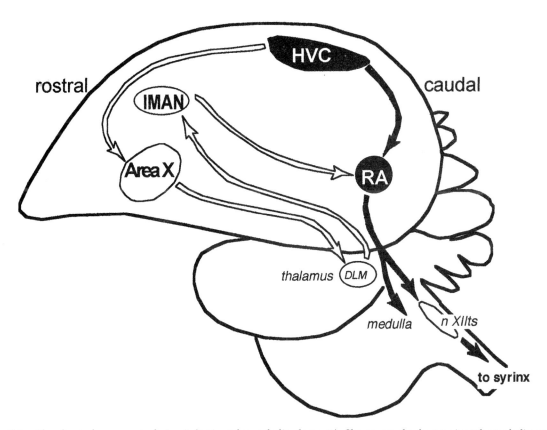

Figure 7.2. The classical song control circuit (major telencephalic elements). Shown are the four major telencephalic nuclei described in the text, and a thalamic relay (DLM, the medial portion of the dorsolateral nucleus). The nuclei are interconnected by two major pathways. A caudal pathway (filled arrows) descends from HVC to RA, and thence to the tracheosyringeal part of the hypoglossal motor nucleus in the brainstem (nXIIts); RA also projects to nuclei in the medulla that control respiratory neurons. A rostral pathway (open arrows) interconnects elements analogous to mammalian basal ganglia (Area X), thalamus (DLM) and cortex (lMAN). The two pathways intersect at the level of individual neurons in RA. Nuclei afferent to HVC and efferent to RA are summarized elsewhere (Brenowitz *et al.*, 1997; Wild, 1997). See text for full names of brain regions.

(i)   HVC (high vocal center; for discussion of nomen-
       clature, see Fortune and Margoliash, 1995);
(ii) RA (robust nucleus of the archistriatum);
(iii) lMAN (lateral portion of the magnocellular
       nucleus of the anterior neostriatum); and
(iv) Area X, which sits within the avian homolog of the
       mammalian basal ganglia (lobus parolfactorius).

Tract analysis has shown that these four major
nuclei are organized into two branching and merging
pathways in the forebrain (Figure 7.2). One pathway
extends from HVC to RA in the caudal telencephalon,
and by a variety of criteria it appears to be the principle circuit element responsible for the actual performance of song. Axons from RA innervate the motor
neurons in the brainstem that control the muscles of
the vocal organ, the syrinx (Nottebohm *et al.*, 1976;
Vicario, 1991; Fortune and Margoliash, 1992; Wild,
1997; Foster and Bottjer, 1998). Lesion of either HVC
or RA results in immediate disruption of vocal behavior in singing adults, with minimal effect on other
observable behaviors (Nottebohm *et al.*, 1976).

Electrophysiological studies using chronically implanted electrodes in awake zebra finches showed that
neurons in HVC and RA are active during singing
(McCasland, 1987; Vu *et al.*, 1994; Yu and Margoliash,
1996), and perform in a functional relationship that
reflects their anatomical hierarchy (Yu and Margoliash,
1996). Zebra finch songs are composed of a set of
several 'syllables,' each lasting 100–200 ms, separated
by brief pauses and typically repeated in a particular
sequence so that the song as a whole lasts 1–2 s. Each
syllable may in turn contain internal frequency transitions, to define one or more separate 'notes.' RA
neurons, which directly drive the motor neurons of the
brainstem, fire in short phasic bursts (<100 ms) that
are correlated most closely with the appearance of
individual notes in the song. HVC neurons, which
project onto RA neurons, fire tonically across the entire
song, but the firing probability is modulated subtly in
a way that is correlated broadly with the transitions
between syllables (but not individual notes). Hence
the structure of HVC activity is predictive of the
overall organization of the song (the sequence of syllables), whereas RA activity is predictive of the momen-
tary acoustic content (the identity of individual notes)
(Yu and Margoliash, 1996). Consistent with this, direct
electrical stimulation of RA during singing distorts
ongoing syllables, whereas HVC stimulation alters the
ensuing song pattern (Vu *et al.*, 1994).

The other two nuclei of the telencephalic control
system, lMAN and Area X, participate in a more
rostral pathway which is discussed further below
(System 3). Lesion of these nuclei has little or no effect
on singing behavior when applied in adult zebra
finches, but greatly disrupts the development of song
when applied in juveniles before song learning is
completed (Bottjer *et al.*, 1984; Sohrabji *et al.*, 1990;
Scharff and Nottebohm, 1991).

SYSTEM 2: SONG PERCEPTION AND DISCRIMINATION

Identification of systems directly involved in song
perception as opposed to production was hampered
by the lack of good behavioral assays for perception,
and by the obscurity of auditory pathways in the
avian brain beyond the primary auditory thalamo-
recipient area of the telencephalon, Field L2 (see
Figure 7.3). Early electrophysiological studies of
neural activity within HVC and RA (Katz and Gurney,
1981; McCasland and Konishi, 1981; McCasland, 1987)
led to an intense focus on the song control nuclei
themselves as possible sites for formation and storage
of auditory memories of song. In anesthetized birds,
many neurons in all four major song control nuclei
increase their firing rate in response to playbacks of
tape-recorded song. Moreover, a small percentage of
these neurons respond selectively to playbacks of the
bird's own song—their responses are reduced or abolished when the song is played in reverse or when
other conspecific songs are presented (Margoliash,
1983, 1986; Williams and Nottebohm, 1985; Doupe
and Konishi, 1991; Vicario and Yohay, 1993; Volman,
1993; Doupe and Solis, 1997).

Yet the functional significance of these auditory
responses in the major song control nuclei remains to
be clearly defined. Assays based on gene responses in
awake behaving birds (below) typically do not detect
any physiological activation of the song motor nuclei
during auditory stimulation (Mello and Clayton,
1994; Jin and Clayton, 1997a). Recent electrophysiological studies using chronically implanted electrodes
found that some of the established auditory responses
are evident only when the bird is either anesthetized
or asleep (Dave *et al.*, 1998; Schmidt and Konishi,
1998). Behavioral tests indicate that young zebra
finches are able to store specific tutor song memories
at an early age (Böhner, 1990; Slater and Jones, 1995),
yet song-selective auditory responses in the motor
nuclei only emerge later, with the gradual development of the bird's own singing (Volman, 1993; Doupe,

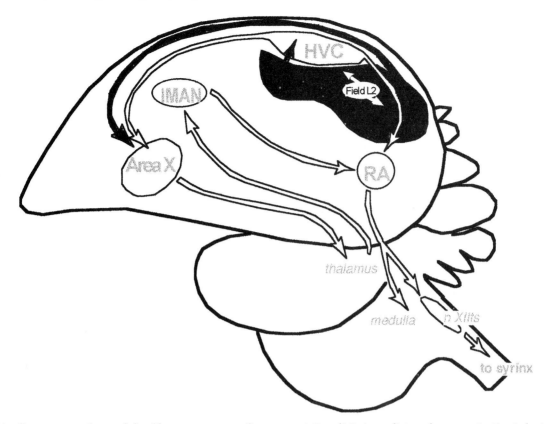

Figure 7.3. Song perceptual areas defined by gene responses. Song presentation elicits immediate early gene activation in brain regions concentrated especially in the caudal and medial portions of the neostriatum (NCM) and hyperstriatum ventrale (CMHV), shown schematically as the filled area superimposed onto the classical song circuit from Figure 7.2, and described in the text as System 2. These responsive areas are not bounded by clear cytoarchitectonic borders and thus have not been identified as specific nuclei. Gene responses to song playbacks have not been observed within the major song nuclei nor within Field L2. Field L2 is the site of auditory inputs from the thalamus and provides a rich innervation to the auditory gene-responsive region.. The gene-responsive region has complex internal interconnections, and includes both the shelf underlying HVC (which provides auditory input to HVC) and a region called paraHVC (which sends a projection to Area X) (Vates *et al.*, 1996; Foster and Bottjer, 1998). Two additional areas of gene response not shown are within the caudal paleostriatum, and immediately adjacent to RA (Mello and Clayton, 1994).

1997; Solis and Doupe, 1997). Adult male zebra finches with lesions of Area X or lMAN are still able to discriminate behaviorally between conspecific and heterospecific songs (although these lesions may have some specific effects on discriminative responses to playbacks of the bird's own song) (Scharff *et al.*, 1998). In addition, female zebra finches (which lack a functional projection from HVC to RA) still respond to and discriminate between conspecific and heterospecific songs, and do so even after selective lesions of HVC (Macdougall-Shackleton *et al.*, 1998). Clearly, systems apart from the vocal motor nuclei must also play major roles in song perception.

Insight into the nature of song perceptual systems came from an unexpected direction in the early 1990s,

when it was observed that song playbacks will induce robust genomic responses in discrete telencephalic regions distinct from the motor control nuclei (Mello *et al.*, 1992; Nastiuk *et al.*, 1994; reviewed in Clayton, 1997). In these experiments, the technique of *in situ* hybridization was used to monitor the local amounts of mRNA from a gene known by the acronym ZENK. Rapid and transient activation of ZENK and other so-called 'immediate early genes' (IEGs) has now been correlated widely with circumstances that elicit functional change in a particular brain circuit or system (for a synthetic review, see Clayton, 2000). Apart from the potential functional and theoretical significance of this genomic response, IEG activation is useful as a tool for mapping sites of significant neurophysiological activity in awake, behaving animals (cf. McCabe and Horn, 1994; Chaudhuri, 1997; Horn, 1998; O'Donovan *et al.*, 1999; see also Brennan and Keverne, Chapter 6; Smulders and DeVoogd, Chapter 8; Horn, Chapter 19).

Using ZENK mRNA levels as a guide, intense physiological responses to song were observed to occur mainly in the most caudal and medial portions of the telencephalon, including parts of the neostriatum (NCM) and the hyperstriatum ventrale (CMHV; Mello and Clayton, 1994). The brain regions that show genomic responses to song presentation are almost entirely distinct from the previously characterized song motor control centers (Figure 7.3), and they also exclude the site of primary auditory input to the telencephalon, Field L2. (Unlike the song control nuclei, these song-responsive areas are not defined by sharp cytoarchitectonic borders, presenting a challenge for nomenclature still to be met.) Further analyses confirmed that song induces not only genomic but also electrophysiological responses in these regions (Chew *et al.*, 1995, 1996; Stripling *et al.*, 1997), and showed that NCM and CMHV are interconnected intimately with Field L2 and with the motor pathways for song control (Vates *et al.*, 1996; Mello *et al.*, 1998b; see also Foster and Bottjer, 1998).

Interestingly, most cells in NCM and CMHV of zebra finches do not show intrinsic selectivity for specific songs, including the bird's own song (Stripling *et al.*, 1997), yet they undergo highly specific changes in both genomic and electrophysiological responses to individual songs based on recent experience (Chew *et al.*, 1995; Mello *et al.*, 1995; Stripling *et al.*, 1997). Single auditory neurons in NCM initially will respond to virtually any song presented to the bird (Stripling *et al.*, 1997). With repetition of a single song, gene responses to that song but not others are completely abolished (Mello *et al.*, 1995), and electrophysiological responses undergo a change that has been described as habituation (Chew *et al.*, 1995) or loss of modulation (Stripling *et al.*, 1997). These observations are indicative of a role for NCM/CMHV in the formation of auditory representations of current experience, but probably not as the long-term storage site for any single auditory memory. The auditory coding mechanisms at work are obscure, although some insight into this has come from study of canaries. Canary songs typically contain many single-frequency elements, unlike the complex harmonic stacks characteristic of zebra finch song. Presentation of pure tones activates gene expression in many neurons in canary NCM, but they are typically concentrated in bands or fields

within the structure, and mixtures of two tones elicit responses in additional fields not activated by either tone alone (Ribeiro *et al.*, 1998). This suggests that NCM may retain some parallels to the tonotopic organization of Field L2, but it may also be integrating across frequencies to represent more complex combinations of acoustic and/or temporal information.

SYSTEM 3: TEMPLATE MATCHING AND ERROR CORRECTION

The sensorimotor phase of song learning is often described as a process of template matching (Marler, 1976), i.e. the bird gradually alters its motor performance until the auditory result comes to match a memory of the song model (Figure 7.1). Thus a neural 'comparator' must exist to detect error between auditory performance and goal. If error is present, the motor control system must change or adjust its performance, until error is no longer detected. The evidence reviewed above implicates the caudal pathway of the song system (HVC–RA) in primary motor control (Figure 7.2), and suggests that primary auditory representations may be generated in cell populations in NCM, CMHV and other sites where gene responses occur during auditory stimulation (Figure 7.3). How is this auditory information brought to bear on the pattern of song motor activity generated by HVC and RA?

Several re-entrant loops have now been demonstrated within the major backbone of the song control network (Figure 7.4), any or all of which could contribute to the comparison that must be made between 'what I just sang' and 'what I remember I should sound like' (Okuhata and Saito, 1987; Bottjer *et al.*, 1989; Wild, 1993; Vates and Nottebohm, 1995; Foster *et al.*, 1997; Vates *et al.*, 1997; Foster and Bottjer, 1998). The most obvious and promising candidate for a template-matching role is the rostral song control pathway itself, running through Area X and lMAN (Figure 7.2). Area X sits within a region homologous to the mammalian basal ganglia (Casto and Ball, 1994; Bottjer and Alexander, 1995). In mammals, the basal ganglia have been strongly implicated in processes of motor skill learning and template matching (Graybiel *et al.*, 1994; Graybiel, 1995; Jueptner *et al.*, 1997). Area X receives inputs from HVC (Nottebohm *et al.*, 1982; Bottjer *et al.*, 1989) and lMAN (Okuhata and Saito, 1987; Vates and Nottebohm, 1995), from ZENK-responsive auditory areas (Clayton, 1997; Foster and

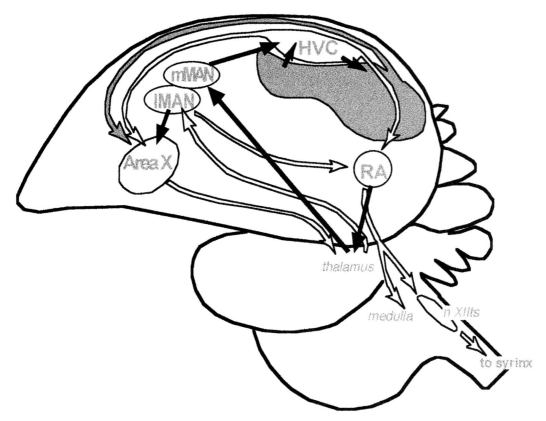

Figure 7.4. Reafferent pathways in the song control circuit. Black arrows indicate projections found since the original demonstration of the classical song control circuit (Figure 7.2), and which potentially allow feedback that could be used in template matching (Okuhata and Saito, 1987; Bottjer *et al.*, 1989; Wild, 1993; Vates and Nottebohm, 1995; Foster *et al.*, 1997; Vates *et al.*, 1997; Foster and Bottjer, 1998). The rostral song control pathway itself (Figure 7.2) may contribute to this function, as described in the text (System 3).

Bottjer, 1998) and from the dopaminergic neuro-modulatory system (Lewis *et al.*, 1981; Sakaguchi and Saito, 1989; Bottjer, 1993; Casto and Ball, 1994; Soha *et al.*, 1996). Following the general vertebrate plan of cortical–striatal organization, Area X projects to the thalamus (DLM) which returns projections to the song motor control pathway via a nucleus (lMAN) in the neostriatum, part of the avian analog of the mammalian neocortex (Okuhata and Saito, 1987; Bottjer *et al.*, 1989; Bottjer and Johnson, 1997). Lesion of nuclei in this rostral pathway disrupts the acquisition and modification of song by juvenile zebra finches, but has minimal effects if administered in adulthood after song production has matured (Bottjer *et al.*, 1984; Sohrabji *et al.*, 1990; Scharff and Nottebohm, 1991).

As in most other parts of the dedicated song control network (including the syringeal muscles themselves; Williams and Nottebohm, 1985); passive listening in anesthetized birds results in electrophysiological responses in both Area X and lMAN, and these responses increase in selectivity for the bird's own song as production of that song is perfected (Doupe and Solis, 1997; Solis and Doupe, 1997). Information about electrophysiological activities that occur in lMAN and Area X during singing is still emerging (McCasland, 1987; Hessler and Doupe, 1999). Recent studies using assays of IEG expression have revealed significant genomic activation in all four of the telencephalic song nuclei during singing but not passive listening, with the greatest response in Area X (Jarvis and Nottebohm, 1997; Jin and Clayton, 1997a). The subject of IEG responses in the rostral pathway is developed further in the next section.

In juvenile male zebra finches, the rostral forebrain pathway also undergoes a variety of molecular changes coincident with the progress of song rehearsal and stabilization (Clayton, 1997). For example, early in the sensorimotor phase (by ~35 days of age, when a functional song template has first been acquired), synuclein/synelfin gene expression in lMAN declines, followed by a loss of the protein in synaptic terminals at lMAN's target, nucleus RA (George *et al.*, 1995; Jin and Clayton, 1997b). Synuclein/synelfin is a presynaptic protein possibly involved in supporting membrane structure and plasticity, and its loss could contribute to synaptic stabilization during song learning (Clayton and George, 1998). With a somewhat slower time course, NMDA receptor binding capacity in lMAN also declines (Aamodt *et al.*, 1992, 1995). Gradual increases in dopaminergic and cholinergic terminals (Sakaguchi and Saito, 1991; Bottjer, 1993; Soha *et al.*, 1996; Li and Sakaguchi, 1997; Harding *et al.*, 1998) and androgen binding capacity (Bottjer, 1987) might be important in later phases of the song learning process that are sensitive to social context (Jones *et al.*, 1996), and/or may contribute to the eventual stabilization of the song in adults.

The ultimate point of intersection between this putative error detection system and the motor output control pathway is at nucleus RA, the sole output nucleus of the telencephalic song control network (Figure 7.2). Neurons in RA receive two known extrinsic inputs, both glutamatergic, from HVC and from lMAN. The inputs from lMAN (unlike HVC) are mediated primarily by *N*-methyl-D-aspartate (NMDA) receptors (Kubota and Saito, 1991; Mooney and Konishi, 1991; Mooney, 1992). In many systems, NMDA receptor activity has been associated with synaptic plasticity (Cotman *et al.*, 1988; Constantine-Paton *et al.*, 1990; see also Dudai and Morris, Chapter 9; Winder and Kandel, Chapter 10; Horn, Chapter 19). NMDA receptor activation requires coincident receptor binding and postsynaptic depolarization, and thus the receptors in RA presumably are activated only during coincident activity in both the caudal and rostral song control pathways. Thus any error signal reaching RA from lMAN might be most effective at promoting plastic changes in motor synapses that were active just before the bird heard its own immature (or mismatched) song. This model for integrative circuit design makes two predictions confirmed by experiment (cf. Brainard and Doupe, 2000).

(i) Lesion of the output nucleus of the error detection system (lMAN) should decrease the bird's capacity to modify its song. This appears to be the case in juvenile male zebra finches (Bottjer

et al., 1984; Scharff and Nottebohm, 1991), and also in adults adapting to unilateral tracheosyringeal nerve injury (Williams and Mehta, 1999).

(ii) Since Area X has inhibitory outputs onto the thalamus (Bottjer and Johnson, 1997), lesion of it might be expected to disinhibit the signal generation capacity of the thalamocortical output through lMAN, and thus result in a chronic 'error' signal onto RA. Indeed, zebra finches with Area X lesions fail to crystallize a stable song (Scharff and Nottebohm, 1991)

THE GENOME AS AN AGENT OF CIRCUIT INTEGRATION

Thus far in this chapter, we have considered the evidence suggesting three discrete systems involved in the process of song learning. For each system, progress is being made in understanding where and how the appropriate representations are lodged. Song motor patterns are generated through the hierarchical actions of HVC and RA (System 1). Sensory images of songs heard are encoded in the patterns of distributed populations of neurons in NCM/CMHV (System 2). Finally, a rostral forebrain loop analogous to the mammalian cortico-striato-cortical pathway may subserve the function of comparing immediate song performance with the stored memory of a song performance (System 3). Many details remain to be worked out for each system alone, but perhaps no issue is more fundamental than understanding how the patterns of activity in these different systems are integrated, to result in an appropriate functional change in the specific output of the HVC–RA pathway during an age-limited period in development.

Fresh clues to this issue of functional integration may be emerging once again from the study of IEG expression. As reviewed earlier, the sound of conspecific bird song elicits an IEG response in NCM/CMHV in adult birds, whereas the act of singing induces a genomic response in the motor nuclei, especially HVC and Area X. Although the functional significance of IEG responses is a full subject in its own right (Clayton, 2000), these observations beg the question of whether there are any differences in IEG response patterns in young birds actively engaged in song learning, as compared with the adult birds where the responses were first observed. For all three of the proposed functional systems, the answer appears to be 'yes.'

Regarding the motor system, age-related differences in ZENK gene induction during singing have been reported for RA, but not for the other nuclei (Jin and Clayton, 1997a). Throughout most of RA, little induction was seen in adult zebra finches following song. In young birds producing immature song, however, robust gene induction occurred throughout the nucleus. Intriguingly, robust induction throughout the whole of RA was reported for canaries (Jarvis and Nottebohm, 1997), a species in which song modification occurs into adulthood. Thus, using ZENK expression again as an indicator for information storage capacity, these results would identify RA as the critical node at which song plasticity may be constrained or released in at least these two species of songbird.

Regarding the sensory system (NCM), zebra finches at 20 days of age (just prior to the onset of song learning) do not yet show any inducible ZENK response to song stimuli (Jin and Clayton, 1997a), although their electrophysiological responses to songs are equivalent to those of adults (Stripling and Clayton, unpublished data). Even without song stimulation, however, the basal level of ZENK expression is quite high at these young ages. Elevated ZENK expression levels often have been correlated with an increased capacity for long-term memory storage (O'Donovan et al., 1999; Clayton, 2000). Thus in birds just beginning to learn a song model, high constitutive levels of ZENK mRNA may indicate a high but non-selective capacity for storage of any new auditory representations—exactly what one would expect for a bird about to form a deep memory of the song to which it currently is exposed the most (i.e. its tutor's). With increasing experience, basal levels of ZENK then decline, increasing the selectivity of new information storage. In adults, high ZENK expression will only occur after exposure to songs that are deemed 'significant' by their novelty or context (Mello et al., 1995). (Another example of ZENK response modulation by context may be seen in the augmentation of ZENK responses when the song is paired to a foot shock; Jarvis et al., 1995.)

Regarding the error correction system (Area X and lMAN), ZENK induction occurs in adult birds when they sing, but the response seems to vary profoundly depending upon the context in which the song is being produced (Jarvis et al., 1998). Zebra finches sing in at least two contexts. When alone, and often at the beginning of the day, a male finch will sing spontaneously, producing 'undirected' song. Song may also be 'directed' to another bird, for example during courtship of a female. Despite the fact that female-directed song is arguably the more arousing context, undirected song was found to be the more effective stimulus for ZENK induction, especially in Area X, the nucleus in the putative basal ganglia (Jarvis et al., 1998). If undirected song represents a form of song rehearsal, then the active monitoring and error correction processes that presumably occur during undirected rehearsal may be responsible for the elevation of ZENK at these times.

Together, these observations suggest that the neuronal genome may be responding selectively to particular combinations of signals impinging on the cell, effectively integrating information present in multiple neural channels. In RA, for example, neither song production nor passive listening to song is always sufficient to induce a genomic response, even though both of these behavioral contexts result in acute electrophysiological activity apparently via HVC afferents. Although direct evidence remains to be gathered, a parsimonious explanation is that genomic activation in RA also requires an appropriate complement of activity in the lMAN afferent pathway. If so, RA's genomic response could be serving effectively as a gatekeeper, enhancing or inhibiting synaptic information storage dependent on the global pattern of activation each neuron receives. The context-dependent variations in NCM and Area X likewise may reflect an integration of representational information and neuromodulatory pathways (Sakaguchi and Saito, 1989; Soha et al., 1996; Harding et al., 1998; Mello et al., 1998a).

A similar integrative role for the genome could underlie other examples where information storage in a neural system or network depends on an appropriate integration of activities in multiple channels. The neural network model developed to account for aspects of filial imprinting in chicks is an interesting case in point (Bateson and Horn, 1994; Bolhuis, 1999). In this model, information storage depends on the timing and balance of activities in different sensory modules, brought together in part through the action of processing layers for representation, analysis and execution (for discussion, see Bateson, Chapter 15). It would be interesting to determine whether gene responses during filial imprinting to compound stimuli vary with the sequencing of stimulus presentation, which has been shown to have defined effects on the success of imprinting (Van Kampen and Bolhuis, 1993; Bolhuis and Honey, 1994; Bolhuis, 1999).

CONCLUSIONS

When the telencephalic song control nuclei were first identified (Nottebohm *et al.*, 1976), it galvanized interest in the song bird as a model for fundamental neurobiology in part because it seemed plausible that a complex set of behaviors could be 'mapped' and explained by reference to a small set of defined and dedicated brain structures. With more study, it has become apparent that avian song learning involves more than just a couple of dedicated brain nuclei. With hindsight, this is hardly surprising—song is central to the social life and adaptive evolution of literally thousands of species, and it is a complex behavior that probably draws on virtually every functional system in the brain. Nevertheless (or perhaps even because of this complexity), the songbird has emerged as one of the most powerful models for studying the neural bases of behavior and perception. The song control pathways are a paradigm for neural circuit design, and the richness and accessibility of the behavior provide experimental opportunities that have only begun to be tapped. A deeper understanding of basic brain function promises to follow from concerted application of molecular, cellular, physiological and ethological approaches to this system.

REFERENCES

Aamodt, S.M., Kozlowski, M.R., Nordeen, E.J. and Nordeen, K.W. (1992) Distribution and developmental change in [³H]MK-801 binding within zebra finch song nuclei. *Journal of Neurobiology*, 23, 997–1005.

Aamodt, S.M., Nordeen, E.J. and Nordeen, K.W. (1995) Early isolation from conspecific song does not affect the normal developmental decline of *N*-methyl-D-aspartate receptor binding in an avian song nucleus. *Journal of Neurobiology*, 27, 76–84.

Bateson, P. and Horn, G. (1994) Imprinting and recognition memory: a neural net model. *Animal Behaviour*, 48, 695–715.

Beecher, M.D., Stoddard, P.K., Campbell, S.E. and Horning, C.L. (1996) Repertoire matching between neighbouring song sparrows. *Animal Behaviour*, 51, 917–923.

Böhner, J. (1990) Early acquisition of song in the zebra finch, *Taeniopygia guttata*. *Animal Behaviour*, 39, 369–374.

Bolhuis, J.J. (1999) Early learning and the development of filial preferences in the chick. *Behavioural Brain Research*, 98, 245–252.

Bolhuis, J.J. and Honey, R.C. (1994) Within-event learning during filial imprinting. *Journal of Experimental Psychology: Animal Behavior Processes*, 20, 240–248.

Bottjer, S.W. (1987) Ontogenetic changes in the pattern of androgen accumulation in song-control nuclei of male zebra finches. *Journal of Neurobiology*, 18, 125–139.

Bottjer, S.W. (1993) The distribution of tyrosine hydroxylase immunoreactivity in the brains of male and female zebra finches. *Journal of Neurobiology*, 24, 51–69.

Bottjer, S.W. and Alexander, G. (1995) Localization of met-enkephalin and vasoactive intestinal polypeptide in the brains of male zebra finches. *Brain, Behavior and Evolution*, 45, 153–177.

Bottjer, S.W. and Johnson, F. (1997) Circuits, hormones and learning—vocal behavior in songbirds. *Journal of Neurobiology*, 33, 602–618.

Bottjer, S.W., Miesner, E.A. and Arnold, A.P. (1984) Forebrain lesions disrupt development but not maintenance of song in passerine birds. *Science*, 224, 901–903.

Bottjer, S.W., Halsema, K.A., Brown, S.A. and Meisner, E.A. (1989) Axonal connections of a forebrain nucleus involved with vocal learning in zebra finches. *Journal of Comparative Neurology*, 379, 312–326.

Brainard, M.S. and Doupe, A.J. (2000). Interruption of a basal ganglia-forebrain circuit prevents plasticity of learned vocalizations. *Nature*, 404, 762–766.

Brenowitz, E.A. (1991) Evolution of the vocal control system in the avian brain. *Seminars in Neuroscience*, 3, 399–407.

Brenowitz, E.A. (1997) Comparative approaches to the avian song system. *Journal of Neurobiology*, 33, 517–531.

Brenowitz, E.A., Arnold, A.P. and Levin, R. (1985) Neural correlates of female song in tropical duetting birds. *Brain Research*, 343, 104–112.

Brenowitz, E.A., Margoliash, D. and Nordeen, K.W. (1997) An introduction to birdsong and the avian song system. *Journal of Neurobiology*, 33, 495–500.

Casto, J.M. and Ball, G.F. (1994) Characterization and localization of D1 dopamine receptors in the sexually dimorphic vocal control nucleus, area X and the basal ganglia of european starlings. *Journal of Neurobiology*, 25, 767–780.

Catchpole, C.K. (1982) The evolution of bird sounds in relation to mating and spacing behaviour. In: Kroodsma, D.E. and Miller, E.H. (eds), *Acoustic Communication in Birds*. Academic Press, New York, pp. 297–319.

Chaudhuri, A. (1997) Neural activity mapping with inducible transcription factors. *Neuroreport*, 8, R5–R9.

Chew, S.J., Mello, C., Nottebohm, F., Jarvis, E. and Vicario, D.S. (1995) Decrements in auditory responses to a repeated conspecific song are long-lasting and require two periods of protein synthesis in the songbird forebrain. *Proceedings of the National Academy of Sciences of the United States of America*, 92, 3406–3410.

Chew, S.J., Vicario, D.S. and Nottebohm, F. (1996) A large-capacity memory system that recognizes calls and songs of individual birds. *Proceedings of the National Academy of Sciences of the United States of America*, 93, 1950–1955.

Clayton, D.F. (1997) Role of gene regulation in song circuit development and song learning. *Journal of Neurobiology*, 33, 549–571.

Clayton, D.F. (2000) The genomic action potential. *Neurobiology of Learning and Memory*, in press.

Clayton, D.F. and George, J.M. (1998) The synucleins: a family of proteins involved in synaptic function, plasticity, neurodegeneration and disease. *Trends in Neurosciences*, 21, 249–254.

Constantine-Paton, M., Cline, H.T. and Debski, E.A. (1990) Patterned activity, synaptic convergence and the NMDA receptor in developing visual pathways. *Annual Review of Neuroscience*, 13, 129–154.

Cotman, C.W., Monaghan, D.T. and Ganong, A.H. (1988) Excitatory amino acid neurotransmission: NMDA receptors and Hebb-type synaptic plasticity. *Annual Review of Neuroscience*, 11, 61–80.

Dave, A.S., Yu, A.C. and Margoliash, D. (1998) Behavioral state modulation of auditory activity in a vocal motor system. *Science*, 282, 250–254.

Doupe, A.J. (1997) Song- and order-selective neurons in the songbird anterior forebrain and their emergence during vocal development. *Journal of Neuroscience*, 17, 1147–1167.

Doupe, A.J. and Konishi, M. (1991) Song-selective auditory circuits in the vocal control system of the zebra finch. *Proceedings of the National Academy of Sciences of the United States of America*, 88, 11339–11343.

Doupe, A.J. and Solis, M.M. (1997) Song- and order-selective neurons develop in the songbird anterior forebrain during vocal learning. *Journal of Neurobiology*, 33, 694–709.

Fortune, E. and Margoliash, D. (1992) Cytoarchitectonic organization and morphology of cells of the Field L complex in male zebra finches (*Taenopygia guttata*). *Journal of Comparative Neurology*, 325, 388–404.

Fortune, E.S. and Margoliash, D. (1995) Parallel pathways and convergence onto HVc and adjacent neostriatum of adult zebra finches (*Taeniopygia guttata*). *Journal of Comparative Neurology*, 360, 413–441.

Foster, E.F. and Bottjer, S.W. (1998) Axonal connections of the high vocal center and surrounding cortical regions in juvenile and adult male zebra finches. *Journal of Comparative Neurology*, 397, 118–138.

Foster, E.F., Mehta, R.P. and Bottjer, S.W. (1997) Axonal connections of the medial magnocellular nucleus of the anterior neostriatum in zebra finches. *Journal of Comparative Neurology*, 382, 364–381.

Gahr, M., Guttinger, H.-R. and Kroodsma, D. (1993) Estrogen receptors in the avian brain: survey reveals general distribution and forebrain areas unique to songbirds. *Journal of Comparative Neurology*, 327, 112–122.

George, J.M., Jin, H., Woods, W.S. and Clayton, D.F. (1995) Characterization of a novel protein regulated during the critical period for song learning in the zebra finch. *Neuron*, 15, 361–372.

Graybiel, A.M. (1995) Building action repertoires: memory and learning functions of the basal ganglia. *Current Opinion in Neurobiology*, 5, 733–741.

Graybiel, A.M., Aosaki, T., Flaherty, A.W. and Kimura, M. (1994) The basal ganglia and adaptive motor control. *Science*, 265, 1826–1831.

Harding, C.F., Barclay, S.R. and Waterman, S.A. (1998) Changes in catecholamine levels and turnover rates in hypothalamic, vocal control and auditory nuclei in male zebra finches during development. *Journal of Neurobiology*, 34, 329–346.

Hessler, N.A. and Doupe, A.J. (1999). Singing-related neural activity in a dorsal forebrain-basal ganglia circuit of adult zebra finches. *Journal of Neuroscience*, 19, 10461–10481.

Horn, G. (1998) Visual imprinting and the neural mechanisms of recognition memory. *Trends in Neurosciences*, 21, 300–305.

Immelmann, K. (1969) Song development in the zebra finch and other estrilid finches. In: Hinde, R.A. (ed.), *Bird Vocalizations*. Cambridge University Press, Cambridge, pp. 61–74.

Jarvis, E.D. and Nottebohm, F. (1997) Motor-driven gene expression. *Proceedings of the National Academy of Sciences of the United States of America*, 94, 4097–4102.

Jarvis, E.D., Mello, C.V. and Nottebohm, F. (1995) Associative learning and stimulus novelty influence the song-induced expression of an immediate early gene in the canary forebrain. *Learning and Memory*, 2, 62–80.

Jarvis, E.D., Scharff, C., Grossman, M.R., Ramos, J.A. and Nottebohm, F. (1998) For whom the bird sings—context-dependent gene expression. *Neuron*, 21, 775–788.

Jin, H. and Clayton, D.F. (1997a) Localized changes in immediate-early gene regulation during sensory and motor learning in zebra finches. *Neuron*, 19, 1049–1059.

Jin, H. and Clayton, D.F. (1997b) Synelfin regulation during the critical period for song learning in normal and isolated juvenile zebra finches. *Neurobiology of Learning and Memory*, 68, 271–284.

Jones, A.E., Ten Cate, C. and Slater, P.J.B. (1996) Early experience and plasticity of song in adult male zebra finches (*Taeniopygia guttata*). *Journal of Comparative and Physiological Psychology*, 110, 354–369.

Jueptner, M., Frith, C.D., Brooks, D.J., Frackowiak, R.S.J. and Passingham, R.E. (1997) Anatomy of motor learning. II. Subcortical structures and learning by trial and error. *Journal of Neurophysiology*, 77, 1325–1337.

Katz, L.C. and Gurney, M. (1981) Auditory responses in the zebra finch's motor system for song. *Brain Research*, 12, 192–197.

Konishi, M. (1965) The role of auditory feedback in the control of vocalizations in the white-crowned sparrow. *Zeitschrift für Tierpsychologie*, 22, 770–783.

Kroodsma, D.E. and Byers, B.E. (1991) The function(s) of birdsong. *American Zoologist*, 31, 318–328.

Kroodsma, D.E. and Konishi, M. (1991) A suboscine bird (Eastern phoebe, Sayornis-Phoebe) develops normal song without auditory feedback. *Animal Behaviour*, 42, 477–487.

Kubota, M. and Saito, N. (1991) NMDA receptors participate differentially in two different synaptic inputs in neurons of the zebra finch robust nucleus of the archistriatum *in vitro*. *Neuroscience Letters*, 125, 107–109.

Lewis, J.W., Ryan, S.M., Arnold, A.P. and Butcher, L.L. (1981) Evidence for a catecholaminergic projection to area X in the zebra finch. *Journal of Comparative Neurology*, 196, 347–354.

Li, R. and Sakaguchi, H. (1997) Cholinergic innervation of the song control nuclei by the ventral paleostriatum in the zebra finch—a double-labeling study with retrograde fluorescent tracers and choline acetyltransferase immuno-histochemistry. *Brain Research*, 763, 239–246.

Macdougall-Shackleton, S.A., Hulse, S.H. and Ball, G.F. (1998) Neural bases of song preferences in female zebra finches (*Taeniopygia guttata*). *Neuroreport*, 9, 3047–3052.

Margoliash, D. (1983) Acoustic parameters underlying the responses of song-specific neurons in the white-crowned sparrow. *Journal of Neuroscience*, 3, 1039–1057.

Margoliash, D. (1986) Preference for autogenous song by auditory neurons in a song system nucleus of the white-crowned sparrow. *Journal of Neuroscience*, 6, 1643–1661.

Marler, P. (1976) Sensory templates in species-specific behavior. In: Fentress, J. (ed.), *Simpler Networks and Behavior*. Sinauer, Sunderland, Massachusetts, pp. 314–329.

Marler, P. (1997) Three models of song learning—evidence from behavior. *Journal of Neurobiology*, 33, 501–516.

Marler, P. and Peters, S. (1977) Selective vocal learning in a sparrow. *Science*, 198, 519–527.

Marler, P. and Peters, S. (1982) Developmental overproduction and selective attrition: new processes in the epigenesis of birdsong. *Developmental Psychobiology*, 15, 369–378.

Marler, P. and Peters, S. (1987) A sensitive period for song acquisition in the song sparrow, *Melospiza melodia*: a case of age-limited learning. *Ethology*, 76, 89–100.

Marler, P. and Waser, M. (1977) The role of auditory feedback in canary song development. *Journal of Comparative and Physiological Psychology*, 91, 8–16.

McCabe, B.J. and Horn, G. (1994) Learning-related changes in Fos-like immunoreactivity in the chick forebrain after imprinting. *Proceedings of the National Academy of Sciences of the United States of America*, 91, 11417–11421.

McCasland, J.S. (1987) Neuronal control of birdsong production. *Journal of Neuroscience*, 7, 23–39.

McCasland, J.S. and Konishi, M. (1981) Interaction between auditory and motor activities in an avian song control nucleus. *Proceedings of the National Academy of Sciences of the United States of America*, 78, 7815–7819.

Mello, C.V. and Clayton, D.F. (1994) Song-induced ZENK gene expression in auditory pathways of songbird brain and its relation to the song control system. *Journal of Neuroscience*, 14, 6652–6666.

Mello, C.V., Vicario, D.S. and Clayton, D.F. (1992) Song presentation induces gene expression in the songbird forebrain. *Proceedings of the National Academy of Sciences of the United States of America*, 89, 6818–6822.

Mello, C.V., Nottebohm, F. and Clayton, D.F. (1995) Repeated exposure to one song leads to a rapid and persistent decline in an immediate early gene's response to that song in zebra finch telencephalon. *Journal of Neuroscience*, 15, 6919–6925.

Mello, C.V., Pinaud, R. and Ribeiro, S. (1998a) Noradrenergic system of the zebra finch brain—immunocytochemical study of dopamine-beta-hydroxylase. *Journal of Comparative Neurology*, 400, 207–228.

Mello, C.V., Vates, G.E., Okuhata, S. and Nottebohm, F. (1998b) Descending auditory pathways in the adult male zebra finch (*Taeniopygia guttata*). *Journal of Comparative Neurology*, 395, 137–160.

Mooney, R. (1992) Synaptic basis for developmental plasticity in a birdsong nucleus. *Journal of Neuroscience*, 12, 2464–2477.

Mooney, R. and Konishi, M. (1991) Two distinct inputs to an avian song nucleus activate different glutamate receptor subtypes on individual neurons. *Proceedings of the National Academy of Sciences of the United States of America*, 88, 4075–4079.

Nastiuk, K.L., Mello, C.V., George, J.M. and Clayton, D.F. (1994) Immediate-early gene responses in the avian song control system: cloning and expression analysis of the canary c-*jun* cDNA. *Molecular Brain Research*, 27, 299–309.

Nottebohm, F. (1968) Auditory experience and song development in the chaffinch, *Fringilla coelebs*. *Ibis*, 110, 549–568.

Nottebohm, F. and Arnold, A. (1976) Sexual dimorphism in vocal control areas of the songbird brain. *Science*, 194, 211–213.

Nottebohm, F., Stokes, T. and Leonard, C.M. (1976) Central control of song in the canary. *Journal of Comparative Neurology*, 165, 457–486.

Nottebohm, F., Kelley, D.B. and Paton, J.A. (1982) Connections of vocal control nuclei in the canary telencephalon. *Journal of Comparative Neurology*, 207, 344–357.

Nowicki, S., Searcy, W.A. and Hughes, M. (1998) The territory defense function of song in song sparrows—a test with the speaker occupation design. *Behaviour*, 135, 615–628.

O'Donovan, K.J., Tourtellotte, W.G., Milbrandt, J. and Baraban, J.M. (1999) The EGR family of transcription-regulatory factors: progress at the interface of molecular and systems neuroscience. *Trends in Neurosciences*, 22, 167–173.

Okuhata, S. and Saito, N. (1987) Synaptic connection of thalamo-cerebral vocal nuclei of the canary. *Brain Research Bulletin*, 18, 35–44.

Price, P. (1979) Developmental determinants of structure in zebra finch song. *Journal of Comparative and Physiological Psychology*, 93, 260–277.

Ribeiro, S., Cecchi, G.A., Magnasco, M.O. and Mello, C.V. (1998) Toward a song code—evidence for a syllabic representation in the canary brain. *Neuron*, 21, 359–371.

Sakaguchi, H. and Saito, N. (1989) The acetylcholine and catecholamine contents in song control nuclei of zebra finch during song ontogeny. *Developmental Brain Research*, 47, 313–317.

Sakaguchi, H. and Saito, N. (1991) Developmental change of cholinergic activity in the forebrain of the zebra finch during song learning. *Developmental Brain Research*, 62, 223–228.

Scharff, C. and Nottebohm, F. (1991) A comparative study of the behavioral deficits following lesions of various parts of the zebra finch song system: implications for vocal learning. *Journal of Neuroscience*, 11, 2896–2913.

Scharff, C., Nottebohm, F. and Cynx, J. (1998) Conspecific and heterospecific song discrimination in male zebra finches with lesions in the anterior forebrain pathway. *Journal of Neurobiology*, 36, 81–90.

Schmidt, M.F. and Konishi, M. (1998) Gating of auditory responses in the vocal control system of awake songbirds. *Nature Neuroscience*, 1, 513–518.

Slater, P.J.B. and Jones, A.E. (1995) The timing of song and distance call learning in zebra finches. *Animal Behaviour*, 49, 548–550.

Soha, J.A., Shimizu, T. and Doupe, A.J. (1996) Development of the catecholaminergic innervation of the song system of the male zebra finch. *Journal of Neurobiology*, 29, 473–489.

Sohrabji, F., Nordeen, E.J. and Nordeen, K.W. (1990) Selective impairment of song learning following lesions of a forebrain nucleus in juvenile zebra finches. *Behavioral and Neural Biology*, 53, 51–63.

Solis, M.M. and Doupe, A.J. (1997) Anterior forebrain neurons develop selectivity by an intermediate stage of birdsong learning. *Journal of Neuroscience*, 17, 6447–6462.

Stripling, R., Volman, S. and Clayton, D. (1997) Response modulation in the zebra finch caudal neostriatum: relationship to nuclear gene regulation. *Journal of Neuroscience*, 17, 3883–3893.

Thorpe, W.H. (1958) The learning of song patterns by birds, with especial reference to the song of the chaffinch, *Fringilla coelebs*. *Ibis*, 100, 535–570.

Van Kampen, H.S. and Bolhuis, J.J. (1993) Interaction between auditory and visual learning during imprinting. *Animal Behaviour*, 45, 623–625.

Vates, G.E. and Nottebohm, F. (1995) Feedback circuitry within a song-learning pathway. *Proceedings of the National Academy of Sciences of the United States of America*, 92, 5139–5143.

Vates, G.E., Broome, B.M., Mello, C.V. and Nottebohm, F. (1996) Auditory pathways of caudal telencephalon and their relation to the song system of adult male zebra finches (*Taeniopygia guttata*). *Journal of Comparative Neurology*, 366, 613–642.

Vates, G.E., Vicario, D.S. and Nottebohm, F. (1997) Reafferent thalamo-cortical loops in the song system of oscine songbirds. *Journal of Comparative Neurology*, 380, 275–290.

Vicario, D.S. (1991) Organization of the zebra finch song control system: II. Functional organization of outputs from nucleus robustus archistriatalis. *Journal of Comparative Neurology*, 309, 486–494.

Vicario, D.S. and Yohay, K.H. (1993) Song-selective auditory input to a forebrain vocal control nucleus in the zebra finch. *Journal of Neurobiology*, 24, 488–505.

Volman, S.F. (1993) Development of neural selectivity for birdsong during vocal learning. *Journal of Neuroscience*, 13, 4737–4747.

Vu, E.T., Mazurek, M.E. and Kuo, Y.-C. (1994) Identification of a forebrain motor programming network for the learned song of zebra finches. *Journal of Neuroscience*, 14, 6924–6934.

Wild, J.M. (1993) Descending projections of the songbird nucleus robustus archistriatalis. *Journal of Comparative Neurology*, 338, 225–241.

Wild, J.M. (1997) Neural pathways for the control of birdsong production. *Journal of Neurobiology*, 33, 653–670.

Wiley, R., Tatchwell, B. and Davis, N. (1991) Recognition of individual males' songs by female dunnocks: a mechanism increasing the number of copulatory partners and reproductive success. *Ethology*, 88, 145–153.

Williams, H. and Mehta, N. (1999) Changes in adult zebra finch song require a forebrain nucleus that is not necessary for song production. *Journal of Neurobiology*, 39, 14–28.

Williams, H. and Nottebohm, F. (1985) Auditory responses in avian vocal motor neurons: a motor theory for song perception in birds. *Science*, 229, 279–282.

Yu, A.C. and Margoliash, D. (1996) Temporal hierarchical control of singing in birds. *Science*, 273, 1871–1185.

8 THE AVIAN HIPPOCAMPAL FORMATION AND MEMORY FOR HOARDED FOOD: SPATIAL LEARNING OUT IN THE REAL WORLD

Tom V. Smulders and Timothy J. DeVoogd

INTRODUCTION

Any organism that navigates through its environment needs spatial information. This can be as simple as knowing where obstacles are, so that they can be avoided, and as complicated as knowing how to migrate half way across the globe. For most species, this information is specific to any given situation and needs to be acquired by learning. Thus, spatial learning and memory are of fundamental importance to those interested in the mechanisms of learning in general. Moreover, since spatial knowledge is universally relevant, it lends itself extremely well to investigation using a comparative approach to behavioral neurobiology. The study of how different species approach similar navigation problems can help us to understand better the neural mechanisms of spatial memory, and of learning mechanisms in general (discussed by Capaldi *et al.*, 1999). In this chapter, we will focus on birds. Many bird species perform prominent feats of spatial navigation, on both a local and a long-distance level. Birds are observed easily in the field and their phylogeny is fairly well studied, making them ideal for comparative analyses. They also generally adapt well to captivity. These features make birds a particularly appropriate group in which to study the neural basis of naturally occurring types of spatial navigation.

In the first half of this chapter, we will discuss what we know about the avian hippocampal formation (HF). In mammals, the hippocampus has been suggested to play an important role in the processing of spatial information. Rats with hippocampal lesions perform less well at tasks that require them to process spatial information (Olton *et al.*, 1979; Jarrard, 1995)

and many hippocampal neurons encode the location of the animal in their environment, as well as other information (O'Keefe and Dostrovsky, 1971; O'Keefe and Nadel, 1978; Eichenbaum *et al.*, 1987; Muller and Kubie, 1987; Muller *et al.*, 1987). The avian HF is believed to be homologous to the mammalian hippocampus and parahippocampal regions. We will show that, like its mammalian counterpart, the avian HF is also implicated in processing spatial navigation information.

In the second half of the chapter, we will focus on a fairly well studied avian behavior in which spatial information processing plays an important role: food hoarding. Bird species in several families of songbirds are known to scatter hoard food items (Vander Wall, 1990). This means that instead of hoarding all their food in one central location, the animals scatter their hoards across their home range in small caches of one to 20 or so items. Because the food is widely distributed, retrieving this food for later consumption poses an interesting spatial challenge. One of the strategies used by many of these species is to learn and remember the exact locations of their caches (Tomback, 1980; Sherry *et al.*, 1981; Shettleworth and Krebs, 1982). To relocate many caches with such accuracy requires a very detailed representation of the environment. The avian HF plays an important role in processing this form of spatial memory (reviewed by Krebs *et al.*, 1996). We will describe what is known about the function of the HF in the memory for the location of food caches, and discuss this knowledge in the broader context of the ecology and evolution of food hoarding. We will end with some suggestions for future avenues of research in this system that are needed to elucidate the many outstanding questions.

A BRIEF HISTORY OF AVIAN HIPPOCAMPUS RESEARCH: ANATOMY AND FUNCTION

Anatomy

History

In a seminal paper comparing the forebrains of several different bird species, Rose (1914) described the medio-dorsal cortical area of the avian telencephalon (Figure 8.1) as the 'Area Entorhinalis' or 'Hippokampusrinde' (hippocampus cortex). In his first description of this region in the great tit (*Parus major*), he writes:

'The upper half of the medial wall of the ventricle shows the four-layered organization which we have already described

in the previous two sections: we are clearly dealing with the hippocampal cortex here.' (p. 294, translation from the original German by T.V.S.)

Later in the same paper, he also remarks on the conserved nature of this structure, noting that next to the olfactory bulb, it is the most constant cortical structure in the avian brain. His findings agreed with those of Johnston (1913), who described a similar structure in the reptilian brain, and drew the same conclusions about its identity. All other authors after him, studying bird species from diverse avian radiations (from kiwi to hummingbird), have adopted the identification of this structure with the mammalian hippocampal formation or some subpart of it (e.g. Huber and Crosby, 1929; Craigie, 1930, 1932, 1935, 1940;

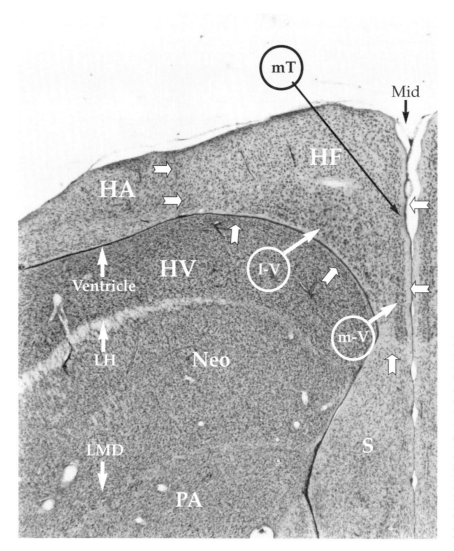

Figure 8.1. Photomicrograph of a coronal section through the left hemisphere HF of a black-capped chickadee. Open white arrows delineate the boundaries of the HF. Circled structures are within the HF (mT, medial fiber tract; m-V, medial arm of the cell-dense 'V'; l-V, lateral arm of the 'V'). Other abbreviations: Mid, midline of the brain; HA, hyperstriatum accessorium; HV, hyperstriatum ventrale; Neo, neostriatum, S, septum; PA, paleostriatum augmentatum; LH, lamina hyperstriatica; LMD, lamina medullaris dorsalis.

Durward, 1932). They often disagreed on questions of exact homologies with both mammalian and reptilian structures, especially when discussing subdivisions of the hippocampal complex or its neighboring cortical areas. This question of one-to-one homologies with the mammalian hippocampal formation (and whether they exist at all) remains a point of contention among present-day researchers (e.g. Erichsen *et al.*, 1991; Krebs *et al.*, 1991; Montagnese *et al.*, 1996; Székely, 1999).

In a study of the embryonic development of the chick brain, Källén (1962) argued that the developmental origins of brain structures can be used to determine homologies between different species. He used the hippocampus and parahippocampus (the region bordering the hippocampus proper) as clear examples of pallial structures that develop from the same layers in the embryo and migrate to relatively similar positions in both mammals and birds. Based on the overwhelming agreement in the literature on what is called the hippocampus (and the area parahippocampalis) in birds, Karten and Hodos (1967) included this nomenclature in their atlas of the pigeon brain.

Any meaningful understanding of the functional morphology of the avian HF (which includes both hippocampus proper and parahippocampus) requires detailed knowledge of its connections with other brain areas. In the 1970s, several studies examined the connections of the avian HF. Bouillé and colleagues (Bons *et al.*, 1976; Bouillé *et al.*, 1977) were interested in hippocampal influences on hypothalamic–adrenocortical interactions and described the projection from the HF to the nucleus posterior medialis hypothalami. Benowitz and Karten (1976) looked for homologies with the mammalian hippocampus, in particular trying to locate the avian version of the fornix longus. No such major fiber tract could be identified, however. Krayniak and Siegel (1978a) published a study on the efferent connections of the pigeon hippocampus. Since then, others have also studied the connectivity of the HF in several bird species in more detail (Casini *et al.*, 1986; Székely and Krebs, 1996). We will now summarize the main results from these studies.

Connectivity

The HF has reciprocal connections with the contralateral HF, the area corticoidea dorsolateralis, the hyperstriatum dorsale and the piriform cortex, as well as with the archistriatum and nucleus taeniae, and the diagonal band of Broca, the nucleus mammilaris lateralis and the area ventralis of Tsai (Figure 8. 2). In addition, the HF sends projections to the ipsi- and contralateral septum in a somewhat topographical projection (rostral HF to rostral septum, and caudal HF to caudal septum) (Krayniak and Siegel, 1978a,b; Casini *et al.*, 1986; Bingman *et al.*, 1994; Székely and Krebs, 1996; Székely, 1999). In domestic chicks, Bradley *et al.* (1985) found a projection from the HF to the intermediate and medial part of the hyperstriatum ventrale, a projection for which there is some evidence in pigeons as well (Casini *et al.*, 1986). In zebra finches, Székely and Krebs (1996) found additional projections to the lobus parolfactorius (LPO), the preoptic area and several thalamic areas (most notably the nucleus dorsomedialis posterior and the subhabenular region). Veenman *et al.* (1995) found projections from the most rostral part of the HF in pigeons to the ventral part of the LPO, part of which they suggest is homologous to the mammalian nucleus accumbens.

In addition to the connections mentioned above as being reciprocal, inputs to the HF are received from the hyperstriatum accessorium, situated just lateral to the area parahippocampalis, and from the dorsal neostriatum. Inputs also come from several thalamic nuclei, such as the nucleus lateralis mammilaris (mentioned above), the stratum cellulare internum, nucleus lateralis hypothalami, nucleus paramedianus internus thalami, nucleus superficialis parvicellularis, nucleus dorsolateralis anterior thalami, nucleus subrotundus medialis and an area ventral to the nucleus ovoidalis (Casini *et al.*, 1986). Projections from the brainstem are mostly monoaminergic in nature (area ventralis of Tsai, raphe nucleus, nucleus linearis caudalis and locus ceruleus), but some also come from the nucleus reticularis pontis oralis and the nucleus centralis superior of Bechterew (Casini *et al.*, 1986). The inputs from the area ventralis of Tsai carry self-motion information from the accessory optic system (Wylie *et al.*, 1999). All the major inputs and outputs that have been described in the mammalian system (reviewed by Amaral and Witter, 1995) are represented in this list of connections of the avian HF (summarized in Figure 8.2). This similarity is a strong indication that, overall, the dorsomedial pallium of birds is indeed homologous to the mammalian hippocampal formation.

Subdivisions

Major questions still remain about whether homologies can be found between subdivisions of the avian and mammalian hippocampal formations. Even

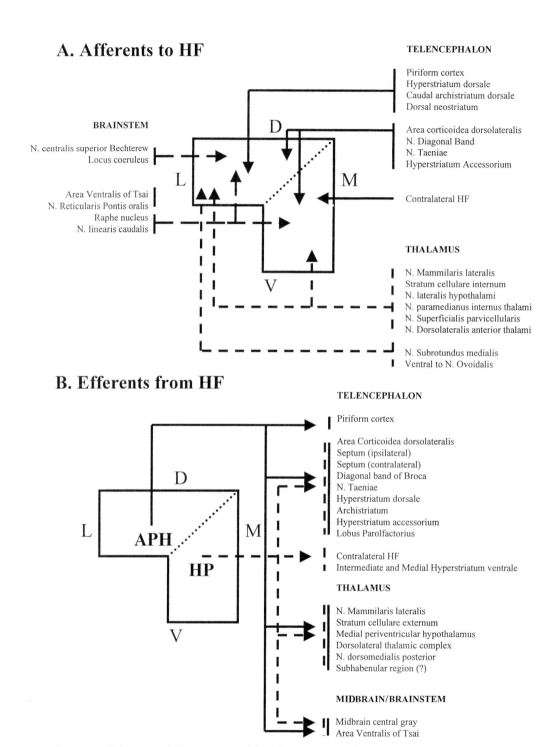

Figure 8.2. Overview of the inputs (**A**) and outputs (**B**) of the avian HF, split into two major subdivisions: the dorsolateral 'parahippocampal area' (APH) and the ventromedial 'hippocampal area' (HP). See text for the sources of the information.

though the avian HF is easily outlined in coronal sections (Figure 8.1), birds do not have the clearly defined internal cytoarchitecture with which neuro-anatomists and neurophysiologists who study mammals are so familiar (see also Brown, Chapter 11). While there are some subdivisions of the avian HF, they do not correspond in any obvious way to the major subdivisions of the mammalian hippocampus, such as the dentate gyrus and Ammon's horn. Well-defined fiber tracts such as the fimbria-fornix cannot be found (Benowitz and Karten, 1976), nor are there mossy fibers or Schaffer's collaterals. Yet despite the apparent lack of this structured connectivity, the avian hippocampus seems to serve much the same function as it does in mammals, as we will describe below. This fact in itself makes a comparative analysis of avian and mammalian hippocampus a valuable tool in understanding structure–function relationships in the brain. In the search for subdivisions of the avian hippocampus, researchers to date have taken three major approaches: differential connectivity, Golgi stain and immunohistochemistry.

Székely (1999) uses the results of her tract-tracing studies to propose a rough subdivision of the HF. She recognizes three subdivisions (dorsolateral, dorso-medial and ventral) of the HF, based on different projection patterns. The dorsolateral part of the HF is the main output to other parts of the brain, as described above (Figure 8.2). The dorsomedial part projects mostly inside the HF, to the other subdivisions, but also sends some projections to the septum and the hyperstriatum accessorium. The ventral part projects mainly to the septum and the contralateral HF. Her rough subdivision is mostly corroborated by the other techniques, as described below, while they add more detail to the emerging picture.

Golgi-stained tissue allows a closer investigation of the distribution of different cell types in the HF. It also allows a peek at the internal connectivity, when the axons can be followed to their terminals. Mollà *et al.* (1986) described several neuronal morphologies in the dorsomedial cortex of the adult chicken, and Montagnese *et al.* (1996) found similar cell classes in the zebra finch. These authors split the cells into two major classes: projection neurons and aspinous neurons, distributed differentially throughout the HF. The projection neurons are characterized by long axons, which project to distant areas of the HF or outside it. The aspinous neurons seem to be part of local circuitry, with short and widely branching axons, rather than long projecting ones. Montagnese

et al. (1996) proposed that the most dorsomedial corner of the HF (which they called the crescent field) receives a large input from outside the structure through the fiber tract that runs along the medial wall of the brain (Figure 8.1). It, in turn, projects exclusively to other parts of the HF. The major output of the HF seems to come from a region they described as the central field of the parahippocampus, in the dorsolateral part of the HF (Figure 8.2). The multipolar projection neurons in this region have large dendritic fields and thick axons which all project in a 'plexus of parallel fibers' that runs ventromedially to the medial fiber tract (Figure 8.1; Montagnese *et al.*, 1996). The other areas of the HF (lateral hippocampus, medial hippocampus and the rest of the para-hippocampal area) are closely interconnected, but the pattern is not yet understood.

The third approach (Erichsen *et al.*, 1991; Krebs *et al.*, 1991) has been to visualize the distribution of as many neurochemicals as possible, and to use this as a basis for subdivision of the HF and of putative homologies with the mammalian system. These studies find that the major afferents to the avian HF are very similar to those in the mammalian HF. Fibers in the medial fiber tract in the pigeon can be choli-nergic (from the septum), serotonergic (from the raphe nucleus) or catecholaminergic (from the locus coeruleus and other brainstem nuclei). This neuro-chemical evidence of homology corroborates the connectivity data discussed earlier. All six of the neuropeptides examined by Erichsen *et al.* (1991) [substance P (SP), somatostatin (SS), leucine enke-phalin (LENK), neuropeptide Y (NPY), vasoactive intestinal peptide (VIP) and cholecystokinin (CCK)] are also found in the medial fiber tract. In addition, NPY-, SS- and VIP-like staining can be found in the hippocampal commissure. Cell bodies stained for NPY and SS are found in a specific region in the center of the ventral and medial part of the HF. This co-localization is reminiscent of the mammalian hilar region. VIP-positive cells are located in an area dorsal to this region. CCK-immunoreactive neuropil sur-rounds the cells of the V area that runs along the medial wall and the ventricle wall of the ventral HF. CCK reactivity in a basket-like pattern surrounding neuronal cell bodies also occurs in Ammon's horn in the mammalian hippocampus (Nunzi *et al.*, 1985, cited by Erichsen *et al.*, 1991). Finally, all across the HF, small GABAergic cells can be found, which seem to constitute local inhibitory circuitry, again very much like in the mammalian system.

Hormones

All avian species investigated to date have estrogen receptors in their HF (Gahr *et al.*, 1993). Recently, it has become clear that this is another characteristic shared between birds and mammals (Maggi *et al.*, 1989; Bettini *et al.*, 1992; Li *et al.*, 1997; Weiland *et al.*, 1997; Register *et al.*, 1998). The importance of estrogens in cognitive processing in both males and females only recently has become a topic of intense investigation (reviewed by McEwen *et al.*, 1997). Interestingly, even though all bird species seem to express estrogen receptors in their HF, in studies to date, only songbirds (Passeriformes) also express aromatase (the enzyme that converts testosterone into estradiol) in the same area (Saldanha *et al.*, 1998). The significance of this finding for the role of estrogens in the functioning of the HF, and how it may be different in songbirds, is still an open question.

Function

Neurophysiology and neurochemistry

Even though we do not know nearly as much about the anatomy and internal connectivity of the avian hippocampus as we do about its mammalian counterpart (Amaral and Witter, 1995), it is clear from the evidence presented in the previous section that there are many anatomical similarities between the two systems. Are there functional homologies as well? This has been studied both on a microscopic (electrophysiological) and on a macroscopic (behavioral) level. Wieraszko and Ball (1991, 1993) found that they could induce long-term potentiation (LTP)-like potentiation (see Winder and Kandel, Chapter 10) in hippocampal slices from song sparrows and pigeons. In white carneaux pigeons, this potentiation was not dependent on *N*-methyl-D-aspartate (NMDA) receptors, but it was NMDA receptor dependent in homing pigeons (Shapiro and Wieraszko, 1996). Apparently different mechanisms can be involved in the induction of LTP, even between different strains of the same species. Margrie *et al.* (1998) studied LTP in chicken hippocampal slices, and found that LTP was robust and long lasting, but was dependent neither on NMDA receptors nor on adenylyl cyclase, the two most commonly described forms of LTP in mammalian systems. From this physiological work, it is clear that there are forms of LTP in the avian hippocampus, but that their mechanisms may, in some cases, be different from those in mammals.

Based on the differential effects of NMDA blockers on LTP in homing versus non-homing pigeons, Meehan (1996) compared homing and non-homing pigeons on a spatial memory task (radial arm maze). Both breeds performed equally well when injected with saline vehicle. MK-801 (a non-competitive NMDA antagonist) had effects on spatial reference memory performance in non-homing pigeons, but not in homing pigeons. Spatial working memory was not affected in either breed. This result seems counter to the *in vitro* physiology results of Shapiro and Wieraszko (1996). MK-801 does have an effect on a natural form of spatial memory in homing pigeons (Riters and Bingman, 1994). Normal homing pigeons improve their homeward orientation on the second release from a particular location. MK-801 prevents this improvement in orientation. In both these experiments, the drugs were administered systemically. Therefore, brain structures other than the HF were probably also affected by the treatment. This could account for the inconsistencies among the *in vivo* and the *in vitro* experiments, as well as the differences between tasks. More detailed experiments using electrophysiology and functional neurochemistry are needed before we can fully understand the many subtleties of the functioning of the avian HF.

Lesion studies

Other investigations of the function of the avian hippocampus have taken the more classical approach of lesioning the structure and investigating which behavioral tasks are affected. This has been done both in a traditional laboratory situation, typically using pigeons and trying to replicate lesion effects observed in rats, and in more naturalistic situations, using a variety of bird species and their species-specific behaviors. Lesions of the HF in birds tend to affect those tasks that rely strongly on spatial information processing, but not those that do not. HF-lesioned pigeons are impaired on a reversal of position discrimination in a T-maze and on the acquisition of a conditional discrimination of position, but not on a pure pattern discrimination in the same apparatus (Good, 1987). They are also impaired on a forced-choice spatial alternation in a T-maze (Reilly and Good, 1987). They suffer from deficits in a delayed match to position task, but only with delays of 2 s and up (Good and Macphail, 1994a). Delayed match to sample tasks using color, non-match tasks using natural scenes (Good and Macphail, 1994a) and a non-spatial six-pair concurrent discrimination task (Colombo *et al.*, 1997b) are not affected by lesions of the HF. Acquisition of a radial arm maze equivalent is impaired (Colombo *et al.*, 1997a), as is the acquisition of the spatial version of a dry water maze equivalent, but not the cued version (Fremouw *et al.*, 1997). Excitotoxic lesions of a small part of the HF (up to 2.9%) in zebra finches (*Taeniopygia guttata*) result in impairment on a spatial memory task, as well as a less robust impairment on a color-cued version of the same task. Transplantation of embryonic HF tissue (but not anterior telencephalic tissue) into the lesion site was able to reverse the lesion effect on the spatial memory task (Patel *et al.*, 1997a).

HF lesions have no effect on some of the typical phenomena in classical conditioning in which one conditioned stimulus prevents the formation of an association with a different conditioned stimulus (overshadowing, blocking) (Good and Macphail, 1994b). They do, however, affect another classical conditioning phenomenon: the autoshaping of a keypeck (Good, 1987; Reilly and Good, 1989; Good and Macphail, 1994a,b). In this paradigm, the pigeon learns to peck a lighted key purely by association with the delivery of a reward. HF lesions also affect performance on a Differential Reinforcement of Low rates of responding (DRL) task. In this task, the animal has to withhold responding for a given period of time in order to receive a reward. Depending on the previous experience of the birds, they would either over-respond (Reilly and Good, 1989), or under-respond (i.e. improve performance) (Reilly and Good, 1987). The effects on autoshaping and DRL have been interpreted by the authors to be due to an inability to incorporate context into the learned representation, something that has been shown to be necessary in both autoshaping and DRL (Reilly and Good, 1989). Dependence on context has also been considered as a form of spatial information processing (see Brown, Chapter 11). Thus, in broad terms, the results of HF lesions found to date in birds are very similar to those found in mammals, in that they affect tasks in which spatial information processing is important, but not those in which it is not.

In mammals, several authors have proposed a role for the hippocampal formation in the processing of relational information, of which spatial information is a subcategory (Rudy and Sutherland, 1995; Eichenbaum *et al.*, 1996; for a discussion of the role of the mammalian hippocampus in memory, see also Brown, Chapter 11; Buckley and Gaffan, Chapter 16).

Strasser and Bingman (1997) found that HF-lesioned pigeons cannot encode the relationships between several different stimuli, but remember the stimuli separately from each other. The relationships between the stimuli in their task can be interpreted as being spatial in nature (e.g. 'food is in the blue cup next to the big landmark on the far side of the room'). Hippocampally lesioned pigeons would solve it as a single cue task (e.g. 'food is in the blue cup'). Bingman *et al.* (1998) directly tested the hypothesis that the HF in pigeons is involved in non-spatial relational encoding of paired associates (e.g. 'A' is rewarded when preceded by 'B', but not by 'C', 'D' or 'E'). They found that, unlike in rats (Rudy and Sutherland, 1995), hippocampal lesions do *not* disrupt this type of learning in the pigeon. Although the mammalian and avian hippocampus are obviously homologous, 300 million years of separate evolution may have led to differences in the types of information processed by this structure. The encoding of spatial information (which is inherently relational in nature) may be the ancestral function of this part of the brain. However, in different lineages, control of other distinct or unique types of relational information may have been adopted in the time since (Bingman *et al.*, 1998).

Natural behaviors
Several avian systems have been studied for the role of the HF in naturally occurring behaviors. Horn and colleagues have studied the neural basis of imprinting in newly hatched chicks (*Gallus gallus domesticus*). They found that exposure to an imprinting stimulus increased expression of the immediate early gene product Fos (see Clayton, Chapter 7) in the dorsolateral HF of chicks (McCabe and Horn, 1994), compared with controls that were kept in the dark. This expression was not related to how well the chick imprinted on the stimulus, however. The number of neurons expressing Fos in the ventrolateral HF correlated positively with the amount of approach activity the chick had shown towards the imprinting stimulus during training (McCabe and Horn, 1994). Electrophysiological recording showed that many neurons in the chick HF respond differentially to different distances between the chick and the imprinted stimulus (Nicol *et al.*, 1998). Sandi *et al.* (1992) showed that left (but not right) HF lesions in chicks impaired learning a passive avoidance task in which the animal learns not to peck at beads of a certain color. Both imprinting and avoidance of certain food items are adaptive and

natural learning behaviors for young galliforms. Though the involvement of the HF in these behaviors is not quite clear yet, these experiments eventually will help us to understand better the role of the avian HF in general.

Several laboratories have studied the role of HF in migration or long-distance navigation. Healy and colleagues have made use of the fact that many small songbirds migrate long distances, but nest in virtually the same area year after year. This feat requires a good memory for the local landmarks of the breeding and the wintering areas, as well as the various stopover locations along the way. In general, migratory birds do not appear to have a larger HF relative to brain size than do other, non-migratory birds (Krebs *et al.*, 1989; Healy *et al.*, 1991). Nevertheless, Healy *et al.* (1996) showed that garden warblers (*Sylvia borin*) which have experienced migration have a larger relative HF size than younger, pre-migration birds or age-matched birds kept in captivity for the first year, so they could not experience migration. This suggests not only an involvement of the HF in this kind of spatial navigation, but also an influence of experience on the size of the structure relative to the rest of the telencephalon.

This same involvement of the HF in navigation over longer distances has been studied in homing pigeons. Rehkämper *et al.* (1988) found that the HF in homing pigeons is larger than it is in non-homing breeds of pigeons. Bingman and colleagues showed in a series of studies that the HF in homing pigeons plays a role in navigation in the final phases of homing, when the bird has to navigate through familiar terrain to locate its own home loft (Bingman *et al.*, 1987, 1988; Bingman and Mench, 1990; Bingman and Yates, 1992). While the early stages of homing can be learned by birds with HF lesions, they do so by remembering a compass heading rather than by remembering relationships between landmarks (Gagliardo *et al.*, 1999). The HF is also involved in the development of the navigational map, which the birds use later in life to navigate home from unknown release locations. Once this map is established, the HF is not necessary any more for its use (Bingman *et al.*, 1990). Long-distance navigation is an example of an extreme form of spatial information processing that can only be studied in natural or semi-natural conditions. The involvement of the HF in this set of behaviors allows us to study its structure–function relationship under circumstances that would never be possible in a normal laboratory environment.

Variation in relative HF volume is related to another avian spatial behavior as well: remembering nest sites. The brownheaded cowbird (*Molothrus ater*) is a brood-parasitic species in which the female looks for possible host nests for her eggs. She monitors nests until they are at the appropriate stage in the host's breeding cycle, at which point she lays an egg in them. To do this, she must remember the location of all possible host nests. The male does not participate in this behavior. Sherry *et al.* (1993) found a sexual dimorphism in the relative size of the HF in this species, with the female having a relatively larger HF volume than the male. No such dimorphism was found in two closely related, non-parasitic species, the red-winged blackbird (*Agelaius phoeniceus*) and the common grackle (*Quiscalus quiscula*). Reboreda *et al.* (1996) expanded on this work by comparing three species of South American cowbirds with different patterns of reproductive behaviors. In one species (the shiny cowbird, *M. bonariensis*), females search for host sites as in the brown-headed cowbird. In the second species (the screaming cowbird, *M. rufoaxilaris*), both males and females look for host nests, while the third species (the bay-winged cowbird, *M. badius*) is not brood parasitic. The volumes of the HF followed the predicted pattern, being larger in the brood parasites than in the non-brood parasites, and only showing a sexual dimorphism in the species that was sexually dimorphic in its behavior. Clayton *et al.* (1997) found that brood parasites had a smaller HF outside the breeding season, while there was no seasonal variation in the HF of non-parasitic species. This model system illustrates how sex differences, interspecific differences and seasonal patterns in behavior can be reflected in the underlying neuroanatomy. The study of the mechanisms underlying these differences will contribute significantly to our knowledge of how the HF processes spatial information.

Conclusion

Because of the similarities in embryology, connectivity, neurochemistry and function, the avian HF can be considered homologous to its mammalian counterpart. However, 300 million years of independent evolution have also resulted in many differences, most prominently in cytoarchitecture. The HF of many bird species plays an important role in behaviors that have spatial characteristics. In some of these species, a behavioral specialization for spatial information processing (such as long-distance navigation or nest searching) is accompanied by a larger relative volume of the HF. This link between spatial information processing, the size of the HF and its function has been particularly well studied in food-hoarding birds and will be reviewed in detail in the next part of this chapter.

INVOLVEMENT OF THE AVIAN HIPPOCAMPAL FORMATION IN THE MEMORY FOR HOARDED FOOD

Behavior

Animals from many different lineages hoard food to buffer temporary food shortages. Different forms of this behavior can be classified along a continuum from 'larder hoarding' to 'scatter hoarding' (Vander Wall, 1990). At the one extreme, all food reserves are stored in one central larder (usually in a nest or burrow), and defended from possible thieves. This strategy is employed by species as diverse as bees, hamsters and acorn woodpeckers. At the other extreme, scatter hoarders hide each food item in a different location. They cannot physically defend their caches against thieves but, by distributing them across a wide range, they are able to distribute the risk of losing their entire hoard (Sherry *et al.*, 1982; Vander Wall, 1990). This strategy is employed by many rodents (e.g. squirrels and kangaroo rats) and bird species (e.g. chickadees, jays and nuthatches).

Retrieving scatter-hoarded food items poses an interesting spatial challenge to the individuals that employ this strategy. Any obvious external markings indicating the location of caches would alert potential thieves to their presence and would diminish their benefit to the hoarding individual. One strategy that allows a hoarder to retrieve scattered caches months later is to only hoard in its own foraging niche, which can be different even from that of conspecific group members (Pravosudov, 1986; Brodin, 1994b; Smulders, 1998). Another strategy is to remember exactly where each of the caches has been stored. Species from both the Corvidae (crows and jays) and Paridae (chickadees and titmice) have been shown to be able to remember the exact locations of their caches, either in the laboratory or in the field (Tomback, 1980; Sherry *et al.*, 1981; Shettleworth and Krebs, 1982; Hitchcock and Sherry, 1990). Whereas for the parid species studied, the maximum duration for this memory does not seem to exceed 4–6 weeks (Hitchcock and Sherry, 1990; Brodin, 1994a), Clark's nutcracker (*Nucifraga columbiana*, a corvid) has been

shown to remember the location of buried seeds for up to 9 months (Balda and Kamil, 1992). Remembering locations of up to many thousands of cached food items (Pravosudov, 1985) clearly requires a very detailed and long-lasting representation of spatial information. Because of this, scatter-hoarding birds have become the model of choice to study the role of the avian HF in adaptively specialized spatial processing.

The strength of the food-hoarding system as a model for spatial memory in general lies in the fact that it is a naturally occurring behavior, shaped by natural selection. We can therefore assume that the underlying neural mechanisms have been optimized by evolution to perform the required behavior better or more efficiently. To elucidate exactly which aspects of both behavior and its neural underpinnings have been affected by such selective pressures, it is necessary to conduct comparative studies. In this type of experiment, food-hoarding species are compared with non-hoarding species on the feature of interest, be it brain or behavior. It is important that the non-hoarding species chosen for these comparisons are as similar to the hoarding species as possible, with the exception of the hoarding behavior. This means that, ideally, they should be matched for such characteristics as preferred habitat, social system, ecological niche and phylogeny. This is possible to a large degree in the European parid species: non-hoarding blue tits (*Parus caeruleus*) and great tits (*P. major*) are sympatric with hoarding species such as marsh tits (*P. palustris*) and coal tits (*P. ater*) and exploit similar resources. In North America, however, no non-hoarding parid species can be found, and compromises have to be made. Because species never differ only on food-hoarding behavior, only by comparing many different species on many different aspects of brain and behavior can we identify characteristics that are specific to the food-hoarding life-style (Kamil, 1988). Many of these experiments will be in the laboratory, because of the experimental control allowed in this environment. However, it is important eventually to test laboratory findings against the litmus test of the animals' natural environment if we want to be sure that our findings are relevant to the natural behavior we are studying.

Comparative neuroanatomy

Volumes
In 1989, Sherry, Krebs and colleagues (Krebs *et al.*, 1989; Sherry *et al.*, 1989) compared HF volume among

several families of songbirds, including North American and European species. When they controlled HF size for body size and the size of the rest of the brain, they found that species in food-hoarding families had a larger HF than did those in non-hoarding families. Since one of the food-hoarding families in question (the Paridae) consists of two branches, one of which is made up of non-hoarders and the other of hoarding species (Figure 8.3), they split that family in two. Within this family, the hoarding species had a larger HF than the non-hoarders. For example, marsh tits (a hoarding species) have a larger absolute HF than great tits (a non-hoarder), even though the great tit is twice as heavy as the marsh tit and has a larger brain (Krebs *et al.*, 1989).

This basic finding—that food-hoarding species having a larger relative HF than non-hoarding species—has since been replicated several times (Shettleworth *et al.*, 1995; Hampton and Shettleworth, 1996b). Across different hoarding species, relative HF size is related to the intensity with which the species hoards, its dependence on hoarded food during its life cycle and/or its manner of hoarding. Healy and Krebs (1992, 1996) compared different species of corvids and parids and classified them as (i) storing little or not at all, (ii) storing tens to hundreds of food items and (iii) storing thousands of food items and being very dependent on these for survival. They found that relative HF volume correlated positively with their classification of hoarding intensity. Hampton *et al.* (1995) found similar results when comparing three species of North American parids [black-capped chickadee (*Parus atricapillus*), Mexican chickadee (*P. clateri*) and bridled titmouse (*P. wollweberi*)]. The black-capped chickadees stored more seeds in a laboratory experiment than did the other two species, and they also had the largest HF. Basil *et al.* (1996) compared four species of food-hoarding corvids, and again found that HF volume correlated with the intensity of hoarding by these species in the field. Finally, Volman *et al.* (1997) compared brain structure across four woodpecker species: red-bellied woodpeckers (*Melanerpes carolinus*) that scatter hoard, redheaded woodpeckers (*M. erythrocephalus*) that larder hoard and hairy (*Picoides villosus*) and downy woodpeckers (*P. pubescens*) that do not hoard. They found that the scatter-hoarding species has a larger HF than the congeneric larder-hoarding species, as would be predicted from its need to retain more items in spatial memory. The non-hoarding species they studied (which are more distantly related), however,

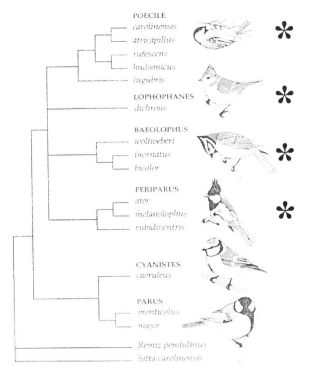

Figure 8.3. Phylogeny of the family Paridae. Asterisks indicate food-hoarding branches. Note that food-hoarding behavior seems to be a monophyletic trait in this family. (Adapted from Slikas *et al.* 1996, courtesy of the *Journal of Avian Biology*).

also have a larger HF than the larder hoarder. This discrepancy still remains to be explained. In summary, scatter-hoarding species seem to have a larger relative HF than closely related non-scatter hoarders. We believe that this reflects their need for better spatial information processing involved in hoarding and retrieving their caches.

Neurochemistry
Several studies have investigated neurochemical differences in the HF between hoarding and non-hoarding species. Montagnese *et al.* (1993) found that there are calbindin-immunoreactive neurons in the HF of two unrelated species of food-storing birds [marsh tit and magpie (*Pica pica*)] and two unrelated species of non-storing birds [great tits and jackdaws (*Corvus monedula*)], but the cells are larger in the food storers. Further work is needed to determine whether this difference is related specifically to enhanced spatial processing. In addition, food-hoarding birds have more nitric oxide (NO) synthase in their HF than do non-hoarding birds (Székely and Krebs, 1993;

Székely, 1999). NO is a molecule that some authors claim is important for certain forms of synaptic plasticity in the hippocampus of mammals (Holscher, 1997). Stewart *et al.* (1999) report that food-hoarding marsh tits have a (24%) lower density of NMDA receptors in the HF than do non-hoarding blue tits. If we expect NMDA receptors to be involved in neuronal plasticity, this result is counterintuitive. It is reminiscent, however, of the results obtained by Meehan (1996) comparing homing and non-homing pigeons, as discussed in the first section of this chapter. Clearly, much remains to be discovered about the anatomy and physiology of the avian HF before such findings can be related to HF function in birds generally, and before neurochemical differences between storing and non-storing species can be related to differences in behavior.

Development

The previous section shows that there are substantial differences in relative HF volume between hoarding and non-hoarding bird species. Do these differences occur with maturation or are they experience dependent? A series of experiments by Clayton, Healy, Krebs and co-workers have shed light on this question. Healy (Healy and Krebs, 1993; Healy *et al.*, 1994) investigated volume, cell number and density in the HF of hoarders (h) and non-hoarders (nh) from two families [parids: marsh tit (h) and blue tit (nh); corvids: magpie (h) and jackdaw (nh)]. Within families, there is no difference in relative HF volume between nestlings of the hoarding and non-hoarding species, but there is in the adults (hoarders>non-hoarders; Figure 8.4). The difference in HF volume in the adults is due to fewer neurons in the HF of the non-hoarders together with a slightly higher cell density (i.e. less neuropil). Both hoarders and non-hoarders of comparable sizes start off with the same number of neurons in the HF as nestlings. The HF attains its adult morphology slowly in comparison with other telencephalic structures. During this prolonged development, non-hoarding birds undergo a net loss of neurons compared with the hoarders. We have found that juvenile black-capped chickadees (~30–90 days post-hatch) have a smaller HF than adults caught at the same time of the year (Smulders *et al.*, 1995). These juveniles have much higher cell densities than adults, resulting in similar total cell numbers between juveniles and adults in the late spring and summer (Smulders *et al.*, 2000). By the mid-fall, this difference in cell density between adults

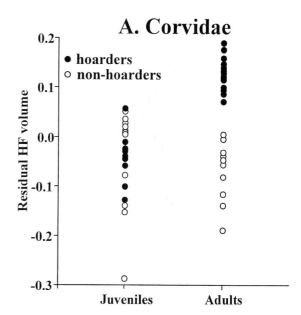

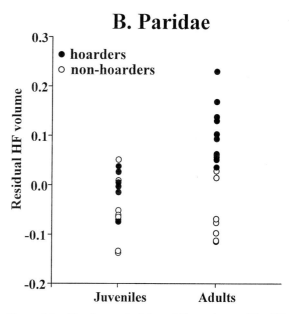

Figure 8.4. Development of the relative volume of the HF in hoarding and non-hoarding species in two families of songbirds: Corvidae (**A**) and Paridae (**B**). Closed symbols represent the hoarding species [(magpie (*Pica pica*; A) and marsh tit (*Parus palustris*; B)] and open symbols the non-hoarding species [jackdaw (*Corvus monedula*; A) and blue tit (*Parus caeruleus*; B)]. (Adapted from Healy and Krebs, Copyright 1993 and Healy *et al.*, Copyright 1994, with permission from Elsevier Science.)

and juveniles has mostly disappeared (see Figure 8.7, below). Thus, attaining adult HF volume coincides with the development of independent foraging and hoarding. Could this experience affect HF development?

Clayton investigated the neural and behavioral development of food hoarding in parids in some detail (Clayton, 1992, 1994, 1995a,b, 1996; Clayton and Krebs, 1994a). She found that food-hoarding behavior in marsh tits develops as a combination of effects of maturation and experience. Food-hoarding behavior starts abruptly at about 6 weeks after hatching. The actual handling of seeds for storage improves with experience, as does the use of memory to retrieve previously stored items (Clayton, 1992, 1994). Hippocampal volume is larger in birds that are allowed to store than in those that never have an opportunity to do so, indicating that experience also plays a role in the rate and extent of HF development (at least within the window of the experiment, which went up to 138 days post-hatch) (Clayton and Krebs, 1994a). Experienced birds have more neurons in the HF, while deprived birds have more apoptotic cells (Clayton, 1995b, 1996; Clayton and Krebs, 1994a) and/or fewer newly generated neurons (Patel *et al.*, 1997b). The same effect of experience with storing on HF volume can be obtained by using a non-hoarding spatial memory task, such as a one-trial associative memory task (Clayton, 1995a). In this task, the birds are required to return to a feeder which they earlier had found to be baited. Exposing non-hoarding blue tits to this same task has no effect on their adult HF volume. The two species differ not only in their neural response to solving this task, but also in the way they solve it. Whereas marsh tits remember exactly which of the feeders was baited in the exploration phase, blue tits seem to remember which feeders they had visited, but not whether they were baited or not. It is possible that this difference in strategy is related to the differences in how the brain responds to the spatial memory experience. Whether it is directly responsible for these differences, however, is not yet clear. What is clear is that whatever the underlying mechanism, the marsh tit HF responds to experience with forming spatial memories, while the blue tit HF does not.

In summary, food-hoarding birds obtain their larger HF relative to non-hoarders by maintaining more neurons from fledging to adulthood. Both hoarding and non-hoarding species overproduce neurons and then later discard a proportion of them, but hoarders discard fewer. Experience with the use of spatial memory seems to be crucial in this process for hoarders, but does not make a difference for non-hoarders. Further comparative studies are needed to investigate which features of the HF allow spatial memory experience to influence neuronal survival in one group, but have no effect in the other.

The function of the HF in memory for spatial locations

Lesion studies

Krushinskaya (1966) lesioned the HF in Eurasian nutcrackers and found that they were unable to retrieve previously stored nuts in their outdoor aviary. Approximately 20 years later, Sherry and Vaccarino (1989) performed the same manipulation in black-capped chickadees. Their HF-lesioned birds continued to cache seeds. However, they did not retrieve them except at chance levels of accuracy (Figure 8.5). The control lesioned group (in the hyperstriatum accessorium) retrieved previously stored caches with the same accuracy as sham-lesioned animals. When tested on a task in which baited sites were marked with cue cards, the HF-lesioned animals performed well on the (non-spatial) reference memory part of the task (knowing that the cards indicated food), but poorly on the (spatial) working memory part (remembering which of the visually identical cards they had already visited). These results suggest again that, as for homing pigeons (discussed earlier), an intact HF is necessary for spatial information processing.

HF lesions also cause deficits in other forms of spatial cognition. Large neurotoxic lesions of the HF in black-capped chickadees had a deleterious effect on re-acquiring a spatial reference memory task, but not on a simple cue version of the same task (Rice, 1992). Hampton and Shettleworth (1996a) found similar results in an operant task. They trained black-capped chickadees and dark-eyed juncos (*Junco hyemalis*) on a delayed match to sample task in which either the color or the location of the stimuli on a touch screen was the relevant dimension for obtaining a reward. HF lesions in both species affected performance on the spatial aspect of the task, but not on the color aspect. It is interesting to note in this context that food-hoarding parids prefer to use spatial cues over local color cues when the two are dissociated experimentally (Brodbeck, 1994; Clayton and Krebs, 1994b; Brodbeck and Shettleworth, 1995). Non-hoarders (who have a smaller HF relative to the rest of the

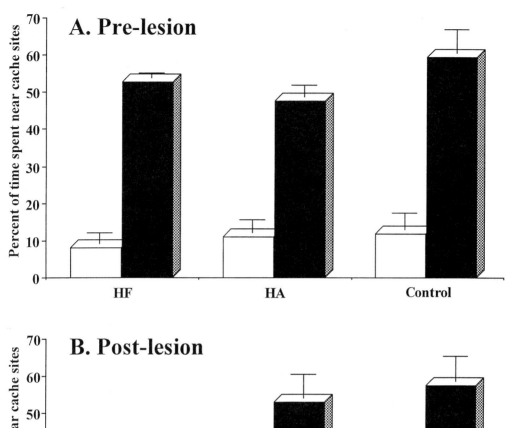

Figure 8.5. Recovery accuracy of black-capped chickadees before (**A**) and after (**B**) surgery. The open bars represent the amount of time spent (during a pre-cache phase) near the sites in which the birds will have cached later during the cache phase. Closed bars represent the amount of time spent near these same sites during the recovery phase (seeds had been removed). After HF lesion [but not after hyperstriatum accessorium (HA) lesion or sham lesion], birds performed at chance levels. Error bars represent the standard error of the mean. (From Sherry and Vaccarino, Copyright 1989 by the American Psychological Association. Adapted with permission.)

brain) show no preference of spatial cues over color ones when tested on the same task. They were equally likely to choose either cue when confronted with an experimental dissociation of the two.

In summary, lesions of the HF disrupt cache recovery in food-hoarding birds. From the experiments discussed here, it is not clear whether the impairment is the consequence of an encoding deficit, a retrieval deficit or both. To address this question, more subtle manipulations need to be used, such as temporary inactivation of the HF only during hoarding or only during retrieval. Other spatial memory tasks were also impaired by HF lesions, but not memory performance on non-spatial tasks. This is consistent with the data for other avian species, discussed in the first half of this chapter.

Immediate early gene expression
Another approach to understanding the function of the HF in food hoarding is the use of molecular markers of neural activity, such as immediate early genes (Clayton and Krebs, 1995; Smulders and De Voogd, 2000; for a discussion of immediate early gene techniques, see also Clayton, Chapter 7). Clayton

and Krebs (1995) found that food-hoarding experience causes an up-regulation of Fos expression in the left (but not the right) HF of marsh tits, and a down-regulation of Fos in the right LPO, a region known to be connected to the HF (Veenman *et al.*, 1995; Székely and Krebs, 1996). Smulders and DeVoogd (2000) found that black-capped chickadees that had just stored seeds, or retrieved previously stored items, had fewer Fra-1-like immunoreactive cells in the dorsal part of the HF than did control birds that just flew around the room without storing or retrieving (Figure 8.6). This shows that the HF is involved during both the storing and the retrieval phase of the food-hoarding behavior. Closer examination of the birds in the retrieval condition revealed that the number of HF cells expressing ZENK was positively related to the accuracy with which the birds retrieved their seeds. In addition, birds that had stored, and consequently retrieved, more items, had more Fos-like immunoreactive cells in the HF (Smulders and DeVoogd, 2000). These results suggest that more neurons are activated, or recruited into the active circuit, as more items are remembered successfully. Extrapolated to a larger scale, this may explain why food-hoarding birds have

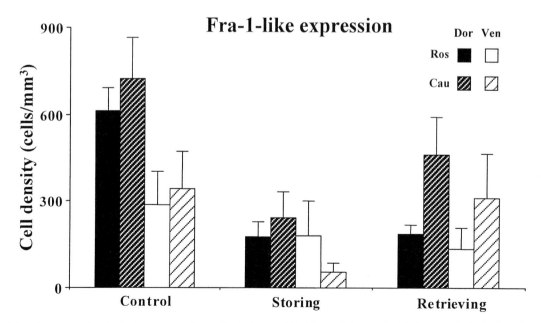

Figure 8.6. Density of Fra-1-like immunoreactive cells in four subdivisions of the HF in black-capped chickadees that were exposed to three different treatments: controls, storing and retrieving. Density is higher in the dorsal HF of control birds, compared with the other two groups. Dark bars represent dorsal regions and striped bars represent caudal regions. Error bars represent the standard error of the mean. (From Smulders and DeVoogd, 2000.)

a larger HF with more neurons than non-hoarders. A larger circuit containing more neurons is necessary simply to remember accurately the many different locations these animals need to keep in memory.

Smulders *et al.* (1997) also found suggestive evidence (*P*-values varied between 0.04 and 0.07 depending on the location of the counting grid) of a reduction of the number of Fos-immunoreactive cells in the intermediate area of the medial hyperstriatum ventrale in the retrieval group compared with both the hoarding and control groups. This area is very similar in location to the intermediate and medial hyperstriatum ventrale (IMHV) of chicks, which is known to be involved in imprinting and passive avoidance learning (Horn *et al.*, 1979; Rose, 1991; McCabe and Horn, 1994; Honey *et al.*, 1995; see also Horn, Chapter 19) and receives input from the HF (Bradley *et al.*, 1985). Both LPO (mentioned earlier) and IMHV are brain areas that are involved in forms of visual learning and that are downstream from the HF. It is possible that they play a role in remembering some aspect of the caches, such as their location, appearance or content. Here again, more research is needed to investigate the neural basis for sensory integration in this form of spatial learning.

Seasonal changes in food hoarding and the HF

In all parid species studied in detail, food hoarding is a seasonal behavior. The animals show a clear peak in hoarding during fall, when the seed crop is abundant and winter shortages are imminent (Odum, 1942; Ludescher, 1980; Pravosudov, 1985; Nakamura and Wako, 1988; Vander Wall, 1990). Smulders *et al.* (1995) investigated whether this peak in behavior was accompanied by a peak in HF anatomy. They found that the HF in free-living black-capped chickadees is larger, relative to the rest of the brain, in the mid-fall than at any other time of the year. By early winter, the HF is back down to the same size as during the rest of the year (Figure 8.7A). The increase in HF volume is due mainly to an increase in cell number in the late summer and fall, followed by a net cell loss towards early winter (Figure 8.7B; Smulders *et al.*, 2000). Barnea and Nottebohm (1994) found a peak of neurogenesis in the HF of free-living black-capped chickadees around this same time of year (fall), but they did not find a seasonal change in overall cell number. The discrepancy between their results and those of Smulders *et al.* (2000) may be due to differences in the exact timing of the collection of the brains. Both juvenile (first year) birds and adults undergo an increase in cell number toward fall

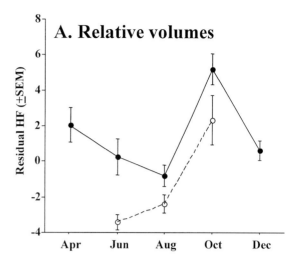

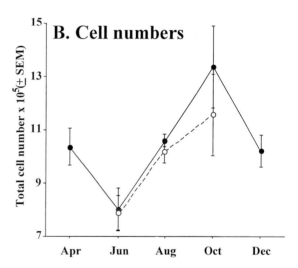

Figure 8.7. Seasonal changes in relative HF volume (**A**) and estimated total cell number (**B**) in the HF of wild-caught black-capped chickadees. Closed symbols represent adult animals and open symbols represent juvenile birds. Error bars represent the standard error of the mean. (Adapted from Smulders *et al.*, 1995 and Smulders *et al.*, 2000)

(Smulders *et al.*, 2000). Barnea and Nottebohm (1996) found that juvenile black-capped chickadees in the early fall have more newly generated neurons as well as more total neurons than adult birds. Smulders *et al.* (2000) did not find evidence for this, but, again, he did not sample the exact same time period as did Barnea and Nottebohm (1996). It is therefore possible that the increase in cell number happens earlier in juveniles than in adults. Studies on a more detailed time scale are necessary to resolve these discrepancies.

At first, it seems strange that the increase in HF volume should only be maintained during the fall season, while hoarded seeds are used throughout winter. Some corvid species (such as Clark's nut-cracker, *Nucifraga columbiana*) have been shown to remember their caches for up to 9 months (Balda and Kamil, 1992). These corvids cache their seeds far away from their summer time foraging range, and need to retrieve them from under thick layers of snow, buried in the soil. However, both in the laboratory (Hitchcock and Sherry, 1990) and in the field (Brodin, 1994a), the estimate of the maximum memory duration for a parid species is only of the order of 4 weeks. Most parids cache their food in the same foraging niche they will be using all winter, such as on branches or between twigs high up in the trees (Pravosudov, 1985, 1986; Brodin, 1994a,b; Lens *et al.*, 1994). They will come across these same food items during their foraging all winter long, and have no need to remember all locations for months on end (Brodin and Clark, 1997; Smulders, 1998). During winter, these birds do still hoard and retrieve smaller numbers of food items over a time period of hours to days but, presumably, the normal, year-round size of the HF is sufficient to accommodate this smaller memory load.

So why do chickadees have an enlarged HF in the fall at all? During the peak in food hoarding, the animals need to distribute their caches as optimally as possible. Badly distributed caches are more prone to loss to heterospecific thieves, such as other small songbirds and squirrels. Sherry *et al.* (1982) placed artificial caches in typical marsh tit cache locations, at different densities, and showed that there is an optimal density of caches. They also showed that marsh tits store their food items at approximately that optimum. Not only should the caches be placed at a certain density, but the distribution should be as uniform as possible. A more patchy distribution makes it easier for other animals to steal more of the caches, using a local search pattern. All these require-ments for cache distribution make it important for the bird to remember where it has stored previous caches while distributing new ones. Thus, we infer that having to remember the many thousands of cache locations made during the fall for the duration of the hoarding peak would be the reason for the increase in HF volume at that time of year (Smulders and Dhondt, 1997). This hypothesis could be tested in certain corvid species. Because many corvid species need to remember all their caches throughout winter, we would predict an increase in HF volume that lasts through the hoarding as well as the retrieval period. No studies have yet been conducted on seasonal changes in the HF of any corvid species, so this issue remains to be addressed.

Is the observed seasonal increase in HF volume dependent on the experience of actually hoarding seeds? Cristol (1996) provided one group of willow tits (*Parus montanus*) with the opportunity to store many seeds for the duration of a month, while depriving another group of any hoarding experience at all. Afterward, the two groups did not differ in HF volume. These birds, however, had been in captivity for many years and the amount of storing that they did in captivity was nowhere near the normal amount observed in the field. It is also possible that seasonal cues, such as day length and temperature, trigger the change in HF volume directly. Krebs *et al.* (1995) induced hoarding behavior in the laboratory by housing birds on decreasing day length and tempera-ture. Their birds hoarded in a wooden block in the home cage, so they did not need to use memory to retrieve their caches. This study also did not find a difference in the volume of HF between birds that were induced to hoard in this way and birds that were kept on long days.

It is clear that whichever cue triggers the addition of new cells and the consequent increase in HF volume in the wild, these two laboratory studies were not able to replicate it. A more detailed inspection of the seasonal data from the wild-caught birds reveals an increase in cell density in the rostral part of the HF in the late summer, before the increase in HF volume (Smulders *et al.*, 2000). This is the same region of the HF in which Barnea and Nottebohm (1994) observed most of the newly generated neurons. This may indi-cate that the onset of cell addition starts around this time of year. Since this is presumably slightly before the start of the hoarding peak, it suggests that non-experiential factors play a role at least in initiating the process. It is possible that only an interplay of both environmental (day length and temperature) and experiential factors can obtain the full effect observed in the wild caught birds.

To summarize, in parids, the HF is larger and con-tains more neurons during the peak in hoarding behavior that takes place in the fall, but is back down to year-round levels in early winter. This pattern probably reflects the need for high memory capacity during the hoarding peak, when the birds have to keep track of a large inventory of caches. In winter, the caches can be retrieved by random foraging in the birds' own niches and there is no more need for increased memory capacity. The mechanisms underlying the increase and later decrease in HF morphology are still unknown.

Future directions

Research on food-hoarding birds has yielded some important information about the role of the HF in spatial cognition. A better understanding of the importance of anatomical specializations such as increased cell number or larger calbindin-immunoreactive cells, relative to non-hoarders, may contribute to our knowledge of how memory systems work in general. In order to put these differences in the proper context, however, a better knowledge is needed of the basic anatomy of the avian HF. Even though its external connections have been fairly well described, little is known about its internal connectivity and functional subdivision. More detailed tracing studies inside the HF of both hoarding and non-hoarding birds will be necessary to fill this gap.

The difference in the role that memory may play in long-term hoarding in the corvids, but not in the parids, will prove to be an important insight upon which studies of the more basic processes of memory can be based. It seems that most food-hoarding parids have been adapted for a large memory capacity, especially during the fall. Corvids such as Clark's nutcracker, however, are adapted both for capacity and duration of memory. A more detailed anatomical and physiological investigation of the differences between the HF of the two types of food hoarders should yield clues as to the (possibly different) neural mechanisms underlying memory duration and memory capacity.

A direction of investigation that has hardly been touched upon in this field is the use of electrophysiological techniques. If the avian HF is indeed homologous to its mammalian counterpart, we would expect to find neurons that respond selectively to the animal's current location in the environment ('place cells') (O'Keefe and Dostrovsky, 1971; Muller and Kubie, 1987; Muller *et al.*, 1987). Comparative studies of how these cells react to manipulations of the environment in hoarders and non-hoarders should give us a deeper insight into how spatial information is processed, and how this processing can be modified to meet the specialized needs of hoarding species. The *in vitro* approach, using slice preparations, should also be expanded, as it allows a more detailed comparison of cellular and molecular processes in hippocampal

physiology between the different groups of birds. Both these approaches promise to contribute significantly to our knowledge and understanding of spatial information processing in birds, and possibly in mammals as well.

The regulation of the seasonal increase in cell number, as well as its behavioral implications, is another important avenue of exploration. Clayton and Cristol (1996) found that marsh tits perform slightly (but significantly) better at a spatial memory task during decreasing day length than they do during increasing or long day length. It would be interesting to see if the way in which information is processed by this 'augmented' HF is different from information processing with a 'non-enlarged' HF. Again, an interaction of neuroanatomical, physiological and behavioral experiments with food-hoarding birds could shed light on such basic questions of the structure–function relationship in memory processing.

Finally, even though the HF is the only structure studied in any detail in this context to date, it should be evident that it is not the only brain structure involved in the memory for cache locations. As we mentioned earlier, there is some suggestive evidence to implicate parts of the LPO and the hyperstriatum ventrale in remembering locations of hoarded food. Neither piece of evidence was conclusive, such that further directed research will be necessary in order to investigate whether these (and possibly other) brain areas play a role in this system. The fact that both areas receive inputs from the HF, and that both play a role in visual learning in chicks, would make them prime candidates, even if they had not been implicated by other experiments.

GENERAL CONCLUSIONS

The research summarized above raises far more questions than it answers. Clearly the HF is required in birds for processing spatial information, as it is in mammals. Clearly, too, adding 'more' hippocampus, whether through evolutionary selection or through plastic processes within an animal, augments the animal's capacity for behaviors that require spatial skills. However, we know almost nothing of the neural processes responsible for these capacities. We do not know which attributes of hippocampal anatomy and physiology allow it to play an important role in the analysis and storage of spatial information. Does the hippocampus form spatial maps or, more broadly, index classes of information, as has been suggested for mammals? Research is underway in several laboratories that will describe hippocampal connectivity, physiology and biochemistry in birds in greater detail, and that will work out plausible mechanisms of synaptic plasticity.

What sets aside the comparative approach to neurobiology are questions of natural function. How does the avian hippocampus carry out the high demands naturally placed on it by birds that evolved the specialized spatial behaviors mentioned above? To date, research on this system has used experimental designs so much more limited than the animals' natural capacities as to be almost of a different category. As we write this, we watch a phoebe bring insects to its young in a nest over the doorway to the house. This phoebe has nested in this exact site now for 3 years and, in between, has migrated to and from South America three times. What sort of neural algorithm can seamlessly blend the scales of intercontinental maps, regional geography and local landmarks, resulting in this accurate, precisely timed commuting? Similarly, what sort of neural database can keep track either of the thousands of items needed for the survival of a Siberian tit, or of dozens of miles of changing landscape over many months of retention experienced by Clark's nutcracker? Choosing between a handful of feeders in a laboratory over an interval of hours or pecking computer keys would seem to tap abilities that are radically simpler. As we begin to design experiments that go beyond present laboratory studies toward investigating these natural capacities, we may not only discover how plastic changes occur in a brain structure designed for spatial analysis, but we may also discover novel algorithms for efficient coding that mammals have never evolved.

ACKNOWLEDGEMENTS

We are grateful to Johan Bolhuis, Kristy Gould-Beierle, Saleem Nicola and Tora Smulders-Srinivasan for their constructive criticism of earlier drafts of this manuscript.

REFERENCES

Amaral, D.G. and Witter, M.P. (1995) Hippocampal formation. In: Paxinos, G. (ed.), *The Rat Nervous System*, 2nd edn. Academic Press, San Diego, pp. 443–493.

Balda, R.P. and Kamil, A.C. (1992) Long-term spatial memory in Clark's nutcracker, *Nucifraga columbiana*. *Animal Behaviour*, 44, 761–769.

Barnea, A. and Nottebohm, F. (1994) Seasonal recruitment of hippocampal neurons in adult free-ranging black-capped chickadees. *Proceedings of the National Academy of Sciences of the United States of America*, 91, 11217–11221.

Barnea, A. and Nottebohm, F. (1996) Recruitment and replacement of hippocampal neurons in young and adult chickadees: an addition to the theory of hippocampal learning. *Proceedings of the National Academy of Sciences of the United States of America*, 93, 714–718.

Basil, J.A., Kamil, A.C., Balda, R.P. and Fite, K.V. (1996) Differences in hippocampal volume among food storing corvids. *Brain, Behavior and Evolution*, 47, 156–164.

Benowitz, L.I. and Karten, H.J. (1976) The tractus infundibuli and other afferents to the parahippocampal region of the pigeon. *Brain Research*, 102, 174–180.

Bettini, E., Pollio, G., Santagati, S. and Maggi, A. (1992) Estrogen receptor in rat brain: presence in the hippocampal formation. *Neuroendocrinology*, 56, 502–508.

Bingman, V.P. and Mench, J.A. (1990) Homing behavior of hippocampus and parahippocampus lesioned pigeons following short-distance releases. *Behavioural Brain Research*, 40, 227–238.

Bingman, V.P. and Yates, G. (1992) Hippocampal lesions impair navigational learning in experienced homing pigeons. *Behavioral Neuroscience*, 106, 229–232.

Bingman, V.P., Ioale, P., Casini, G. and Bagnoli, P. (1987) Impaired retention of preoperatively acquired spatial reference memory in homing pigeons following hippocampal ablation. *Behavioural Brain Research*, 26, 147–156.

Bingman, V.P., Ioale, P., Casini, G. and Bagnoli, P. (1988) Hippocampal ablated homing pigeons show a persistent impairment in the time taken to return home. *Journal of Comparative Physiology A*, 163, 559–563.

Bingman, V.P., Ioale, P., Casini, G. and Bagnoli, P. (1990) The avian hippocampus: evidence for a role in the development of the homing pigeon navigational map. *Behavioral Neuroscience*, 104, 906–911.

Bingman, V.P., Casini, G., Nocjar, C. and Jones, T.J. (1994) Connections of the piriform cortex in homing pigeons (*Columba livia*) studied with fast blue and WGA–HRP. *Brain, Behavior and Evolution*, 43, 206–218.

Bingman, V.P., Strasser, R., Baker, C. and Riters, L.V. (1998) Paired-associate learning is unaffected by combined hippocampal and parahippocampal lesions in homing pigeons. *Behavioral Neuroscience*, 112, 533–540.

Bons, K., Bouillé, C., Baylé, J.D. and Assenmacher, I. (1976) Light and electron microscopic evidence of hypothalamic afferences originating from the hippocampus in the pigeon. *Experientia*, 32, 1443–1445.

Bouillé, C., Raymond, J. and Baylé, J.D. (1977) Retrograde transport of horseradish peroxidase from the nucleus posterior medialis hypothalami to the hippocampus and the medial septum in the pigeon. *Neuroscience*, 2, 435–439.

Bradley, P., Davies, D.C. and Horn, G. (1985) Connections of the hyperstriatum ventrale of the domestic chick (*Gallus domesticus*). *Journal of Anatomy*, 140, 577–589.

Brodbeck, D.R. (1994) Memory for spatial and local cues: a comparison of a storing and a nonstoring species. *Animal Learning and Behavior*, 22, 119–133.

Brodbeck, D.R. and Shettleworth, S.J. (1995) Matching location and color of a compound stimulus: comparison of a food-storing and a nonstoring bird species. *Journal of Experimental Psychology: Animal Behavior Processes*, 21, 64–77.

Brodin, A. (1994a) The disappearance of caches that have been stored by naturally foraging willow tits. *Animal Behaviour*, 47, 730–732.

Brodin, A. (1994b) Separation of caches between individual willow tits hoarding under natural conditions. *Animal Behaviour*, 47, 1031–1035.

Brodin, A. and Clark, C.W. (1997) Long-term hoarding in the *Paridae*: a dynamic model. *Behavioral Ecology*, 8, 178–185.

Capaldi, E.A., Robinson, G.E. and Fahrbach, S.E. (1999) Neuroethology of spatial learning: the birds and the bees. *Annual Review of Psychology*, 50, 651–682.

Casini, G., Bingman, V.P. and Bagnoli, P. (1986) Connections of the pigeon dorsomedial forebrain studied with WGA–HRP and ^{3}H-proline. *Journal of Comparative Neurology*, 245, 454–470.

Clayton, N.S. (1992) The ontogeny of food-storing and retrieval in marsh tits. *Behaviour*, 122, 11–25.

Clayton, N.S. (1994) The role of age and experience in the behavioural development of food-storing and retrieval in marsh tits, *Parus palustris*. *Animal Behaviour*, 47, 1435–1444.

Clayton, N.S. (1995a) Development of memory and the hippocampus: comparison of food-storing and nonstoring birds on a one-trial associative memory task. *Journal of Neuroscience*, 15, 2796–2807.

Clayton, N.S. (1995b) The neuroethological development of food-storing memory: a case of use it, or lose it! *Behavioural Brain Research*, 70, 95–102.

Clayton, N.S. (1996) Development of food-storing and the hippocampus in juvenile marsh tits (*Parus palustris*). *Behavioural Brain Research*, 74, 153–159.

Clayton, N.S. and Cristol, D.A. (1996) Effects of photoperiod on memory and food storing in captive marsh tits, *Parus palustris*. *Animal Behaviour*, 52, 715–726.

Clayton, N.S. and Krebs, J.R. (1994a) Hippocampal growth and attrition in birds affected by experience. *Proceedings of the National Academy of Sciences of the United States of America*, 91, 7410–7414.

Clayton, N.S. and Krebs, J.R. (1994b) Memory for spatial and object-specific cues in food-storing and non-storing birds. *Journal of Comparative Physiology A*, 174, 371–379.

Clayton, N.S. and Krebs, J.R. (1995) Lateralization in memory and the avian hippocampus in food-storing birds. In: Alleva, E., Fasolo, A., Lipp, H.-P., Nadel, L. and Ricceri, L. (eds), *Behavioural Brain Research in Naturalistic and Semi-naturalistic Settings*. Kluwer Academic Publishers, Dordrecht, pp. 139–157.

Clayton, N.S., Reboreda, J.C. and Kacelnik, A. (1997) Seasonal changes of hippocampus volume in parasitic cowbirds. *Behavioural Processes*, 41, 237–243.

Colombo, M., Cawley, S. and Broadbent, N. (1997a) The effects of hippocampal and area parahippocampalis lesions in pigeons: II. Concurrent discrimination and spatial memory. *Quarterly Journal of Experimental Psychology*, 50B, 172–189.

Colombo, M., Swain, N., Harper, D. and Alsop, B. (1997b) The effects of hippocampal and area parahippocampalis lesions in pigeons: I. Delayed matching to sample. *Quarterly Journal of Experimental Psychology*, 50B, 149–171.

Craigie, E.H. (1930) Studies on the brain of the kiwi (*Apteryx australis*). *Journal of Comparative Neurology*, 49, 223–357.

Craigie, E.H. (1932) The cell structure of the cerebral hemisphere of the humming bird. *Journal of Comparative Neurology*, 56, 135–168.

Craigie, E.H. (1935) The hippocampal and parahippocampal cortex of the emu (*Dromiceius*). *Journal of Comparative Neurology*, 61, 563–591.

Craigie, E.H. (1940) The cerebral cortex of palaeognathine and neognathine birds. *Journal of Comparative Neurology*, 73, 179–234.

Cristol, D.A. (1996) Food storing does not affect hippocampal volume in experienced adult willow tits. *Behavioural Brain Research*, 81, 233–236.

Durward, A. (1932) Observations on the cell masses in the cerebral hemisphere of the New Zealand kiwi (*Apteryx australis*). *Journal of Anatomy*, 66, 437–477.

Eichenbaum, H., Kuperstein, M., Fagan, A. and Nagode, J. (1987) Cue-sampling and goal-approach correlates of hippocampal unit activity in rats performing an odor-discrimination task. *Journal of Neuroscience*, 7, 716–732.

Eichenbaum, H., Dusek, J., Young, B. and Bunsey, M. (1996) Neural mechanisms of declarative memory. *Cold Spring Harbor Symposia on Quantitative Biology*, 61, 197–206.

Erichsen, J.T., Bingman, V.P. and Krebs, J.R. (1991) The distribution of neuropeptides in the dorsomedial telencephalon of the pigeon (*Columba livia*): a basis for regional subdivisions. *Journal of Comparative Neurology*, 314, 478–492.

Fremouw, T., Jackson-Smith, P. and Kesner, R.P. (1997) Impaired place learning and unimpaired cue learning in hippocampal-lesioned pigeons. *Behavioral Neuroscience*, 111, 963–975.

Gagliardo, A., Ioalé, P. and Bingman, V.P. (1999) Homing in pigeons: the role of the hippocampal formation in the representation of landmarks used for navigation. *Journal of Neuroscience*, 19, 311–315.

Gahr, M., Güttinger, H.-R. and Kroodsma, D.E. (1993) Estrogen receptors in the avian brain: survey reveals general distribution and forebrain areas unique to songbirds. *Journal of Comparative Neurology*, 327, 112–122.

Good, M. (1987) The effects of hippocampal-area parahippocampalis lesions on discrimination learning in the pigeon. *Behavioural Brain Research*, 26, 171–184.

Good, M. and Macphail, E.M. (1994a) The avian hippocampus and short-term memory for spatial and non-spatial information. *Quarterly Journal of Experimental Psychology*, 47B, 293–317.

Good, M. and Macphail, E.M. (1994b) Hippocampal lesions in pigeons (*Columba livia*) disrupt reinforced preexposure but not overshadowing or blocking. *Quarterly Journal of Experimental Psychology*, 47B, 263–291.

Hampton, R.R. and Shettleworth, S.J. (1996a) Hippocampal lesions impair memory for location but not color in passerine birds. *Behavioral Neuroscience*, 110, 831–835.

Hampton, R.R. and Shettleworth, S.J. (1996b) Hippocampus and memory in a food-storing and in a nonstoring bird species. *Behavioral Neuroscience*, 110, 946–964.

Hampton, R.R., Sherry, D.F., Shettleworth, S.J., Khurgel, M. and Ivy, G. (1995) Hippocampal volume and food-storing behavior are related in parids. *Brain, Behavior and Evolution*, 45, 54–61.

Healy, S.D. and Krebs, J.R. (1992) Food storing and the hippocampus in corvids: amount and volume are correlated. *Proceedings of the Royal Society of London Series B*, 248, 241–245.

Healy, S.D. and Krebs, K.R. (1993) Development of hippocampal specialisation in a food-storing bird. *Behavioural Brain Research*, 53, 127–131.

Healy, S.D. and Krebs, J.R. (1996) Food storing and the hippocampus in Paridae. *Brain, Behavior and Evolution*, 47, 195–199.

Healy, S.D., Krebs, J.R. and Gwinner, E. (1991) Hippocampal volume and migration in passerine birds. *Naturwissenschaften*, 78, 424–426.

Healy, S.D., Clayton, N.S. and Krebs, J.R. (1994) Development of hippocampal specialisation in two species of tit (*Parus* spp). *Behavioural Brain Research*, 61, 23–28.

Healy, S.D., Gwinner, E. and Krebs, J.R. (1996) Hippocampal volume in migratory and non-migratory warblers: effects of age and experience. *Behavioural Brain Research*, 81, 61–68.

Hitchcock, C.L. and Sherry, D.F. (1990) Long-term memory for cache sites in the black-capped chickadee. *Animal Behaviour*, 40, 701–712.

Holscher, C. (1997) Nitric oxide, the enigmatic neuronal messenger: its role in synaptic plasticity. *Trends in Neurosciences*, 20, 298–303.

Honey, R.C., Horn, G., Bateson, P. and Walpole, M. (1995) Functionally distinct memories for imprinting stimuli: behavioral and neural dissociations. *Behavioral Neuroscience*, 109, 689–698.

Horn, G., McCabe, B.J. and Bateson, P.P.G. (1979) An autoradiographic study of the chick brain after imprinting. *Brain Research*, 168, 361–373.

Huber, G.C. and Crosby, E.C. (1929) The nuclei and fiber paths of the avian diencephalon, with consideration of telencephalic and certain mesencephalic centers and connections. *Journal of Comparative Neurology*, 48, 1–225.

Jarrard, L.E. (1995) What does the hippocampus really do? *Behavioural Brain Research*, 71, 1–10.

Johnston, J.B. (1913) The morphology of the septum, hippocampus and pallial commissures in reptiles and mammals. *Journal of Comparative Neurology*, 23, 371–474.

Källén, B. (1962) Embryogenesis of brain nuclei in the chick telencephalon. *Ergebnisse der Anatomie und Entwicklungsgeschichte*, 36, 62–82.

Kamil, A.C. (1988) A synthetic approach to the study of animal intelligence. In: Leger, D.W. (ed.), *Comparative Perspective in Modern Psychology. Nebraska Symposium on Motivation 1987.* University of Nebraska Press, Lincoln, Nebraska, pp. 257–308.

Karten, H. and Hodos, W. (1967) *A Stereotaxic Atlas of the Brain of the Pigeon (Columba livia).* Johns Hopkins University Press, Baltimore, Maryland.

Krayniak, P.F. and Siegel, A. (1978a) Efferent connections of the hippocampus and adjacent regions in the pigeon. *Brain, Behavior and Evolution*, 15, 372–388.

Krayniak, P.F. and Siegel, A. (1978b) Efferent connections of the septal area in the pigeon. *Brain, Behavior and Evolution*, 15, 389–404.

Krebs, J.R., Sherry, D.F., Healy, S.D., Perry, V.H. and Vaccarino, A.L. (1989) Hippocampal specialization of food-storing birds. *Proceedings of the National Academy of Sciences of the United States of America*, 86, 1388–1392.

Krebs, J.R., Erichsen, J.T. and Bingman, V.P. (1991) The distribution of neurotransmitters and neurotransmitter-related enzymes in the dorsomedial telencephalon of the pigeon (*Columba livia*). *Journal of Comparative Neurology*, 314, 467–477.

Krebs, J.R., Clayton, N.S., Hampton, R.R. and Shettleworth, S.J. (1995) Effects of photoperiod on food-storing and the hippocampus in birds. *NeuroReport*, 6, 1701–1704.

Krebs, J.R., Clayton, N.S., Healy, S.D., Cristol, D.A., Patel, S.N. and Joliffe, A.R. (1996) The ecology of the avian brain: food-storing memory and the hippocampus. *Ibis*, 138, 34–46.

Krushinskaya, N.L. (1966) Some complex forms of feeding behaviour of the nut-cracker *Nucifraga caryocatactes*, after removal of old cortex. *Zhurnal Evoliutsionnoi Biokhimii i Fisiologii*, 11, 563–568.

Lens, L., Adriaensen, F. and Dhondt, A.A. (1994) Age-related hoarding strategies in the crested tit *Parus cristatus*: should the cost of subordination be re-assessed? *Journal of Animal Ecology*, 63, 749–755.

Li, X., Schwartz, P.E. and Rissman, E.F. (1997) Distribution of estrogen receptor-beta-like immunoreactivity in rat forebrain. *Neuroendocrinology*, 66, 63–67.

Ludescher, F.B. (1980) Fressen und Verstecken von Sämereien bei der Weidenmeise *Paraus montanus* im Jahresverlauf unter konstanten Ernährungsbedingungen. *Ökologie der Vögel*, 2, 135–144.

Maggi, A., Susanna, L., Bettini, E., Mantero, G. and Zucchi, I. (1989) Hippocampus: a target for estrogen action in mammalian brain. *Molecular Endocrinology*, 3, 1165–1170.

Margrie, T.W., Rostas, J.A.P. and Sah, P. (1998) Long-term potentiation of synaptic transmission in the avian hippocampus. *Journal of Neuroscience*, 18, 1207–1216.

McCabe, B.J. and Horn, G. (1994) Learning-related changes in Fos-like immunoreactivity in the chick forebrain after imprinting. *Proceedings of the National Academy of Sciences of the United States of America*, 91, 11417–11421.

McEwen, B.S., Alves, S.E., Bulloch, K. and Weiland, N.G. (1997) Ovarian steroids and the brain: implications for cognition and aging. *Neurology*, 48, S8–S15.

Meehan, E.F. (1996) Effects of MK-801 on spatial memory in homing and nonhoming pigeon breeds. *Behavioral Neuroscience*, 110, 1487–1491.

Mollà, R., Rodriguez, J., Calvet, S. and Garcia-Verdugo, J.M. (1986) Neuronal types of the cerebral cortex of the adult chicken (*Gallus gallus*). A Golgi study. *Journal für Hirnforschung*, 27, 381–390.

Montagnese, C.M., Krebs, J.R., Szekely, A.D. and Csillag, A. (1993) A subpopulation of large calbindin-like immunopositive neurones is present in the hippocampal formation in food-storing but not in non-storing species of bird. *Brain Research*, 614, 291–300.

Montagnese, C.M., Krebs, J.R. and Meyer, G. (1996) The dorsomedial and dorsolateral forebrain of the zebra finch, *Taeniopygia guttata*: a Golgi study. *Cell and Tissue Research*, 283, 263–282.

Muller, R.U. and Kubie, J.L. (1987) The effects of changes in the environment on the spatial firing of hippocampal complex-spike cells. *Journal of Neuroscience*, 7, 1951–1968.

Muller, R.U., Kubie, J.L. and Ranck, J.B., Jr (1987) Spatial firing patterns of hippocampal complex-spike cells in a fixed environment. *Journal of Neuroscience*, 7, 1987.

Nakamura, H. and Wako, Y. (1988) Food storing behavior of willow tit *Parus montanus*. *Kenkyusho Kenkyu Hokoku*, 20, 21–36.

Nicol, A.U., Brown, M.W. and Horn, G. (1998) Hippocampal neuronal activity and imprinting in the behaving domestic chick. *European Journal of Neuroscience*, 10, 2738–2741.

Nunzi, M.G., Gorio, A., Milan, F., Freund, T.F., Somogyi, P. and Smith, A.D. (1985) Cholecystokinin-immunoreactive cells form symmetrical synaptic contacts with pyramidal and nonpyramidal neurons in the hippocampus. *Journal of Comparative Neurology*, 237, 485–505.

Odum, E.P. (1942) Annual cycle of the black-capped chickadee-3. *Auk*, 59, 499–531.

O'Keefe, J. and Dostrovsky, J. (1971) The hippocampus as a spatial map. Preliminary evidence from unit activity in the freely moving rat. *Brain Research*, 34, 171–175.

O'Keefe, J. and Nadel, L. (1978) *The Hippocampus as a Cognitive Map*. Clarendon Press, Oxford.

Olton, D.S., Becker, J.T. and Handelmann, G.E. (1979) Hippocampus, space and memory. *Behavioral and Brain Sciences*, 2, 313–365.

Patel, S.N., Clayton, N.S. and Krebs, J.R. (1997a) Hippocampal tissue transplants reverse lesion-induced spatial memory deficits in zebra finches (*Taeniopygia guttata*). *Journal of Neuroscience*, 17, 3861–3869.

Patel, S.N., Clayton, N.S. and Krebs, J.R. (1997b) Spatial learning induces neurogenesis in the avian brain. *Behavioural Brain Research*, 89, 115–128.

Pravosudov, V.V. (1985) Search for and storage of food by *Parus cinctus lapponicus* and *P.montanus borealis* (Paridae). *Zoologicheskii Zhurnal*, 64, 1036–1043.

Pravosudov, V.V. (1986) Individual differences in foraging and storing behaviour in Siberian tit *Parus cinctus* Bodd. and Willow tit *Parus montanus* Bald. *Soviet Journal of Ecology*, 4, 60–64.

Reboreda, J.C., Clayton, N.S. and Kacelnik, A. (1996) Species and sex differences in hippocampus size in parasitic and non-parasitic cowbirds. *NeuroReport*, 7, 505–508.

Register, T.C., Shively, C.A. and Lewis, C.E. (1998) Expression of estrogen receptor alpha and beta transcripts in female monkey hippocampus and hypothalamus. *Brain Research*, 788, 320–322.

Rehkämper, G., Haase, E. and Frahm, H.D. (1988) Allometric comparison of brain weight and brain structure volumes in different breeds of the domestic pigeon *Columba livia f.d.* (Fantails, homing pigeons, Strassers). *Brain, Behavior and Evolution*, 31, 141–149.

Reilly, S. and Good, M. (1987) Enhanced DRL and impaired forced-choice alternation performance following hippocampal lesions in the pigeon. *Behavioural Brain Research*, 26, 185–197.

Reilly, S. and Good, M. (1989) Hippocampal lesions and associative learning in the pigeon. *Behavioral Neuroscience*, 103, 731–742.

Rice, H.N. (1992) Food-caching, simple association and spatial memory in the black-capped chickadee. Unpublished MA thesis, University of Western Ontario.

Riters, L.V. and Bingman, V.P. (1994) The NMDA-receptor antagonist MK-801 impairs navigational learning in homing pigeons. *Behavioral and Neural Biology*, 62, 50–59.

Rose, M. (1914) Über die cytoarchitektonische Gliederung des Vorderhirns der Vögel. *Journal für Psychologie und Neurologie*, 21, 278–352.

Rose, S.P.R. (1991) How chicks make memories: the cellular cascade from c-*fos* to dendritic remodelling. *Trends in Neurosciences*, 14, 390–397.

Rudy, J.W. and Sutherland, R.J. (1995) Configural association theory and the hippocampal formation: an appraisal and reconfiguration. *Hippocampus*, 5, 375–389.

Saldanha, C.J., Popper, P., Micevych, P.E. and Schlinger, B.A. (1998) The passerine hippocampus is a site of high aromatase: inter- and intraspecies comparisons. *Hormones and Behavior*, 34, 85–97.

Sandi, C., Rose, S.P.R. and Patterson, T.A. (1992) Unilateral hippocampal lesions prevent recall of a passive avoidance task in day-old chicks. *Neuroscience Letters*, 141, 255–258.

Shapiro, E. and Wieraszko, A. (1996) Comparative, *in vitro*, studies of hippocampal tissue from homing and non-homing pigeon. *Brain Research*, 725, 199–206.

Sherry, D.F. and Vaccarino, A.L. (1989) Hippocampus and memory for food caches in black-capped chickadees. *Behavioral Neuroscience*, 103, 308–318.

Sherry, D.F., Krebs, J.R. and Cowie, R.J. (1981) Memory for the location of stored food in marsh tits. *Animal Behaviour*, 29, 1260–1266.

Sherry, D.F., Avery, M. and Stevens, A. (1982) The spacing of stored food by marsh tits. *Zeitschrift für Tierpsychologie*, 58, 153–162.

Sherry, D.F., Vaccarino, A.L., Buckenham, K. and Herz, R.S. (1989) The hippocampal complex of food-storing birds. *Brain, Behavior and Evolution*, 34, 308–317.

Sherry, D.F., Forbes, M.R.L., Khurgel, M. and Ivy, G.O. (1993) Females have a larger hippocampus than males in the brood-parasitic brown-headed cowbird. *Proceedings of the National Academy of Sciences of the United States of America*, 90, 7839–7843.

Shettleworth, S.J. and Krebs, J.R. (1982) How marsh tits find their hoards: the roles of site preference and spatial memory. *Journal of Experimental Psychology: Animal Behavior Processes*, 8, 354–375.

Shettleworth, S.J., Hampton, R.R. and Westwood, R.P. (1995) Effects of season and photoperiod on food storing by black-capped chickadees, *Parus atricapillus*. *Animal Behaviour*, 49, 989–998.

Slikas, B., Sheldon, F.H. and Gill, F.B. (1996) Phylogeny of titmice (Paridae): I. Estimate of relationships among subgenera based on DNA–DNA hybridization. *Journal of Avian Biology*, 27, 70–82.

Smulders, T.V. (1998) A game theoretical model of the evolution of food hoarding: applications to the Paridae. *American Naturalist*, 151, 356–366.

Smulders, T.V. and DeVoogd, T.J. (2000) Expression of immediate early genes in the hippocampal formation of the black-capped chickadee (*Poecile atricapillus*) during a food-hoarding task. *Behavioural Brain Research*, in press.

Smulders, T.V. and Dhondt, A.A. (1997) How much memory do tits need? *Trends in Ecology and Evolution*, 12, 417–418.

Smulders, T.V., Sasson, A.D. and Devoogd, T.J. (1995) Seasonal variation in hippocampal volume in a food-storing bird, the black-capped chickadee. *Journal of Neurobiology*, 27, 15–25.

Smulders, T.V., Newman, S.W. and DeVoogd, T.J. (1997) Expression of immediate early genes during a food-hoarding task. *Society for Neuroscience Abstracts*, 23, 2127.

Smulders, T.V., Shiflett, M.W., Sperling, A.J. and DeVoogd, T.J. (2000) Seasonal changes in neuron numbers in the hippocampal formation of a food-hoarding bird: the black-capped chickadee. *Journal of Neurobiology*, 44, in press.

Stewart, M.G., Cristol, D., Philips, R., Steele, R.J., Stamatakis, A., Harrison, E. *et al.* (1999) A quantitative autoradiographic comparison of binding to glutamate receptor subtypes in hippocampus and forebrain regions of a food-storing and a non-food-storing bird. *Behavioural Brain Research*, 98, 89–94.

Strasser, R. and Bingman, V.P. (1997) Goal recognition and hippocampal formation in the homing pigeon (*Columba livia*). *Behavioral Neuroscience*, 111, 1245–1256.

Székély, A.D. (1999) The avian hippocampal formation: subdivisions and connectivity. *Behavioural Brain Research*, 98, 219–225.

Székély, A.D. and Krebs, J.R. (1993) More hippocampal nitric oxide synthase in food-storing than in non-storing birds. *Society for Neuroscience Abstracts*, 19, 1448.

Szekely, A.D. and Krebs, J.R. (1996) Efferent connectivity of the hippocampal formation of the zebra finch (*Taenopygia guttata*): an anterograde pathway tracing study using *Phaseolus vulgaris* leucoagglutinin. *Journal of Comparative Neurology*, 368, 198–214.

Tomback, D.F. (1980) How nutcrackers find their seed stores. *Condor*, 82, 10–19.

Vander Wall, S.B. (1990) *Food Hoarding in Animals*. The University of Chicago Press, Chicago.

Veenman, C.L., Wild, J.M. and Reiner, A. (1995) Organization of the avian 'corticostriatal' projection system: a retrograde and anterograde pathway tracing study in pigeons. *Journal of Comparative Neurology*, 354, 87–126.

Volman, S.F., Grubb, T.C. and Schuett, K.C. (1997) Relative hippocampal volume in relation to food-storing behavior in four species of woodpeckers. *Brain, Behavior and Evolution*, 49, 110–120.

Weiland, N.G., Orikasa, C., Hayashi, S. and McEwen, B.S. (1997) Distribution and hormone regulation of estrogen receptor immunoreactive cells in the hippocampus of male and female rats. *Journal of Comparative Neurology*, 388, 603–612.

Wieraszko, A. and Ball, G.F. (1991) Long-term enhancement of synaptic responses in the songbird hippocampus. *Brain Research*, 538, 102–106.

Wieraszko, A. and Ball, G.F. (1993) Long-term potentiation in the avian hippocampus does not require activation of the *N*-methyl-D-aspartate (NMDA) receptor. *Synapse*, 13, 173–178.

Wylie, D.R.W., Glover, R.G. and Aitchison, J.D. (1999) Optic flow input to the hippocampal formation from the accessory optic system. *Journal of Neuroscience*, 19, 5514–5527.

9 TO CONSOLIDATE OR NOT TO CONSOLIDATE: WHAT ARE THE QUESTIONS?

Yadin Dudai and Richard G.M. Morris

INTRODUCTION

The concept of memory consolidation was introduced into the scientific discourse over a century ago (Muller and Pilzecker, 1900). However, its consolidation into the collective memory of the neuroscience community remains incomplete. For, although extensively discussed, the term consolidation means different things to different people. In its most general meaning, it refers to the idea that recently formed memories can sometimes be subject to stabilization over time, rendering them less susceptible to disruption by both new information and brain dysfunction. This process of stabilization manifests itself at different levels of brain organization and at multiple time windows. It is both conceptually and methodologically useful to distinguish between cellular consolidation and system consolidation (Dudai, 1996). The first refers to processes that take place locally, in individual nodes of neuronal circuits, i.e. synapses and neurons, during the first hours or days after learning. The second refers to processes that occur at a circuit level, may involve the progressive reorganization of memory traces throughout the brain and seem to last, in some cases, weeks or longer. In the simplest of circuits, cellular and system consolidation may be isomorphic. In more complex circuits, system consolidation probably involves additional mechanisms that reflect the selective activity of different circuits; a consequence of this selectivity is the potential, after consolidation, to retrieve memory using neural circuits different from those encoding memory traces at an earlier stage of their existence (Squire and Zola, 1996; Shadmehr and Holocomb, 1997).

In the present chapter, we restrict our discussion to cellular consolidation. It is this facet of consolidation that has, in recent years, benefited most from exciting developments at the cutting edge of cellular and molecular biology. Hence, from now on, whenever we say 'consolidation', unless otherwise specified, we are referring to events that take place in synapses and individual neurons within the first hours after training. The field of system consolidation, which is being rapidly pushed into new vistas by sophisticated neuropsychology and neuroimaging, is not discussed.

In spite of the recent developments in understanding mechanisms of neuronal plasticity, which potentially relate to consolidation, many questions remain unsettled. These include basic issues such as *how*, *where* and *when* consolidation takes place in local nodes in the neuronal circuits that encode experience-dependent internal representations. (On learning and memory defined in terms of experience-dependent internal representations, and on the advantages of defining them in these terms, see Dudai, 1989, 1992.) One approach that we will discuss makes reference to the idea that local 'synaptic tags' set at the time of memory formation have the job of capturing diffusely targeted gene products to consolidate otherwise unstable synaptic connections (Frey and Morris, 1997). This concept raises the specter of the potential for consolidation without, necessarily, setting in train at the locus of consolidation all the neural events that would inexorably lead to it. In the present context, it is noteworthy that Gabriel Horn himself proposed a similar idea in the context of his work on filial imprinting (Horn, 1998).

COMMON THEMES

Experimental data from a variety of species, memory systems and preparations are often crystallized to yield a number of common themes concerning consolidation. It is useful to start by listing those that epitomize the Zeitgeist in this dynamic field:

(i) Over time, new memories become resistant to certain kinds of interference. These include behavioral distractors, drugs, seizures and brain lesions. The time window of susceptibility depends on the task and type of interference. It may range from seconds to minutes (e.g. electro-convulsive shocks in associative conditioning, McGaugh, 1966), through hours (distractor tasks in motor skills, Shadmehr and Holcomb, 1997; macromolecular synthesis inhibition in a variety of tasks, Davis and Squire, 1984), up to weeks or more (hippocampal lesions in so-called declarative memory tasks, Squire and Zola-Morgan, 1991; Winocur, 1990). The latter, longer time windows of susceptibility are usually considered to reflect system consolidation, and will not be discussed further here.

(ii) The application of drugs that are known to inhibit the synthesis of RNA or of proteins during a time window of up to a few hours after training blocks the formation of memories that last for longer than a day (Davis and Squire, 1984; Montarolo *et al.*, 1986; Rosenblum *et al.*, 1993; Freeman *et al.*, 1995). In the behaving animal, drug doses that result in massive reduction in protein synthesis (>90–95%) are required to achieve such an effect. Often, a similar transient reduction in macromolecular synthesis does not significantly affect perception, short-term memory or either the retention or the retrieval of long-term memory once relevant traces have been established. (The claim that retention is unaffected must be qualified since, in the limit, broad-spectrum and long-lasting protein synthesis inhibition is expected to result in neuronal malfunction and ultimately death.)

(iii) The transformation of short- into long-term memory is not a step-like function, and various drugs or mutations can be used to dissect it further into what appear to be intermediate phases (e.g. Grecksch and Matthies, 1980; Rosenzweig *et al.*, 1993; DeZazzo and Tully, 1995; Ghirardi *et al.*, 1995; Winder *et al.*, 1998). However, it recently became evident that the time course of such phases is not a given, and might be altered (Frey and Morris, 1997). Moreover, it is not clear whether intermediate phases of memory consolidation must take place in a prescribed order, or even that the creation of long-term memory traces requires a short-term one; the processes may occur in parallel (e.g. Emptage and Carew, 1993).

(iv) Signal transduction cascades, and specifically the cAMP-response element (CRE)-mediated modulation of gene expression by such cascades, are thought to be important players in the consolidation of short- into long-term memory. This has been established in behaving animals as well as in neuronal models of plasticity (e.g. Kaang *et al.*, 1993; Frank and Greenberg, 1994; Yin *et al.*, 1994; Deisseroth *et al.*, 1996; Lamprecht *et al.*, 1997). An example is the cAMP cascade (Kaang *et al.*, 1993; Frank and Greenberg, 1994; Deisseroth *et al.*, 1996). It involves activation of a cAMP-dependent kinase, which phosphorylates and activates isoforms of cAMP-response element-binding proteins (CREBs); the balance between activator and repressor forms of CREB may be critical in triggering long-term information storage (Bourtchuladze *et al.*, 1994; Yin *et al.*, 1994). CREB modulates the expression of CRE-regulated genes, including a number of immediate-early genes (IEGs such as transcription factors that, in turn, regulate the expression of late response genes). Other IEGs identified so far include ubiquitin C-terminal hydrolase (Hegde *et al.*, 1997), extracellular protease plasminogen activator (Frey *et al.*, 1996) and neural cell adhesion molecule (NCAM; Fields and Itoh, 1996). Gabriel Horn and his colleagues have also reported evidence implicating NCAMs in long-term memory (Solomonia *et al.*, 1998). Compared with immediate and early response genes, much less currently is known about late response genes, though candidates have been suggested (Kennedy *et al.*, 1992; Kuhl *et al.*, 1992; Cavallaro *et al.*, 1997).

(v) There is evidence suggesting that long-term synaptic plasticity and long-term memory are correlated with morphological changes in synapses (e.g. Horn *et al.*, 1985; Bailey and Kandel, 1993; Weiler *et al.*, 1995).

THE ANALOGY WITH DEVELOPMENT

The aforementioned themes are usually fitted into a conceptual paradigm that depicts the cellular manifestations of memory consolidation as growth or developmental processes. This paradigm exerts a marked influence on current research in molecular and cellular neurobiology, and is behind much of the striking merger of the concepts of developmental neurobiology and the molecular biology of memory (e.g. Corfas and Dudai, 1991; Davis *et al.*, 1996; Martin and Kandel, 1996). As such, it is probably the most influential in current research on consolidation.

The notion that neural remodeling subserves behavioral plasticity (James, 1890) and that experience-dependent cellular growth processes take place in the mature brain (Cajal, 1911; Hebb, 1949) are tenets of neurobiology at large. The response of neural tissue to stimulation was shown long ago to be accompanied by alteration in proteins (Hamberger and Hyden, 1945). Soon after, the suggestive data and the aforesaid dogma combined to yield a proposal that new memory traces depend on proteins (Monne, 1949), and paved the way for the reports that synthesis of brain RNA (Dingman and Sporn, 1961) and protein (Flexner *et al.*, 1963; Agranoff and Klinger, 1964) are obligatory for the formation of long-term memory.

At its outset, the role of macromolecular synthesis in memory consolidation was embedded in two radically different conceptual frameworks. The first was the 'macromolecular code' hypothesis. It stated that neuronal memory, similarly to genetic memory, is encoded in the primary structure of nucleic acids and proteins, and hence that learning is an experience-dependent modification in the structure of these macromolecules (Dingman and Sporn, 1961; Hyden and Egyhazi, 1962). The macromolecular code hypothesis stimulated work which contributed valuable data on the metabolism of brain nucleic acids and proteins (Hyden and Egyhazi, 1962; Hyden and Lange, 1965), but it also resulted in some dead ends. These included attempts to transfer specific memories from one individual to another—attempts that followed directly from the supposition that memories were encoded in the primary structure of the molecules (e.g. Ungar, 1970). The appeal of the macromolecular code dwindled as these experiments failed or, in some cases, where apparently positive results were shown to be artifactual (e.g. Byrne *et al.*, 1966). Consequently, the second conceptual framework—the 'macromolecular synthesis' hypothesis—came to dominate the field. In brief, it states that newly synthesized gene products do not themselves encode memory, but rather promote and sustain modifications in neuronal circuits that encode internal representations (Dudai, 1989). Over the years, two types of methods have been used to reveal the possible roles that RNA and protein synthesis might play in memory. The first is interventional, based on inference of function from dysfunction. The second is cor-relative, involving direct measurement of macromolecular synthesis in brain during or after learning and/or artificial models of neural plasticity.

Initially, antibiotics that specifically inhibit RNA or protein synthesis were used to determine the necessary role of macromolecular synthesis in behavior (reviewed in Davis and Squire, 1984), this approach being complemented by the gene targeting techniques of today (Winder and Kandel, Chapter 10). Despite occasional worries about the exact site of action of the drugs used (e.g. Kyriakis *et al.*, 1994), the overwhelming conclusion was that protein synthesis during or shortly after training is required for consolidation of long-term memory but not for acquisition, short-term memory or retrieval once long-term memory had been formed (Davis and Squire, 1984). However, injection of inhibitors into the brain could not provide definitive evidence that their critical effect was on neurons. This problem was resolved only in the mid-1980s, when preparations were developed which allowed both the isolation of individual memory-subserving neurons in relatively simple nervous systems and, separately, the analysis of cellular experience-dependent modifications in discrete pathways in the mammalian brain. Application of antibiotics to these preparations confirmed the general approach, showing macromolecular synthesis to be required for long-term heterosynaptic facilitation of the sensory-to- motor synapse in the *Aplysia* defensive reflexes circuits (Montarolo *et al.*, 1986), conditioning in *Hermissenda* photoreceptors (Crow and Forrester, 1990), long-term potentiation (LTP) in various fields of the hippocampal formation (dentate gyrus, Krug *et al.*, 1984; Otani *et al.*, 1989; hippocampal area CA1, Stanton and Sarvey, 1984; Nguyen *et al.*, 1994) and long-term depression (LTD) in the cerebellum (Linden, 1996). In parallel, local microinjection of antibiotics into circumscribed brain areas known to subserve specific experience-dependent behaviors also confirmed that protein synthesis is required for various kinds of memory in the brain of the behaving organism (Grecksch and Matthies, 1980; Horn *et al.*, 1985, Chapter 19; Mizumori *et al.*, 1985; Rosenblum *et al.*, 1993; Brennan and Keverne, Chapter 6). More recently, novel variants of perturbational methodology have been deployed to investigate the role of gene expression in memory consolidation; these include local microinjection of oligodeoxynucleotides antisense to transcription factors into the brain (Guzowski and McGaugh, 1997; Lamprecht *et al.*, 1997), local application of antibodies to transcription factors (Bartsch *et al.*, 1995) and the use of transgenes and knockouts of genes that encode such factors (Bourtchuladze *et al.*, 1994; Yin *et al.*, 1994; Blendy *et al.*, 1996).

The second and complementary approach, based on looking for correlations between macromolecular synthesis in the brain and parameters of learning or memory, was also applied early but with only limited success (Hyden and Egyhazi, 1962; Zemp *et al.*, 1966; Shashua, 1979). The development of cellular preparations and the improved sophistication of cellular and molecular neurobiology [including, for example, the single-cell polymerase chain reaction (PCR) techniques] have opened new vistas for the correlative approach. This has led to the identification of experience-dependent modulation of protein synthesis in both invertebrate and vertebrate nervous systems (Mayford *et al.*, 1992; Kaang *et al.*, 1993; Meberg *et al.*, 1995; Impey *et al.*, 1996; Hegde *et al.*, 1997; Martin *et al.*, 1997a; Casadio *et al.*, 1999).

On the basis of the above and similar findings, a picture thus is commonly portrayed of cellular consolidation being analogous to a developmental process. In both cases, gene expression is regulated by extracellular signals via intracellular signal transduction cascades and, in both cases, similar ubiquitous signaling cascades, such as the cAMP (see above) and mitogen-activated protein kinase cascades (MAPKs; Hill and Treisman, 1995; Martin *et al.*, 1997b; Berman *et al.*, 1998; Crow *et al.*, 1998), are recruited, culminating in cellular remodeling and growth. However, at this stage, the scenes in this picture justify a closer look. We will consider the questions of *how*, *where* and *when* does cellular consolidation takes place in turn, turning toward the end of this chapter to the more speculative issue of *why* it takes place at all.

HOW?

A birds-eye view of the current data on cellular consolidation may lead one to conclude that the process is triggered in a step-function-like manner depending upon the availability of an input signal, and that it later unfolds as an orderly, multiple phase cascade of 'developmental decisions' culminating in the modulation of gene expression. Is this an adequate account?

Let us start with the trigger. Experimental protocols used to elicit consolidation in both *Aplysia* and LTP are usually based on increasing the intensity of input.

For example, one pulse of serotonin is used to induce short-term facilitation in the sensory-to-motor synapse in *Aplysia*, whereas five spaced pulses are required to elicit the long-term facilitation (Montarolo *et al.*, 1986). However, the notion that consolidation is a function of the intensity of a single input might well be too simplistic. It also is not in accord with the natural situation, in which much of the information that we consolidate frequently is distinguished from the non-consolidated by virtue of context and association rather than intensity. We therefore favor the notion that a time-dependent convergence of two or more events usually is required.

To illustrate this latter possibility, let us take a closer look at mechanisms of LTP in hippocampal area CA1. It has long been thought that *N*-methyl-D-aspartate (NMDA) receptor-dependent LTP is a homosynaptic event, i.e. glutamatergic synapses are capable of inducing and maintaining all processes required to enhance the efficacy at the particular synapse. However, activation of ionotropic glutamatergic receptors alone leads only to a short- (<1 h) but not a long-term potentiation, provided that the extracellular ion concentrations are not manipulated (Kullmann *et al.*, 1992). Further, it has been shown that late-LTP in CA1 and dentate gyrus can be prevented or stimulated by inhibitors and activators, respectively, of aminergic, opioid or metabotropic glutamate receptors coupled to the cAMP cascade (for a review, see Frey and Morris, 1998). We therefore suggest that late-LTP requires concomitant activation of multiple extracellular signaling systems. The typical LTP experiment, involving a brief period of high-frequency stimulation (or, with intracellular recording, the pairing of pre- and postsynaptic activation), overlooks the more likely situation in the behaving organism where the synaptic population of an individual CA1 cell is likely to have a unique history and change dynamically with time. Potentiation will occur at some sites matched by heterosynaptic and homosynaptic decreases in synaptic efficacy elsewhere. The artificial massive stimulation, involving simultaneous activation of hundreds of fibers, probably activates more than one kind of neurotransmitter input, and it is that cooperative action of inputs that, experimentally, enables late-LTP. The main 'take-home' message is that consolidation is not a function merely of more-of-the-same (i.e. a single transmitter), but also of coincidence (i.e. external stimuli, internal states or both).

Having set the process in motion, two main classes of scenarios can be considered for the conversion of this short- into a more long-term synaptic change (though others can also be envisaged—see Lisman and Fallon, 1999):

(i) the same molecular species and cellular processes that subserve the short-term changes, also subserve the long-term change;

(ii) some of the molecular species and cellular processes subserving the short- might also subserve the long-term changes, but additional molecular species and processes must be recruited with time.

The first scenario is theoretically possible, and can be subserved, for example, by a durable shift in the kinetics of autocatalytic protein kinase–protein phosphatase cascades in the synapse (Crick, 1984; Lisman, 1985; Buxbaum and Dudai, 1989). In this scenario, macromolecular synthesis is not expected to have a causal role in establishing the persistence of traces over time, but rather to have a role in supplying the synapse with resources for enhanced molecular turnover, in expanding synaptic space for future plasticity, and in homeostatic functions. Using a simplistic metaphor of the synapse as a motor vehicle, it has the engine required for a very long ride, but will evidently stop running in the absence of an appropriate supply of fuel and spare parts.

The second scenario regards modulation of macromolecular synthesis as causally required for retention of memory over time. This may be done locally at or near the synapse, or cell wide. Adhering to the above metaphor, the non-consolidated synapse does not have an engine, merely a starter. The combustion engine, powerful enough to travel for years, must be assembled during consolidation from new parts that are either manufactured on the spot, or shipped from the main factory, i.e. the nucleus and cytoplasm.

What macromolecules might be involved in each of the above scenarios? If we focus on the synapse as the critical (and most thoroughly investigated) locus of change, both pre- and postsynaptic changes could be entertained. Presynaptic modifications are expected to consist of alterations in the efficacy of transmitter release. These might be induced either by changes in the availability of Ca^{2+} (from external as well as from internal stores, Reyes and Stanton, 1996) or directly in the release machinery. There are various ways of realizing such processes. Experience-dependent phosphorylation of ion channels, for which there is experimental evidence, is one of them (Kandel and Schwartz, 1982). So is, potentially, a direct modi-

fication in the release machinery. An appealing memory-keeping step is persistent activation of the appropriate protein kinase(s), resulting in continuous phosphorylation and rephosphorylation of the relevant substrate proteins in the synapse (Schwartz, 1993; Chain *et al.*, 1995). Postsynaptic mechanisms are expected to involve alterations in receptors for neurotransmitters and their coupled intracellular signal transduction cascades. Examples are α-amino-3-hydroxy-5-methyl-4-isoxazole propionic acid (AMPA) receptors in LTP, modulated by phosphorylation (Barria *et al.*, 1997); here again, persistent activation of protein kinases is one of the candidates for the memory-keeping devices. Calcium/calmodulin-dependent protein kinase II is a prime suspect, but definitely not the only one (Otmakhov *et al.*, 1997; Ouyang *et al.*, 1997). Modulation of kinases and receptors need not be expressed only in altered receptor responsiveness to an incoming stimulus; it can also involve modification in the interfacing of a membrane-associated receptor with the cytoskeleton and intracellular signal transduction cascades (e.g. Niethammer *et al.*, 1996; Otmakhov *et al.*, 1997), and in the availability of receptor molecules (Hayashi *et al.*, 2000).

So what might consolidation be in each of the above scenarios? In the first scenario, the initiation of long-term memory actually coincides with the short-term process, and consolidating consists of recruiting supportive mechanisms. In the second scenario, macromolecular synthesis might be required to generate more of the same or new variants or types of protein that augment and extend the function of the those modified in the short term—such as proteases that degrade the inhibitory, regulatory subunit of cAMP-dependent protein kinase (Hegde *et al.*, 1993). In addition, mechanisms not required in the short term might be called into service, e.g. intra- and extracellular proteolysis for synaptic remodeling, and alterations in intra- and extracellular architecture brought about by members of the large family of cell adhesion molecules (Fields and Itoh, 1996; Martin and Kandel, 1996; Solomonia *et al.*, 1998). This scenario indeed depicts consolidation as including mechanisms similar if not identical to those recruited in growth and differentiation (Davis *et al.*, 1996). However, since most cellular preparations used to investigate experience-dependent modifications in synaptic efficacy use rather strong, non-physiological stimulation protocols, it is not unlikely that they reveal molecular events that *in vivo* are recruited only in response to stress and injury. The specificity of the transcriptional modulation in such preparations to trace formation in the behaving animal must therefore be regarded with some caution. Whatever is the case, in the long term, the synapse, whether strengthened by proliferation or not, is still expected to harbor modified channels, enzymes or receptors of the kinds mentioned above (Martin and Kandel, 1996). Again, this hints at the notion that too much emphasis on the nucleus, an understandable outcome of the impressive success of developmental cell biology, might be luring us away from mechanisms specific to representational changes in the circuit which operate over a much faster time scale (Dudai, 1997b; Singer, Chapter 3).

WHERE?

The discussion so far leads to the inevitable conclusion that consolidation proceeds at multiple sites within neurons. Consider in this respect the engineering problem that neurons face in determining where consolidated changes in neuronal function are to occur. Cortical pyramidal cells have many thousands of excitatory glutamatergic synapses receiving afferent input from a large number of other cells. An individual cell functions, therefore, in numerous distinct but overlapping circuits, and the spatial distribution of synaptic weights on such a cell will reflect this at any one time. It follows that any decision to consolidate or not to consolidate the synaptic strength of an individual synapse is not likely to be taken in the cell body exclusively if the desired change is to be specific to a subset of inputs onto that cell. What the cell body can do, however, is to effect a change that creates the potential for consolidation, but allow the final decision as to whether and where this is to occur to be determined locally. This solution is attractive, but it requires a potentially complex interaction between local and central mechanisms within a neuron.

One engineering solution for avoiding this complexity would be to allow all decision making to be done locally, once the relevant permissive or instructive information is available. Individual synapses could not only have the machinery for changing synaptic efficacy, but also all the machinery for ensuring that this change is persistent in the face of protein turnover (e.g. Davis *et al.*, 1987; Feig and Lipton, 1993; Ouyang *et al.*, 1999). In this view, the cell body would have only the housekeeping role of synthesizing the mRNAs and proteins required at the periphery, but play no part in determining whether or where local

consolidation occurred. Such an arrangement is, however, wasteful, for at least two reasons. First, the neuron is an integrative computing element that, in addition to summating excitatory postsynaptic potentials (EPSPs) and enabling action potential propagation (over a fast time scale), could also maintain a record of its own recent history of activation. This history could play a part in making decisions about consolidation. To take advantage of this opportunity, aspects of the decision making cannot be only at the local elements of connectivity, but must also be at either the cell body or, allowing one further level of complexity, within individual dendritic domains. The key concept here is to remove part (but not all) of the decision making from sites where only limited information is available to sites where afferent information can accumulate. Secondly, an exclusively local mechanism of consolidation may be biochemically wasteful. If macromolecules are necessary for consolidation, and similar if not identical molecules are required at all synapses, it may make no sense to endow each of the thousands of synapses on a cell with the intricate machinery for achieving persistent change. Thus, irrespective of the specific mechanisms involved, a distributed process has the merits of intraneuronal integration and biochemical economy—subject to the eventual necessity for achieving input specificity.

The aforementioned reference to dendritic domains deserves further comment. In the cerebral cortex, inputs are received in particular cortical layers that correspond to specific domains of a pyramidal cell's architecture (Creutzfeld, 1995). This state of affairs allows the possibility that synapse formation and/or synaptic change and consolidation may be required in these domains of the cell but not others. Under these circumstances, the question arises of the efficiency of having only the options of local or central decision making; it may be advantageous to traffic cellular machinery to intermediate locales, i.e. those cellular domains where it will be used most intensively. By way of illustration, it may be advantageous to have specific types of RNA or protein synthesis in layer IV of the neocortex where thalamic inputs are received; or in specific segments of the medial perforant path where entorhinal input to the dentate gyrus terminates. It should be recognized, however, that this gain in efficiency cannot be at the expense of the necessity for shared decision making by the synapse and the cell body, and the advantages it confers upon the neuron.

For a process involving decision making at distributed loci in a neuron to be effective and to evade catastrophes, it is essential that there is appropriate overall cellular coordination. Furthermore, this co-ordination may enrich and optimize the metabolic and computational repertoire of the neuron. This is one of the ideas behind the concept of 'synaptic tagging' (Frey and Morris, 1997), whereby local sites at which consolidation is presumed to occur (i.e. individual synapses) can sequester the products of consolidation processing elsewhere. The first experiment to illustrate this point established that it is possible to induce protein synthesis-dependent late-LTP during the inhibition of protein synthesis provided that the macromolecules required for this local consolidation have been synthesized earlier. Moreover, weak stimulation, that ordinarily gives rise only to transient changes in synaptic efficacy, can also result in a lasting change if this stimulation follows much stronger prior activation of the neuron by stimulus patterns that are sufficient for triggering macromolecular synthesis. Consolidation at local sites in a neuronal domain (such as a small population of synapses) is therefore determined in a dual fashion—by the cell-wide availability of macromolecules that may (and often will) have been synthesized in response to other events, and by local postsynaptic 'tags' that sequester or 'hijack' these proteins and so render permissive the 'final common path' of synaptic consolidation. Frey and Morris (1998) have also reported that there is an appealing symmetry about these dual-location arrangements—persistent synaptic change can also occur if the weak stimulation on a pathway (that sets a local synaptic tag) precedes the stronger stimulation of a population of neurons on another pathway, provided that the interval between the two patterns of stimulation is quite short (<1–2 h). The success of both the original 'strong-before-weak' and the newer 'weak-before-strong' protocols in inducing persistent change on the weakly stimulated pathway offers strong evidence that consolidation is a consequence of two or more neuronal processes operating at different loci within cells. Each creates the potential for persistent change; neither can induce it alone.

These experiments were conducted using extracellular recording techniques and stimulation of large numbers of afferent fibers and neurons. Striking evidence for synaptic tagging occurring within individual cells has been obtained in *Aplysia* cell cultures. In a preparation in which one sensory cell was afferent onto two motor neurons, weak facilitatory activation of one synaptic terminal following prior strong activation of the other revealed a lasting presynaptic facilitation at both (Martin *et al.*, 1997a). Furthermore, whereas repeated application of serotonin to an individual synapse produced a CREB-mediated, synapse-specific long-term facilitation, repeated pulses of serotonin to the cell soma produced a CREB-dependent cell-wide facilitation that, alas, was only short lived. However, if a single pulse of serotonin, which by itself produced only transient synaptic facilitation, was then applied to an individual synapse, that synapse acquired persistent facilitation and synapse-specific growth. The effect of the single serotonin pulse on the synapse and its priming for capturing and locally stabilizing the cell-wide facilitation involves cAMP-induced post-translational modifications as well as local protein synthesis (Casadio *et al.*, 1999). All in all, the results from *Aplysia* extend our understanding of synaptic tagging in several important respects: it establishes that tag–macromolecule interactions occur within single cells, it indicates that this can happen presynaptically (as well as postsynaptically), it shows that the local synaptic processes involve both protein synthesis-dependent and protein synthesis-independent mechanisms, and it firmly establishes that dual control of cellular consolidation by the synapse and the nucleus occurs in both invertebrate and vertebrate nervous systems.

WHEN?

A frequent claim is that consolidation involves a series of discrete phases. This way of thinking invites the notion of critical periods at which it is feasible to interfere with specific players in this cascade of events. In this view, consolidation may be said to have both a start- and an end-point, with each of its component processes having characteristic durations after some unique triggering event. Several factors will determine the time course of these constituent elements of the machinery, including the typical half-life of synaptic proteins, the speed with which molecules are transported to and from the nucleus, rates of protein synthesis, and so forth (e.g. Huh and Wentfold, 1999; Xu and Sapleter, 1999). Knowledge of these time courses, coupled with the assumption that they occur in a prescribed sequence, would enable one to work out the important time points of consolidation including the duration of critical periods after learning has taken place.

However, if, as discussed previously, decision making in a neuronal domain is distributed, it seems to us more likely that different triggers will be responsible for different elements of the consolidation machinery. Temporal intersection of the products of these different mechanisms at local sites presumably will be both necessary and sufficient for consolidation to occur, but there may then be no rigorously prescribed time course or critical periods at which interference with consolidation will always be successful. To spell out this quite radical suggestion more precisely, suppose local consolidation involved the utilization of somatically synthesized plasticity-related proteins at sites at which specific receptor proteins recently had been phosphorylated (e.g. AMPA receptors, Wyllie and Nicoll, 1994; Barria *et al.*, 1997). If these plasticity proteins were to be synthesized in advance, perhaps in response to neuromodulatory input elsewhere on the cell, there is no *a priori* reason why consolidation could not occur very rapidly after the local phosphorylation events had taken place. The time-consuming cycle of translocation to and from the nucleus would be finessed by virtue of the prior history of activation of the neuron. Thus, a phase of consolidation usually described as being a 'late' phase could often occur quite early. In the case of 'late-LTP', for example, the prior induction of early-LTP may still be a necessary condition, but the local changes at synapses that characterize a consolidated alteration to receptor proteins may nonetheless occur very soon thereafter. This suggestion does, incidentally, have the immediate practical importance that it could enable techniques such as intracellular or patch-clamp electrophysiology to be deployed in the analysis of 'phases' of memory formation that have hitherto seemed beyond its reach.

A final aspect of the 'when' question has to do with whether consolidation ever ends. We suspect not. A typical pedagogical scenario is the supposition that a labile memory trace is established and it is then subject to consolidation beginning at time t_1 and ending at time t_2. Consolidation complete, it can now survive the winds and waves of any brainstorm that the nervous system may throw at it. Some memories may be like this—being dredged up years after they supposedly were forgotten. However, everyday reality is likely to be a more dynamic process of storage, consolidation, retrieval, integration with other new information, re-storage, a new cycle of consolidation, and so on (e.g. Roullet and Sara, 1998). This more dynamic perspective sees memory traces assuming a status where they acquire both persistence and resistance to interference, yet somehow maintain the capacity to be resculpted and so transformed. There is a mystery embedded in such a state of affairs, but one which our present understanding of how internal representations are retained, reactivated or reconstructed in retrieval is still poorly equipped to address.

WHY?

We do not intend to ask the metaphysical question of why is there long-term memory to start with, but rather why it does not stabilize instantaneously. Though well aware of the teleological nature of the question and the speculative nature of any answers, we deem it useful to delve into the game, because, apart from its mere theoretical interest, it could pinpoint potential experimental avenues.

One potential explanation to be kept in the back of one's mind is that the gradual nature of the maturation of synaptic changes that subserve memory traces arises, in part at least, by virtue of the mechanistic constraints imposed on the nervous system by phylogenesis. These could be of two types. First, synapses and neurons, having to react quickly to incoming stimuli, must rely in their detection and immediate registration machinery on fast biophysical and post-translational modifications. However, alas, the latter are also short lived and, additional mechanisms, more immune to molecular turnover, must therefore be engaged to keep the trace going (e.g. Crick, 1984; Goelet *et al.*, 1986; Lisman and Fallon, 1999). This transition establishes consolidation by definition. Secondly, the possibility should be considered that it was phylogenetically parsimonious for evolving phyla to utilize in memory systems the same cellular building blocks used in development, growth and response to injury. The resemblance of cellular processes of growth and learning and the overlap of the molecular machinery between the two have already been mentioned above (see also Carew *et al.*, 1998). It has also been suggested specifically, for example, that behavioral plasticity stems from a more primitive compensatory plasticity (e.g. Walters *et al.*, 1991). The reliance on primitive mechanisms may have imposed some basic constraints on neurons, and shaped them to function in certain ways which might not necessarily be optimal.

Mechanistic and phylogenetic constraints notwithstanding, one could envisage theoretically a situation in which newly formed memories do stabilize instantaneously, evading the risk of erasure by confounding input and metabolic interference. This indeed may happen occasionally, as in certain instances of flashbulb memory (Brown and Kulik, 1977), but, routinely, there are good reasons not to have such a step-function change. Contemplating such hypothetical rationales must take into account not merely cellular consolidation but also system consolidation, which the former is postulated to subserve. One of the reasons to assume that instantaneous stabilization of memory is a counterproductive routine is that immediate conversion of information into a long-term store might waste brain space on events that have to be retained for intermediate periods but can then be safely forgotten. Presumably, most of the sensory information that impinges on our senses does not culminate in lasting traces, for, if it were to do so, it would impede our ability to construe the world efficiently and react to it (Dudai, 1997a). Another potential drive may have to do with the way in which the brain constructs narratives to construe the world and react to it. The construction of such internal narratives may take the form of pruning and rearrangement of mental items, a process that takes time and has to be performed against the background of ongoing brain activity. Consolidation, including cellular consolidation immediately after learning, may allow such processes to take place. Furthermore, while reconstructing internal narratives, consolidation may promote generalization and categorization (McClelland *et al.*, 1995), without which the perceived world may become confusing and the reaction to it ineffective (Luria, 1968). Finally, the reason for the gradual stabilization of memories in brain systems may be an algorithmic one; for example, gradual interweaving of new information can, with certain learning algorithms, avoid catastrophic interference (McClelland *et al.*, 1995).

Turning again from the circuit to the cellular processes, and refocusing on cellular consolidation and its mechanisms, what might be the functional advantage of having cell-wide in addition to synaptic changes in cellular consolidation? The following possibilities could be entertained.

Cell-wide changes might fulfill a storehouse function, needed because synapses do not have sufficient metabolic assets. More than 20 years ago, Squire and Barondes (1976) concluded, based on kinetic argumentation and on data from systemic inhibition of protein synthesis, that the effect of macromolecular synthesis inhibition on consolidation is not due to the depletion of constitutively expressed proteins. This might

indeed hold for the critical initial period, but does not reflect the synaptic need for protein supplies over longer time periods. Despite the theoretical ability of neurites and synapses to sustain long-term change autonomously (Crick, 1984; Lisman, 1985; Buxbaum and Dudai, 1989; Friedrich, 1990), and their possibility of sustaining some degree of protein synthesis locally (e.g. Davis *et al.*, 1987; Feig and Lipton, 1993; Ouyang *et al.*, 1997; Casadio *et al.*, 1999), it is plausible to assume that nuclear transcriptional changes must be invoked to supplement and replenish the synapse with housekeeping and building material. Furthermore, the fact that a synapse is active might signal to the nucleus that it should be strengthened properly and supplied to withstand the demands of extensive use. It reminds one of the instantaneous recruitment of blood to activated brain areas, so successfully exploited in functional neuroimaging (Cohen and Bookheimer, 1994). The capillary blood flow is not part of the computational machinery, but rather fuels the machinery to keep the computations going. This raises issues of causality and specificity. Though obligatory for sustaining the process over time, modulation of transcription might be neither causal nor sufficient for determining the specificity of changes in a neuronal circuit; specificity could be determined locally and autonomously. If this is true, one should not expect to elucidate mechanisms of specificity, so critical to learning and memory, by analyzing cell-wide transcriptional alterations alone.

A quite separate issue has to do with some facets of integration, context and generalization of information. Additional dissociations emerge from recent studies on hippocampus and *Aplysia*. One is spatial—between the hijacker and the hijacked—namely the dissociation between the local tag (enabling spatial specificity and some measure of temporal specificity) and the proteins captured from other components of the neuron (reinforcing the embodiment of the long-term change at the specific tagged location). Another is definitively temporal, between the event marking specificity (and leading to the creation of the local tag) and the time window surrounding it (during which activity-dependent proteins can be captured by the tagged synapse). At the cellular level, these spatial and the temporal linkages might subserve binding and encoding of context over time and space (Frey and Morris, 1997). Hence it might be advantageous to 'inform' other synapses on a neuron that a salient event has occurred, and to have a cellular mechanism of 'local attention' that—provided the context signifies saliency—permits mild stimuli to be construed as important ones (and ultimately resulting in a more permanent record of their occurrence). Such a mechanism might also contribute to generalization and categorization, mirroring at the cellular level functional drives that operate at the system level (e.g. McClelland *et al.*, 1995). What is unveiled here could be regarded as an additional manifestation of an elementary property of perceptual, mnemonic and cognitive systems, namely the ability to bind representational elements into a coherent whole over time and space. This is realized in the brain at different levels of resolution. For example, perceptual binding of instantaneous events in the sub-second range by some sort of fast coincidence detection in neuronal assemblies (which refers to the current popular usage of 'binding' in the neurosciences, see also Singer, Chapter 3); binding of context and events on a time scale of minutes to hours which might be subserved among others at the cellular level by local consolidation; and binding of events into narratives and categories over weeks to years in system consolidation (Dudai, 1996, 1997b). It should also be noted that local, cellular processes of integration and generalization, embodied in the interdependency of remote synapses on the same neuron in cellular consolidation, may pose as yet unknown constraints on computations made over elements of internal representations.

A third factor is metaplasticity. In both vertebrate (Kirkwood *et al.*, 1996) and invertebrate (Fischer *et al.*, 1997) nervous systems, the induction of synaptic plasticity also results in a modulation of the ability of synapses to induce or maintain plasticity subsequently. This form of higher order plasticity is dubbed metaplasticity (Abraham and Bear, 1996). The induction by activated synapses of cell-wide waves of protein synthesis, and the resulting effects of these waves on synapses in which local protein synthesis had not been triggered, could be another example of metaplasticity.

CONCLUSIONS

We have focused on a number of open questions concerning local, cellular consolidation in neuronal circuits. Recent evidence suggests that consolidation need not be triggered in an abrupt, step-like function manner by intensive input, and does not necessarily unfold in a predetermined, fixed cascade of developmental decisions. Rather, it appears to involve decision making at multiple sites in the neuronal domain,

and an intricate interaction between local and central mechanisms within the neuron. It may, *in vivo*, need coincident inputs in order to start rolling. Its time course depends on the history of the neuron and the circuit, and is not expected to follow rigid time windows and phases. Whereas macromolecular synthesis appears obligatory for the process to proceed, the possibility that it does not play a causal role in altering representational properties and does not contribute to the specificity of the change, but rather fulfills post-factum supportive, homeostatic and possibly preparatory functions, should not be ignored. In spite of its appeal, the analogy to developmental processes, which emerges from the cellular analysis of consolidation, should not blur the search for the unique representational properties of synapses and neurons in the brain and their stabilization over time. A developing neuromuscular junction may use molecular cascades similar to those that are detected in a consolidating synapse but, for all their capacity to move minds, muscles did not think up *Hamlet*.

Consolidation is not only indispensable for some types of memory; it is also a potential window into the functions of memory at large, the processes that subserve these functions, the mechanisms that embody these processes and the interaction between levels of organization and function in the brain. Recent investigations of the cellular biology of consolidation begin to expose fine distinctions between the specific and the general, the local and the global, the tokens and the types of the cellular processes and mechanisms that subserve the conversion of precepts into long-lasting internal representations. These processes and mechanisms now become definable in a molecular language. This makes it attractive to consider the formulation of rudimentary correspondence rules (Nagel, 1979) for the translation of certain aspects of behavioral and physiological phenomena related to consolidation, such as attention, association and generalization, into cellular and molecular events, and vice versa.

ACKNOWLEDGEMENTS

Preparation of this chapter was made possible by a Programme Grant from the Medical Research Council to R.G.M.M. which provided funds for a visit by Y.D. to Edinburgh, and funds from the Dominic Center, the Weizmann Institute of Science to Y.D.

REFERENCES

Abraham, W.C. and Bear, M.F. (1996) Metaplasticity: the plasticity of synaptic plasticity. *Trends in Neurosciences*, 19, 126–130.

Agranoff, B.W. and Klinger, P.D. (1964) Puromycin effect on memory fixation in the goldfish. *Science*, 146, 952–953.

Bailey, C.H. and Kandel, E.R. (1993) Structural changes accompanying memory storage. *Annual Review of Physiology*, 55, 397–426.

Barria, A., Muller, D., Derkach, V., Griffith, L.C. and Soderling, T.R. (1997) Regulatory phosphorylation of AMPA-type glutamate receptors by CaM-KII during long-term potentiation. *Science*, 276, 2042–2045.

Bartsch, D., Ghirardi, M., Skehel, P.A., Karl, K.A., Herder, S.P., Chen, M., Bailey, C.H. and Kandel, E.R. (1995) *Aplysia* CREB2 represses long-term facilitation: relief of repression converts transient facilitation into long-term functional and structural change. *Cell*, 83, 979–992.

Berman, D.E., Hazvi, S., Rosenblum, K., Seger, R. and Dudai, Y. (1998) Specific and differential activation of mitogen-activated protein kinase cascades by unfamiliar taste in the insular cortex of the behaving rat. *Journal of Neuroscience*, 18, 10037–10044.

Blendy, J.A., Kaestner, K.H., Schmid, W., Gass, P. and Schutz, G. (1996) Targeting of the CREB gene leads to up-regulation of a novel CREB mRNA isoform. *EMBO Journal*, 15, 1098–1106.

Bourtchuladze, R., Frenguelli, B., Blendy, J., Cioffi, D., Schutz, G. and Silva, A.J. (1994) Deficient long-term memory in mice with a targeted mutation of the cAMP-repsonsive element-binding protein. *Cell*, 79, 59–68.

Brown, R. and Kulik, J. (1977) Flashbulb memories. *Cognition*, 5, 73–99.

Buxbaum, J. and Dudai, Y. (1989) A quantitative model for the kinetics of cAMP-dependent protein kinase (type II) activity: long-term activation of the kinase and its possible relevance to learning and memory. *Journal of Biological Chemistry*, 264, 9344–9351.

Byrne, W.L., Samuel, D., Bennett, E.L., Rosenzweig, M.R., Wasserman, E., Wagner, A.R. *et al.* (1966) Memory transfer. *Science*, 153, 658–659.

Cajal, R.Y. (1911) *Histologie du Systeme Nerveux de l'Homme et des Vertebres*. Tipografica Artistica, Madrid.

Carew, T.J., Menzel, R. and Shatz, C.J. (1998) Points of contact between development and learning. In: Carew, T.J., Menzel, R. and Shatz, C.H. (eds), *Mechanistic Relationships between Development and Learning*. Wiley, Chichester, UK, pp. 1–15.

Casadio, A., Martin, K., Giustetto, M., Zhu, H., Chen, M., Bartsch, D., Bailey, C.H. and Kandel, E.R. (1999) A transient, neuron-wide form of CREB-mediated long-term facilitation can be stabilized at specific synapses by local protein synthesis. *Cell*, 99, 221–237.

Cavallaro, S., Meiri, N., Yi, C.-L., Musso, S., Ma, W., Goldberg, J. and Alkon, D.L. (1997) Late memory-related genes in the hippocampus revealed by RNA fingerprinting. *Proceedings of the National Academy of Sciences of the United States of America*, 94, 9669–9673.

Chain, D.G., Hegde, A.N., Yamamoto, N., Liu-Marsh, B. and Schwartz, J.H. (1995) Persistent activation of cAMP-dependent protein kinase by regulated proteolysis suggests a neuron-specific function of the ubiquitin system in *Aplysia*. *Journal of Neuroscience*, 15, 7592–7603.

Cohen, M.S. and Bookheimer, S.Y. (1994) Localization of brain function using magnetic resonance imaging. *Trends in Neurosciences*, 17, 268–277.

Corfas, G. and Dudai, Y. (1991) Memory mutations and age affect the fine structure of an identified sensory neuron in *Drosophila*. *Proceedings of the National Academy of Sciences of the United States of America*, 88, 7252–7256.

Creutzfeld, O.D. (1995) *Cortex Cerebri: Performance, Structure and Functional Organization of the Cortex*. Oxford University Press, Oxford.

Crick, F. (1984) Memory and molecular turnover. *Nature*, 312, 101.

Crow, T. and Forrester, J. (1990) Inhibition of protein synthesis blocks long-term enhancement of generator potentials produced by one-trial *in vivo* conditioning in *Hermissenda*. *Proceedings of the National Academy of Sciences of the United States of America*, 87, 4490–4494.

Crow, T., Xue-Bian, J.J., Siddiqi, V., Kang, Y. and Neary, J.T. (1998) Phosphorylation of mitogen-activated protein kinase by one-trial and multi-trial classical conditioning. *Journal of Neuroscience*, 18, 3480–3487.

Davis, G.W., Schuster, C.M. and Goodman, C.S. (1996) Genetic dissection of structural and functional components of synaptic plasticity. 3. CREB is necessary for presynaptic functional plasticity. *Neuron*, 17, 669–679.

Davis, H.P. and Squire, L.R. (1984) Protein synthesis and memory: a review. *Psychological Bulletin*, 96, 518–559.

Davis, L., Banker, G.A. and Steward, O. (1987) Selective dendritic transport of RNA in hippocampal neurons in culture. *Nature*, 330, 477–479.

Deisseroth, K., Bito, H. and Tsien, R.W. (1996) Signaling from synapse to nucleus: postsynaptic CREB phosphorylation during multiple forms of hippocampal synaptic plasticity. *Neuron*, 16, 89–101.

DeZazzo, J. and Tully, T. (1995) Dissection of memory formation: from behavioral pharmacology to molecular genetics. *Trends in Neurosciences*, 18, 212–218.

Dingman, W. and Sporn, M.B. (1961) The incorporation of 8-azaguanine into rat brain RNA and its effect on maze-learning by the rat: an inquiry into the biochemical basis of memory. *Journal of Psychiatric Research*, 1, 1–11.

Dudai, Y. (1989) *The Neurobiology of Memory. Concepts, Findings, Trends*. Oxford University Press, Oxford.

Dudai, Y. (1992) Why should 'learning' and 'memory' be redefined (or, an agenda for focused reductionism). *Concepts in Neuroscience*, 3, 99–121.

Dudai, Y. (1996) Consolidation: fragility on the road to the engram. *Neuron*, 17, 367–370.

Dudai, Y. (1997a) How big is human memory, or, on being just useful enough. *Learning and Memory*, 3, 341–365.

Dudai, Y. (1997b) Time to remember. *Neuron*, 18, 179–182.

Emptage, N.J. and Carew, T.J. (1993) Long-term synaptic facilitation in the absence of short-term facilitation in *Aplysia* neurons. *Science*, 262, 253–256.

Feig, S. and Lipton, D. (1993) Pairing the cholinergic agonist carbachol with patterned Schaffer collaterals stimulation initiates protein synthesis in hippocampal CA1 pyramidal cell dendrites via a muscarinic NMDA-dependent mechanism. *Journal of Neuroscience*, 13, 1010–1021.

Fields, R.D. and Itoh, K. (1996) Neural cell adhesion molecules in activity-dependent development and synaptic plasticity. *Trends in Neurosciences*, 19, 473–480.

Fischer, T.M., Blazis, D.E.J., Priver, N.A. and Carew, T.J. (1997) Metaplasticity at identified inhibitory synapses in *Aplysia*. *Nature*, 389, 860–865.

Flexner, J.B., Flexner, L.B., and Stellar, E. (1963) Memory in mice as affected by intracerebral puromycin. *Science*, 141, 57–59.

Frank, D.A. and Greenberg, M.E. (1994) CREB: a mediator of long-term memory from mollusks to mammals. *Cell*, 79, 5–8.

Freeman, F.M., Rose, S.P.R. and Scholey, A.B. (1995) Two time windows of anisomycin-induced amnesia for passive avoidance training in the day-old chick. *Neurobiology of Learning and Memory*, 63, 291–295.

Frey, U. and Morris, R.G.M. (1997) Synaptic tagging and long-term potentiation. *Nature*, 385, 533–536.

Frey, U. and Morris, R.G.M. (1998) Synaptic tagging: implications for late maintenance of hippocampal long-term potentiation. *Trends in Neurosciences*, 21, 181–187.

Frey, U., Müller, M. and Kuhl, D. (1996) A different form of long- lasting potentiation revealed in tissue plasminogen activator mutant mice. *Journal of Neuroscience*, 16, 2057–2063.

Friedrich, P. (1990) Protein structure: the primary substrate for memory. *Neuroscience*, 35, 1–7.

Ghirardi, M., Montarolo, P.G. and Kandel, E.R. (1995) A novel intermediate stage in the transition between short- and long-term facilitation in the sensory to motor neuron synapse of *Aplysia*. *Neuron*, 14, 413–420.

Goelet, P., Castellucci, V.F., Schacher, S. and Kandel, E.R. (1986) The long and the short of long-term memory—a molecular framework. *Nature*, 322, 419–422

Grecksch, G, and Matthies, H. (1980) Two sensitive periods for the amnesic effect of anisomycin. *Pharmacology, Biochemistry and Behavior*, 12, 663–665.

Guzowski, J.F. and McGaugh, J.L. (1997) Antisense oligodeoxynucleotide-mediated disruption of hippocampal cAMP response element binding protein levels impairs consolidation of memory for water maze training. *Proceedings of the National Academy of Sciences of the United States of America*, 94, 2693–2698.

Hamberger, C.A. and Hyden, H. (1945) Cytochemical changes in the cochlear ganglion caused by acoustic stimulation and trauma. *Acta Oto-Laryngology*, 61 (Suppl.), 5–89.

Hayashi, Y., Shi, S.H., Esteban, J.A., Piccini, A., Poncer, J.C. and Malinow, R. (2000) Driving AMPA receptors into synapses by LTP and CaMKII: Requirement for GluR1 and PDZ domain interaction. *Science*, 287, 2262–2267.

Hebb, D.O. (1949) *The Organization of Behavior: A Neuropsychological Theory*. Wiley, New York.

Hegde, A.N., Goldberg, A.L. and Schwartz, J.H. (1993) Regulatory subunits of cAMP-dependent protein kinases are degraded after conjugation to ubiquitin: a molecular mechanism underlying long-term synaptic plasticity. *Proceedings of the National Academy of Sciences of the United States of America*, 90, 7436–7440.

Hegde, A.N., Inokuchi, K., Pei, W.Z., Casadio, A., Ghirardi, M., Chain, D.G., Martin, K.C., Kandel, E.R. and Schwartz, J.H. (1997) Ubiquitin C-terminal hydrolase is an immediate-early gene essential for long-term facilitation in *Aplysia*. *Cell*, 89, 115–126.

Hill, C.S. and Treisman, R. (1995) Transcriptional regulation by extracellular signals: mechanisms and specificity. *Cell*, 80, 199–211.

Horn, G. (1998) Visual imprinting and the neural mechanisms of recognition memory. *Trends in Neurosciences*, 21, 300–305.

Horn, G.., Bradley, P. and McCabe, B.J. (1985) Changes in the structure of synapses associated with learning. *Journal of Neuroscience*, 5, 3161–3168.

Huh, K.-H. and Wenthold, R.J. (1999) Turnover analysis of glutamate receptors identifies a rapidly degraded pool of the *N*-methyl-D-aspartate receptor subunit, NR1, in cultured cerebellar granule cells. *Journal of Biological Chemistry*, 274, 151–157.

Hyden, H. and Egyhazi, E. (1962) Nuclear RNA changes of nerve cells during a learning experiment in rats. *Proceedings of the National Academy of Sciences of the United States of America*, 48, 1366–1373.

Hyden, H. and Lange, P. (1965) A differentiation in RNA response in neurons early and late in learning. *Proceedings of the National Academy of Sciences of the United States of America*, 53, 946–952.

Impey, S., Mark, M., Villacres, E.C., Poser, S., Chavkin, C. and Storm, D.R. (1996) Induction of CRE-mediated gene expression by stimuli that generate long-lasting LTP in area CA1 of the hippocampus. *Neuron*, 16, 973–982.

James, W. (1890/1950) *The Principles of Psychology*. Dover, New York.

Kaang, B.-K., Kandel, E.R. and Grant, S.G.N. (1993) Activation of cAMP-responsive genes by stimuli that produce long-term facilitation in *Aplysia* sensory neurons. *Neuron*, 10, 427–435.

Kandel, E.R. and Schwartz, J.H. (1982) Molecular biology of learning: Modulation of transmitter release. *Science*, 218, 433–443.

Kennedy, T.E., Kuhl, D., Barzilai, A., Sweatt, J.D. and Kandel, E.R. (1992) Long-term sensitization training in *Aplysia* leads to an increase in calreticulin, a major presynaptic calcium-binding protein. *Neuron*, 9, 1013–1024.

Kirkwood, A., Rioult, M.G. and Bear, M.F. (1996) Experience-dependent modification of synaptic plasticity in visual cortex. *Nature*, 381, 526–528.

Krug, M., Lossner, B. and Ott, T. (1984) Anisomycin blocks the late phase of long-term potentiation in the dentate gyrus of freely moving rats. *Brain Research Bulletin*, 13, 39–42.

Kuhl, D., Kennedy, T.E., Barzilai, A. and Kandel, E.R. (1992) Long-term sensitization training in *Aplysia* leads to an increase in the expression of BiP, the major protein chaperon of the ER. *Journal of Cell Biology*, 119, 1069–1076.

Kullmann, D.M., Perkel, D.J., Manabe, T. and Nicoll, R.A. (1992) Calcium entry via postsynaptic voltage-sensitive calcium channels can transiently potentiate excitatory synaptic transmission in the hippocampus. *Neuron*, 9, 1175–1183.

Kyriakis, J.M., Banerjee, P., Nikolakai, E., Dai, T., Rubie, E.A., Ahmad, M.F., Avruch, J. and Woodgett, J.R. (1994) The stress-activated protein kinase subfamily of c-Jun kinases. *Nature*, 369, 156–160.

Lamprecht, R., Hazvi, S. and Dudai, Y. (1997) cAMP response element-binding protein in the amygdala is required for long- but not short-term conditioned taste aversion memory. *Journal of Neuroscience*, 17, 8443–8450.

Linden, D.J. (1996) A protein synthesis-dependent late phase of cerebellar long-term depression. *Neuron*, 17, 483–490.

Lisman, J.E. (1985) A mechanism for memory storage insensitive to molecular turnover: a bistable autophosphorylating kinase. *Proceedings of the National Academy of Sciences of the United States of America*, 82, 3055–3057.

Lisman, J.E. and Fallon, J.R. (1999) What maintains memories? *Science*, 283, 339–340.

Luria, A.R. (1968) *The Mind of a Mnemonist*. Jonathan Cape, London.

Martin, K.C. and Kandel, E.R. (1996) Cell adhesion molecules, CREB, and the formation of new synaptic connections. *Neuron*, 17, 567–570.

Martin, K.C., Casadio, A., Zhu, H.X., E, Y., Rose, J.C., Chen, M., Bailey, C.H. and Kandel, E.R. (1997a) Synapse-specific, long-form facilitation of *Aplysia* sensory to motor synapses: a function for local protein synthesis in memory storage. *Cell*, 91, 927–938.

Martin, K.C., Michael, D., Rose, J.C., Barad, M., Casadio, A., Zhu, H.X. and Kandel, E.R. (1997b) MAP kinase translocates into the nucleus of the presynaptic cell and is required for long-term facilitation in *Aplysia*. *Neuron*, 18, 899–912.

Mayford, M., Barzilai, A., Keller, F., Schacher, S. and Kandel, E.R. (1992) Modulation of an NCAM-related adhesion molecular with long-term synaptic plasticity in *Aplysia*. *Science*, 256, 638–644.

McClelland, J.L., McNaughton, B.L. and O'Reilly, R.C. (1995) Why there are complementary learning systems in the hippocampus and neocortex: insights from the successes and failures of connectionist models of learning and memory. *Psychological Review*, 102, 419–457.

McGaugh, J.L. (1966) Time-dependent processes in memory storage. *Science*, 153, 1351–1358.

Meberg, P.J., Valcourt, E.G. and Routtenberg, A. (1995) Protein F1/GAP-43 and PKC gene expression patterns in hippocampus are altered 1–2 h after LTP. *Molecular Brain Research*, 34, 343–346.

Mizumori, S.J.Y., Rosenzweig, M.R. and Bennett, E.L. (1985) Long-term working memory in the rat: effects of hippocampally applied anisomycin. *Behavioral Neuroscience*, 99, 220–232.

Monne, L. (1949) Structure and function of neurones in relation to mental activity. *Biological Reviews*, 24, 297–315.

Montarolo, P.G., Goelet, P., Castellucci, V.F., Morgan, J., Kandel, E.R. and Schacher, S. (1986) A critical period for macromolecular synthesis in long-term heterosynaptic facilitation in *Aplysia*. *Science*, 234, 1249–1254.

Muller, G.E. and Pilzecker, A. (1900) Experimentelle Beitrage zur Lehre von Gedachtnis. *Zeitschrift für Psychologie*, 1, 1–300.

Nagel, E. (1979) *The Structure of Science. Problems in the Logic of Scientific Explanation*. Hackett, Indianapolis.

Nguyen, P.V., Abel, T. and Kandel, E.R. (1994) Requirement of a critical period of transcription for induction of a late phase of LTP. *Science*, 265, 1104–1107.

Niethammer, M., Kim, E. and Sheng, M. (1996) Interaction between the C terminus of NMDA receptor subunits and multiple members of the PSD-95 family of membrane-associated guanylate kinases. *Journal of Neuroscience*, 16, 2157–2163.

Otani, S., Marshall, C.J., Tate, W.P., Goddard, G.V. and Abraham, W.C. (1989) Maintenance of long-term potentiation in rat dentate gyrus requires protein synthesis but not messenger RNA synthesis immediately post-tetanization. *Neuroscience*, 28, 519–526.

Otmakhov, N., Griffith, L.C. and Lisman, J.E. (1997) Postsynaptic inhibitors of calcium/calmodulin-dependent protein kinase type II block induction but not maintenance of pairing-induced long-term potentiation. *Journal of Neuroscience*, 17, 5357–5365.

Ouyang, Y., Kantor, D., Harris, K.M., Schuman, E.M. and Kennedy, M.B. (1997) Visualization of the distribution of autophosphorylated calcium/calmodulin-dependent protein kinase II after tetanic stimulation in the CA1 area of the hippocampus. *Journal of Neuroscience*, 17, 5416–5427.

Ouyang, Y., Rosenstein, A., Kreiman, G., Schuman, E.M. and Kennedy, M.B. (1999) Tetanic stimulation leads to increased accumulation of Ca^{2+}/calmodulin-dependent protein kinase II via dendritic protein synthesis in hippocampal neurons. *Journal of Neuroscience*, 19, 7823–7833

Reyes, M. and Stanton, P.K. (1996) Induction of hippocampal long-term depression requires release of Ca^{2+} from separate presynaptic and postsynaptic intracellular stores. *Journal of Neuroscience*, 16, 5951–5960.

Rosenblum, K., Meiri, N. and Dudai, Y. (1993) Taste memory: the role of protein synthesis in gustatory cortex. *Behavioral and Neural Biology*, 59, 49–56.

Rosenzweig, M.R., Bennett, E.L., Colombo, P.J., Lee, D.W. and Serrano, P.A. (1993) Short-term, intermediate-term, and long-term memories. *Behavioural Brain Research*, 57, 193–198.

Roullet, P. and Sara, S.J. (1998) Consolidation of memory after its re-activation: involvement of beta-noradregernic receptors in the late-phase. *Neural Plasticity*, 6, 63–68.

Schwartz, J.H. (1993) Cognitive kinases. *Proceedings of the National Academy of Sciences of the United States of America*, 90, 8310–8313.

Shadmehr, R. and Holcomb, H.H. (1997) Neural correlates of motor memory consolidation. *Science*, 277, 821–825.

Shashua, V. (1979) Brain metabolism and the acquisition of new behaviors. III. Evidence for secretion of two proteins into the brain extracellular fluid after training. *Brain Research*, 166, 349–358.

Solomonia, R.O., McCabe, B.J. and Horn, G. (1998) Neural cell-adhesion molecules, learning and memory in the domestic chick. *Behavioral Neuroscience*, 112, 1–10.

Squire, L.R. and Barondes, S.H. (1976) Amnesic effect of cycloheximide not due to depletion of a constitutive brain protein with short half-life. *Brain Research*, 103, 183–189.

Squire, L.R. and Zola-Morgan, S. (1991) The medial temporal lobe memory system. *Science*, 253, 1380–1386.

Squire, L.R. and Zola, S.M. (1996) Structure and function of declarative and non-declarative memory systems. *Proceedings of the National Academy of Sciences of the United States of America*, 93, 13515–13522.

Stanton, P.K. and Sarvey, J.M. (1984) Blockade of long-term potentiation in rat hippocampal CA1 region by inhibitors of protein synthesis. *Journal of Neuroscience*, 4, 3080–3088.

Ungar, G (1970) Molecular mechanisms in information processing. *International Review of Neurobiology*, 13, 223–250.

Walters, E.T., Alizadeh, H. and Castro, G.A. (1991) Similar neuronal alterations induced by axonal injury and learning in *Aplysia*. *Science*, 253, 797–799.

Weiler, I.J., Hawrylak, N. and Greenough, W.T. (1995) Morphogenesis in memory formation: synaptic and cellular mechanisms. *Behavioural Brain Research*, 66, 1–6.

Winder, D.G., Mansuy, I.M., Osman, M., Moallem, T.M. and Kandel, E.R. (1998) Genetic and pharmacological evidence for a novel, intermediate phase of long-term potentiation suppressed by calcineurin. *Cell*, 92, 25–37.

Winocur, G. (1990) Anterograde and retrograde amnesia in rats with dorsal hippocampal or dorsomedial thalamic lesions. *Behavioural Brain Research* 38, 145–154.

Wyllie, D.J. and Nicoll, R.A. (1994) A role for protein kinases and phosphatases in the Ca^{2+}-induced enhancement of hippocampal AMPA receptor-mediated synaptic responses. *Neuron*, 13, 635–643.

Xu, R. and Salpeter, M.M. (1999) Rate constants of acetylcholine receptor internalization and degradation in mouse muscles. *Journal of Cell Physiology*, 181, 107–112

Yin, J.C.P., Wallach, J.S., Del Vecchio, M., Wilder, E.L., Zhou, H., Quinn, W.G, and Tully, T. (1994) Induction of a dominant negative CREB transgene specifically blocks long-term memory in *Drosophila*. *Cell*, 79, 49–58.

Zemp, J.W., Wilson, J.E., Schlesinger, K., Boggan, W.O. and Glassman, E. (1966) Brain function and macromolecules. I. Incorporation of uridine into RNA of mouse brain during short-term training experience. *Proceedings of the National Academy of Sciences of the United States of America*, 55, 1423–1431.

10 GENETIC STRATEGIES FOR THE STUDY OF HIPPOCAMPAL-BASED MEMORY STORAGE

Danny G. Winder and Eric R. Kandel

INTRODUCTION

Memory is a remarkable mental faculty, one that is distinguished for both its importance and its variability. Under some circumstances, memory can persist reliably for decades. Under other circumstances, it can fade or become unreliable, or even distorted. The same person that might vividly recall in minute details the events surrounding their wedding 20 years ago can forget the details of a breakfast they had a few hours ago. Such variability in memory storage is important for our day-to-day lives. It is in part the variability of memory that helps in prioritizing the information that we do store. Indeed, a reasonable balance of memory storage and memory loss may be one of the essential requirements of a well-functioning free and independent mind. Memory storage that is either too detailed or too feeble would be detrimental to optimal functioning.

What then are the basic mechanisms of memory storage? Also what factors impart variability on the storage of memory? Since Ramon Y Cajal in his Croonian lecture to the Royal Society in 1894 first proposed that memory formation must involve a lasting modification in neuronal connections, neuroscientists (Gabriel Horn among them; see, for example, Horn, 1998, Chapter 19) have been pursuing the cellular substrate for learning and memory.

In the 1970s, Bliss and Lømo (1973) discovered long-term potentiation (LTP) of glutamatergic synaptic transmission. LTP is a robust enhancement of synaptic transmission, and currently is a leading candidate for the cellular substrate for hippocampal-based learning and memory in mammals. Thus, for the last 30 years, neuroscientists have been trying to unravel the molecular mechanisms underlying LTP and attempting to determine the relevance of LTP to memory storage (see Dudai and Morris, Chapter 9).

In this chapter, we will briefly describe those aspects of LTP that make it an appealing candidate for a cellular substrate for memory formation. We then describe new genetic approaches for studying LTP that have begun to delineate the signal cascades necessary for distinct phases of LTP and the relationship of these cellular physiological phases to the phases of memory storage.

BASIC PROPERTIES OF LTP: A CELLULAR SUBSTRATE FOR LEARNING AND MEMORY?

LTP is a lasting enhancement of synaptic transmission in response to a brief high-frequency stimulus that shares several properties with hippocampal-based learning and memory (Figure 10.1).

(i) LTP occurs at synapses that, based on lesion studies, are thought to play a role in learning and memory. Studies ranging from rodents, monkeys and humans with temporal lobe damage all suggest that the hippocampus plays a key role in long-term memory formation. The hippocampus is a rudimentary cortical structure with a basic trisynaptic organization in which each of the main cell types is glutamatergic (Figure 10.1A). Each of the synapses in this structure can undergo LTP. The Schaffer collateral–CA1 pyramidal cell pathway is thought to be particularly important for memory storage, since selective lesions of this pathway in humans and in experimental animals produce significant interference in memory storage (Zola-Morgan *et al.*, 1986).

(ii) LTP is associative, like some forms of memory. This associativity is imparted by the unique properties of the N-methyl-D-aspartate (NMDA)

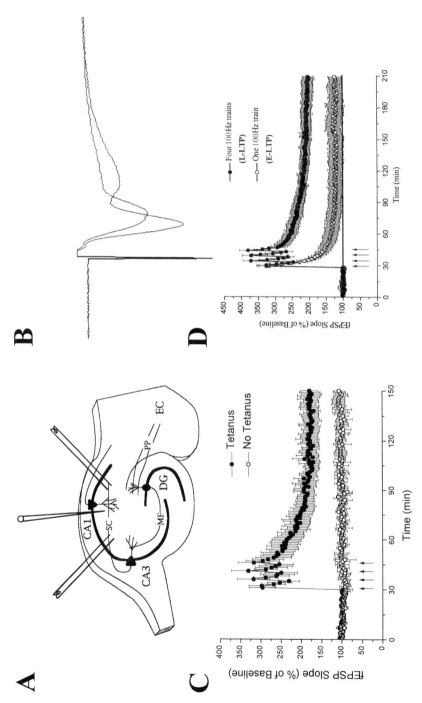

Figure 10.1. (A) Hippocampal slice schematic including two stimulating electrodes and a central recording micropipet (adapted from a schematic kindly provided by Dr Robert Gereau, IV). (B) Typical fEPSPs recorded before and after the induction of LTP at the Schaffer collateral–CA1 pyramidal cell synapse in a mouse hippocampal slice. (C) Two-pathway experiment demonstrating the pathway specificity of LTP. Upward arrows in (C) and (D) represent timing of LTP. (D) Multiple trains of tetanization recruit a non-decremental late phase of LTP.

subclass of glutamate receptor. Calcium influx through this receptor is required for NMDA receptor-dependent forms of LTP, yet this receptor is tonically blocked at resting membrane potentials by magnesium. Thus, the simultaneous presence of glutamate at postsynaptic NMDA receptors and postsynaptic depolarization is required to activate the NMDA receptor and to induce LTP.

(iii) LTP is pathway specific (Figure 10.1C). One can record from one CA1 pyramidal cell and stimulate two independent inputs onto that cell that synapse on distinct populations of dendritic spines. If one of these pathways is tetanized so that it undergoes NMDA receptor-dependent LTP, the second pathway will not show LTP unless the synapses happen to be extremely close to one another (<70 μm) (Engert and Bonhoeffer, 1997).

(iv) LTP, like memory, exists in distinct temporal and biochemical phases (Huang *et al.*, 1996). Thus, while short-term memory and short-lasting forms of LTP do not require protein or RNA synthesis, both long-term memory and a long-lasting form of LTP referred to as late-phase LTP require both RNA and protein synthesis (Figure 10.1D). These phases will be discussed in more detail later in this chapter.

(v) Like memory, LTP is quite susceptible to modulation, so that stimuli which elicit little if any LTP in one context might elicit robust LTP in another context. For example, as we will discuss in more detail later, the neuromodulator noradrenaline can convert stimuli that normally never elicit LTP to stimuli that produce robust LTP. Paralleling these data, noradrenaline has been suggested to play facilitatory roles in learning and memory (McGaugh *et al.*, Chapter 13).

INITIAL APPROACHES TO THE STUDY OF LTP AND THE LINK TO MEMORY STORAGE

While these five properties of LTP make it an attractive candidate for a cellular substrate for memory storage, it has proven extremely difficult to test this idea. There are two key problems. First, LTP is not unique to the Schaffer collateral pathway, but can be elicited at many synaptic sites within the brain, making it difficult to know where to begin to study the relationship between LTP and memory. Even within the hippocampus, a structure strongly implicated in memory formation, LTP can be generated at each of the glutamatergic synapses in the hippocampal trisynaptic circuit. Secondly, there remains a great deal of controversy about mechanisms required for the initiation and maintenance of LTP.

The bulk of experiments assessing mechanisms underlying LTP, and the link between LTP and memory, have been pharmacological in nature until recently (e.g. Morris, 1989). Pharmacological approaches, while providing good temporal resolution, are limited in scope and specificity. First, many molecules, such as transcription factors, that are interesting candidates as part of the LTP cascade are not tractable to pharmacological interventions. Secondly, pharmacological reagents often suffer from nonspecific actions, which can be quite insidious in the study of LTP and memory. For example, one controversial aspect of the induction of LTP in the hippocampus is the possible involvement of metabotropic glutamate receptors (mGluRs). Several groups have demonstrated that mGluR antagonists reduce NMDA receptor-dependent LTP (Bashir *et al.*, 1993; Riedel and Reymann, 1993; Richter-Levin *et al.*, 1994). However, an approximately equal number of groups working under quite similar conditions have failed to replicate these findings (Bordi and Ugolini, 1995; Selig *et al.*, 1995; Thomas and O'Dell, 1995). One possible explanation for this controversy was provided recently by Contractor *et al.* (1998) who demonstrated that the antagonists utilized in these studies bind not only to mGluRs but also to the glycine-binding site of the NMDA receptor (Contractor *et al.*, 1998).

In this chapter, we will review a parallel genetic approach to the study of synaptic plasticity and memory that has emerged recently, and rapidly is becoming an extremely useful adjunct approach to pharmacological studies as well as allowing the study of targets that previously were inaccessible.

GENETIC APPROACHES TO THE STUDY OF LTP AND MEMORY STORAGE

Studying LTP and memory storage with a genetic approach, deleting or overexpressing specific genes within an animal's genome, has a number of advantages. (i) This approach allows the study of some genes and their encoded proteins for which no pharmacological inhibitors exist. Moreover, in the case where pharmacological inhibitors do exist, genetic approaches provide converging lines of data. (ii) By altering the expression of a single gene, genetic approaches provide precise and specific experimental manipulations. (iii) Mice in which genes have been knocked out or overexpressed can be bred to produce large numbers of identical genetically modified animals, greatly reducing experimental variability. (iv) Once created, genetically modified animals can be backcrossed onto different strains with distinctive characteristics (such as fast and slow learners). (v) Genetically modified mice allow direct correlations between biochemical, morphological and electrophysiological data on the one hand, and intact animal behavioral data on the other.

First genetic approaches to the study of LTP and memory

Genetic approaches have had a major impact on the study of LTP and its relationship to hippocampal-based memory storage. For example, while it was clear from pharmacological studies that protein kinases are key signaling elements in LTP, it was not clear which particular kinases are involved. Leading candidates from early pharmacological studies included protein kinase C (PKC), calcium/calmodulin-dependent protein kinase IIα (CaMKIIα) and tyrosine kinases. To test these possibilities further, through targeted homologous recombination in embryonic stem (ES) cells, genes encoding specific isoforms of these kinases were deleted in mice. Briefly, the strategy for generating a knockout mouse involves the creation of a targeting vector that will undergo site-specific recombination in ES cells. ES cells that undergo this site-specific recombination, and thus have incorporated a portion of the targeting vector into the genome at the expense of a portion of the gene to be deleted, are then cloned and injected into blastocysts to produce chimeric animals that have a mosaic pattern of expression of the targeting vector. Chimeric animals that incorporate the targeting construct into the genome of stem cells are then mated to appropriate inbred mouse strains to produce non-mosaic mutant animals in which every cell in their body has the targeting construct integrated into the genome (for a more detailed description, see Soriano, 1995).

Studies from mice lacking the genes encoding CaMKIIα, PKCγ and the tyrosine kinase Fyn have provided critical converging data to those from pharmacological studies. Consistent with previous pharmacological studies, in mice lacking CaMKIIα, virtually no NMDA receptor-dependent LTP could be evoked, suggesting that CaMKIIα is an intrinsic signaling molecule in the minimal pathway necessary to elicit LTP (Silva *et al.*, 1992b). Mice lacking Fyn had a dramatic reduction of LTP elicited by high-frequency tetanization similar to that seen in tyrosine kinase inhibitor experiments, but did not have deficits in NMDA receptor-dependent LTP induced by saturating postsynaptic depolarization (Grant *et al.*, 1992). Interestingly, in mice lacking PKCγ, LTP was dramatically impaired, but could be restored through prior administration of prolonged low-frequency stimulation (Abeliovich *et al.*, 1993a). Thus, these data suggest the possibility that Fyn and PKCγ play important regulatory roles in the induction of LTP, or are more critically involved in later stages of LTP. Consistent with a role in the regulation of the induction of LTP, recent studies with Fyn knockout mice show that tyrosine phosphorylation of the NR2A subunit of the NMDA receptor is reduced compared with wild-type mice (Tezuka *et al.*, 1999).

Because these animals were deficient in hippocampal LTP, the performance of these animals was assessed on tasks that are thought to exploit hippocampal-dependent memory. One such task is the Morris water maze (Figure 10.2B). In this task, mice are placed in a pool of opaque water in which a hidden platform is positioned. The mice are trained over several trial blocks to find the hidden platform under conditions in which the location of the hidden platform and distal visual cues are held constant. Wild-type mice with an intact hippocampus can learn the location of the platform, as shown by a decreased latency to finding the platform and a greater than chance amount of time spent swimming in the quadrant that contained the platform when it is removed (for example, see left panel of Figure 10.2B). However, CaMKIIα and Fyn knockout mice were unable to perform this task successfully (Grant *et al.*, 1992; Silva *et al.*, 1992a). In contrast, PKCγ knockouts performed normally and were virtually indistinguishable from controls in Morris maze performance (Abeliovich *et al.*, 1993b). Thus while the CaMKIIα and Fyn knockout data seem to support a role for LTP in spatial memory formation, the PKCγ knockouts do not, although the argument can be made that *in vivo* LTP may be elicited in these mice during maze training. Further, while the PKCγ knockout mice did not show deficits in performance on the Morris water maze,

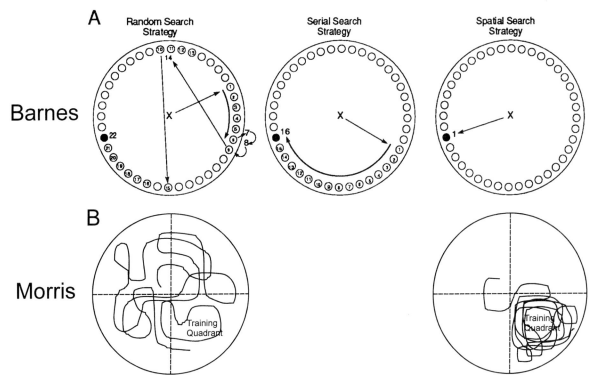

Figure 10.2. Morris and Barnes mazes for the study of learning and memory in rodents. (**A**) Schematic of Barnes maze apparatus with examples of distinct search strategies employed by mice. (**B**) Schematic of Morris maze apparatus illustrating the similarities between the two mazes.

they performed poorly in fear-conditioning paradigms that are thought to require the hippocampus.

Limitations of traditional knockout techniques

Using the conventional knockout approach to create genetically modified mice has provided important new data both for the molecular basis of LTP and for the correlation between LTP and behavior. However, there are significant problems inherent in these genetic approaches. These include: (i) a lack of spatial control of the mutation; (ii) lack of temporal control of the mutation; (iii) the genetic background on which the mutation is made; and (iv) gene compensation.

(i) In a conventional knockout, every cell in the animal's body lacks the gene of interest. Because of this, it is difficult to relate alterations in cell function in a particular region of the brain to whole animal behavior. It is possible, in fact likely, that unanticipated effects of the genetic alteration in other body regions could at least partially account for the behavioral phenotype. For example, a somatic or central nervous system (CNS) effect on motor coordination would seriously impair interpretation of learning and memory assays that require movement through space.

(ii) In addition to each cell lacking the gene, each cell carries this modification for the lifetime of the organism. Thus, it becomes difficult to distinguish whether a particular phenotype observed in an adult animal is the result of the acute effect of that genetic modification in the adult animal or whether it is a consequence of the prolonged genetic alteration throughout development. For example, in the Fyn knockout mouse, in addition to the defect in LTP in the hippocampus, hippocampal anatomy was also altered, making it difficult to know what the locus of the LTP deficit is (see below).

(iii) The genetic background of a strain of mice on which the genetic manipulation is made can contribute to the observed phenotype. Several studies have demonstrated that different inbred strains of mice perform quite distinctly on various behavioral paradigms (Crawley *et al.*, 1997). For example, two different mice lacking mGluR1 have been produced (Aiba *et al.*, 1994; Conquet *et al.*, 1994). While the mouse produced by Aiba *et al.* exhibits defective LTP at the Schaffer collateral–CA1 pyramidal cell synapse, the one produced by Conquet *et al.* is normal. Similarly, in two distinct lines of mice lacking the neurotrophin brain-derived neurotrophic factor (BDNF), deficits in LTP are seen in both lines, but deficits in basal synaptic transmission are seen in only one line (Korte *et al.*, 1995; Patterson *et al.*, 1996). Although there are other possibilities, one likely one is that the difference in phenotype represents different interactions between the mutation and the genetic background. To compound this problem, in many cases, genetically modified mice are bred as hybrids between different strains, resulting in a variable background from animal to animal.

(iv) There is also the problem of compensation. The ability to delete selectively specific isoforms of various enzymes is both a blessing and a curse. In most cases, pharmacological tools are not available to discriminate the contributions of distinct isoforms of an enzyme such as a kinase, so targeted deletion represents dramatically increased specificity. However, in many cases, the effects of deleting one isozyme are obscured by the compensatory up-regulation of complementary isozymes, as in the case of the RIβ protein kinase A (PKA) subunit knockout (Amieux *et al.*, 1997).

Thus, while in combination with other approaches the data from these mice provide powerful converging lines of evidence for the role of particular molecules both in LTP and memory formation, additional genetic approaches are required to deal with these problems. One approach has been to use antisense technology or viral vectors to alter gene expression. While these techniques show promise, significant problems are associated with them that have slowed their development as techniques for altering gene expression in a temporally controllable fashion selectively within the CNS (for reviews, see Nicot and Pfaff, 1997; Wim *et al.*, 1998). Our laboratories have therefore been interested in modifying genetic approaches in a variety of ways to compensate for the

deficiencies which emerged from the first-generation studies of genetically modified mice.

Rescue of genetic defects by restoration of recombinant protein in knockout mouse

In an attempt to differentiate between chronic and acute effects of the lack of a given gene in a knockout animal, one potentially successful strategy would be to resupply the recombinant protein that the gene encodes. For example, as mentioned earlier, mice lacking the gene encoding the neurotrophin BDNF exhibit reduced LTP (Korte *et al.*, 1995; Patterson *et al.*, 1996) and basal synaptic transmission (Patterson *et al.*, 1996). To determine whether this reflected a need for the protein during development of the hippocampus, Patterson *et al.* supplied recombinant BDNF to hippocampal slices from knockout mice. Interestingly, they found that pre-incubation of slices for 6–12 h with BDNF was sufficient to restore basal transmission and LTP back to wild-type levels. In an independent study, similar results were obtained by resupplying the BDNF gene by viral-mediated transfection (Korte *et al.*, 1996). Thus, these data suggest that in the hippocampus BDNF has a relatively acute role in synaptic transmission and modification of that transmission.

Unfortunately, while this was a compelling strategy for the study of neurotrophins in the hippocampus, resupplying recombinant protein is only useful for a limited subset of genes that encode extracellular signaling molecules such as BDNF. Thus this strategy would not be viable in cases where intracellular proteins are targeted.

Overexpression of transgenes in mouse CNS

As an alternative to targeted deletion of genes of interest, another possibility is the overexpression of genes within the CNS. Briefly, in gene overexpression experiments, linearized cDNA constructs encoding the gene of interest are microinjected into pronuclei of fertilized eggs to allow for random insertion into the genome. These eggs are then injected into pseudo-pregnant females. Offspring from these mothers are then analyzed by Southern blot or polymerase chain reaction (PCR) to determine in which mice the DNA construct underwent random insertion, and these 'founder' mice are backcrossed to inbred mouse strains. Founder mice and their offspring express the transgene according to several factors, mainly determined by the specific promoter utilized to drive transgene expression, the number of copies of the transgene that integrated into the genome and the chromosomal integration site (for a more detailed description, see Hogan *et al.*, 1986).

There are several advantages to the use of gene overexpression. Historically, to determine which regions of the brain participate in memory formation, chemical or electrolytic lesions have been used. These lesion experiments, however, suffer from several problems contributed by the induction of the lesion, the lack of reversibility of the lesion and verification of the extent of the lesion. In addition, such lesions often destroy fibers of passage in the region of interest that are not necessarily involved integrally in the function of that nucleus. By overexpression, one potentially can express a gene within a specific brain region. This represents a great advantage over traditional lesion experiments in that axons of passage are not affected, and the region of interest need not be destroyed but, rather, synaptic plasticity can be up- or down-regulated selectively in that region. Secondly, by using promoters that drive expression postnatally, the developmental consequences of the genetic manipulation are less than those achieved with targeted recombination.

There are, however, several cautions that need to be exercised in interpreting data from random integration-mediated overexpression. For example, while a knockout is an all-or-none modification of the expression of a gene, overexpressed transgenes can vary widely in their level of expression from line to line, depending on the site of integration, the promoter used to direct transgene expression and the number of copies inserted. Secondly, random integration experiments may be affected differentially from line to line by insertion site artifacts. On the other hand, differences in the levels of expression between different lines allow comparisons of an allelic series which aids in the comparison of multiple lines of mice carrying the same transgene and in the clear determination of the extent to which the insertion site contributes to the phenotype. In contrast, knockout animals carry the same linked genes regardless of line, making this determination more difficult, but no less critical, as exhibited by the mGluR1 and BDNF knockout mice.

In an effort to restrict the expression of transgenes spatially, several different promoters have been utilized to limit expression of transgenes to CNS alone, or to some subset of neural structures. One of the most successfully utilized promoters is the CaMKIIα pro-

moter. This promoter is advantageous for two reasons. First, it limits expression of transgenes primarily to forebrain and the limbic system. Secondly, the expression of CaMKIIα is postnatal, reducing the problems associated with transgene effects on development.

With overexpression, one can generate mice that overexpress a wild-type form of a given gene, or a mutated form that acts as a dominant-negative or constitutively activated form. Mayford *et al.* were the first to use this promoter to overexpress a mutated, constitutively active form of CaMKIIα (CaMKIIT286) to test further the roles of CaMKIIα in LTP (Mayford *et al.*, 1995). If activation of CaMKIIα is sufficient to induce LTP, then synaptic transmission should be saturated in mice overexpressing CaMKIIα. Mayford *et al.* actually found that while there was an approximate doubling of calcium-independent kinase activity in mutant mice expressing the transgene, LTP elicited by high-frequency stimulation was normal. However, overexpression of CaMKIIT286 shifted the frequency curve for stimuli that induce LTP versus long-term depression. In particular, 10 Hz stimuli near the endogenous theta frequency (3–7 Hz) firing range evokes LTP in wild-type animals but not in mutant mice. Thus these studies suggest that the roles of CaMKIIα in LTP may be more complex than was appreciated previously.

Although these animals showed no detectable decrease in LTP elicited by high-frequency stimulation traditionally used in the study of plasticity, they were nonetheless severely impaired in performance on a hippocampus-dependent task known as the Barnes maze (Barnes, 1979; Figure 10.2A). This task is a useful variant of the Morris water maze. The Barnes maze consists of a large circular platform around the periphery of which are spaced multiple holes. Under one of these holes is an escape chamber. Mice are trained to learn the location of the chamber by placing them in the center of the platform in a brightly lit room and applying a loud tone. These aversive stimuli compel the mouse to seek shelter. As in the Morris maze, in the spatial version of this task the position of the escape chamber and distal visual cues are kept constant across training trials. An advantage of this task compared with the Morris maze is the ease with which one can determine whether hippocampal- or non-hippocampal-based search strategies are employed. Bach *et al.* (1995) found that mice overexpressing the CaMKIIT286 transgene are selectively impaired in their ability to utilize the hippocampus-dependent spatial search strategy. Thus these studies nicely illustrate that it is insufficient to evaluate LTP only at high frequencies of stimulation. One needs also to consider the effects of a genetic manipulation on LTP elicited by lower frequency, more physiologically relevant stimuli when comparing LTP phenotypes in the hippocampal slice with memory phenotypes in the awake behaving animal. Further, these findings demonstrated that overexpression of transgenes in the CNS with the CaMKIIα promoter is a useful means of obtaining information about the contribution of a particular gene to LTP.

Another use for overexpression strategies is to resupply a gene deleted through targeted recombination. For example, while mice lacking Fyn exhibited defective LTP, they also had quite dramatic anatomical defects in their hippocampi that could contribute to the LTP deficit. To examine this possibility, Kojima *et al.* (1997) overexpressed a Fyn transgene under the control of the CaMKIIα promoter in mice lacking the Fyn gene. Since the transgene was not expressed until day 10 postnatally, the anatomical defects in the Fyn knockouts were not rescued by Fyn transgene overexpression. However, LTP was much greater in the knockouts that expressed the transgene than in those that did not, suggesting a clear dissociation between the anatomical and electrophysiological defects of Fyn deletion.

Finally, overexpressed transgenes can be very useful as reporters of biological activity. For example, mice overexpressing the reporter gene β-galactosidase under the direction of either cAMP-regulated element (CRE) sites that can be bound by the transcription factor CRE-binding protein (CREB) or the GAP-43 promoter have been useful in determining the physiological stimuli that activate these promoters (Impey *et al.*, 1996; Namgung *et al.*, 1997). In addition, one could overexpress a protein tagged with green fluorescent protein to study subcellular targeting of that protein in real time.

Temporal control of genetic manipulations in the CNS

The overexpression technique suffers from many of the same problems as the traditional knockout technique, and a few unique ones. Thus, a second generation of genetically modified animals has begun to be employed. One attractive model is to regulate temporally the expression of transgenes incorporated through random insertion. While the CaMKIIα promoter provides some level of spatial and temporal

restriction, one cannot turn the expression of the transgene on and off at will. Temporally regulated expression addresses two of the problems listed above. First, by being able to manipulate the timing of transgene expression, one can begin to differentiate between effects of a transgene during development versus acute effects in adult animals. Secondly, the reversal of a phenotype by turning off transgene expression argues against insertion site artifacts contributing to that phenotype. While several different inducible systems are in various stages of development, such as systems based on the insect ecdysone response (No *et al.*, 1996) as well as tamoxifen-regulated systems (Feil *et al.*, 1996; Zhang *et al.*, 1996; Brocard *et al.*, 1997; Schwenk *et al.*, 1998), by far the most successfully utilized system for the inducible overexpression of transgenes in the adult mouse brain to date is the tetracycline transactivator system developed by Bujaard and colleagues (Figure 10.3).

Tetracycline transactivator system

The tetracycline transactivator system utilizes a tetracycline-controlled transactivator protein (tTA), containing the repressor from the tetracycline resistance operon and the transactivating domain of the viral protein VP16 (Furth *et al.*, 1994). This mutant transactivator binds to the tet operator (*tetO*) and initiates transcription of the downstream gene. This system has the advantage that administration of tetracycline analogs displaces tTA from *tetO*, and thus suppresses transcription of the transgene. Since many tetracycline analogs have excellent bioavailability, this system is attractive as an inducible expression system in mouse. Thus, Mayford *et al.* generated mice overexpressing this transactivator using the CaMKIIα promoter. By crossing these mice with mice overexpressing the CaMKIIT286 transgene under the direction of *tetO*, they were able to obtain the same biochemical, electrophysiological and behavioral phenotypes observed in the first line of CaMKIIT286 mice, and demonstrate that the effects of the activated CaMKIIT286 transgene at each of these levels was reversed in mutant mice by administration of 1 mg/ml of the tetracycline analog doxycycline in the animals' drinking water for 2–3 weeks (Mayford *et al.*, 1996). Thus these data demonstrate that the phenotype observed is not a function of an insertion artifact, and suggest that the effect on LTP is not due to the chronic presence of the transgene during animal development. This system has also been utilized

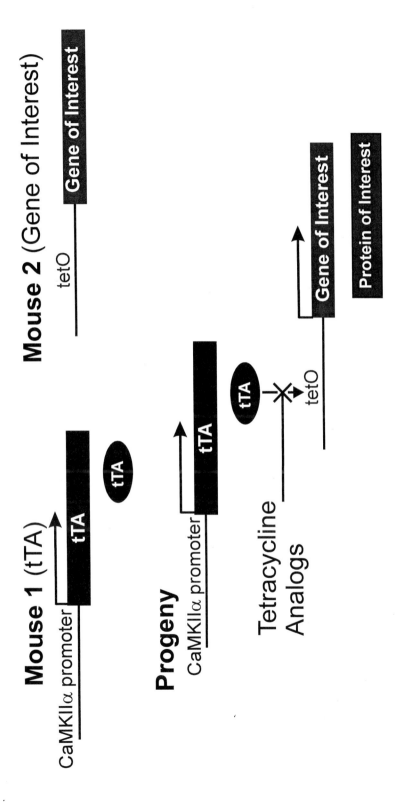

Figure 10.3. Second-generation gene overexpression strategies in mice: Schematic for the tTA system.

recently to overexpress an activated form of calcineurin (Mansuy *et al.*, 1998a; Winder *et al.*, 1998).
The phenotype of these mice, which will be discussed
below, was also reversed by the administration of
doxycycline in the animals' drinking water.

Reverse tetracycline transactivator system

While the tTA system is a major step forward in the
development of inducible gene expression systems in
mouse, it nonetheless still has weaknesses. For
example, it would be advantageous to be able to turn
a transgene on, rather than off, with the tetracycline
analog. One could consider administering the analogs
during gestation and then removing them during
adulthood, but this must be done very carefully since
tetracycline analogs in high doses can interfere with
normal development, and can be taken up into bone
where they then slowly leach out over an extended
period of time (although see Chen *et al.*, 1998).

In an attempt to circumvent some of these problems, Bujaard and colleagues performed chemical
mutagenesis of tTA. One of these mutants, referred to
as reverse tTA, or rtTA, had the unique feature that
rather than tetracycline analogs inhibiting binding of
the transactivator to *tetO*, these analogs are *required* to
facilitate this binding (Kistner *et al.*, 1996). Thus the
rtTA system can, in principle, be utilized as a forward
inducible system (Figure 10.4).

One of the problems originally associated with the
rtTA system was leakiness (see, for example, No *et al.*,
1996). Several laboratories have reported that there is
a high level of basal expression of transgenes in the
absence of tetracycline analogs in mice utilizing this
system, and particularly in transient transfection
systems. However, we recently have utilized the rtTA
system successfully for overexpression of two different transgenes in the CNS, the reporter gene β-galac-
tosidase and the phosphatase calcineurin (Mansuy *et
al.*, 1998b). In these mice, we found that administration of doxycycline at 6 mg/kg in the animal's food
for 2 weeks was sufficient to initiate expression of the
transgene in both lines, and that removal of doxycycline for 2 weeks was sufficient to return the level of
expression back to uninduced levels. Thus, through
utilization of the rtTA system, one can obtain relatively rapid induction and reversal of transgene
expression (although turnover rate is probably transgene specific), allowing for more creative experimental designs (see below). It is likely that the leakiness of
the rtTA system seen in other reports is a product of

positional effects of the insertion sites and, in the case
of transient transfections, an unusually high number
of copies inserted into the genome. One way to reduce
these problems would be to sequence the insertion site
in one of the lines of rtTA that does not give high
levels of basal transgene expression, and 'knock in'
rtTA into that locus using targeted recombination.

The convergence of overexpression and knockouts: Cre–*lox* system for spatially restricted gene knockout

In addition to the inducible, spatially localized overexpression strategies we have already considered, it
would be extremely useful to have similarly restricted
methods for gene ablation. This possibility has become
viable with the recent successful application of the
Cre–*loxP* system in mouse brain (Figure 10.5). In this
two-mouse system, *loxP* sites are inserted into the gene
through standard targeting techniques in one line of
mice. In the second line of mice, Cre recombinase is
overexpressed under the direction of a tissue-specific
promoter such as that for CaMKIIα. In double-positive
progeny of the matings of these two mice, the Cre
recombinase clips out DNA sequences between the
loxP sites, generating a knockout. Through the utilization of specific promoters to drive expression of Cre
recombinase, one can generate knockouts with some
degree of temporal and spatial regulation. In the
amazing extreme case, the Kandel and Tonegawa laboratories utilized the CamKIIα promoter to drive expression of Cre recombinase, and found that in some
lines of mice they were able to limit the knockout to the
CA1 region. The Tonegawa laboratory then used this
strategy to generate CA1-specific knockouts of the
NMDAR1 subunit of the NMDA receptor that did not
occur until about 3 weeks postnatally (Tsien *et al.*,
1996a,b). In these animals, NMDA receptor-dependent
LTP in area CA1 was abolished, while NMDA receptor-dependent LTP at the perforant path–dentate
granule cell synapse was unaltered. Although the LTP
deficit apparently was restricted to area CA1, there was
nonetheless a dramatic impairment of performance on
the spatial version of the Morris water maze. Since
basal synaptic transmission and briefer, NMDA recep-
tor-independent forms of plasticity were unaltered in
these animals, these experiments are some of the
strongest to date suggesting a direct link between
NMDA receptor-dependent LTP in area CA1 of the
hippocampus and learning and memory.

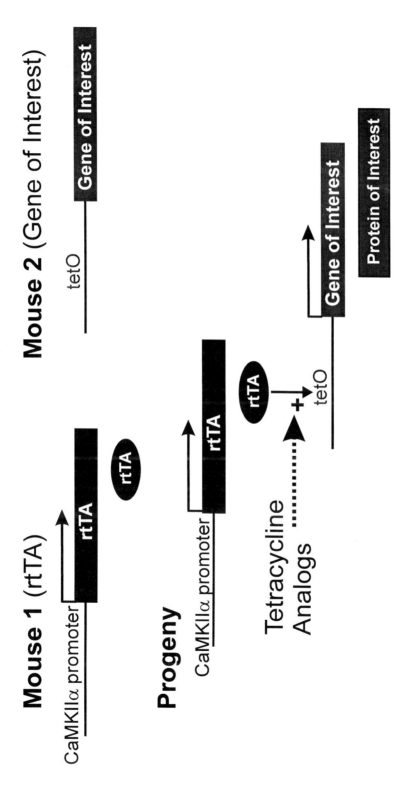

Figure 10.4. Second-generation gene overexpression strategies in mice: Schematic for the rtTA system.

174

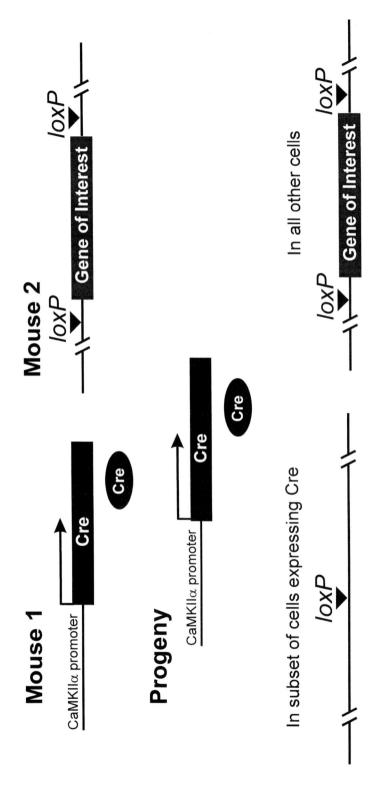

Figure 10.5. Second-generation Cre–*lox*-mediated gene knockout strategy in mice.

Future directions with second-generation genetic models

The development of more temporally and spatially restricted genetic modifications now allows the pursuit of many avenues of investigation that would have been difficult with the first generation of genetically modified mice. For example, one can imagine administering doxycycline to brain slice preparations after dissection from mice expressing transgenes under the rtTA system to carry out intra-animal gene/no gene comparisons of LTP. Further, one could examine the effects of different levels of transgene expression by utilizing doxycycline dose–response curves. Indeed, Chen *et al.* have shown recently that several orders of magnitude lower concentrations of doxycycline (25 μg/ml in drinking water) can still fully suppress transgene expression in the CNS under the tTA system (Chen *et al.*, 1998). This finding should greatly improve the kinetics of the tTA system by allowing more rapid reversal of the effects of doxycycline. Further, by using such a low dose, the toxic effects of doxycycline on development apparently are removed, allowing for experiments in which animals can be raised on doxycycline to suppress transgene expression through development. This should allow the development of mice overexpressing CRE recombinase under the tTA system to achieve temporally inducible knockouts in the CNS.

By utilizing the reversibility of regulatable systems, in particular the rtTA system, one can now begin to dissect the distinct components of learning and memory disrupted by a given transgene. For example, Mansuy *et al.* found that by overexpressing a calcineurin transgene in mouse brain, they could impair both LTP induced by two 100 Hz trains and performance on the spatial version of the Morris water maze (Figure 10.4; Mansuy *et al.*, 1998b). However, mutant animals utilizing the rtTA system that were not administered doxycycline, and thus did not express the transgene, were able to navigate this task successfully. When these mice were now administered doxycycline for 2 weeks, and then tested again for their memory of the location of the hidden platform, they spent a chance amount of time in each of the four quadrants, while their control counterparts show a strong preference for the quadrant that contained the hidden platform. This apparent deficit in the retrieval of spatial information was reversible, since these mice could be removed from doxycycline and tested a third time, at which time they then again showed a memory of the location of the hidden platform.

Thus these studies demonstrate that one effectively can manipulate the expression of the transgene during discrete periods of a behavioral experiment.

UTILIZATION OF GENETIC APPROACHES FOR THE STUDY OF SIGNALING CASCADES AND THEIR RELEVANCE TO LTP, NEUROMODULATION AND MEMORY STORAGE

With the array of genetic tools outlined above, neuroscientists are now in a position to test hypotheses that previously were very difficult to address. One area in which genetic approaches to the study of LTP are proving particularly useful is in the unraveling of signaling cascades that are required. Since it would be beyond the scope of this chapter to give a comprehensive review of the genetic approaches used to target signaling cascades involved in LTP and memory, we will focus on the genetic and pharmacological evidence suggesting the existence of multiple phases of NMDA receptor-dependent LTP and the implications for the function of the PKA signaling pathway in plasticity and memory.

LTP at the Schaffer collateral–CA1 pyramidal cell synapse exists in biochemically and stimulus-dependent distinct phases

As mentioned earlier, one of the attractive aspects of LTP as a cellular substrate of memory storage is that it exists in distinct temporal and biochemical phases. Thus, protein and RNA synthesis inhibitors reduce a late component of LTP elicited by strong stimulation, but do not affect LTP elicited by weak stimulation. For example, administration of a single 100 Hz train to the Schaffer collateral–CA1 pyramidal cell synapse results in a decremental form of LTP that lasts 2–3 h (Figure 10.1D). In contrast, administration of three to four 1 s 100 Hz trains spaced by 5 min elicits a non-decremental form of LTP that lasts as long as a healthy slice preparation can be maintained. While the LTP elicited by one train is unaffected by protein and RNA synthesis inhibitors, LTP elicited by 3–4 trains is reduced 2–4 h after the tetanus by these inhibitors. This difference led to the discrimination between early and late phases of LTP (for a review, see Huang *et al.*, 1996).

The finding that inhibitors of RNA synthesis reduce LTP elicited by multiple high-frequency trains suggests that this LTP involves one or more transcription factors. In the invertebrates *Aplysia* and *Drosophila*, the transcription factor CREB has been found to play a critical role in the generation of long-term facilitation of synaptic transmission and long-term memory (for a review, see Abel and Kandel, 1998). Thus it has been suggested that CREB plays a role in late-phase LTP in hippocampus. Unfortunately, to date, knockout mice have provided ambiguous results, in large part due to isozyme compensation by other CREB isoforms.

However, using a reporter mouse in which multiple CREs drive the expression of β-galactosidase, Impey *et al.* (1996) have demonstrated that stimuli that elicit late-phase LTP, but not early-phase LTP, elicit the initiation of CRE-dependent transcription.

What kinases initiate this transcriptionally dependent late phase of LTP? In the invertebrates *Aplysia* and *Drosophila*, previous studies have demonstrated a role for the PKA signaling cascade in long-term facilitation of synaptic transmission and long-term

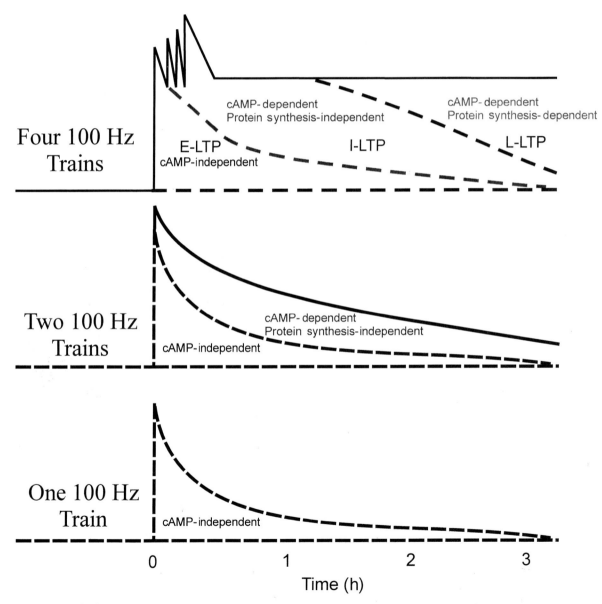

Figure 10.6.   Cartoon of LTP elicited by phases underlying one, two and four trains of 100 Hz stimulation.

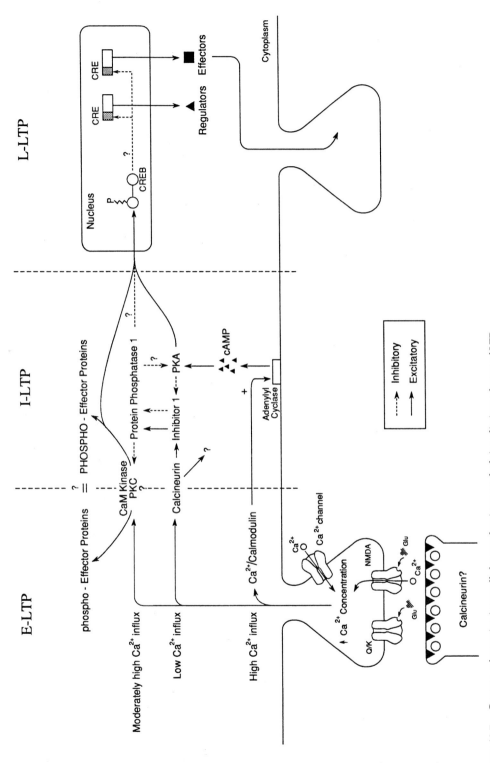

Figure 10.7. Cartoon of putative intracellular mechanisms underlying distinct phases of LTP.

memory, both of which are dependent on macro-molecular synthesis. Consistent with a role for PKA in the late phase of LTP, pharmacological activation of the PKA signaling cascade elicits a macromolecular synthesis-dependent enhancement of transmission that is mutually occlusive with tetanus-evoked late-phase LTP (Frey *et al.*, 1993). Conversely, inhibitors of PKA block the induction of late-phase LTP by repeated high-frequency tetanization. Just as with protein and RNA synthesis inhibitors in area CA1, PKA inhibitors were not effective in inhibiting LTP evoked by a single high-frequency train, but only LTP evoked by multiple high-frequency trains.

These data suggest that one of the distinctions between early- and late-phase LTP is that stronger stimuli that elicit late-phase LTP evoke the activation of additional second messenger systems (Figures 10.6 and 10.7). For example, a simple model for evoking more persistent LTP with repeated trains would be the stronger recruitment of a given kinase. If this were the case, it would be predicted that the kinase inhibitor would be more effective at inhibiting LTP evoked by a single high-frequency train, and less effective at inhibit-ing LTP evoked by repeated high-frequency trains. The fact that the opposite result was found with PKA inhibitors suggests that there is a threshold for the recruitment of PKA or a PKA-associated protein for the induction of late-phase LTP. Consistent with this idea, administration of a single high-frequency tetanus to hippocampal slices does not evoke the detectable activa-tion of PKA, accumulation of cAMP or initiation of CRE-dependent transcription, while administration of multiple high-frequency trains does in an NMDA-receptor dependent manner (Chetkovich *et al.*, 1991; Chetkovich and Sweatt, 1993; Frey *et al.*, 1993; Roberson and Sweatt, 1996).

Data from genetically modified mice provide con-verging evidence that PKA has a role in late-phase LTP at the Schaffer collateral–CA1 pyramidal cell synapse. Constitutive overexpression of a dominant-negative regulatory subunit of PKA [R(AB)] results in a modest reduction of total hippocampal PKA activity and a reduction in LTP elicited by four 100 Hz trains but not by a single 100 Hz train. Again, if the establishment of late-phase LTP was simply the result of the ramping up of PKA activity as the number of trains is increased, it would be predicted that LTP elicited by a single 100 Hz train would be reduced to a greater extent than LTP elicited by four 100 Hz trains.

In addition to providing genetic verification of pharmacological data, the R(AB) mice also allow comparisons to be made between the physiological phenotype and memory formation. Consistent with a proposed role for late-phase LTP in long-term memory storage, mice overexpressing the R(AB) transgene have deficient long-term memory, as they seem to learn spatial memory tasks such as the Morris water maze with the same time course as wild-types but, 24 h after the last training trial, probe trial analysis of memory in these animals showed that the R(AB) mutants could no longer remember the location of the hidden platform, while the wild-types did.

Interestingly, mice in which individual RIβ or CIβ subunits of the regulatory and catalytic subunits of PKA have been removed by targeted deletion do not show decreases in total PKA activity in hippocampal homogenates (Brandon *et al.*, 1995; Qi *et al.*, 1996). However, late-phase LTP was nonetheless reduced in area CA1 in the CIβ mice, although not to the degree seen in the R(AB) knockout mice. These findings suggest that specific isoforms of PKA play unique roles in LTP. Further, this provides an example of how, in some cases, overexpression of dominant-negative con-structs can be a more effective strategy than targeted deletion, depending on the specific question being addressed.

Evidence for an intermediate phase intervening between the early and late phases

One interesting result that is not explained by a simple division of LTP into early and late phases at the Schaffer collateral–CA1 pyramidal cell synapse is the finding that LTP evoked by multiple (3–4) high-frequency trains decays much more rapidly in the presence of PKA inhibitors than in the presence of protein synthesis inhibitors. This suggests that in addition to initiating a macromolecular synthesis-dependent late phase, PKA may participate in an intermediate, macromolecular synthesis-independent phase of LTP. A convergence of pharmacological and genetic data is consistent with this hypothesis. First, in contrast to LTP elicited by four 100 Hz trains, LTP elicited by two 100 Hz trains is independent of protein synthesis, yet still requires the activation of PKA. PKA inhibitors reduce LTP elicited by two 100 Hz trains in area CA1, and LTP induced by this protocol is reduced in R(AB) mice. Thus there exists a stimulus that can induce a form of PKA-dependent LTP that is macromolecular synthesis independent.

What role does PKA play in this intermediate phase of LTP? A growing body of evidence suggests that phosphatases may play roles in constraining synaptic enhancement, and mediating long-term depression of transmission (Mulkey *et al.*, 1993, 1994; Blitzer *et al.*, 1995, 1998; Thomas *et al.*, 1996; Winder *et al.*, 1998). Several mechanisms have been proposed as determinants of the balance of activity between kinases and phosphatases. In particular, the Ca^{2+}-activated phosphatase calcineurin (PP2B) has been a focus of attention because it is activated by calcium at concentrations that have little or no effect on Ca^{2+}-activated kinases. In addition to potentially dephosphorylating key molecules mediating synaptic plasticity, calcineurin can dephosphorylate a family of small molecular weight proteins such as inhibitor-1 and DARPP-32 that regulate the activity of protein phosphatase-1 (PP1). PKA can inactivate this phosphatase cascade by phosphorylation of these small molecular weight proteins, resulting in the inhibition of PP1. Thus, it has been suggested that one role for PKA in LTP is to suppress phosphatase cascades to allow the full expression of LTP.

Both pharmacological and genetic evidence suggest that the role of PKA in this intermediate phase is to suppress an endogenous phosphatase cascade. First, inhibition of phosphatases pharmacologically removes the ability of PKA inhibitors to reduce LTP evoked by strong stimuli (Blitzer *et al.*, 1995; Thomas *et al.*, 1996). Secondly, injection into pyramidal neurons of mutated forms of the small molecular weight protein inhibitor-1, a point of convergence of PKA and the phosphatase calcineurin, disrupts LTP (Blitzer *et al.*, 1998). Finally, overexpression of the phosphatase calcineurin, either constitutively with the CaMKIIα promoter or regulated with the tTA or rtTA systems, selectively inhibits PKA-dependent forms of LTP at the Schaffer collateral–CA1 pyramidal cell synapse (Mansuy *et al.*, 1998a,b; Winder *et al.*, 1998). Interestingly, however, pharmacologically evoked late-phase LTP that bypasses the earlier phases was not decreased by overexpression of calcineurin. Thus, in total, a convergence of pharmacological data suggests that PKA plays multiple roles in mediating LTP through both macromolecular synthesis-independent and -dependent means (Figures 10.6 and 10.7). One of these roles appears to involve suppression by PKA of an endogenous phosphatase cascade to allow for the more effective phosphorylation of effector molecules by kinases such as CaMKIIα. A second role is to initi-ate a macromolecular synthesis-dependent long-lasting late-phase potentiation.

Multiple sources of cAMP: neuromodulation in the hippocampus

The apparent involvement of distinct kinases in distinct phases of LTP has potentially important implications. In particular, while CaMKIIα is activated primarily by influx of calcium from the extracellular space, the cAMP signaling cascade can be regulated by a myriad of stimuli, including Ca^{2+}-, PKC, G-protein-coupled receptors, etc. Thus, it is conceivable that a wider variety of initiating stimuli could participate in the induction of PKA-dependent forms of LTP at the Schaffer collateral–CA1 pyramidal cell synapse than in the NMDA receptor-dependent initiation of the early phase through activation of CaMKIIα. This is particularly interesting given previous studies showing that there are a large number of neuromodulatory inputs into the hippocampus and that the modulators can regulate learning and memory on the one hand, and cAMP levels on the other. In addition to intrinsic modulation of these glutamatergic synapses by NMDA and mGlu receptors, the hippocampus receives extrinsic neuromodulatory input from several sources. For example, it receives noradrenergic input from the locus ceruleus, serotonergic input from the dorsal raphe, cholinergic input from the lateral septal nucleus and dopaminergic input from the ventral tegmentum. Activation of receptors for these neuromodulatory inputs in the hippocampus regulates glutamatergic transmission through the hippocampal circuit through activation of G-proteins that regulate various second messenger cascades, including the cAMP signaling cascade.

Previous pharmacological studies have suggested that many neuromodulators important in memory storage also have a role in LTP in the hippocampus. Antagonists of D1/D5 dopamine receptors reduce the tetanus-induced increase in cAMP levels as well as LTP induced by these strong tetani (Frey *et al.*, 1993; Huang and Kandel, 1995; Otmakhova and Lisman, 1996, 1998). In addition, a long-lasting increase in synaptic transmission that appears to share properties of late-phase LTP can be generated in a manner that bypasses electrical stimulation by application of agents that directly increase cAMP levels in area CA1, in particular D1/D5 dopamine receptor agonists (Huang and Kandel, 1995). Thus, these data suggest that D1/D5 dopamine receptors may play a role in the late phase of LTP by increasing cAMP levels.

In addition to dopaminergic receptor modulation of LTP, recent evidence suggests that β-adrenergic receptors can regulate LTP in a cAMP-dependent manner as well. For example, activation of the cAMP cascade by β-adrenergic receptor stimulation in area CA1 enables prolonged low-frequency stimulation, which normally elicits little change in synaptic transmission, to elicit robust LTP (Thomas *et al.*, 1996; Katsuki *et al.*, 1997, Winder *et al.*, 1999).

cAMP as a key messenger for modulation of neuronal signaling

What is the particular role of PKA in these later phases of LTP? Although regulation of endogenous phosphatases is one apparent mechanism, as discussed below, the cAMP signaling cascade plays an important role in a number of aspects of hippocampal neuronal function, and its levels are regulated by a diverse array of mechanisms. In fact, as will be detailed below, increasing evidence exists for PKA-independent roles for cAMP in the hippocampus, necessitating the need for genetic approaches specifically to target PKA-dependent versus independent roles in LTP.

Rapid modulation of cellular excitability

Activation of the neuronal cAMP signaling cascade has almost exclusively excitatory effects on CA1 and CA3 pyramidal cell excitability. Application of agents that enhance the cAMP signaling pathway at a gross level increases input resistance and to some degree depolarizes these neurons from their resting membrane potential. In addition, either directly or indirectly, cAMP elevations result in a decrease in the slow afterhyperpolarization (sAHP) that is thought to be responsible for limiting firing frequency, induce an inhibitory shift in the activation–inactivation kinetics of the A-current, enhance an inwardly rectifying chloride current, decrease the conductance of sodium channels, enhance L-type calcium channel availability and enhance currents elicited from P-type calcium channels (Madison and Nicoll, 1986; Gray and Johnston, 1987; Staley, 1994; Cantrell *et al.*, 1997, Kavalali *et al.*, 1997, Hoffman and Johnston, 1998). Data also suggest that cAMP may modulate hippocampal neuron excitability directly, without requiring PKA, through its actions on Ih and CNG channels (Pedarzani and Storm, 1995).

Rapid regulation of synaptic transmission

In addition to acute regulation of postsynaptic excitability, the cAMP signaling cascade can also regulate transmitter release from both glutamatergic and GABAergic synapses in the hippocampus. For example, activation of β-adrenergic receptors elicits a transient enhancement of synaptic transmission that is associated with an increased frequency of mini amplitudes but not frequency, and is associated with a decrease in paired-pulse facilitation (Gereau and Conn, 1994). Application of the adenylyl cyclase activator forskolin also results in a rapid enhancement of glutamatergic transmission that is associated with an increase in mini frequency but not amplitude (Chavez-Noriega and Stevens, 1992). Similar results have been obtained with γ-aminobutyric acid (GABA) release (Capogna *et al.*, 1995; Trudeau *et al.*, 1996).

Current evidence suggests that multiple mechanisms may underlie the acute enhancement of synaptic transmission elicited by the cAMP signaling cascade. For example, both presynaptic calcium channels and synaptic vesicle release machinery are phosphorylated in response to activation of PKA (Parfitt *et al.*, 1992; Hell *et al.*, 1995).

Rapid regulation of postsynaptic responsiveness

Activation of the PKA signaling cascade can regulate postsynaptic responsiveness to released glutamate and GABA. Activation of this cascade selectively enhances glutamate responsiveness in cultured hippocampal neurons, probably through phosphorylation of GluR6, although similar results have not been obtained in slice preparations (Greengard *et al.*, 1991; Wang *et al.*, 1991). PKA can also regulate NMDA receptor function by reducing the desensitization elicited by calcineurin. Further, PKA phosphorylates a serine residue on the C-terminus of GluR1, and the phosphorylation state of this site is decreased after low-frequency stimulation that induces long-term depression of transmission (Kameyama *et al.*, 1998). Finally, GABA responsiveness is reduced in a PKA-dependent manner in CA1 pyramidal cells (Poisbeau *et al.*, 1999).

Future directions: genetic approaches to neuromodulation and cAMP-dependent plasticity

Given the large array of effects of the cAMP system on neuronal function, how does one determine which of these particular targets is important? The availability of new genetic strategies should help in this regard. First, by expressing transgenes that regulate the cAMP cascade pre- and postsynaptically, one may be able to eliminate the contribution of one side of the synapse. Secondly, by genetically altering target molecules, one can tease out their contributions to PKA-dependent forms of LTP systematically. For example, if PKA-mediated phosphorylation of GluR1 is important, then a 'knock in' of GluR1 lacking the PKA phosphorylation site should impair PKA-dependent forms of LTP.

In addition, we need to know more about the temporal and spatial dynamics of the activation of the cAMP signaling cascade. While evidence suggests that tetanus-evoked increases in cAMP levels and PKA activity are transient in nature, it is likely that the increases in cAMP generated by the neuromodulators released during behavioral tasks could be more prolonged. Thus, one possibility is that tonic levels of PKA activity can influence PKA-dependent forms of LTP differently from transiently increased levels of cAMP. Recent experiments have shown that concentrations of a cAMP phosphodiesterase inhibitor that do not affect basal synaptic transmission of basal cAMP levels nonetheless facilitate cAMP responses evoked by forskolin, and LTP evoked by early-phase LTP-inducing stimuli (Barad *et al.*, 1998). One could test this possibility genetically by comparing the effects of overexpression of an activated adenylyl cyclase or PKA with that of perhaps a dominant-negative form of a phosphodiesterase. Finally, given such a diverse array of possible effects elicited by the cAMP signaling cascade, the possibility must be considered that compartmentalized subcellular increases in cAMP levels may regulate distinct subsets of these effects. One approach to test this idea is to target these neuromodulatory systems genetically, for example by the generation of CA1-specific knockouts of the β_1-adrenergic receptor and the D5 dopamine receptor, or by the overexpression of regulatable transgenes in noradrenaline- and dopamine-producing neurons that can be used to manipulate the endogenous release of these catecholamines. These types of genetically modified mice would then allow the determination of both the specific effects mediated by these modulators and the behavioral consequences of manipulation of these systems.

CONCLUSIONS

While the initial demonstration that mice in which kinases had been knocked out by targeted recombina-

tion enticed the scientific community with its remarkable specificity, the problems associated with those strategies at the time seemed severe and hard to overcome. In only a few years, however, significant progress has been made in addressing these problems. The speed with which this progress has been made suggests that further advances in these techniques are not far away. Examination of the literature shows that we are already at a point where problems in LTP and memory storage can be seriously addressed with these techniques.

REFERENCES

Abel, T. and Kandel, E.R. (1998) Positive and negative regulatory mechanisms that mediate long-term memory storage. *Brain Research Reviews*, 26, 360–378.

Abeliovich, A., Chen, C., Goda, Y., Silva, A.J., Stevens, C.F. and Tonegawa, S. (1993a) Modified hippocampal long-term potentiation in PKCγ-mutant mice. *Cell*, 75, 1253–1262.

Abeliovich, A., Paylor, R., Chen, C., Kim, J.J., Wehner, J.M. and Tonegawa, S. (1993b) PKCγ mutant mice exhibit mild deficits in spatial and contextual learning. *Cell*, 75, 1263–1271.

Aiba, A., Chen, C., Herrup, K., Rosenmund, C., Stevens, C.F. and Tonegawa, S. (1994) Reduced hippocampal long-term potentiation and context-specific deficit in associative learning in mGluR1 mutant mice. *Cell*, 79, 365–375.

Amieux, P.S., Cummings, D.E., Motamed, K., Brandon, E.P., Wailes, L.A., Le, K., Idzerda, R.L. and McKnight, G.S. (1997) Compensatory regulation of RIα protein levels in protein kinase A mutant mice. *Journal of Biological Chemistry*, 272, 3993–3998.

Bach, M.E., Hawkins, R.D., Osman, M., Kandel, E.R. and Mayford, M. (1995) Impairment of spatial but not contextual memory in CaMKII mutant mice with a selective loss of hippocampal LTP in the range of the theta frequency. *Cell*, 81, 905–915.

Barad, M., Bourtchouladze, R., Winder, D.G., Golan, H. and Kandel, E.R. (1998) Rolipram, a type IV-specific phosphodiesterase inhibitor, facilitates the establishment of long-lasting long-term potentiation and improves memory. *Proceedings of the National Academy of Sciences of the United States of America*, 95, 15020–15025.

Barnes, C. (1979) Memory deficits associated with senescence: a neurophysiological and behavioral study in the rat. *Journal of Comparative and Physiological Psychology*, 93, 74–104

Bashir, Z.I., Bortolotto, Z.A., Davies, C.H., Berretta, N., Irving, A.J., Seal, A.J., Henley, J.M., Jane, D.E., Watkins, J.C. and Collingridge, G.L. (1993) Induction of LTP in the hippocampus needs synaptic activation of glutamate metabotropic receptors. *Nature*, 363, 347–350.

Bliss, T.V. and Lømo, T. (1973) Long-lasting potentiation of synaptic transmission in the dentate area of the anaesthetized rabbit following stimulation of the perforant path. *Journal of Physiology*, 232, 331–356.

Blitzer, R.D., Wong, T., Nouranifar, R., Iyengar, R. and Landau, E.M. (1995) Postsynaptic cAMP pathway gates early LTP in hippocampal CA1 region. *Neuron*, 15, 1403–1414.

Blitzer, R.D., Connor, J.H., Brown, G.P., Wong, T., Shenolikar, S., Iyengar, R. and Landau, E.M. (1998) Gating of CaMKII by cAMP-regulated protein phosphatase activity during LTP. *Science*, 280, 1940–1942.

Bordi, F. and Ugolini, A. (1995) Antagonists of the metabotropic glutamate receptor do not prevent induction of long-term potentiation in the dentate gyrus of rats. *European Journal of Pharmacology*, 273, 291–294.

Brandon, E.P., Zhuo, M., Huang, Y.Y., Qi, M., Gerhold, K.A., Burton, K.A., Kandel, E.R., McKnight, G.S. and Idzerda, R.L. (1995) Hippocampal long-term depression and depotentiation are defective in mice carrying a targeted disruption of the gene encoding the RIβ subunit of cAMP-dependent protein kinase. *Proceedings of the National Academy of Sciences of the United States of America*, 92, 8851–8855.

Brocard, J., Warot, X., Wendling, O., Messaddeq, N., Vonesch, J.L., Chambon, P. and Metzger, D. (1997) Spatio-temporally controlled site-specific somatic mutagenesis in the mouse. *Proceedings of the National Academy of Sciences of the United States of America*, 94, 14559–14563.

Cantrell, A.R., Smith, R.D., Goldin, A.L., Scheuer, T., Catterall, W.A. (1997) Dopaminergic modulation of sodium current in hippocampal neurons via cAMP-dependent phosphorylation of specific sites in the sodium channel alpha subunit. *Journal of Neuroscience*, 17, 7330–7338.

Capogna, M., Gahwiler, B.H. and Thompson, S.M. (1995) Presynaptic enhancement of inhibitory synaptic transmission by protein kinases A and C in the rat hippocampus *in vitro*. *Journal of Neuroscience*, 15, 1249–1260.

Chavez-Noriega, L.E. and Stevens, C.F. (1992) Modulation of synaptic efficacy in field CA1 of the rat hippocampus by forskolin. *Brain Research*, 574, 85–92.

Chen, J., Kelz, M.B., Zeng, G., Sakai, N., Steffen, C., Shockett, P.E., Picciotto, M.R., Duman, R.S. and Nestler, E.J. (1998) Transgenic animals with inducible, targeted gene expression in brain. *Molecular Pharmacology*, 54, 495–503.

Chetkovich, D.M. and Sweatt, J.D. (1993) NMDA receptor activation increases cyclic AMP in area CA1 of the hippocampus via calcium/calmodulin stimulation of adenylyl cyclase. *Journal of Neurochemistry*, 61, 1933–1942.

Chetkovich, D.M., Gray, R., Johnston, D. and Sweatt, J.D. (1991) N-Methyl-D-aspartate receptor activation increases cAMP levels and voltage-gated Ca^{2+} channel activity in area CA1 of hippocampus. *Proceedings of the National Academy of Sciences of the United States of America*, 88, 6467–6471.

Conquet, F., Bashir, Z.I., Davies, C.H., Daniel, H., Ferraguti, F., Bordi, F. *et al.* (1994) Motor deficit and impairment of synaptic plasticity in mice lacking mGluR1. *Nature*, 372, 237–243.

Contractor, A., Gereau, R.W.T., Green, T. and Heinemann, S.F. (1998) Direct effects of metabotropic glutamate receptor compounds on native and recombinant N-methyl-D-aspartate receptors. *Proceedings of the National Academy of Sciences of the United States of America*, 95, 8969–8974.

Crawley, J.N., Belknap, J.K., Collins, A., Crabbe, J.C., Frankel, W., Henderson, N. *et al.* (1997) Behavioral phenotypes of inbred mouse strains: implications and recommendations for molecular studies. *Psychopharmacology*, 132, 107–124.

Engert, F. and Bonhoeffer, T. (1997) Synapse specificity of long-term potentiation breaks down at short distances. *Nature*, 388, 279–284.

Feil, R., Brocard, J., Mascrez, B., LeMeur, M., Metzger, D. and Chambon, P. (1996) Ligand-activated site-specific recombination in mice. *Proceedings of the National Academy of Sciences of the United States of America*, 93, 10887–10890.

Frey, U., Huang, Y.Y. and Kandel, E.R. (1993) Effects of cAMP simulate a late stage of LTP in hippocampal CA1 neurons. *Science*, 260, 1661–1664.

Furth, P.A., St Onge, L., Boger, H., Gruss, P., Gossen, M., Kistner, A., Bujard, H. and Hennighausen, L. (1994) Temporal control of gene expression in transgenic mice by a tetracycline-responsive promoter. *Proceedings of the National Academy of Sciences of the United States of America*, 91, 9302–9306.

Gereau, R.W.T. and Conn, P.J. (1994) Presynaptic enhancement of excitatory synaptic transmission by β-adrenergic receptor activation. *Journal of Neurophysiology*, 72, 1438–1442.

Grant, S.G., O'Dell, T.J., Karl, K.A., Stein, P.L., Soriano, P. and Kandel, E.R. (1992) Impaired long-term potentiation, spatial learning, and hippocampal development in fyn mutant mice. *Science*, 258, 1903–1910.

Gray, R. and Johnston, D. (1987) Noradrenaline and β-adrenoceptor agonists increase activity of voltage-dependent calcium channels in hippocampal neurons. *Nature*, 327, 620–622.

Greengard, P., Jen, J., Nairn, A.C. and Stevens, C.F. (1991) Enhancement of the glutamate response by cAMP-dependent protein kinase in hippocampal neurons. *Science*, 253, 1135–1138.

Hell, J.W., Yokoyama, C.T., Breeze, L.J., Chavkin, C. and Catterall, W.A. (1995) Phosphorylation of presynaptic and postsynaptic calcium channels by cAMP-dependent protein kinase in hippocampal neurons. *EMBO Journal*, 14, 3036–3044.

Hoffman, D.A., Johnston, D. (1998) Downregulation of transient K$^+$ channels in dendrites of hippocampal CA1 pyramidal neurons by activation of PKA and PKC. *Journal of Neuroscience*, 18, 3521–3528.

Hogan, B., Constantini, F. and Lacy, E. (1986) *Manipulating the Mouse Embryo: A Laboratory Manual*. Cold Spring Harbor Press, Cold Spring Harbor, New York.

Horn, G. (1998) Visual imprinting and the neural mechanisms of recognition memory. *Trends in Neurosciences*, 21, 300–305.

Huang, Y.Y. and Kandel, E.R. (1995) D1/D5 receptor agonists induce a protein synthesis-dependent late potentiation in the CA1 region of the hippocampus. *Proceedings of the National Academy of Sciences of the United States of America*, 92, 2446–2450.

Huang, Y.-Y., Nguyen, P.V., Abel, T. and Kandel, E.R. (1996) Long-lasting forms of synaptic potentiation in the mammalian hippocampus. *Learning and Memory*, 3, 74–85.

Impey, S., Mark, M., Villacres, E.C., Poser, S., Chavkin, C. and Storm, D.R. (1996) Induction of CRE-mediated gene expression by stimuli that generate long-lasting LTP in area CA1 of the hippocampus. *Neuron*, 16, 973–982.

Kameyama, K., Lee, H.-K., Bear, M.F. and Huganir, R.L. (1998) Involvement of a postsynaptic protein kinase A substrate in the expression of homosynaptic long-term depression. *Neuron*, 21, 1163–1175.

Katsuki, H., Izumi, Y. and Zorumski, C.F. (1997) Noradrenergic regulation of synaptic plasticity in the hippocampal CA1 region. *Journal of Neurophysiology*, 77, 3013–3020.

Kavalali, E.T., Hwang, K.S. and Plummer, M.R. (1997) cAMP-dependent enhancement of dihydropyridine-sensitive calcium channel availability in hippocampal neurons. *Journal of Neuroscience*, 17, 5334–5348.

Kistner, A., Gossen, M., Zimmermann, F., Jerecic, J., Ullmer, C., Lubbert, H. and Bujard, H. (1996) Doxycycline-mediated quantitative and tissue-specific control of gene expression in transgenic mice. *Proceedings of the National Academy of Sciences of the United States of America*, 93, 10933–10938.

Kojima, N., Wang, J., Mansuy, I.M., Grant, S.G., Mayford, M. and Kandel, E.R. (1997) Rescuing impairment of long-term potentiation in fyn-deficient mice by introducing Fyn transgene. *Proceedings of the National Academy of Sciences of the United States of America*, 94, 4761–4765.

Korte, M., Carroll, P., Wolf, E., Brem, G., Thoenen, H. and Bonhoeffer, T. (1995) Hippocampal long-term potentiation is impaired in mice lacking brain-derived neurotrophic factor. *Proceedings of the National Academy of Sciences of the United States of America*, 92, 8856–8860.

Korte, M., Griesbeck, O., Gravel, C., Carroll, P., Staiger, V., Thoenen, H. and Bonhoeffer, T. (1996) Virus-mediated gene transfer into hippocampal CA1 region restores long-term potentiation in brain-derived neurotrophic factor mutant mice. *Proceedings of the National Academy of Sciences of the United States of America*, 93, 12547–12552.

Madison, D.V. and Nicoll, R.A. (1986) Cyclic adenosine 3′,5′-monophosphate mediates β-receptor actions of noradrenaline in rat hippocampal pyramidal cells. *Journal of Physiology (London)*, 372, 245–259.

Mansuy, I.M., Mayford, M., Jacob, B., Kandel, E.R. and Bach, M.E. (1998a) Restricted and regulated overexpression reveals calcineurin as a key component in the transition from short-term to long-term memory. *Cell*, 92, 39–49.

Mansuy, I.M., Winder, D.G., Moallem, T.M., Osman, M., Mayford, M., Hawkins, R.D. and Kandel, E.R. (1998b) Inducible and reversible gene expression with the rtTA system for the study of memory. *Neuron*, 21, 257–265.

Mayford, M., Bach, M.E., Huang, Y.Y., Wang, L., Hawkins, R.D. and Kandel, E.R. (1996) Control of memory formation through regulated expression of a CaMKII transgene. *Science*, 274, 1678–1683.

Mayford, M., Wang, J., Kandel, E.R. and O'Dell, T.J. (1995) CaMKII regulates the frequency-response function of hippocampal synapses for the production of both LTD and LTP. *Cell*, 81, 891–904.

Morris, R.G. (1989) Synaptic plasticity and learning: selective impairment of learning in rats and blockade of long-term potentiation *in vivo* by the *N*-methyl-D-aspartate receptor antagonist AP5. *Journal of Neuroscience*, 9, 3040–3057.

Mulkey, R.M., Herron, C.E. and Malenka, R.C. (1993) An essential role for protein phosphatases in hippocampal long-term depression. *Science*, 261, 1051–1055.

Mulkey, R.M., Endo, S., Shenolikar, S. and Malenka, R.C. (1994) Involvement of a calcineurin/inhibitor-1 phosphatase cascade in hippocampal long-term depression. *Nature*, 369, 486–488.

Namgung, U., Matsuyama, S. and Routtenberg, A. (1997) Long-term potentiation activates the GAP-43 promoter: selective participation of hippocampal mossy cells. *Proceedings of the National Academy of Sciences of the United States of America*, 94, 11675–11680.

Nicot, A. and Pfaff, D.W. (1997) Antisense oligodeoxynucleotides as specific tools for studying neuroendocrine and behavioral functions: some prospects and problems. *Journal of Neuroscience Methods*, 71, 45–53.

No, D., Yao, T.P. and Evans, R.M. (1996) Ecdysone-inducible gene expression in mammalian cells and transgenic mice. *Proceedings of the National Academy of Sciences of the United States of America*, 93, 3346–3351.

Otmakhova, N.A. and Lisman, J.E. (1996) D1/D5 dopamine receptor activation increases the magnitude of early long-term potentiation at CA1 hippocampal synapses. *Journal of Neuroscience*, 16, 7478–7486.

Otmakhova, N.A. and Lisman, J.E. (1998) D1/D5 dopamine receptors inhibit depotentiation at CA1 synapses via cAMP-dependent mechanism. *Journal of Neuroscience*, 18, 1270–1279.

Parfitt, K.D., Doze, V.A., Madison, D.V. and Browning, M.D. (1992) Isoproterenol increases the phosphorylation of the synapsins and increases synaptic transmission in dentate gyrus, but not in area CA1, of the hippocampus. *Hippocampus*, 2, 59–64.

Patterson, S.L., Abel, T., Deuel, T.A., Martin, K.C., Rose, J.C. and Kandel, E.R. (1996) Recombinant BDNF rescues deficits in basal synaptic transmission and hippocampal LTP in BDNF knockout mice. *Neuron*, 16, 1137–1145.

Pedarzani, P. and Storm, J.F. (1995) Protein kinase A-independent modulation of ion channels in the brain by cyclic AMP. *Proceedings of the National Academy of Sciences of the United States of America*, 92, 11716–11720.

Poisbeau, P., Cheney, M.C., Browning, M.D. and Mody, I. (1999) Modulation of synaptic GABAA receptor function by PKA and PKC in adult hippocampal neurons. *Journal of Neuroscience*, 19, 674–683.

Qi, M., Zhuo, M., Skalhegg, B.S., Brandon, E.P., Kandel, E.R., McKnight, G.S. and Idzerda, R.L. (1996) Impaired hippocampal plasticity in mice lacking the Cβ1 catalytic subunit of cAMP-dependent protein kinase. *Proceedings of the National Academy of Sciences of the United States of America*, 93, 1571–1756.

Richter-Levin, G., Errington, M.L., Maegawa, H. and Bliss, T.V. (1994) Activation of metabotropic glutamate receptors is necessary for long-term potentiation in the dentate gyrus and for spatial learning. *Neuropharmacology*, 33, 853–857.

Riedel, G. and Reymann, K. (1993) An antagonist of the metabotropic glutamate receptor prevents LTP in the dentate gyrus of freely moving rats. *Neuropharmacology*, 32, 929–931.

Roberson, E.D. and Sweatt, J.D. (1996) Transient activation of cyclic AMP-dependent protein kinase during hippocampal long-term potentiation. *Journal of Biological Chemistry*, 271, 30436–30441.

Schwenk, F., Kuhn, R., Angrand, P.O., Rajewsky, K. and Stewart, A.F. (1998) Temporally and spatially regulated somatic mutagenesis in mice. *Nucleic Acids Research*, 26, 1427–1432.

Selig, D.K., Lee, H.K., Bear, M.F. and Malenka, R.C. (1995) Reexamination of the effects of MCPG on hippocampal LTP, LTD, and depotentiation. *Journal of Neurophysiology*, 74, 1075–1082.

Silva, A.J., Paylor, R., Wehner, J.M. and Tonegawa, S. (1992a) Impaired spatial learning in α-calcium–calmodulin kinase II mutant mice. *Science*, 257, 206–211.

Silva, A.J., Stevens, C.F., Tonegawa, S. and Wang, Y. (1992b) Deficient hippocampal long-term potentiation in α-calcium–calmodulin kinase II mutant mice. *Science*, 257, 201–206.

Soriano, P. (1995) Gene targeting in ES cells. *Annual Review of Neuroscience*, 18, 1–18.

Staley, K. (1994) The role of an inwardly rectifying chloride conductance in postsynaptic inhibition. *Journal of Neurophysiology*, 72, 273–284.

Tezuka, T., Umemori, H., Akiyama, T., Nakanishi, S. and Yamamoto, T. (1999) PSD-95 promotes Fyn-mediated tyrosine phosphorylation of the *N*-methyl-D-aspartate receptor subunit NR2A. *Proceedings of the National Academy of Sciences of the United States of America*, 96, 435–440.

Thomas, M.J. and O'Dell, T.J. (1995) The molecular switch hypothesis fails to explain the inconsistent effects of the metabotropic glutamate receptor antagonist MCPG on long-term potentiation. *Brain Research*, 695, 45–52.

Thomas, M.J., Moody, T.D., Makhinson, M. and O'Dell, T.J. (1996) Activity-dependent β-adrenergic modulation of low frequency stimulation induced LTP in the hippocampal CA1 region. *Neuron*, 17, 475–482.

Trudeau, L.E., Emery, D.G. and Haydon, P.G. (1996) Direct modulation of the secretory machinery underlies PKA-dependent synaptic facilitation in hippocampal neurons. *Neuron*, 17, 789–797.

Tsien, J.Z., Chen, D.F., Gerber, D., Tom, C., Mercer, E.H., Anderson, D.J., Mayford, M., Kandel, E.R. and Tonegawa, S. (1996a) Subregion- and cell type-restricted gene knock-out in mouse brain. *Cell*, 87, 1317–1326.

Tsien, J.Z., Huerta, P.T. and Tonegawa, S. (1996b) The essential role of hippocampal CA1 NMDA receptor-dependent synaptic plasticity in spatial memory. *Cell*, 87, 1327–1338.

Wang, L.Y., Salter, M.W. and MacDonald, J.F. (1991) Regulation of kainate receptors by cAMP-dependent protein kinase and phosphatases. *Science*, 253, 1132–5.

Wim, T.J., Hermens, M.C. and Werhaagen, J. (1998) Viral vectors, tools for gene transfer in the nervous system. *Progress in Neurobiology*, 55, 399–432.

Winder, D.G., Mansuy, I.M., Osman, M., Moallem, T.M. and Kandel, E.R. (1998) Genetic and pharmacological evidence for a novel, intermediate phase of long-term potentiation suppressed by calcineurin. *Cell*, 92, 25–37.

Winder, D.G., Martin, K.C., Muzzio, I.A., Rohrer, D., Chruscinski, A., Kobilka, B. Kandel, E.R. (1999) ERK plays a regulatory role in induction of LTP by theta frequency stimulation and its modulation by beta-adrenergic receptors. *Neuron*, 24, 715–726.

Zhang, Y., Riesterer, C., Ayrall, A.M., Sablitzky, F., Littlewood, T.D. and Reth, M. (1996) Inducible site-directed recombination in mouse embryonic stem cells. *Nucleic Acids Research*, 24, 543–548.

Zola-Morgan, S., Squire, L.R. and Amaral, D.G. (1986) Human amnesia and the medial temporal region: enduring memory impairment following a bilateral lesion limited to field CA1 of the hippocampus. *Journal of Neuroscience*, 6, 2950–2967.

11 NEURONAL CORRELATES OF RECOGNITION MEMORY

Malcolm W. Brown

INTRODUCTION

Tests of human visual recognition memory have demonstrated its great facility and enormous capacity (Standing, 1973). Indeed, recognition memory is so much a part of everyday living that it can easily be taken for granted. Yet it requires the brain to solve complex problems of stimulus identification together with judgements concerning the previous occurrence of what has been identified. The present chapter is concerned with neuronal responses that carry information relating to the previous occurrence of visual stimuli.

Introspection and growing experimental evidence indicate that recognition memory is not a unitary process but has a variety of different component features. Thus, for example, should you meet someone in the street, you will normally rapidly know whether or not they are someone you have met before. Further, if you have met them before, you will be able to judge whether they are highly familiar or relatively unfamiliar to you and, independently of this judgement, whether you have seen them recently or not for a long time. Not uncommonly, you may feel that the person is familiar but, at least initially, be unable to remember their name, other details about them or indeed the place or other circumstances of your previous meeting. Thus one aspect of recognition memory involves judgements of familiarity and of recency of occurrence, while, more generally, it additionally involves associative and recollective recall. Moreover, recognition memory is not restricted to one person or thing at a time; it can be for particular arrangements of collections of individual items in addition to being for the individual items themselves. For instance, if you walk into your own living room, you will rapidly register either the presence of a new item of furniture or a new re-arrangement of the old, familiar items of furniture.

It seems probable that the recollective aspects of recognition memory are dependent on a system that involves the hippocampus of the temporal lobe (Aggleton and Brown, 1999). Moreover, recent findings indicate that the hippocampus is involved in assessing the novelty or familiarity of spatial arrangements of items (Wan et al., 1999a). In contrast, there is much evidence that judgements of the familiarity of individual items are dependent on a system that involves parahippocampal, notably perirhinal, cortex (Brown et al., 1987; Brown, 1996; Brown and Xiang, 1998; Aggleton and Brown, 1999; Wan et al., 1999a). This chapter concentrates on what is known of neuronal responses within this perirhinal system and their potential relationships to familiarity and recency discrimination for individual items.

BACKGROUND

Much research into recognition memory was stimulated by the profound memory loss that followed the bilateral removal of parts of the medial temporal lobe in patient H.M. (Scoville and Milner, 1957; Corkin et al., 1997). Eventually, after numerous unsuccessful attempts, a monkey model for H.M.'s loss of recognition memory was found (Mishkin, 1978; see also Buckley and Gaffan, Chapter 16). Monkeys were trained on a delayed non-matching to sample task using a large set of objects so that all the objects were relatively unfamiliar. The delayed non-matching to sample task comprises an acquisition and a choice phase separated by a delay period. During acquisition, the subject is shown an object. After the delay, the subject is required to choose between the object seen in the acquisition phase and another object, the correct choice being the object that does not match that shown at acquisition. (Contrastingly, in delayed matching, the subject has to choose the previously encountered stimulus.) Correct performance therefore requires accurate judgement of prior occurrence for individual items. Monkeys with bilateral temporal lobe lesions that included the hippocampus, amygdala and adjacent cortex were found to be severely impaired (Mishkin, 1978). Subsequent ablation studies have established that it is lesions of this adjacent cortex that are critical. Within this parahippocampal cortex, the perirhinal cortex (Figure 11.1) that is found adjacent to the rhinal (or, in humans, collateral) sulcus on the under surface of the temporal lobe is of particular importance. Lesions of the perirhinal cortex produce major impairment of delayed non-matching to sample tasks, with the contributions of the hippocampus and amygdala being relatively minor (Zola-Morgan *et al.*, 1989; Gaffan and Murray, 1992; Meunier *et al.*, 1993, 1996; Alvarez *et al.*, 1995; Murray, 1996; Murray and Mishkin, 1998). Although most of these studies have been performed using monkeys, findings consistent with these have been reported for human amnesic patients and for rats (Mumby and Pinel, 1994; Aggleton and Shaw, 1996; Ennaceur *et al.*, 1996; Aggleton and Brown, 1999).

Perirhinal cortex receives inputs from all the sensory systems (Jones and Powell, 1970; Felleman and Van Essen, 1991; Burwell *et al.*, 1995; Shi and Cassell, 1997). It is close to the top of the hierarchy of sensory processing areas within the cerebral cortex (Felleman and Van Essen, 1991; Burwell *et al.*, 1995; Shi and Cassell, 1997). Hence perirhinal cortex receives highly processed sensory information. Accordingly, it is well placed to take part in perceptual processes concerning the identification of stimuli and mnemonic processes concerning the prior history of these stimuli in relation to the individual. Perirhinal cortex is a major source of inputs to the entorhinal cortex and hippocampus (for a review, see Burwell *et al.*, 1995).

REPETITION-SENSITIVE RESPONSES

A change in a neuron's response when a stimulus is repeated indicates that that neuron has access to information concerning the prior occurrence of the stimulus. This information may be held totally or in part in that neuron or its afferent synapses, or may be held in neurons afferent to it, with the neuron itself passively reflecting changes produced elsewhere. In either case, one simple way of potentially judging the prior occurrence of a stimulus is to compare responses of a population of neurons whose responses change on stimulus repetition (repetition-sensitive responses) with those of a population of neurons whose responses do not change consistently with stimulus repetition (repetition-invariant responses).

The potential to make such comparisons concerning prior occurrence exists in the cortex of the anterior temporal lobe, including the perirhinal cortex, where neurons with repetition-sensitive responses and those with repetition-invariant responses are found intermingled. Neurons with repetition-sensitive responses (see, for example, Figures 11.2–11.4) are found commonly in the anterior inferior temporal cortex—in the perirhinal cortex and the medially adjacent entorhinal cortex and laterally adjacent part of the inferior temporal cortex (the anterior part of area TE); they are relatively uncommon in the hippocampus (Brown *et al.*, 1987; Brown and Xiang, 1998; Rolls *et al.*, 1993; Xiang and Brown, 1998c). Their distribution is thus consistent with the major effects of ablations of perirhinal cortex and relatively minor effects of hippocampal lesions on delayed matching or non-matching to sample tasks mentioned previously.

Such response changes with stimulus repetition have been confirmed in several laboratories (Brown *et al.*, 1987; Eskandar *et al.*, 1992; Li *et al.*, 1993; Miller *et al.*, 1993; Sobotka and Ringo, 1993; Desimone, 1996; Ringo, 1996; Brown and Xiang, 1998; Xiang and Brown, 1998c). They have been studied most commonly during the performance by monkeys of variants of delayed non-matching to sample or of serial recognition memory tasks. In a serial recognition memory task, a single stimulus is presented on each trial; after a variable number of intervening trials, a stimulus will be presented again, the animal being required to make a different response to first than to subsequent presentations of each stimulus. The neuronal response changes can thus be found under behavioral conditions that are closely controlled. Such conditions indicate that the response changes cannot be explained as simple or artifactual consequences of alterations in alertness, attention, eye movements, pupillary diameter, behavioral responses or the reward value of stimuli (Fahy *et al.*, 1993b; Miller *et al.*, 1993; Sobotka and Ringo, 1993; Wilson and Goldman-Rakic, 1994; Xiang and Brown, 1998c), or ordinary habituation (see below).

The repetition-sensitive responses of neurons recorded in anterior inferior temporal cortex (including perirhinal cortex) have properties that might be expected of neurons involved in processes underlying

(a) Monkey brain (ventral view)

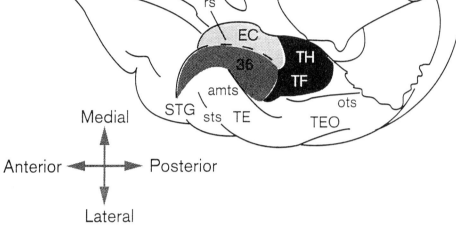

(b) Rat brain (lateral view)

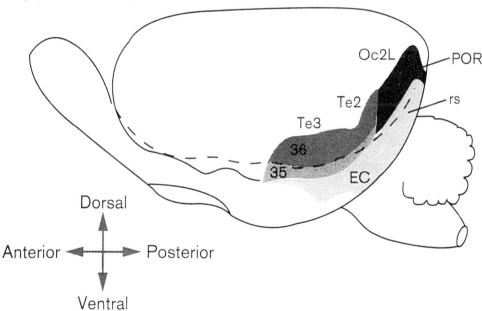

Figure 11.1. The position of perirhinal cortex (areas 35 and 36) is shown by dark shading in (**A**) the monkey and (**B**) the rat brain. There is still some dispute as to the boundaries of the perirhinal cortex. Those used here follow Burwell *et al.* (1995). Recent studies have indicated that this region is important for paired associate learning and fear conditioning as well as visual recognition memory (Suzuki, 1996). Entorhinal cortex (EC) is shown in light shading and areas TF and TH of the parahippocampal gyrus of the monkey and postrhinal cortex (POR) in the rat in black. Other abbreviations: (A) TE = area TE; TEO = area TEO; amts = anterior medial temporal sulcus; ots = occipitotemporal sulcus; STG = superior temporal gyrus; sts = superior temporal sulcus. (B) rs = rhinal sulcus; Te2, Te3 = temporal cortex; Oc2L = lateral occipital visual association cortex. Reproduced with permission from Suzuki (1996).

that part of recognition memory concerned with familiarity and/or recency discrimination for individual items. These properties are listed and explained below.

Signaling of information concerning prior occurrence

Neurons in the cortex of the anterior temporal lobe, including the perirhinal cortex, with repetition-sensitive responses typically respond much less strongly on the second than on the first occasion a stimulus appears (Brown *et al.*, 1987; Brown and Xiang, 1998; see Figures 11.2 and 11.3). Accordingly, the responses of these neurons convey information concerning the prior occurrence of that stimulus.

The incidence of such decremental responses is high. In a recent experiment, recordings were made while monkeys performed a serial recognition memory task (Xiang and Brown, 1998c). Of the neurons recorded in anterior inferior temporal cortex, 63% responded to the visual stimuli presented. For 40% of these visually responsive neurons, the response to previously presented stimuli differed

Novelty neurone
(in perirhinal cortex)

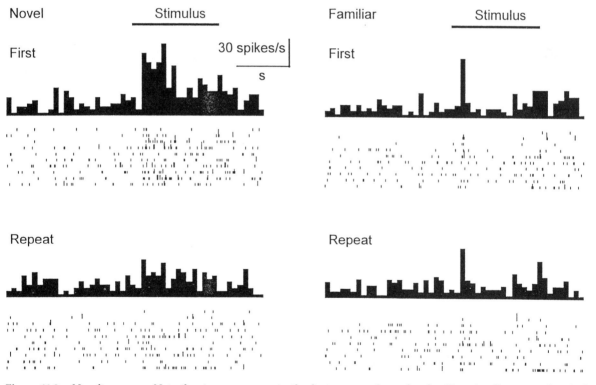

Figure 11.2. Novelty neuron. Note the strong response to the first presentations of unfamiliar stimuli compared with the responses to repeat presentations of those stimuli or presentations of familiar stimuli. In this and the next two figures, responses of individual neurons to the first (top row) and second (bottom row) presentations of unfamiliar ('novel'; left column) and highly familiar (right column) visual stimuli are shown for 10 trials of each type during a monkey's performance of a serial recognition memory task. In each case, a peristimulus time histogram of the cumulated activity is shown above rasters indicating the times of occurrence of action potentials during each of the 10 trials. Repeat presentations are of the same stimuli as first presentations, with the rasters in the same order. Trial types were intermingled during recording. Reproduced with permission from Xiang and Brown (1998c).

Recency neurone
(in entorhinal cortex)

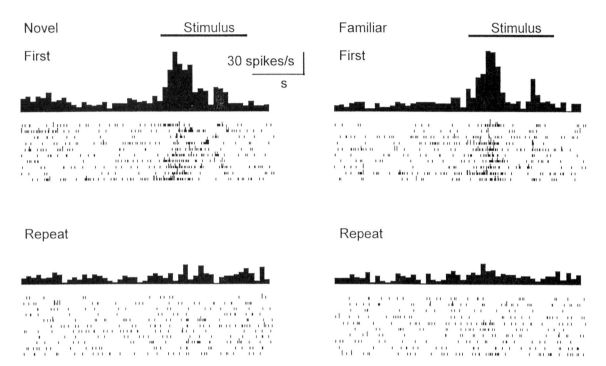

Figure 11.3. Recency neuron. Conventions as for Figure 11.2. Responses to first presentations were stronger than to their repeats regardless of whether novel or familiar stimuli were shown, i.e. the responses signal whether a stimulus has been seen recently but not its relative familiarity. Reproduced with permission from Xiang and Brown (1998c).

significantly from that to first presentations, and for the remaining 60% the response did not differ. The response to repeated stimuli was reduced for 98% of the neurons whose responses changed with repetition. Corresponding incremental changes occurred at less than the incidence expected by chance. Accordingly, under these conditions, the direction of response change with stimulus repetition in anterior inferior temporal cortex is overwhelmingly a reduction. Thus overall, reduced responses for stimuli that had been seen before were found for approximately 25% of the total recorded sample of neurons. This large percentage of neurons with repetition-sensitive responses means that a response decrement can be demonstrated in population measures, as has been exploited in imaging studies in humans using positron emission tomography (PET) (Squire *et al.*, 1992; Vandenberghe *et al.*, 1995) and in rats using

immunohistochemistry to stain activated neurons (Zhu *et al.*, 1995b, 1996; Wan *et al.*, 1999a).

The neurons with repetition-sensitive responses separably signal different types of information of potential importance to recognition memory (Fahy *et al.*, 1993b). In the same neuronal recordings as reported above, the great majority (>90%) of neurons with repetition-sensitive responses could be placed into one of three categories according to the response changes that occurred when either unfamiliar or highly familiar stimuli were repeated (Xiang and Brown, 1998c).

(i) *Novelty neurons* responded most strongly to the first presentations of stimuli that had been seen either rarely (and not during the previous several weeks) or never before. They responded significantly less vigorously when such unfamiliar

Familiarity neurone

(in area TE)

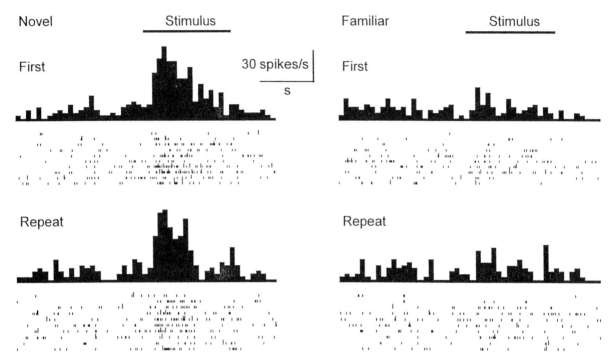

Figure 11.4. Familiarity neuron. Conventions as for Figure 11.2. Responses to the novel stimuli were stronger than to the familiar stimuli regardless of whether a stimulus was appearing for the first or second time in that recording session, i.e. the response signaled the relative familiarity of the stimulus but not whether it had been seen very recently. Reproduced with permission from Xiang and Brown (1998c).

stimuli were repeated or when stimuli were shown that had been seen many times previously so that they were highly familiar (see, for example, Figure. 11.2). Thus these neurons responded best to novel stimuli.

(ii) *Recency neurons* responded strongly to the first presentations during a given recording session of either unfamiliar or familiar stimuli. They responded significantly less well when either unfamiliar or familiar stimuli were shown again (see, for example, Figure 11.3). Accordingly, the responses of these neurons signaled that a stimulus had been seen recently but did not indicate whether that stimulus was unfamiliar or highly familiar.

(iii) *Familiarity neurons* responded strongly to both the first and second presentations of unfamiliar stimuli during a recording session, but responded significantly less strongly to highly familiar stimuli (see Figure 11.4). Thus the responses of these neurons signaled information about the relative familiarity of the stimuli but not about whether the stimuli had been seen very recently.

This double (or rather triple) dissociation of the types of neuronal responses establishes that information concerning the familiarity and recency of presentation of stimuli is encoded separably at the single neuronal level (Fahy *et al.*, 1993b). Collectively, the responses of these neurons signal the types of information upon which judgements of the prior occurrence of individual items can be made.

Single trial learning

For both recency and novelty neurons, the response to the first presentations of unfamiliar stimuli is significantly greater than that to the second presentations of these stimuli (Xiang and Brown, 1998c; see Figures 11.2 and 11.3). Thus a single presentation of a stimulus is sufficient to produce a subsequent response decrement. Accordingly, the change demonstrates learning as a result of a single trial, as is required of any potential recognition memory mechanism.

In the recent study referred to above (Xiang and Brown, 1998c), it has been found that a single presentation of a stimulus is sufficient to produce a response decrement in familiarity neurons—but that this decrement develops slowly over a period of some minutes. If a stimulus is repeated within a few minutes, no noticeable response decrement is observed, even if the stimulus is repeated a few times within this period (Xiang and Brown, 1998c; see Figure 11.5). Thus there are at least two plastic processes—one fast and expressed by recency neurons plus one slow and expressed by familiarity neurons—each of which demonstrates single trial learning (given that sufficient time has elapsed). At present, it is not clear whether the plastic processes underlying the responses of novelty neurons are a complex combination of these two processes or whether their responses imply some additional mechanism.

Novelty, familiarity and recency neurons were named because of the type of information their response changes most obviously signaled under the experimental conditions in which they were discovered (Fahy *et al.*, 1993b; Xiang and Brown, 1998c). However, it should be noted that recent results (Xiang and Brown, 1998c) indicate that these names may not describe accurately the functional significance of these neurons' responses under all conditions: a full description of their functional significance may require further refinement following study under other conditions.

Stimulus selectivity (stimulus identification)

The decremental neuronal responses are selective for particular physical features of the presented stimuli in two ways. First, neurons with decremental responses respond better to the first presentations of certain stimuli than they do to the first presentations of other stimuli, i.e. these neurons selectively respond to certain preferred features or combinations of features. For example, for some neurons, it is possible to establish that the neurons respond to a particular class of stimuli such as red-colored stimuli, or pictures of faces (Riches *et al.*, 1991; Fahy *et al.*, 1993b). The responses thus carry information concerning stimulus identification. Secondly, the response decrement is specific to stimuli that have been seen before. Presentation of a novel stimulus can evoke a strong response even for a neuron that has just responded weakly to a previously encountered stimulus. Accordingly, the response decrements are not produced by generalized fatigue of the neuron or its afferents. In counterpart to this, the response decrements signal identification of a specific previously encountered stimulus.

There is evidence that the response decrements show some stimulus generalization, for example across changes in size—as do non-decremental responses in anterior inferior temporal cortex (Lueschow *et al.*, 1994). As yet there have been no reports of the effects of presenting different views or rotations of objects upon repetition-sensitive responses.

Large storage capacity

Human visual recognition memory capacity is clearly extremely large: subjects can judge accurately the prior occurrence of thousands of visual pictures (Standing, 1973). Similarly, monkeys can perform recognition memory tasks accurately that, across sessions, use many hundreds of pictures. The capacity of the system of neurons with decremental responses seems to be similarly large. Thus stimulus-specific decremental responses are found even after an animal has seen many hundreds of pictures. This finding implies a very high capacity both for stimulus discrimination/identification and for the registration of prior occurrence of the individual stimuli.

Given that about 25% of the neurons in monkey anterior inferior temporal cortex have decremental responses (see above), the number of neurons involved could be approximately 10^7 so that the potential information capacity of the system is indeed very large. It has been calculated that discrimination based on the output of only 25 decrementally responsive neurons can achieve a performance equivalent to a monkey in a modified delayed non-matching to sample task (Miller *et al.*, 1993). Moreover, a simple

Responses of visual differential neurones in serial recognition task

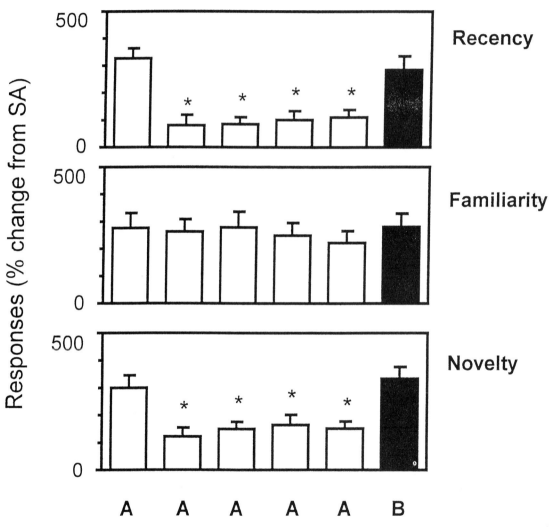

Figure 11.5. Development of a response decrement in recency, familiarity and novelty neurons. (**A**) Mean (±SEM) population responses of recency, familiarity and novelty neurons to multiple presentations on successive trials of a serial recognition memory task of initially novel stimuli ('A'). Also shown is the mean response on the subsequent trial when a novel stimulus was presented ('B'). Means are changes in firing rate (%) relative to the pre-cue level (spontaneous activity, SA = 0%) for 35 neurons of each type. Note the absence of a significant response decrement for a population of familiarity neurons in spite of five successive presentations within a 2–4 min period for each initially novel stimulus. The response decrement for recency and novelty neurons is the same from the second to the fifth trial. *P <0.05 compared with mean response for first presentations. Reproduced with permission from Xiang and Brown (1998c).

Memory span of recency, familiarity and novelty neurones

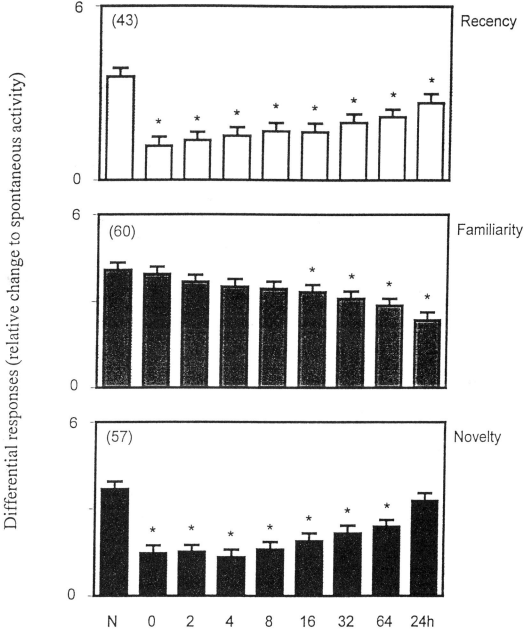

Figure 11.5. (B) Mean population responses for first presentations (N) and second presentations after different intervals (numbers of intervening trials or 24 h) for recency, familiarity and novelty neurons in anterior inferior temporal cortex (Xiang and Brown, 1998c). For these intervals, memory across the population increased with time elapsed for familiarity neurons, but decreased for novelty and recency neurons. The decrement developed rapidly (<10 s) for recency and novelty neurons but took more than about 5 min to become significant for the population of familiarity neurons. *P <0.05 difference in mean response to second presentations compared with first presentations.

neural network model indicates that a network of about 10^7 neurons could remember about 10^8 patterns with an error rate of less than one in a million (Bogacz *et al.*, 1999, 2000).

Long-term memory

Decremental neuronal responses can only provide a viable substrate for recognition memory if the response decrements demonstrate access to memory held for appropriately long periods, i.e. a response decrement must still be found even when a long time has elapsed since a stimulus was encountered previously. In fact, the response decrements persist for a long time even when there is distraction of the animal's attention by the presentation of other stimuli to be remembered. Moreover, when performing a serial recognition task, it is necessary for an animal to remember many (>>7) stimuli at the same time (Fahy *et al.*, 1993b; Xiang and Brown, 1998c). Both these characteristics mean that performance must rely on long-term rather than short-term memory processes.

When considering long-lasting changes, it is convenient to talk about the *memory span* of a neuron (Fahy

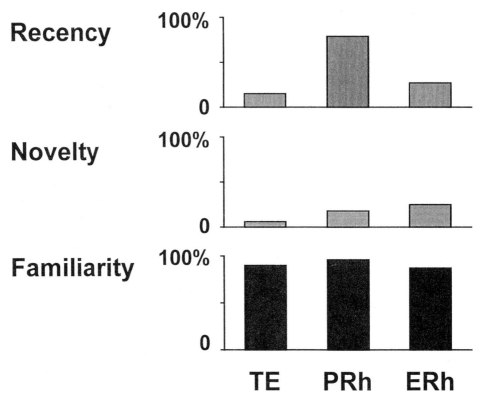

Proportions of recognition-related neurones with 24 hour memory span in anterior temporal cortex

Figure 11.6. The proportions of recency, familiarity and novelty neurons with 24 h memory spans in anterior TE, perirhinal and entorhinal cortex (Xiang and Brown, 1998c). Note the high proportion of 24 h memory spans for recency neurons in perirhinal cortex.

et al., 1993b). The memory span of a neuron is defined as the longest interval over which there is evidence of a significant change in response. Establishing memory spans of up to an hour or so may be accomplished within a single recording session simply by spacing the repetitions of stimuli by the appropriate period. The existence of memory spans longer than a few hours, i.e. longer than a typical recording session, may be established by making use of sets of stimuli that the animal last saw at a known time previously, for example the previous day. By these means, the memory spans of certain neurons have been shown to be at least 24 h, the longest interval routinely tested (Fahy *et al.*, 1993b; Xiang and Brown, 1998c). The incidence of neurons in anterior inferior temporal cortex with memory spans of at least 24 h is illustrated in Figure 11.6. One neuron with a memory span of more than 72 h has been reported (Fahy *et al.*, 1993b). The relatively high incidence of 24 h memory spans suggests that the memory span of the system is considerably longer than 1 day, but longer memory spans have not been sought systematically. Not all memory spans are long, hence the time of last occurrence (recency) of a stimulus is calculable potentially from the variability in memory spans (variation in response decrement with time) across the population of neurons (Fahy *et al.*, 1993b).

Fast processing

Studies of humans making familiarity (old/new) judgements have demonstrated that the discrimination can be made very quickly (Seeck *et al.*, 1997; Hintzman *et al.*, 1998). This speed is paralleled by findings concerning response decrements in monkeys. The first time at which the neuronal activity evoked by the first presentations of visual stimuli differs from that evoked by their second presentations across a recorded population of neurons with decremental responses in the monkey is approximately 75 ms in area TE and approximately 105 ms in perirhinal cortex (Xiang and Brown, 1998c; see Table 11.1). For many cells, these differential latencies are not measurably longer than the latency to respond to a novel visual stimulus (Fahy *et al.*, 1993b; Miller *et al.*, 1993; Xiang and Brown, 1998c), i.e. discrimination of the prior occurrence of a stimulus is as fast as identification of what that stimulus is.

Efficient processing

Although there are still many unanswered questions concerning the mechanisms underlying the response

Table 11.1 Population differential latencies in anterior area TE, perirhinal and entorhinal cortex

	Recency neurons	Familiarity neurons	Novelty neurons a	b
Area TE	75	75	75	75
Perirhinal cortex	105	135	105	75
Entorhinal cortex	135	225	135	135

The latency (in ms) is measured as the mean of the first of successive 30 ms bins for which there was a significant difference in the cumulated spike counts for various types of trial averaged across all the repetition-sensitive neurons recorded in a given area (for further details, see Brown and Xiang, 1998).
Recency neurons, first versus second presentations; familiarity neurons, novel versus familiar stimuli; novelty neurons, a = first versus second presentations; b = novel versus familiar stimuli. Population latencies were shortest in area TE and longest in entorhinal cortex; perirhinal cortex was intermediate between the other two areas.

decrement (see further below), it is possible to design plausible network models (cf. Bateson, Chapter 15) that perform familiarity discrimination using activity-dependent changes in synaptic efficacy. These models turn out to be remarkably efficient: compared with standard associative networks, they have a very high information storage capacity and are very fast in operation (Bogacz *et al.*, 1999, 2000). The implication is that with an architecture even only a fraction as efficient as that of the model, a population of neurons in anterior inferior temporal cortex could perform familiarity discrimination very quickly and with very high accuracy for an enormous number of patterns (stimuli). The number of neurons required in such a facility could be expected to be very small compared with that required for associative learning processes. Accordingly, the cost in terms of space and energy usage of having such a facility is comparatively very low. The ability rapidly and efficiently to discriminate novelty and familiarity would seem to be of major behavioral advantage, so providing an important reason for the evolutionary development of such a facility in addition to associative learning systems (Bogacz *et al.*, 1999, 2000).

Endogenous and automatic registration

As described above, response decrements are found during the performance of explicit recognition memory tasks. However, response decrements are also found when stimuli are repeated even though discrimination of these stimuli is not being used to gain reward (Riches *et al.*, 1991; Fahy *et al.*, 1993b).

Indeed, in the rat, response decrements are found even though the animal has not been trained to perform any explicit recognition memory task (Zhu *et al.*, 1995a,b, 1996; Wan *et al.*, 1999a). Accordingly, the response changes are endogenous and automatic, and do not occur because of any training an animal has received. The implication is that these neurons are part of a system that automatically registers the occurrence of items during ongoing experience (Riches *et al.*, 1991; Brown and Xiang, 1998).

Generality of occurrence

Decremental responses have been described for visual stimuli that are three-dimensional objects and two-dimensional pictures, for pictures of real objects, geometric patterns or complex visual scenes (Riches *et al.*, 1991; Fahy *et al.*, 1993b; Miller *et al.*, 1993). Such responses occur in rats (Zhu *et al.*, 1995a) as well as in monkeys (Brown and Xiang, 1998), and may be inferred from imaging studies of humans where the task is to make a familiarity or recency judgement rather than recognition based on recollective recall (Squire *et al.*, 1992; Vandenberghe *et al.*, 1995). Moreover, detailed analysis of human recognition memory performance is consistent with such an underlying mechanism (Doty and Savakis, 1997; Hintzman *et al.*, 1998; Yonelinas *et al.*, 1998). The response decrements occur during the performance of delayed matching or serial recognition memory tasks that can be solved on the basis of the relative familiarity or recency of presentation of stimuli, as well as when there is no required behavioral contingency (Riches *et al.*, 1991; Miller *et al.*, 1993; Sobotka and Ringo, 1993; Zhu *et al.*, 1995a; Xiang and Brown, 1998c).

Repetition-sensitive neuronal responses have been described in rat perirhinal cortex during performance of a serial olfactory recognition memory task (Young *et al.*, 1997). No recording studies have been published concerning auditory recognition memory, but recent lesion studies in the monkey and dog (Kowalska *et al.*, 1998; Saunders *et al.*, 1998) indicate that auditory association cortex may be more important than perirhinal cortex. Consistent with these findings, a recent study using immunocytochemistry of the immediate early gene product Fos (see also Clayton, Chapter 7) has shown greater activation by novel than familiar sounds of neurons in rat temporal auditory association cortex and perirhinal cortex, but the difference reached significance only in temporal auditory association cortex (Wan *et al.*, 1999b). The differential activ-

ation of neurons in temporal auditory association cortex by novel and familiar sounds is consistent with the differential activation of neurons in temporal visual association cortex (anterior area TE) by novel and familiar pictures (Zhu *et al.*, 1996; Xiang and Brown, 1998c).

The occurrence of repetition-sensitive neuronal responses has not yet been studied as extensively during performance of recognition memory tasks that rely on recall or contextual discrimination, or where the relative familiarity of arrangements of items rather than of single items is required for task solution. However, there is already evidence that the hippocampus and entorhinal cortex are involved when there is a spatial component to the judgement of prior occurrence (Rolls *et al.*, 1989; Suzuki *et al.*, 1997; Wan *et al.*, 1999a; see also Buckley and Gaffan, Chapter 16).

INVOLVEMENT OF OTHER AREAS

Most areas which might be expected to play a role in recognition memory have been explored in the search for appropriate repetition-sensitive neuronal responses. Repetition-sensitive responses potentially related to recognition memory mechanisms (as opposed to responses that gradually habituate over many repetitions of a stimulus) have been described in areas other than the anterior inferior temporal cortex (for a review, see Brown and Xiang, 1998). Such responses have been found in more posterior parts of inferior temporal cortex (Baylis and Rolls, 1987; Miller *et al.*, 1991; Fahy *et al.*, 1993b; Vogels *et al.*, 1995), in entorhinal cortex (Fahy *et al.*, 1993b; Xiang and Brown, 1998c) and in prefrontal cortex (Miller *et al.*, 1996; Xiang and Brown, 1998a). They have also been found in the amygdala (Nishijo *et al.*, 1988; Riches *et al.*, 1991; Wilson and Rolls, 1993), the basal ganglia (Caan *et al.*, 1984; Riches *et al.*, 1991; Brown *et al.*, 1995; Xiang and Brown, 1998b), the medial dorsal (Fahy *et al.*, 1993a) and pregeniculate nuclei (Brown and Xiang, 1997) of the thalamus, the basal forebrain (Rolls *et al.*, 1982; Wilson and Rolls, 1990) and the locus ceruleus (Foote *et al.*, 1980; Vankov *et al.*, 1995). Small numbers of such responses for single stimulus items (as opposed to arrangements of items) have also been reported in the hippocampus in some studies (Rolls *et al.*, 1993), though their incidence is much lower than that in anterior inferior temporal cortex (Riches *et al.*, 1991; Zhu *et al.*, 1995a; Xiang and Brown, 1998c; Wan *et al.*, 1999a). They have not been found in areas TF and TH of the parahippocampal cortex (Riches *et al.*, 1991).

LOCALIZING THE SITE OF CHANGE

It is important to establish where response changes on stimulus repetition are first generated. Clearly, once such a change has been generated, any neuron receiving connections from a neuron generating the change may merely reflect that change passively. Two issues are significant: the earliest time after the appearance of a stimulus at which a neuron's responses to first and subsequent presentations of the stimulus differ, i.e. the differential latency of the response, and the length of the neuron's memory span. Shorter latencies

and longer memory spans cannot reflect longer latencies and shorter memory spans passively. In this context, the chief direction of information flow to and from perirhinal cortex (for simplicity omitting feedback connections) is shown in Figure 11.7.

In the monkey, differential latencies in anterior inferior temporal cortex for novel and familiar stimuli are similar to the visual latencies for many of the neurons, i.e. such neurons differentiate the relative familiarity of the stimuli as quickly as they detect their presence and identify them (Fahy *et al.*, 1993b; Miller *et al.*, 1993; Xiang and Brown, 1998c). This finding has important implications. First, it indicates that the response decrements cannot be being fed back from areas further along the processing stream, nor can they be being produced in these neurons by

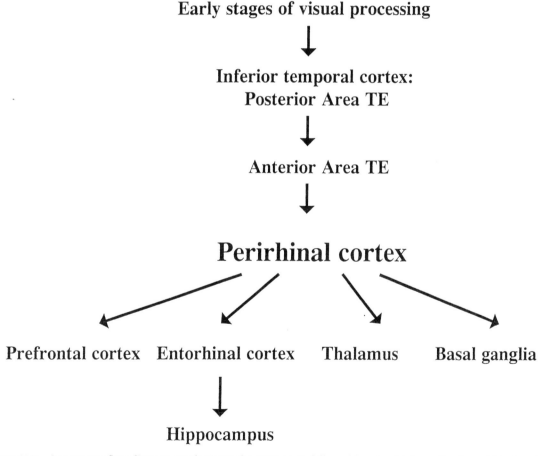

Figure 11.7. A summary flow diagram emphasizing the main route followed by visual information to perirhinal cortex. The diagram includes only a few of the connections of perirhinal cortex. It does not include feedback pathways such as those from the thalamus and prefrontal cortex to perirhinal cortex, nor pathways from perirhinal cortex to and from other parts of association cortex.

interactions over long synaptic loops: in both cases, there would be a lag between the visual and the differential latency. (Note that interactions involving fast, local synaptic loops are not excluded.) Consistent with this suggestion, none of the population of neurons in any of the other areas examined (with the exception of more posterior visual cortex) has a mean differential response latency as short as that in area TE (Wilson and Rolls, 1993; Miller *et al.*, 1996; Brown and Xiang, 1998; Xiang and Brown, 1998a,b,c; see also Table 11.1). Moreover, and adding support to this conclusion, ablation of other such areas (entorhinal cortex, hippocampus, amygdala, basal ganglia, medial dorsal thalamic nucleus and prefrontal cortex) does not cause such a large impairment of delayed non-matching to sample as does perirhinal ablation (Meunier *et al.*, 1993, 1997; Leonard *et al.*, 1995; Parker *et al.*, 1997; Murray and Mishkin, 1998). Accordingly, it is unlikely that such differential responses are generated in any of these other areas, though it remains theoretically possible that the response changes in anterior inferior temporal cortex could passively reflect changes in a small number of neurons with very early changes in some other area. Secondly, it suggests that the anterior part of area TE is the region in which the response decrements originate (for visual stimuli). The reason for this is as follows. Although, in principle, the decrements could be being fed forward to anterior TE by neurons earlier in the processing chain, the number and complexity of the visual stimuli make it unlikely that these stimuli could be differentiated from one another at an earlier stage than area TE. Accordingly, familiarity or recency discrimination for large numbers of such stimuli cannot be being performed at an earlier stage of visual processing (Brown and Xiang, 1998). Consistent with this deduction, recordings from more posterior visual areas have not found response decrements that can account for those in anterior TE: the memory spans of neurons recorded in more posterior areas are far shorter than those found anteriorly—usually lasting only a few seconds or less than five intervening stimuli (Baylis and Rolls, 1987; Miller *et al.*, 1991; Fahy *et al.*, 1993b; Vogels *et al.*, 1995). Thirdly, these conclusions provide a powerful argument that the response decrements in area TE cannot originate as a passive reflection of attentive changes. The attentive changes cannot precede familiarity discrimination and hence cannot occur earlier than changes in area TE. On the contrary, attentive changes may well be initiated by the response decrements.

In summary, in no other area has it been shown that the population differential response latencies are shorter and the memory spans longer than those in anterior inferior temporal cortex. Moreover, lesion effects are in each case less marked than for perirhinal ablation. Accordingly, changes in these other areas may be dependent on those in anterior inferior temporal cortex, but those in anterior inferior temporal cortex cannot be wholly dependent on changes in these other areas.

Within anterior inferior temporal cortex, the mean population differential latency is shorter for area TE than for perirhinal cortex (which, in turn, is shorter than for entorhinal cortex) (Xiang and Brown, 1998c; see Table 11.1). Accordingly, it is unlikely that the response decrements in area TE are passive reflections of those in perirhinal cortex (though because the possibility cannot be excluded that a few fast neurons in perirhinal cortex feed back changes to many neurons in area TE, this argument is persuasive rather than logically water-tight). However, at least for recency neurons, the mean memory span is longer in perirhinal cortex than in area TE (Xiang and Brown, 1998c). Hence (with the same logical weakness concerning extreme cases), the response decrements in perirhinal cortex are probably more than passive reflections of those in area TE. Thus response changes are probably generated in both area TE and perirhinal cortex.

POTENTIAL UNDERLYING MECHANISMS

There is as yet no firm evidence concerning the synaptic plastic mechanisms responsible for the response decrements. Uncovering these mechanisms presents a major experimental challenge. Possibilities for the mechanisms include a build up of inhibition, or processes allied to habituation or to long-term synaptic depression (LTD) or long-term potentiation (LTP; see Dudai and Morris, Chapter 9; Winder and Kandel, Chapter 10; see Figure 11.8). There are at least two processes that require explanation: a fast change that produces the response decrements found in recency neurons and a slow change that produces the response decrements found in familiarity neurons (Brown and Xiang, 1998; Xiang and Brown, 1998c).

Perhaps the initially most obvious parallel for the response decrements seen in anterior inferior temporal cortex is with habituation: habituation is characterized by a decrement in response to a monotonously

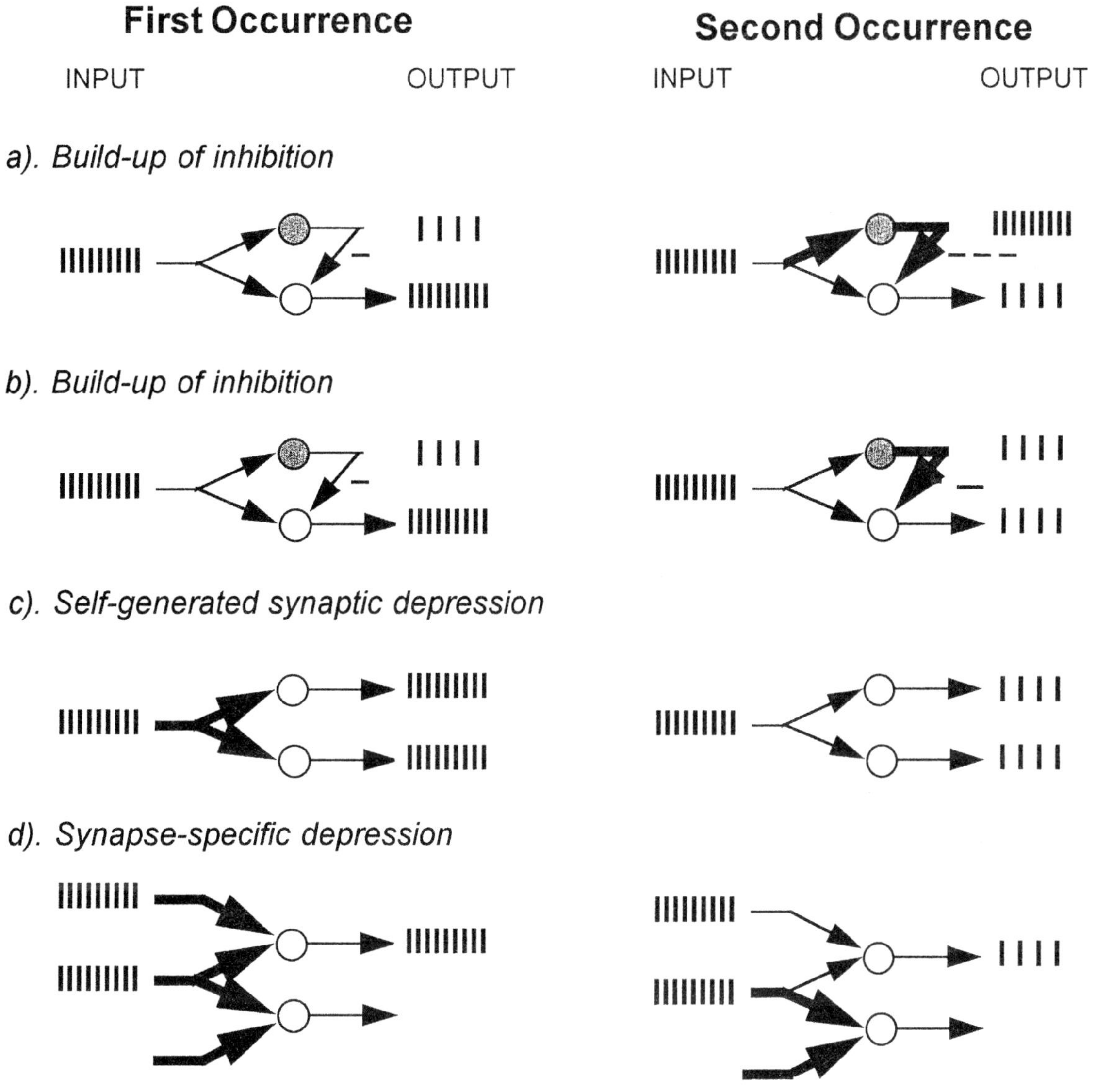

Figure 11.8. Different potential mechanisms that might underlie repetition-sensitive response decrements. (**A**) A build up of inhibition on stimulus repetition results in a reduced response (output: short bars represent notional action potentials) of a principal cell (unshaded) on the second compared with the first occurrence of a stimulus through enhancement of the efficacy of the synapses (shown by thicker arrows) onto the inhibitory neuron (shaded). The response (output) of the inhibitory neuron increments from the first to the second occurrence. (**B**) The build up of inhibition is produced by an increase in the efficacy of the inhibitory synapses onto the principal cell when the stimulus is repeated. In this case, the inhibitory cell does not need to increase its response on the second occurrence of the stimulus. (**C**) Self-generated synaptic depression, if it relies solely on a presynaptic mechanism, will result in weakening of all the synapses of the presynaptic cell (thinner arrows) on stimulus repetition, resulting in non-selectively reduced responses (output) in many cells on the second occurrence of a stimulus. (**D**) Synapse-specific depression, with plasticity being dependent on both a pre- and a postsynaptic condition, can result in a selectively reduced response (output) and synapses (thin arrows) affecting only the active cell when the stimulus occurs a second time.

repeated stimulus. However, there are important differences between the response decrements found in the anterior temporal cortex and those produced by habituation as classically described (Thompson and

Spencer, 1966; Horn, 1967; Kandel and Spencer, 1968; Brown and Xiang, 1998). For the responses of recency neurons to repeated stimuli, the decrement is large (typically >50%) and commonly very long-lasting (often >24 h) after a single exposure (Xiang and Brown, 1998c). Indeed, repeated exposures do not necessarily produce further decrement (Xiang and Brown, 1998c) (Figure 11.5A.). Classically, habituation produces a gradually increasing decrement across a series of exposures, and repeated series of exposures are necessary for the effect to be long lasting (more than minutes). Moreover, habituation is described normally in response to motivationally and emotionally neutral stimuli that are not associated with the obtaining of reward; indeed, recovery of initial responsiveness (dishabituation) is produced by the occurrence of behaviorally arousing stimuli (so-called 'extrastimuli'). The response decrements in anterior inferior temporal cortex occur even with stimuli that the animal is using to obtain reward, and therefore under conditions of continuing alertness. Furthermore, they occur even when the interval between the first and second presentations of a stimulus is filled with many other stimuli to which the animal also attends. Similar arguments apply also for the response decrements of familiarity neurons. Additionally, for familiarity neurons, the time course of the decremental process is quite different from that described in studies of habituation: rapidly repeated presentations of a stimulus (e.g. five times within 1 min) fail to produce a decrement, while a decrement appears after a single presentation if several minutes elapse before the stimulus is repeated (Xiang and Brown, 1998c).

Nevertheless, in spite of the above differences, some elaboration of the synaptic and biochemical processes that produce classical habituation may also be involved in anterior inferior temporal cortex response decrements. However, it appears that this elaboration needs also to include a mechanism that produces synaptic specificity. Habituation can be produced by mechanisms that are presynaptic (for reviews, see Horn, 1967, Chapter 19; Kandel, 1981). If the habituation mechanism is dependent solely on activity of the presynaptic cell, then all the synapses of that cell must habituate in parallel. Such a mechanism makes the change specific to a cell rather than to a synapse, with a large consequent loss of information-storing capacity. The discriminative capacity and hence, by implication, the storage capacity of the anterior inferior temporal cortex system must be very large because the responses discriminate the relative familiarity of very large numbers of complex stimuli. This capacity seems likely to require that the underlying mechanism is synapse specific rather than merely cell specific.

A decremental process that produces a long-term reduction in synaptic efficacy and is known to have such synaptic specificity is homosynaptic long-term depression (LTD). LTD has been much studied in the hippocampus and cerebellum (Ito, 1989; see also King and Thompson, Chapter 12). It can also be induced in slices of rat perirhinal cortex maintained *in vitro* (Ziakopoulos *et al.*, 1997, 1998), though the conditions of its induction are artificial and it is not yet known whether it can be produced by stimulation patterns that mimic the firing of perirhinal cortical neurons *in vivo*. Nevertheless, synaptic and biochemical mechanisms that underlie LTD may also be employed to produce response decrements in anterior inferior temporal cortex *in vivo*.

There is as yet no evidence to support the idea that response decrements in anterior inferior temporal cortex are due to a build up of inhibition, i.e. that the plastic process involves synapses onto or synapses of inhibitory neurons, rather than synapses between excitatory neurons (see also King and Thompson, Chapter 12; Horn, Chapter 19). If the change is a potentiation (e.g. some LTP-like process) of the synapses onto inhibitory neurons, then the firing of such neurons should increase on stimulus repetition. However, incremental responses have been encountered rarely and, moreover, the few increments found have not been large (Xiang and Brown, 1998c). It remains possible that the incrementing neurons are small and therefore are missed because of the sampling bias of the microelectrode technique towards recording larger cells. Nevertheless, if the cells are small or few in number, the discriminative capacity of the system in judging the relative familiarity of many complex stimuli is likely to be compromised. Alternatively, the potentiating synapses might be those of the inhibitory neurons themselves. However, whether the drive to or the drive of inhibitory neurons is increased on stimulus repetition, inhibitory interactions between some simultaneously recorded neurons should increase with stimulus repetition. Again, evidence for such increases being common is lacking (Xiang and Brown, 1997)—though this also may be because of the bias against recording small inhibitory neurons. Nonetheless, even if the synaptic change should prove eventually to involve exclusively or partially connections of inhibitory neurons, the synaptic plastic mechanisms need to have the same specificity and time course as are required should the change depend on connections between excitatory cells—though for synapses of the inhibitory neurons the change will need to be incremental rather than decremental.

Neuronal network modeling indicates that the above arguments require further elaboration. Neuronal firing patterns and decremental responses similar to those observed experimentally in anterior inferior temporal cortex can be generated by quite simple networks that use a mixture of LTP- and LTD-like processes (Bogacz *et al.*, 1999, 2000). As mentioned above, such networks are very fast and efficient at familiarity discrimination. Surprisingly, it is possible to produce a plausible model without any of the neuronal responses showing large incremental changes on stimulus repetition and in which the leading synaptic change is incremental (LTP) rather than decremental (LTD). It is possible to induce LTP as well as LTD in

perirhinal slices (Ziakopoulos *et al.*, 1997, 1998), but again the conditions of the induction are artificial and parallels between the effects of experimental manipulations (e.g. drug effects) on synaptic plasticity, neuronal activity and behavior remain to be established. Moreover, a plausible synaptic substrate has still to be identified for the slow decremental response changes of familiarity neurons.

WHY DECREMENTS?

At first sight, it might seem unexpected for responses in anterior inferior temporal cortex to be reduced when a stimulus is repeated. However, this arrangement means that there is more activity evoked by

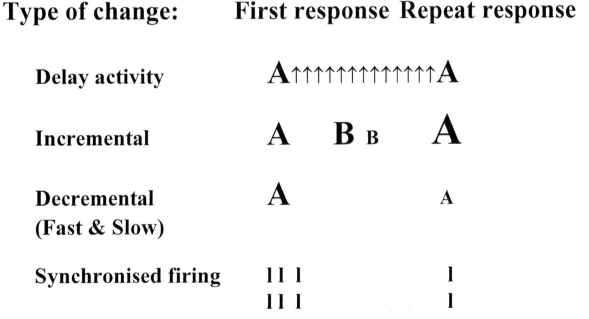

Figure 11.9. Familiarity discrimination substrates: schematic representation of candidate neuronal activity changes found in anterior inferior temporal cortex. Delay activity occurring between the initial and subsequent presentation of a stimulus (A) is represented by arrows. For incremental and decremental changes, the size of the response to a stimulus is represented by the size of the letter. Changes in the synchronization of firing of pairs (groups) of neurons may also transmit information concerning prior occurrence.

novel stimuli, which is appropriate as novel stimuli will in general require more processing and should attract more attention. Furthermore, the majority of stimulus items one meets day by day are the same, i.e. familiar. It is thus more energy efficient if familiar stimuli evoke less neuronal activity than if the activity increases each time a familiar stimulus is encountered. Moreover, the reduction may reflect faster, more nearly optimized processing when a stimulus is encountered more than once. Additionally, modeling suggests that the increased firing to novel stimuli may be used to effect information storage registering their occurrence (Bogacz *et al.*, 1999, 2000). However, that such arguments are not necessarily conclusive is shown by the situation in prefrontal cortex where incremental response changes are more common than decremental ones (Xiang and Brown, 1998a).

POSSIBLE ALTERNATIVE SUBSTRATES

As lesions of perirhinal cortex produce major impairments in the performance of recognition memory tasks, the activity of neurons in this region must in some way be crucial to the task. Several studies have been made of neuronal activity in perirhinal cortex during the performance of recognition memory tasks (for a review, see Brown and Xiang, 1998). In addition to the three types of decremental responses detailed above, three other types of change in activity related to task events have been reported: (i) there are response increments with stimulus repetition; (ii) there is sustained or delay activity related to the previous appearance of a stimulus; and (iii) there is synchronized or near synchronized firing of certain pairs of neurons. These changes are illustrated schematically in Figure 11.9. No other changes that might provide a substrate for recognition memory processes have been described in this critical region.

Response increments

Response increments have been described only when an animal has been trained to discriminate between repetitions of stimuli which require a response in order for a reward to be obtained and repetitions of stimuli which are irrelevant to task solution (Miller and Desimone, 1994). In such a discrimination task, a target picture is shown followed by a series of 1–4 other pictures. To gain reward, the monkey has to press a lever when the target picture appears again.

There is no reward for a press when a non-target picture is repeated. In this task, changes in neuronal responses to a repeated non-target stimulus are always decremental, but for about 30% of the neurons that have a changed response, the response to the repeat of the target is larger than the initial response, i.e. the change is an increment (Miller and Desimone, 1994). It remains to be shown that such response increments occur when more than one stimulus must be held in mind. Moreover, such response increments have not been found in situations other than that of this particular task. Accordingly, although response increments may prove invaluable to the solution of certain recognition tasks, it seems unlikely that they are the normal, general basis for familiarity discrimination.

Delay activity

Delay activity is found following presentation of a target stimulus in situations in which a behavioral decision based on the identity of this stimulus will need to be made within a prescribed time (Fuster and Jervey, 1981; Miyashita and Chang, 1988; Riches *et al.*, 1991; Desimone, 1996). The activity may be sustained throughout the delay period or appear before the anticipated choice time. It may also convey information concerning the identity of the target stimulus. Again, such activity has only been found in situations where the animal has been trained to expect the occurrence of a choice based on the target stimulus, where the choice will occur within a limited time period and when only one stimulus need be held in mind. Such activity has not been observed during performance of a serial recognition memory task where a target stimulus may not re-occur for many trials and where, correspondingly, many stimuli would have to be kept in mind simultaneously (e.g. Xiang and Brown, 1998c). Accordingly, although delay activity may provide an invaluable means for the solution of particular types of recognition memory tasks, it again seems unlikely that it could provide a basis for general familiarity discrimination.

Synchronized firing

It has been suggested that the synchronized or near synchronized firing of neurons may carry important information concerning the identity of a stimulus, and/or information concerning cognitive and behavioral decisions relating to that stimulus (for a review, see Singer and Gray, 1995; Singer, Chapter 3). The firing of many neurons with decremental responses is closely correlated with the firing of neighboring neurons with such responses (Xiang and Brown, 1997). Certain such neuron pairs demonstrate synchronous or near synchronous firing, i.e. the action potentials in one neuron occur within a few milliseconds of the action potentials of another neuron more frequently than could be expected by chance. Accordingly, it is possible that such correlated activity carries important information relating to the relative novelty or familiarity of stimuli. Consistent with this possibility, correlations between such neurons are not random, and the strengths of these correlations are modulated by the relative familiarity of stimuli. Thus when two recency neurons are recorded simultaneously through the same microelectrode, their activity is correlated for most such pairs. Similarly, the activity of most pairs of familiarity neurons and of most pairs of novelty neurons is correlated. In contrast, no correlated firing has been found between pairs of neurons where one is a recency and one a familiarity neuron. The correlations typically are strongest during the presentation of novel stimuli and are reduced during repeat presentations or the presentation of familiar stimuli; they are absent when no stimuli are being shown (Xiang and Brown, 1997; Brown and Xiang, 1998). Hence the correlated firing carries information related to the relative familiarity or recency of presentation of stimuli and to a certain extent parallels the firing rate changes of the responses of the neurons. However, while these data indicate that information is indeed being carried by such correlated firing, it has not yet been shown that this information signals more than is being signaled by the mean firing rate changes of the neurons taken individually. Moreover, there is as yet no evidence that such correlated firing occurs at a latency as short as that of the changes in mean rate (decremental responses). The possible role of synchronized neuronal activity awaits further exploration.

CURRENT AND FUTURE CHALLENGES

Although at present there is no plausible alternative substrate for general familiarity discrimination, the relationship between neuronal response decrements and recognition memory remains to be tested extensively. For example, so far there have been few studies that have tested either the effects on neuronal response decrements of drugs that impair recognition

memory or the effects of drugs that impair response decrements on recognition memory. To provide critical tests of the relationship, it is essential (though not necessarily easy to achieve) that such studies are designed to exclude drug effects that are not due to changes in decremental responses.

One potential challenge to the relationship is provided by the effects of scopolamine. This drug produces an impairment in delayed non-matching to sample performance (Tang *et al.*, 1997). However, given systemically, it does not reduce response decrements on stimulus repetition at short (<5s) delays (Miller and Desimone, 1993; see also Buckley and Gaffan, Chapter 16). Nevertheless, these findings are not necessarily incompatible with the role of decremental responses in recognition memory. Thus, the effect of the drug upon behavior at these short delays does not appear to be delay dependent (Miller and Desimone, 1993) and may well arise from impairment of other processes assisting solution of the task (e.g. a reduction in delay activity) or in other brain regions (e.g. a disruption of normal neuronal activity in prefrontal cortex). At long delays and with lists of items so that delay activity is unlikely to be used to solve the task, infusion of the drug into perirhinal cortex also produces impairment of performance (Tang *et al.*, 1997). This finding therefore suggests an effect upon perirhinal activity other than delay activity. What might be impaired is unknown; in particular, the effect of the drug on response decrements at long delays remains to be investigated. However, preliminary results (Brown *et al.*, 2000) indicate that rats given systemic scopolamine do not show the normal difference in perirhinal Fos counts evoked by exposure to repeatedly seen or never previously seen pictures. The results suggest that following scopolamine treatment there is no response decrement for the previously seen pictures. For a difference in Fos counts to be found, the repeatedly seen pictures must leave a trace (memory) that lasts for at least 3 h. Hence it could be that scopolamine interferes with the persistence (consolidation) of response decrements.

A second potential challenge is provided by work in monkeys with a split optic chiasma so that visual information can be directed initially to the left or right side of the brain independently (Sobotka and Ringo, 1996). Neurons that demonstrate a response decrement when two presentations of a stimulus are made to the same eye do not display such a decrement when the two presentations are made to different eyes. Even so, the animal can still perform (albeit not so well) the recognition memory task. However, the

particular task employed can be solved by using differential delay activity as an alternative substrate to
response decrements. The situation needs to be
explored further using a task that cannot be solved on
the basis of delay activity.

Although there are human brain imaging studies
whose findings are consistent with the response decrement hypothesis of familiarity and recency discrimination (Squire *et al.*, 1992; Vandenberghe *et al.*, 1995),
greater activation by novel than familiar stimuli in
parahippocampal cortex has not been a universal
finding in brain imaging studies during human performance of recognition memory tasks (for a review, see,
for example, Nyberg *et al.*, 1996; cf. Dolan, Chapter 17).
The most reasonable explanation for this discrepancy is
that recollection and associative recall form a very
prominent component of human recognition memory.
Education provides human subjects with extensive
training in making verbal and other associations
(including contextual) of presented material. Thus the
brain processes related to recognition memory performed by a human subject in the unusual environment
of a tomographic brain scanner may differ in crucial
respects from those of a monkey or rat that is presented
with what may be interpretable as no more than
abstract patterns in an apparatus it experiences on a
regular daily basis. Under the present hypothesis, neuronal response decrements are not considered to be substrates of recollective and associative aspects of recall.
Thus brain imaging studies of judgement of prior
occurrence need to establish or constrain carefully the
processes subjects are using during task performance, if
they are to image familiarity discrimination as opposed
to recollective aspects of recognition memory.

IMPLICATIONS FOR STIMULUS
IDENTIFICATION AND FORMATION
OF REPRESENTATIONS

The fact that it is possible to construct a theoretical
model that is based on neuronal response decrements
as found in anterior inferior temporal cortex and which
performs fast, high-capacity and extremely accurate
familiarity discrimination has important implications
for the more general operation of the recognition
system (Bogacz *et al.*, 1999, 2000). It establishes that a
familiarity discrimination network potentially requires
relatively few neurons and hence is operationally
efficient (Bogacz *et al.*, 1999, 2000). The existence of such
a network frees the stimulus categorizing (perceptual

identification) systems from having to perform familiarity discrimination (Brown and Xiang, 1998; Xiang and
Brown, 1998c). (Though note that it does not remove
the need to form new associations for either novel or
familiar stimuli or to create new feature analyzers for
stimuli that cannot be classified adequately.) Hence it is
not necessary to alter the synaptic weights between
neurons of the perceptual categorizing system every
time a novel stimulus is encountered. Not having to
make such changes would assist with achieving perceptual constancy. Moreover, it potentially removes the un-
wanted disruption to such categorization processes that
rule-breaking exemplars have been shown to cause
when adaptive categorization systems are modeled
(McClelland, 1996). Most new stimuli can be classified
as a novel combination of previously known physical
attributes (features). Consider, for example, a new hat:
in general, it will be possible to identify it as an exem-
plar of the class *hat* without regard to whether it is an
object that has been seen before. There is no obvious
problem with the identification (classification) of a
novel or familiar stimulus being encoded as the particular (putatively unique) pattern of activity of the population of neurons activated within feature analysis
networks. Thus there is no need to alter synaptic
weights within the categorization network every time
you encounter, for example, a new hat. However, such a
categorization system would not indicate whether a
pattern of activation had been encountered previously
or not, i.e. whether the stimulus (the hat) was novel or
familiar. This judgement, however, is exactly what is
supplied by the activity of the familiarity discrimination
system. Moreover, this judgement is supplied very
quickly, probably as quickly as that supplied by the
identification system. Thus, modeling suggests that it is
likely to prove efficient to have independent systems
subserving identification and subserving judgement of
prior occurrence. Modeling does not preclude parts of
both systems co-existing in perirhinal cortex; indeed,
such co-existence would be consistent with much
experimental evidence (Brown and Xiang, 1998; see also
Buckley and Gaffan, Chapter 16).

RELATIONSHIP OF RESPONSE
DECREMENTS TO PRIMING MEMORY

In repetition priming, the speed and accuracy of
response are enhanced for a previously encountered
stimulus compared with a novel stimulus. The precise
relationship between this change and the response

decrements of recency neurons is not known. Priming and recognition memory can be dissociated in several ways (Brown *et al.*, 1989; Schacter *et al.*, 1993; Wagner *et al.*, 1998)—though it needs to be noted that there is more than one type of priming and more than one process underlying recognition memory. Most obviously, priming is an essentially unconscious process whereas recognition memory is essentially conscious (Warrington and Weiskrantz, 1968; Jacoby and Witherspoon, 1982; Graf and Schacter, 1985; Schacter *et al.*, 1993; see also Weiskrantz, Chapter 18). Accordingly, repetition priming and recency discrimination cannot have identical neural substrates. However, it remains possible that the two types of memory may share some processing machinery. Such sharing would be evolutionarily efficient. The responses of recency neurons potentially could both provide information necessary for judgement of prior occurrence (recognition memory) and at the same time be a reflection of the more fluent processing of previously encountered stimuli that results in priming. Note that the response changes for familiarity neurons develop too slowly to provide a substrate for repetition priming.

Priming is in most respects normal in amnesic patients with medial temporal lobe lesions (Warrington and Weiskrantz, 1968; Graf *et al.*, 1985; Schacter *et al.*, 1993). In particular, priming is normal but recognition memory is at chance in patient E.P. (Hamann and Squire, 1997). Patient E.P. has bilateral damage that involves the whole of the hippocampal formation (including entorhinal cortex) and perirhinal cortex, though the damage additionally extends to some other temporal cortical areas. Thus priming does not require these temporal lobe regions but recognition memory does. However, recognition memory judgements based on familiarity or recency discrimination do not suffer major impairment following hippocampal lesions in humans or monkeys (Alvarez *et al.*, 1995; Aggleton and Shaw, 1996; Murray and Mishkin, 1998; Aggleton and Brown, 1999). Accordingly, the integrity of the perirhinal cortex is important to some process that underlies recognition memory (familiarity discrimination) as opposed to priming.

CONCLUSIONS

In summary, neurons within a region of the temporal lobe, perirhinal cortex, that is essential to familiarity discrimination respond more strongly to first than to subsequent presentations of visual stimuli. The responses of these neurons thus carry information of potential importance to recognition memory about the prior occurrence of individual visual stimuli. Further, the properties of these neuronal responses are in many respects those required for a substrate of familiarity discrimination (as opposed to recollective or contextual aspects of recognition memory). No other neuronal substrate with properties capable of explaining general familiarity discrimination has yet been discovered. Moreover, neural network modeling establishes that a network with elements having activity similar to that observed experimentally performs familiarity discrimination quickly, economically and accurately. Nevertheless, the relationship between response decrements and recognition memory remains to be tested extensively. In particular, the underlying synaptic changes responsible for the neuronal response decrements have yet to be discovered.

ACKNOWLEDGEMENTS

The author wishes to acknowledge his indebtedness to Gabriel Horn for his instruction, inspiration and assistance over many years. The Wellcome Trust, MRC and BBSRC are thanked for financial support.

REFERENCES

Aggleton, J.P. and Brown, M.W. (1999) Episodic memory, amnesia and the hippocampal–anterior thalamic axis. *Behavioral and Brain Sciences*, 22, 425–498.

Aggleton, J.P. and Shaw, C. (1996) Amnesia and recognition memory: a re-analysis of psychometric data. *Neuropsychologia*, 34, 51–62.

Alvarez, P., Zola-Morgan, S. and Squire, L.R. (1995) Damage limited to the hippocampal region produces long-lasting memory impairment in monkeys. *Journal of Neuroscience*, 15, 3796–3807.

Baylis, G.C. and Rolls, E.T. (1987) Responses of neurons in the inferior temporal cortex in short term and serial recognition memory tasks. *Experimental Brain Research*, 65, 614–622.

Bogacz, R., Brown, M.W. and Giraud-Carrier, C. (2000) Model of familiarity discrimination in perirhinal cortex. *Journal of Computational Neuroscience*, in press

Bogacz, R., Brown, M.W. and Giraud-Carrier, C. (1999) High capacity neural networks for familiarity discrimination. *Proceedings of International Conference on Artificial Neural Networks, Edinburgh*, pp. 773–776.

Brown, M.W. (1996) Neuronal responses and recognition memory. *Seminars in the Neurosciences*, 8, 23–32.

Brown, M.W. and Xiang, J.-Z. (1997) Information processing for novel and familiar visual stimuli in primate pregeniculate nucleus. *Society for Neuroscience Abstracts*, 23, 500.

Brown, M.W. and Xiang, J.Z. (1998) Recognition memory: neuronal substrates of the judgement of prior occurrence. *Progress in Neurobiology*, 55, 149–189.

Brown, M.W., Warburton, E.C. and Duguid, G. (2000) Scopolamine disrupts both differential Fos expression in perirhinal cortex and spontaneous object recognition in rats. *Proceedings of Forum of European Neuroscience*, Brighton, 191, 10.

Brown, M.W., Wilson, F.A.W. and Riches, I.P. (1987) Neuronal evidence that inferomedial temporal cortex is more important than hippocampus in certain processes underlying recognition memory. *Brain Research*. 409, 158–162.

Brown, M.W., Brown, J. and Bowes, J.B. (1989) Absence of priming coupled with substantially preserved recognition in lorazepam-induced amnesia. *Quarterly Journal of Experimental Psychology*, 41A, 599–617.

Brown, V.J., Desimone, R. and Mishkin, M. (1995) Responses of cells in the tail of the caudate nucleus during visual discrimination learning. *Journal of Neurophysiology*, 74, 1083–1094.

Burwell, R.D., Witter, M.P. and Amaral, D.G. (1995) Perirhinal and postrhinal cortices of the rat: a review of the neuroanatomical literature and comparison with findings from the monkey brain. *Hippocampus*, 5, 390–408.

Caan, W., Perrett, D.I. and Rolls, E.T. (1984) Responses of striatal neurons in the behaving monkey. 2. Visual processing in the caudal neostriatum. *Brain Research*, 290, 53–65.

Corkin, S., Amaral, D.G., Gonzalez, R.G., Johnson, K.A. and Hyman, B.T. (1997) H.M.'s medial temporal lobe lesion: findings from magnetic resonance imaging. *Journal of Neuroscience*, 17, 3964–3979.

Desimone, R. (1996) Neural mechanisms for visual memory and their role in attention. *Proceedings of the National Academy of Sciences of the United States of America*, 93, 13494–13499.

Doty, R.W. and Savakis, A.E. (1997) Commonality of processes underlying visual and verbal recognition memory. *Cognitive Brain Research*, 5, 283–294.

Ennaceur, A., Neave, N. and Aggleton, J.P. (1996) Neurotoxic lesions of the perirhinal cortex do not mimic the behavioural effects of fornix transection in the rat. *Behavioural Brain Research*, 80, 9–25.

Eskandar, E.N., Richmond, B.J. and Optican, L.M. (1992) Role of inferior temporal neurons in visual memory: I. Temporal encoding of information about visual images, recalled images and behavioral context. *Journal of Neurophysiology*, 68, 1277–1295.

Fahy, F.L., Riches, I.P. and Brown, M.W. (1993a) Neuronal signals of importance to the performance of visual recognition memory tasks: evidence from recordings of single neurones in the medial thalamus of primates. *Progress in Brain Research*, 95, 401–416.

Fahy, F.L., Riches, I.P. and Brown, M.W. (1993b) Neuronal activity related to visual recognition memory: long-term memory and the encoding of recency and familiarity information in the primate anterior and medial inferior temporal and rhinal cortex. *Experimental Brain Research*, 96, 457–472.

Felleman, D.J. and Van Essen, D.C. (1991) Distributed hierarchical processing in the primate cerebral cortex. *Cerebral Cortex*, 1, 1–47.

Foote, S.L., Aston-Jones, G. and Bloom, F.E. (1980) Impulse activity of locus coeruleus neurons in awake rats and monkeys is a function of sensory stimulation and arousal. *Proceedings of the National Academy of Sciences of the United States of America*, 77, 3033–3037.

Fuster, J.M. and Jervey, J.P. (1981) Inferotemporal neurons distinguish and retain behaviorally relevant features of visual stimuli. *Science*, 212, 952–955.

Gaffan, D. and Murray, E.A. (1992) Monkeys (*Macaca fascicularis*) with rhinal cortex ablations succeed in object discrimination learning despite 24-hr intertrial intervals and fail at matching to sample despite double sample presentations. *Behavioral Neuroscience*, 106, 30–38.

Graf, P. and Schacter, D.L. (1985) Implicit and explicit memory for new associations in normal and amnesic subjects. *Journal of Experimental Psychology: Learning, Memory and Cognition*, 11, 501–518.

Hamann, S.B. and Squire, L.R. (1997) Intact perceptual memory in the absence of conscious memory. *Behavioral Neuroscience*, 111, 850–854.

Hintzman, D.L., Caulton, D.A. and Levitin, D.J. (1998) Retrieval dynamics in recognition and list discrimination: further evidence of separate processes of familiarity and recall. *Memory and Cognition*, 26, 449–462

Horn, G. (1967) Neuronal mechanisms of habituation. *Nature*, 215, 707–711.

Ito, M. (1989) Long-term depression. *Annual Review of Neuroscience*, 12, 85–102.

Jacoby, L.L. and Witherspoon, D. (1982) Remembering without awareness. *Canadian Journal of Psychology*, 36, 300–324.

Jones, E.G. and Powell, T.P.S. (1970) An anatomical study of converging sensory pathways within the cerebral cortex of the monkey. *Brain*, 93, 793–820.

Kandel, E.R. (1981) Calcium and the control of synaptic strength by learning. *Nature*, 293, 697–700.

Kandel, E.R. and Spencer, W.A. (1968) Cellular and neurophysiological approaches to the study of learning. *Physiological Reviews*, 48, 66–134.

Kowalska, D.M., Kusmierek, P. and Kosmal, A. (1998) The effects of auditory association areas lesions on the sound recognition memory in dogs. *Society for Neuroscience Abstracts*, 28, 1305.

Leonard, B.W., Amaral, D.G., Squire, L.R. and Zola-Morgan, S. (1995) Transient memory impairment in monkeys with bilateral lesions of the entorhinal cortex. *Journal of Neuroscience*, 15, 5637–5659.

Li, L., Miller, E.K. and Desimone, R. (1993) The representation of stimulus familiarity in anterior inferior temporal cortex. *Journal of Neurophysiology*, 69 1918–1929.

Lueschow, A., Miller, E.K. and Desimone, R. (1994) Inferior temporal mechanisms for invariant object recognition. *Cerebral Cortex*, 4, 523–531.

McClelland, J.L. (1996) Role of the hippocampus in learning and memory: a computational analysis. In: Ono, T., McNaughton, B.L., Molotchnikoff, S., Rolls, E.T. and Nishijo H. (eds), *Perception, Memory and Emotion: Frontiers in Neuroscience*. Plenum Press, New York, pp. 601–613.

Meunier, M., Bachevalier, J., Mishkin, M. and Murray, E.A. (1993) Effects on visual recognition of combined and separate ablations of the entorhinal and perirhinal cortex in rhesus monkeys. *Journal of Neuroscience*, 13, 5418–5432.

Meunier, M., Hadfield, W., Bachevalier, J. and Murray, E.A. (1996) Effects of rhinal cortex lesions combined with hippocampectomy on visual recognition memory in rhesus monkeys. *Journal of Neurophysiology*, 75, 1190–1205.

Meunier, M., Bachevalier, J. and Mishkin, M. (1997) Effects of orbital frontal and anterior cingulate lesions on object and spatial memory in rhesus monkeys. *Neuropsychologia*, 35, 999–1015.

Miller, E.K. and Desimone, R. (1993) Scopolamine affects short-term memory but not inferior temporal neurons. *NeuroReport*, 4, 81–84.

Miller, E.K. and Desimone, R. (1994) Parallel neuronal mechanisms for short-term memory. *Science*, 263, 520–522.

Miller, E.K., Gochin, P.M. and Gross, C.G. (1991) Habituation-like decrease in the responses of neurons in inferior temporal cortex of the macaque. *Visual Neuroscience*, 7, 357–362.

Miller, E.K., Li, L. and Desimone, R. (1993) Activity of neurons in anterior inferior temporal cortex during a short-term memory task. *Journal of Neuroscience*, 13, 1460–1478.

Miller, E.K., Erickson, C.A. and Desimone, R. (1996) Neural mechanisms of visual working memory in prefrontal cortex of the macaque. *Journal of Neuroscience*, 16, 5154–5167.

Mishkin, M. (1978) Memory in monkeys severely impaired by combined but not by separate removal of amygdala and hippocampus. *Nature*, 273, 297–298.

Miyashita, Y. and Chang, H.S. (1988) Neuronal correlate of pictorial short-term memory in the primate temporal cortex. *Nature*, 331, 68–70.

Mumby, D.G. and Pinel, J.P.J. (1994) Rhinal cortex lesions and object recognition in rats. *Behavioral Neuroscience*, 108, 11–18.

Murray, E.A. (1996) What have ablation studies told us about the neural substrates of stimulus memory? *Seminars in the Neurosciences*, 8, 13–22.

Murray, E.A. and Mishkin, M. (1998) Object recognition and location memory in monkeys with excitotoxic lesions of the amygdala and hippocampus. *Journal of Neuroscience*, 18, 6568–6582.

Nishijo, H., Ono, T. and Nishino, H. (1988) Topographic distribution of modality-specific amygdalar neurons in alert monkey. *Journal of Neuroscience*, 8, 3556–3569.

Nyberg, L., McIntosh, A.R., Cabeza, R., Habib, R., Houles, S. and Tulving, E. (1996) General and specific brain regions involved in encoding and retrieval of events: what, where and when. *Proceedings of the National Academy of Sciences of the United States of America*, 93, 11280–11285.

Parker, A., Eacott, M.J. and Gaffan, D. (1997) The recognition memory deficit caused by mediodorsal thalamic lesion in non-human primates: a comparison with rhinal cortex lesion. *European Journal of Neuroscience*, 9, 2423–2431.

Riches, I.P., Wilson, F.A.W. and Brown, M.W. (1991) The effects of visual stimulation and memory on neurons of the hippocampal formation and the neighboring parahippocampal gyrus and inferior temporal cortex of the primate. *Journal of Neuroscience*, 11, 1763–1779.

Ringo, J.L. (1996) Stimulus specific adaptation in inferior temporal and medial temporal cortex of the monkey. *Behavioural Brain Research*, 76, 191–197.

Rolls, E.T., Perrett, D.I., Caan, A.W. and Wilson, F.A.W. (1982) Neuronal responses related to visual recognition. *Brain*, 105, 611–646.

Rolls, E.T., Miyashita, Y., Cahusac, P.M.B., Kesner, R.P., Niki, H., Feigenbaum, J.D. and Bach, L. (1989) Hippocampal neurons in the monkey with activity related to the place in which a stimulus is shown. *Journal of Neuroscience*, 9, 1835–1845.

Rolls, E.T., Cahusac, P.M.B., Feigenbaum, J.D. and Miyashita, Y. (1993) Responses of single neurons in the hippocampus of the macaque related to recognition memory. *Experimental Brain Research*, 93, 299–306.

Saunders, R.C., Fritz, J.B. and Mishkin, M. (1998) The effects of rhinal cortical lesions on auditory short-term memory in the rhesus monkey. *Society for Neuroscience Abstracts*, 28, 1907.

Schacter, D.L., Chiu, C.Y.P. and Ochsner, K.N. (1993) Implicit memory: a selective review. *Annual Review of Neuroscience*, 16, 183–205.

Scoville, W.B. and Milner, B. (1957) Loss of recent memory after bilateral hippocampal lesions. *Journal of Neurology, Neurosurgery and Psychiatry*, 20, 11–21.

Seeck, M., Michel, C.M., Mainwaring, N., Cosgrove, R. Blume, H., Ives, J., Landis, T. and Schomer, D.L. (1997) Evidence for rapid face recognition from human scalp and intracranial electrodes. *NeuroReport*, 8, 2749–2754.

Shi, C.-J. and Cassell, M.D. (1997) Cortical, thalamic and amygdaloid projections of the rat temporal cortex. *Journal of Comparative Neurology*, 382, 153–175.

Singer, W. and Gray, C.M. (1995) Visual feature integration and the temporal correlation hypothesis. *Annual Review of Neuroscience*, 18, 555–586.

Sobotka, S. and Ringo, J.L. (1993) Investigations of long-term recognition and association memory in unit responses from inferotemporal cortex. *Experimental Brain Research*, 96, 28–38.

Sobotka, S. and Ringo, J.L. (1996) Mnemonic responses of single units recorded from monkey inferotemporal cortex, accessed via transcommissural versus direct pathways: a dissociation between unit activity and behavior. *Journal of Neuroscience*, 16, 4222–4230.

Squire, L.R., Ojemann, J.G., Miezin, F.M., Petersen, S.E., Videen, T.O. and Raichle, M.E. (1992) Activation of the hippocampus in normal humans: a functional anatomical study of memory. *Proceedings of the National Academy of Sciences of the United States of America*, 89, 1837–1841.

Standing, L. (1973) Learning 10,000 pictures. *Quarterly Journal of Experimental Psychology*, 25, 207–222.

Suzuki, W.A. (1996) The anatomy, physiology and functions of the perirhinal cortex. *Current Opinion in Neurobiology*, 6, 179–186.

Suzuki, W.A., Miller, E.K. and Desimone, R. (1997) Object and place memory in the macaque entorhinal cortex. *Journal of Neurophysiology*, 78, 1062–1081.

Tang, Y., Mishkin, M. and Aigner, T.G. (1997) Effects of muscarinic blockade in perirhinal cortex during visual recognition. *Proceedings of the National Academy of Sciences of the United States of America*, 94, 12667–12669.

Thompson, R.F. and Spencer, W.A. (1966) Habituation: a model phenomenon for the study of neuronal substrates of behaviour. *Psychological Review*, 73, 16–43.

Vandenberghe, R., Dupont, P., Bormans, G., Mortelmans, L. and Orban, G. (1995) Blood flow in human anterior temporal cortex decreases with stimulus familiarity. *NeuroImage*, 2, 306–313.

Vankov, A., HerveMinvielle, A. and Sara, S.J. (1995) Response to novelty and its rapid habituation in locus coeruleus neurons of the freely exploring rat. *European Journal of Neuroscience*, 7, 1180–1187.

Vogels, R., Sary, G. and Orban, G.A. (1995) How task-related are the responses of inferior temporal neurons? *Visual Neuroscience*, 12, 207–214.

Wagner, A.D., Stebbins, G.T., Masciari, F., Fleischman, D.A. and Gabrieli, J.D.E. (1998) Neuropsychological dissociation between recognition familiarity and perceptual priming in visual long-term memory. *Cortex*, 34, 493–511.

Wan, H., Aggleton, J.P. and Brown, M.W. (1999a) Different contributions of the hippocampus and perirhinal cortex to recognition memory. *Journal of Neuroscience*, 19, 1142–1148.

Wan, H., Warburton, E., Kowalska, D.M., Aggleton, J.P. and Brown, M.W. (1999b) The involvement of auditory association cortex in auditory recognition memory. *Society for Neuroscience Abstracts*, 29, 91.

Warrington, E.K. and Weiskrantz, L. (1968) New method of testing long-term retention with special reference to amnesic patients. *Nature*, 217, 972–974.

Wilson, F.A.W. and Goldman-Rakic, P.S. (1994) Viewing preferences of rhesus monkeys related to memory for complex pictures, colours and faces. *Behavioural Brain Research*, 60, 79–89.

Wilson, F.A.W. and Rolls, E.T. (1990) Neuronal responses related to the novelty and familiarity of visual stimuli in the substantia innominata, diagonal band of Broca and the periventricular region of the primate basal forebrain. *Experimental Brain Research*, 80, 104–120.

Wilson, F.A.W. and Rolls, E.T. (1993) The effects of stimulus novelty and familiarity on neuronal activity in the amygdala of monkeys performing recognition memory tasks. *Experimental Brain Research*, 93, 367–382.

Xiang, J.-Z. and Brown, M.W. (1997) Processing visual familiarity and recency information: neuronal interactions in area TE and rhinal cortex. *Brain Research Association Abstracts*, 14, 69

Xiang, J.-Z. and Brown, M.W. (1998a) Encoding of relative familiarity and recency information in orbital, ventromedial and dorsolateral prefrontal cortices and anterior cingulate gyrus. *Society for Neuroscience Abstracts*, 28, 1425.

Xiang, J.-Z. and Brown, M.W. (1998b) Neuronal responses to novel and familiar visual stimuli in monkey putamen and caudate nucleus. *European Journal of Neuroscience*, 10, 56.73

Xiang, J.Z. and Brown, M.W. (1998c) Differential neuronal encoding of novelty, familiarity and recency in regions of the anterior temporal lobe. *Neuropharmacology*, 37, 657–676.

Yonelinas, A.P., Kroll, N.E.A., Dobbins, I.G., Lazzara, M. and Knight, R.T. (1998) Recollection and familiarity deficits in amnesia: convergence of remember–know, process dissociation and receiver operating characteristic data. *Neuropsychology*, 12, 323–339.

Young, B.J., Otto, T., Fox, G.D. and Eichenbaum, H. (1997) Memory representation within the parahippocampal region. *Journal of Neuroscience*, 17, 5183–5195.

Zhu, X.O., Brown, M.W. and Aggleton, J.P. (1995a) Neuronal signalling of information important to visual recognition memory in rat rhinal and neighbouring cortices. *European Journal of Neuroscience*, 7, 753–765.

Zhu, X.O., Brown, M.W., McCabe, B.J. and Aggleton, J.P. (1995b) Effects of novelty or familiarity of visual stimuli on the expression of the immediate early gene c-*fos* in rat brain. *Neuroscience*, 69, 821–829.

Zhu, X.O., McCabe, B.J., Aggleton, J.P. and Brown, M.W. (1996) Mapping visual recognition memory through expression of the immediate early gene c-*fos*. *NeuroReport*, 7, 1871–1875.

Ziakopoulos, Z., Brown, M.W. and Bashir, Z.I. (1997) Synaptic depression and long-term potentiation in the rat perirhinal cortex *in vitro*. *Journal of Physiology*, 501P, P8–P9.

Ziakopoulos, Z., C.W. Tillett, Brown, M.W. and Bashir, Z.I. (1999) Input- and layer-dependent synaptic plasticity in the rat perirhinal cortex *in vitro*. *Neuroscience*, 92: 459–472

Zola-Morgan, S., Squire, L.R., Amaral, D.G. and Suzuki, W.A. (1989) Lesions of perirhinal and parahippocampal cortex that spare the amygdala and hippocampal formation produce severe memory impairment. *Journal of Neuroscience*, 9, 4355–4370.

PART THREE LEARNING AND MEMORY: COGNITIVE SYSTEMS IN ANIMALS AND HUMANS

INTRODUCTION

In Part three, the neural mechanisms of learning and memory are analyzed at the systems level (cf. Churchland and Sejnowski, 1980). Here too, however, the allocation of chapters to this part of the book rather than to Part two may sometimes appear arbitrary, as many authors investigate learning and memory at different levels of analysis, ranging from cognitive systems to molecular changes at the level of the synapse.

A good example of such a comprehensive approach is the first chapter of this section, by David King and Richard Thompson. For a long time it was thought that the cerebellum, together with the basal ganglia and the motor cortex, was involved in the moment to moment control of motor functions. However, through the work of Richard Thompson and others, it has become clear that the cerebellum is crucial for motor learning as well. As such, the study of the role of the cerebellum in motor learning is now one of the most prominent paradigms in the search for the neural substrates of learning and memory. King and Thompson provide a thorough review of the work that led to the identification of a restricted region of the cerebellum as the site of the 'engram' for skill learning. Just as in several other contributions to this volume (see, for example McGaugh et al., Chapter 13; Horn, Chapter 19), these authors discuss the criteria that have to be met before one is able to assign a role for a particular region of the brain as a substrate for memory. As Horn (1985) has also pointed out, there is a need for a comprehensive approach involving different techniques, if one wants to arrive at firm conclusions as to the localization of function. King and Thompson confirm that, for example, lesion studies alone are far from conclusive. These authors then discuss how they used a combination of reversible neural inactivation and electrophysiology to establish that the nucleus interpositus and overlying cerebellar cortex contain the neural substrate for eyeblink conditioning in the rabbit. They review other evidence suggesting that this region of the cerebellum is also involved in other forms of motor skill learning, in the rabbit and in other species including humans. Given the high probability that they are actually dealing with the neural substrate of a form of learning, King and Thompson's discussion of the neuronal mechanisms involved is particularly interesting. There is evidence that long-term depresssion (LTD; for a review, see Ito 1989), a long-term reduction in synaptic efficacy, plays an important role.

Chapter 13 by McGaugh et al. is a thorough review of the brain mechanisms underlying the modulation of memory consolidation. The authors provide convincing evidence that noradrenergic systems in the basolateral amygdala (BLA) influence memory by modulating memory storage elsewhere in the brain. The release of norepinephrine (noradrenaline) within the BLA is regulated by stress hormones from the adrenal cortex (glucocorticoids) and medulla (epinephrine or adrenaline). McGaugh et al. suggest that particularly emotionally arousing stimulation is processed by the amygdala. This theme is discussed in detail in the following chapter by Karim Nader and Joseph LeDoux, who concentrate their efforts on fear conditioning in particular. The work of these authors also points to the BLA as being a key structure in this kind of learning. However, in contrast to the modulatory role proposed by McGaugh et al. in the preceding chapter, Nader and Ledoux suggest that the BLA is in fact the site of storage for fear conditioning.

Localization of function is one of the basic themes of this book; McGaugh et al. stress that the BLA itself is not a site of memory storage, but that the BLA modulates memory storage through its effects on other brain regions such as the hippocampus and striatum. However, these authors emphasize that the hippocampus is unlikely to be a site of long-term memory storage and that 'it seems likely that long-term memory ultimately is represented in cortical regions', a view that is shared by Brown in Chapter 11 and by Buckley and Gaffan in Chapter 16. It is clear that Nader and Ledoux have a different view of the role of the amygdala in information storage from that of McGaugh *et al.* in the previous chapter. This issue was addressed in a recent commentary (Cahill *et al.*, 1999) and by the experimental studies of Vazdarja-nova and McGaugh (1998, 1999). Later in this volume, Dolan (Chapter 17) discusses evidence from human imaging studies, suggesting a time-limited role of the amygdala in fear conditioning. Both McGaugh *et al.* and Nader and LeDoux suggest that it cannot be excluded that the amygdala has both a modulatory and a storage function. If anything, the discussion between these two laboratories illustrates the difficulties involved in localizing function in the field of learning and memory.

An alternative approach to the study of the neural mechanisms of learning and memory is to formulate the processing requirements for a system that could subserve information storage, and to construct a model on the basis of these requirements. Numerous such modeling attempts employ the principles of parallel distributed processing (PDP), in which the strength of connections between units in multilayered networks represents stored information (Rumelhart and McClelland, 1986; Morris, 1989). Brown (Chapter 11) illustrates how network simulations of the function of brain regions with known neuronal numbers and connectivity can lead to realistic estimates of the processing capacity of those regions. Patrick Bateson (Chapter 15) reviews recent tests of a neural net model of imprinting that he and Gabriel Horn designed (Bateson and Horn, 1994; see also O'Reilly and Johnson, 1994). The rules governing changes in connectivity of the network include the Hebbian principle that I discussed in the Introduction to Part two, but the network is not 'supervised' and thus does not require 'backpropagation', as many other models do (Rumelhart and McClelland, 1986). It is becoming apparent that Bateson and Horn's neural net model can reliably simulate various aspects of imprinting (Bolhuis, 1991), and, in addition, is a powerful predictor of recent findings concerning the learning processes involved in imprinting (Bolhuis and Honey, 1998).

Scoville and Milner (1957) found that bilateral medial temporal lesions in an epileptic patient, known as H.M., led to severe anterograde amnesia. Ever since their seminal paper, the medial temporal lobe, and particularly the hippocampus, is thought to be important for memory. Accordingly, attempts have been made to find an animal model of medial temporal lobe amnesia, with varying success (e.g. Squire,

1987). As Mark Buckley and David Gaffan discuss in Chapter 16, the best primate approximation of human amnesia was achieved when improved versions of delayed (non-)match to sample tasks were employed, that particularly addressed the animals' recognition memory capacities. The focus on the hippocampus as a possible site of memory storage was so intense that there has been a seemingly unstoppable outpouring of theories of hippocampal function. Only recently it was discovered that in monkeys, the greatest memory impairment was not caused by lesions to the hippocampus, but by damage to adjacent neocortical regions, particularly the perirhinal cortex (Zola-Morgan *et al.*, 1989; Meunier *et al.*, 1993; Murray, 1996). Buckley and Gaffan provide an interesting account of this dramatic switch in this research paradigm, one which I discussed briefly in connection with Chapter 11 by Brown. The authors then proceed with an in depth review of recent work that investigated the roles of the perirhinal cortex and the hippocampus in memory and perception. One important conclusion is that these two structures are part of a larger cerebral complex, with each brain region having a particular role in processing particular aspects of stimuli, depending on the neuroanatomical connections to that region. In this view, no individual part of the temporal lobe is involved specifically in storage of representations of stimuli. Consequently, dense amnesia is a result of brain damage that prevents interaction between a large number of cortical and subcortical structures. Within this neural system, the perirhinal cortex appears to be involved in processing information about objects. The hippocampus proper is thought to be important for processing spatial information. We already saw in the very first chapter of this book (by Graziano *et al.*) that perception and memory are not completely separate, and this overlap may also be true at the neural level. Likewise, another major conclusion from Buckley and Gaffan's review (and one that is shared by Brown in Chapter 11) is that temporal lobe structures such as the perirhinal cortex and the hippocampus have both a perceptual and a memory function. In fact, their findings lead them to suggest that the traditional distinction between perception and memory that is usually made for particular brain regions is 'potentially misleading'.

Raymond Dolan reviews recent work on human imaging of memory in Chapter 17. Essentially, functional magnetic resonance imaging (fMRI) and positron emission tomography (PET) are scanning methods that visualize regional increases in blood flow or oxygen or glucose metabolism. Thus, they are a measure of neural activation during certain behavioral tasks in awake humans. First, Dolan shows that the amygdala is activated in aversive conditioning, which is consistent with the suggestions of McGaugh *et al.* and of Nader and Ledoux in the present volume. Activity in the amygdala is time limited, which is particularly consistent with a modulatory role of this structure in learning and memory (cf. McGaugh *et al.*, Chapter 13). The second paradigm that Dolan and his collaborators have investigated is priming, which is also discussed by Brown (Chapter 11) and by Weiskrantz (Chapter 18). Dolan defines priming as 'a facilitation of recognition or production of a stimulus by prior exposure to a stimulus with which the recognized item has a relationship of physical similarity or associated meaning'. Priming involves activation of the right or left fusiform gyrus for faces and objects, respectively. The fusiform gyrus is in the inferior temporal cortex, caudal to perirhinal cortex. Given the results described by Brown, and by Buckley and Gaffan in the present volume, it is surprising that Dolan and his collaborators did not find activity in the perirhinal cortex itself. Recently, Schacter and Wagner discussed a related issue when they noted that during memory encoding, PET studies showed activation in the anterior temporal lobe, while fMRI studies did not. These authors suggest that the discrepancy may be due to 'a loss of fMRI signal (susceptibility artifact) in the anterior medial temporal lobe' (Schacter and Wagner, 1999, p. 1504).

The last chapter of this part of the book, by Lawrence Weiskrantz, is concerned with arguably the most advanced state of cognition, consciousness. Weiskrantz reviews some of the classic studies of performance without awareness, a field in which he has been a pioneer. For instance, it is now a well known phenomenon in amnesic patients that they can often perform certain tasks (including learning tasks such as Pavlovian conditioning) very well, but they have no recollection of ever having done the task (Weiskrantz and Warrington, 1979). By presenting part of the training stimuli, performance of amnesic patients in recognition tasks can be improved markedly (Warrington and Weiskrantz, 1968), a phenomenon to which I referred earlier and which is now known as 'priming'. Weiskrantz was also the first to discover a phenomenon which he termed 'blindsight' (Weiskrantz, 1986), where patients with extensive damage to their visual cortex nevertheless are able to respond to stimuli in their blind fields. Interestingly, a similar phenomenon has been found in monkeys with lesions to the striate cortex (Cowey and Stoerig, 1995; for a critical discussion of blindsight and animal consciousness, see Macphail, 1998). Weiskrantz discusses the implications of these and related phenomena for our understanding of consciousness.

REFERENCES

Bateson, P. and Horn, G. (1994) Imprinting and recognition memory: a neural net model. *Animal Behaviour*, 48, 695–715.

Bolhuis J.J. (1991) Mechanisms of avian imprinting: a review. *Biological Reviews*, 66, 303–345.

Bolhuis J.J. and Honey R.C. (1998) Imprinting, learning and development: from behaviour to brain and back. *Trends in Neurosciences*, 21, 306–311.

Cahill, L., Weinberger, N.M., Roozendaal, B. and McGaugh, J.L. (1999) Is the amygdala a locus of 'conditioned fear'? Some questions and caveats. *Neuron*, 23, 227–228.

Churchland, P.S. and Sejnowski, T.J. (1988) Perspectives on cognitive neuroscience. *Science*, 242, 741–745.

Cowey, A. and Stoerig, P. (1995) Blindsight in monkeys. *Nature*, 373, 247–249.

Horn, G. (1985) *Memory, Imprinting, and the Brain*. Clarendon Press, Oxford.

Horn, G. (1998) Visual imprinting and the neural mechanisms of recognition memory. *Trends in Neurosciences* 21, 300–305.

Ito, M. (1989) Long-term depression. *Annual Review of Neuroscience*, 12, 85–102.

Macphail, E.M. (1998) *The Evolution of Consciousness*. Oxford University Press, New York.

Meunier, M., Bachevalier, J., Mishkin, M. and Murray, E.A. (1993) Effects on visual recognition of combined and separate ablations of the entorhinal and perirhinal cortex in rhesus monkeys. *Journal of Neuroscience*, 12, 5418–5432.

Morris, R.G.M. (ed.) (1989) *Parallel Distributed Processing: Implications for Psychology and Neurobiology*. Oxford University Press, New York.

Murray, E.A. (1996) What have ablation studies told us about the neural substrates of stimulus memory? *Seminars in the Neurosciences*, 8, 13–22.

O'Reilly R.C. and Johnson, M.H. (1994) Object recognition and sensitive periods: a computational analysis of visual imprinting. *Neural Computation*, 6, 357–389.

Rumelhart, D.E. and McClelland, J.L. (eds) (1986) *Parallel Distributed Processing*, Vol. I. Bradford Books, Cambridge, Massachusetts.

Schacter, D.L. and Wagner, A.D. (1999) Remembrance of things past. *Science*, 285, 1503–1504.

Scoville, W.B. and Milner, B. (1957) Loss of recent memory after bilateral hippocampal lesions. *Journal of Neurology, Neurosurgery and Psychiatry*, 20, 11–21.

Squire, L.R. (1987) *Memory and Brain*. Oxford University Press, Oxford.

Vazdarjanova, A. and McGaugh, J.L. (1998) Basolateral amygdala is not critical for cognitive memory of contextual fear conditioning. *Proceedings of the National Academy of Sciences of the United States of America*, 95, 15003–15007.

Vazdarjanova, A. and McGaugh, J.L. (1999) Basolateral amygdala is involved in modulating consolidation of memory for classical fear conditioning. *Journal of Neuroscience*, 19, 6615–6622.

Warrington, E.K. and Weiskrantz, L. (1968) New method of testing long-term retention with special reference to amnesic patients. *Nature*, 217, 972–974.

Weiskrantz, L.R. (1986) *Blindsight: A Case Study and its Implications*. Clarendon Press, Oxford.

Weiskrantz, L. and Warrington, E.K. (1979) Conditioning in amnesic patients. *Neuropsychologia*, 17, 187–194.

Zola-Morgan, S., Squire, L.R., Amaral, D.G. and Suzuki, W.A. (1989) Lesions of the perirhinal and parahippocampal cortex that spare the amygdala and the hippocampal formation produce severe memory impairment. *Journal of Neuroscience*, 9, 4355–4370.

12 SKILL LEARNING: THE ROLE OF THE CEREBELLUM

David A.T. King and Richard F. Thompson

INTRODUCTION

The cerebellum appears to be critically important for learning a number of motor skill tasks. Possible sites of synaptic plasticity (memory storage or 'engrams') range from known anatomical circuits spanning most of the cerebellum and brainstem (plus cerebral cortical loops) to restricted regions of cerebellar cortex and deep nuclei (including vestibular nuclei).

The first clues to cerebellar function came from cerebellar-lesioned animals and human patients, which display a number of mostly motor-related deficits, including ataxia, disturbed movement timing (especially during rapid and multijoint movements), difficulty in compensating for passive limb displacement and action tremor (a tremor absent during inactivity and most pronounced near the end of a movement). These and similar animal studies have led to the general consensus that the cerebellum receives information from sensory afferents and motor cortical outputs and is crucial for providing coordinated adjustment of all muscle groups such that balance and dexterity are maintained, and the body is rescued from the ongoing perturbations of gravity and the recoil forces of self-generated movements.

Other work argues further that the cerebellum is involved in learning adaptations to skeletomuscular 'problems'—real world problems such as touchtyping or a executing a golf swing as well as simpler skills more easily studied in the laboratory. The critical role of the cerebellum in adaptation of the vestibulo-ocular reflex has been well documented (Ito, 1989, 1993; du Lac et al., 1995). The common theme detectable across cerebellar-dependent forms of motor learning is that simple or complex stimuli, whether of purely somatosensory or proprioceptive or other feedback information, come to be associated with other stimuli or feedback over many trials (stimulus repetitions) such that simple or complex motor movements develop that are adaptive (yet usually not consciously accessible) and very precisely timed, with accuracy of the order of a few milliseconds.

The cerebellum has long been a favored structure for modeling a neuronal learning system, dating from the classic papers of Marr (1969) and Albus (1971). Our empirical work to date on classical conditioning of discrete behavioral responses (see below) has been guided by these models and the related views of Eccles (1977) and Ito (1984), and our results constitute a remarkable verification of the spirit of these theories (see also Thach et al., 1992).

Here we review a selection of studies focusing on cerebellar involvement in classical conditioning of discrete movements, trained reaching and grasping movements, and complex learned skills, and consider possible mechanisms of memory storage in the cerebellum.

THE CEREBELLAR SUBSTRATE OF DISCRETE RESPONSE CLASSICAL CONDITIONING

We begin with classical conditioning of discrete behavioral responses (eyeblink, limb flexion, head turn, etc.) learned to deal with aversive events. The cerebellum is necessary for this basic form of associative learning and the evidence is now very strong that the essential memory traces are formed and stored in the cerebellum. We use eyeblink conditioning as the basic paradigm; the conditioned stimulus (CS) is a neutral tone or light, the unconditioned stimulus (US) is corneal airpuff, and the unconditioned response (UR) and the conditioned response (CR) are external eyelid closure and extension of the nictitating membrane over the nasal portion of the cornea.

The circuitry we hypothesize to be responsible for learning is shown in Figure 12.1. There are two loops bridging sensory input and motor output. The learning circuit provides CS input (in this case a tone) via cochlear nuclei efferents to the pontine nuclei; pontine efferents enter the cerebellum via the middle cerebellar peduncle as mossy fibers, as do some direct projections from auditory relay nuclei, with excitatory synapses onto cortical granule cells and deep nuclear cells. Granule cell axons rise through the cortex and bifurcate as parallel fibers, synapsing (excitatory) on Purkinje cells (and basket, stellate and Golgi cells as well). The inhibitory Purkinje cell axons are the sole output of the cerebellar cortex and synapse on the deep (and vestibular) nuclei. Interpositus cells excite

red nuclear cells in the mesencephalon, which in turn excite motor neurons of premotor nuclei and cranial nuclei, mostly 6, and accessory 6 and 7, producing the learned behavior (CR). The US input is relayed via the trigeminal nucleus to the inferior olive, the efferents of which enter the cerebellum and also synapse on deep nuclear and Purkinje cells (as climbing fibers). The second circuit is a reflex loop responsible for the UR, and connects the trigeminal nucleus directly (or indirectly) to cranial motor nuclei.

We now review briefly the evidence supporting the hypothesis described above and in Figure 12.1. Figure 12.2 is a much simplified diagram of the essential

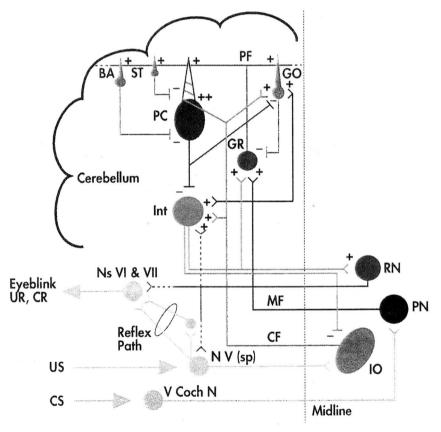

Figure 12.1. The established eyeblink conditioning circuit based on experimental findings and the anatomy of the cerebellum and brainstem. Three pathways involved in acquisition of conditioned responses are illustrated; the fourth, a reflex pathway, does not involve the cerebellum but mediates the unconditioned response (UR). The conditioned stimulus (CS) pathway consists of excitatory mossy fiber (MF) afferents primarily from the pontine nuclei (PN) to the interpositus nucleus (Int) and cerebellar cortex. Within the cortex, mossy fibers synapse on granule cells (GR), the axons of which ascend and bifurcate to form parallel fibers (PF). Parallel fibers form excitatory synapses on Purkinje cells (PC), the sole output of the cerebellar cortex. Purkinje axons make inhibitory synapses on cells of the interpositus and other deep nuclei. Cortical interneurons including Golgi (GO), stellate (ST) and basket (BA) cells make inhibitory synapses on their respective target cells. The unconditioned stimulus (US) pathway consists of strongly excitatory efferents of the inferior olive (IO) projecting to interpositus and Purkinje neurons. The conditioned response (CR) pathway projects from interpositus to red nucleus (RN), which projects directly to motor neurons that generate the eyeblink. V Coch N, ventral cochlear nucleus; N V (sp), spinal fifth cranial nucleus; N VI, sixth and accessory sixth cranial nuclei; N VII, seventh cranial nucleus (from Kim and Thompson, 1997).

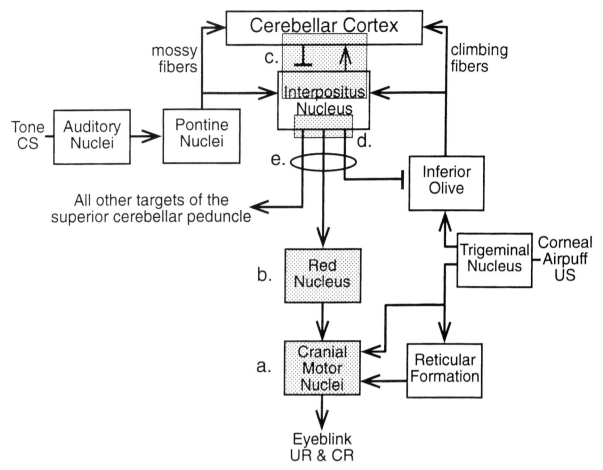

Figure 12.2. Simplified schematic of the essential brain circuitry involved in eyeblink conditioning. Shadowed boxes indicate brain regions that have been inactivated reversibly during training. (a) Inactivation of motor nuclei including facial (seventh) and accessory (sixth). (b) Inactivation of magnocellular red nucleus. (c) Inactivation of the anterior interpositus nucleus and some overlying cerebellar cortex of lobule H VI. (d) Inactivation of ventral anterior interpositus nucleus and associated white matter. (e) Complete inactivation of the superior cerebellar peduncle (scp), essentially all output from the cerebellar hemisphere (from Thompson *et al.*, 1998).

cerebellar circuit, that can serve to summarize our overall results to date. [Laterality is not shown; the critical region of the cerebellum is ipsilateral to the trained eye (or limb), the critical regions of the pontine nuclei, red nucleus and inferior olive are contralateral]. Unless otherwise noted, the data all refer to the basic delay eyeblink CR (Gormezano *et al.*, 1983; standard conditions are 350 ms tone CS, coterminating with a 100 ms corneal airpuff US). We simply note here that with more complex paradigms, e.g. trace conditioning, the hippocampal system also plays a critical role (Solomon *et al.*, 1986b; Moyer *et al.*, 1990; Kim *et al.*, 1995).

THE CR PATHWAY

We first showed that neurons in the cerebellar interpositus nucleus and in cerebellar cortex respond to the CS and US and develop amplitude–time course 'models' of the learned behavioral response that precede and predict the occurrence and form of the CR within trials and over the trials of training using classical conditioning of the eyeblink response in rabbits (McCormick *et al.*, 1982a, 1984a,b; Foy *et al.*, 1984), a result that has been replicated repeatedly (e.g. Berthier and Moore, 1990; Steinmetz, 1990; Tracy *et al.*, 1991). Electrical stimulation in the critical region of the interpositus elicits eyeblink responses in naive animals; the circuit is hard-wired from interpositus to behavior (Chapman *et al.*, 1988). We first showed that lesions of the interpositus abolished the CR and had no effect on the UR (McCormick *et al.*, 1982a). This result has been replicated in more than 15 subsequent studies in several mammalian species (see, for example, Yeo *et al.*, 1985a; for a review, see Thompson and Krupa, 1994; Thompson *et al.*, 1997). Similarly, lesions of the superior cerebellar peduncle and red nucleus can abolish the CR with no effect on the UR (McCormick *et al.*, 1982b; Rosenfeld and Moore, 1983; Rosenfeld *et al.*, 1985). Microinfusion of nanomolar amounts of γ-aminobutyric acid ($GABA_A$) antagonists in the critical region of cerebellar cortex [hemispheric lobule VI (HVI), interpositus or red nucleus completely and reversibly abolish the CR with no effect at all on the UR in a dose-dependent manner (Mamounas *et al.*, 1987; Haley *et al.*, 1988; Chapman *et al.*, 1990). Appropriate cerebellar lesions in humans completely prevent learning of the eyeblink CR and have no effect on the UR (Lye *et al.*, 1988; Solomon *et al.*, 1989; Daum *et al:*, 1993; Schugens *et al.*, 1997). The possibility that effective interpositus lesions abolish the CR by small effects on the UR (the 'performance' argument) has been ruled out decisively (Steinmetz *et al.*, 1992; Ivkovich *et al.*, 1993).

THE US PATHWAY

Lesions of the critical region of the inferior olive, the face representation in the dorsal accessory olive (DAO), completely prevent learning if made before training, and result in extinction/abolition of the CR if made after training [Yeo *et al.*, 1986; McCormick *et al.*, 1985; Voneida *et al.*, 1990 (limb flexion); Mintz *et al.*, 1994]. Unit activity in this critical DAO region does not respond to auditory stimuli (CS), responds only to US onset, shows no learning-related activity and decreases as animals learn (Sears and Steinmetz, 1991). Electrical microstimulation of this region serves as a very effective US (Mauk *et al.*, 1986; Steinmetz *et al.*, 1989; Thompson, 1989), as does stimulation of cerebellar white matter (Swain *et al.*, 1992). All these data argue (i) that the memory trace is not stored in the inferior olive and (ii) that the DAO climbing fiber system is the essential US reinforcing pathway for the learning of discrete responses (Thompson *et al.*, 1998). To our knowledge, this is the only system in the brain, other than reflex afferents, where the exact response

elicited by electrical stimulation can be conditioned to any neutral stimulus. Current evidence suggests that this system, together with the GABAergic projection from interpositus to DAO (Nelson and Mugnoini, 1989), functions as the error-correcting algorithm in classical conditioning (Gluck *et al.*, 1990; Thompson and Krupa, 1994; Kim *et al.*, 1998).

THE CS PATHWAY

The pontine nuclei send axons directly to the cerebellar cortex and interpositus nucleus (Thompson *et al.*, 1985, 1991; Shinoda *et al.*, 1992; Steinmetz and Sengelaub, 1992; Mihaillof, 1993). The pontine nuclei in turn receive projections from auditory, visual and somatosensory systems (Brodal, 1978; Mower *et al.*, 1979; Glickstein *et al.*, 1980; Tusa and Ungerleider, 1988; Schmahmann and Pandya, 1989, 1991, 1993). Several regions of the pontine nuclei exhibit short latency evoked unit responses to auditory stimuli (Aitkin and Boyd, 1978; Steinmetz *et al.*, 1987). Appropriate lesions of the pontine nuclei can abolish the CR established to a tone CS but not a light CS, i.e. can be selective for CS modality (interpositus lesions abolish the CR to all modalities of CS) (Steinmetz *et al.*, 1987). Lesions of the regions of the pons receiving projections from the auditory cortex abolish the CR established with electrical stimulation of auditory cortex as a CS (Knowlton and Thompson, 1992). Infusion of lidocaine into the pontine nuclei in trained animals reversibly attenuates the CR (tone CS) (Knowlton and Thompson, 1988). Extensive lesions of the middle cerebellar peduncle (mcp), which conveys mossy fibers from the pontine nuclei and other sources to the cerebellum, abolish the CR to all modalities of CS (Solomon *et al.*, 1986a; Lewis *et al.*, 1987).

Electrical stimulation of the pontine nuclei serves as a 'supernormal' CS, yielding more rapid learning than does a tone or light CS (Steinmetz *et al.*, 1986; Tracy, 1995; Tracy *et al.*, 1998). With a pontine stimulation CS, lesion of the middle cerebellar peduncle abolishes the CR, thus ruling out the possibility that the pontine CS is activating non-cerebellar pathways, e.g. by stimulating fibers of passage or antidromic activation of sensory afferents (Solomon *et al.*, 1986a). Stimulation of the middle cerebellar peduncle itself is an effective CS, and lesion of the interpositus nucleus abolishes the CR established with a pontine or middle peduncle stimulation CS (Steinmetz *et al.*, 1986). When animals are trained using electrical stimulation of the pontine nuclei as a CS (corneal airpuff US), some animals show immediate and complete transfer of the behavioral CR and of the learning-induced neural responses in the interpositus nucleus to a tone CS. These results suggest that the pontine stimulus and tone must activate a large number of memory circuit elements (neurons) in common (Steinmetz, 1990). In summary, all evidence is consistent with the view that the pontine nuclei–mossy fibers form the necessary CS pathway for all varieties of peripheral stimuli effective as CSs.

Beginning with the classic work of Snyder (e.g. Snyder *et al.*, 1978), there is an extensive literature on sensory projections to the cerebellum (Ito, 1984). In the present context, our own studies and those from other laboratories demonstrate beyond question that the auditory (and visual) stimuli we use as CSs activate a number of Purkinje neurons in cerebellar cortex and many neurons in the interpositus nucleus in naive animals before any training has been given (Foy *et al.*, 1984, 1992; Foy and Thompson, 1986; Berg and Thompson, 1995; Tracy, 1995). There are extensive auditory and visual projections to neurons in the cerebellar cortex and nuclei. Indeed, we and others have recorded Purkinje and interpositus neurons that show convergence of auditory CS and somatosensory (corneal airpuff) US projections prior to any training (e.g. Thompson, 1990; Krupa *et al.*, 1993; Tracy, 1995).

PURKINJE NEURON ACTIVITY

Many Purkinje neurons, particularly in HVI, are responsive to the tone CS and the corneal airpuff US in naive animals, as noted just above. Before training, many Purkinje neurons that are responsive to the tone CS show variable increases in simple spike frequency (parallel fiber activation) in the CS period. After training, many show learning-induced decreases in simple spike frequency in the CS period; however, a significant number show the opposite effect, and still other patterns of learning-induced responses are found (Donegan *et al.*, 1985; Berthier and Moore, 1986; Foy and Thompson, 1986; Thompson, 1990; Foy *et al.*, 1992; Gould and Steinmetz, 1996). Recently, Hesslow and Ivarsson (1994) recorded from Purkinje neurons in the ferret cerebellum using electrical stimulation of the forelimb as the CS and periorbital shock as the US. They reported that Purkinje neurons responded with weak increases or decreases (simple spike) to CS-alone trials before training. In trained animals, a

number of Purkinje neurons showed decreases, sometimes profound, in simple spike discharges in the CS period. In the rabbit eyeblink conditioning preparation, before training, Purkinje neurons that are influenced by the corneal airpuff consistently show an evoked complex spike to US onset (climbing fiber activation). In trained animals, this US-evoked complex spike is virtually absent on paired CS–US trials when the animal gives a CR, but is present and normal on US-alone test trials (Foy and Thompson, 1986; Thompson, 1990; Krupa *et al.*, 1991; Sears and Steinmetz, 1991) (see US pathway above).

An interesting aspect of classical conditioning of discrete behavioral responses (e.g. eyeblink) is the dramatic and almost linear decrease in the ability to learn (e.g. errors or trials to criterion) as a function of age, documented in an important series of studies by Woodruff-Pak and associates (e.g. Woodruff-Pak and Thompson, 1988; Woodruff-Pak and Jaeger, 1998). Importantly, there is a close correlation between decrease in number of cerebellar Purkinje neurons and increased difficulty in learning (Woodruff-Pak *et al.*, 1990).

CEREBELLAR CORTICAL LESIONS

There is a growing consensus that cortical lesions limited to lobule HVI can impair but not abolish the delay eyeblink CR. It is extremely difficult, however, to completely remove the bottom of the sulcus of HVI without damaging the anterior interpositus, which lies directly underneath. Very large cortical lesions that include the anterior as well as posterior lobes (intermediate and lateral zones) can impair acquisition and retention of the delay CR massively and permanently and in some instances prevent acquisition (see, for example, Yeo *et al.*, 1985b; Lavond *et al.*, 1987, 1993; Lavond and Steinmetz, 1989; Logan, 1991; Yeo, 1991). Importantly, large cortical lesions abolish adaptive timing of the CR (Logan, 1991; Perrett *et al.*, 1993) and prevent acquisition of conditioned inhibition (Logan, 1991). In one study, we explored the possible role of the cerebellar cortex and interpositus in retention of the trace CR (Woodruff-Pak *et al.*, 1985). Interpositus lesions abolished the trace CR. Cortical lesions (posterior lobe) caused a transient decrease but recovery of the CR.

Experimentally, it is virtually impossible to remove the entire cerebellar cortex without damaging the nuclei. In a recent study, we made use of the mutant

Purkinje cell degeneration (pcd) mouse strain (Chen *et al.*, 1996; for a review of genetic approaches to the neurobiology of memory, see Winder and Kandel, Chapter 10). In this mutant, Purkinje neurons (and all other neurons studied) are normal throughout pre- and perinatal development. At about 2–4 weeks post-natal, the Purkinje neurons in the cerebellar cortex degenerate and disappear (Landis and Mullen, 1978). For a period of 2–3 months after this time, other neuronal structures appear relatively normal (Goldowitz and Eisenman, 1992). Thus, during this period of young adulthood, the animals have a complete functional decortication of the cerebellum.

We first showed that appropriate lesions of the interpositus nucleus in the wild-type control mice (normal cerebellum) completely prevented learning of the conditioned eyeblink response, as with all other mammals studied. So the cerebellum is completely necessary for learning. We then trained the pcd mice. They learned very slowly and to a much lower level than the wild-type controls, but showed normal extinction with subsequent training to the CS alone. Thus the cerebellar cortex plays a critically important role in normal learning (of discrete behavioral responses), but some degree of learning is possible without the cerebellar cortex. If the interpositus nucleus is lesioned in pcd mice before training, they are completely unable to learn, thus arguing that the residual memories formed by non-lesioned pcd mice are formed in the interpositus nucleus. The fact that extinction appears normal raises questions about a recent report claiming that lesions of the anterior lobe prevent extinction (Perrett and Mauk, 1995).

IMAGING STUDIES IN CLASSICAL CONDITIONING OF DISCRETE RESPONSES

Ample imaging evidence suggests that an analogous cerebellar locus of classical eyeblink conditioning exists in human subjects, consistent with studies in human cerebellar patients (see above). Following paired presentation of tone CS and airpuff US, several brain regions in human cerebellum, hippocampus and striatum underwent significant changes in glucose metabolism, correlated with level of conditioning (Logan and Grafton, 1995). Molchan *et al.* (1994) examined regional cerebral blood flow (rCBF; see also Dolan, Chapter 17) in each of eight normal humans during three phases: unpaired (binaural) tone and

airpuff to the right eye, paired presentations of tone and airpuff, and tone alone. Blood flow decreased significantly in right cerebellar cortex during paired presentations as compared with the unpaired phase. These changes subsequently were found to correlate with the level of conditioning (Schreurs *et al.*, 1997). Other studies also find changes in ipsilateral or bilateral cerebellum following conditioning, with changes that correlate with learning (Blaxton *et al.*, 1996). Human subjects conditioned with a tone CS and plantar nerve shock US demonstrated elevated rCBF in ipsilateral cerebellum as well as in hippocampus and bilateral frontal cortex (Timmann *et al.*, 1996).

THE LOCUS OF THE LONG-TERM MEMORY TRACE IN EYEBLINK CONDITIONING

Overall, the results described to this point demonstrate conclusively that the cerebellum is necessary for learning, retention and expression of classical conditioning of the eyeblink and other discrete responses (e.g. limb flexion, head turn, etc.). The next and more critical issue concerns the locus of the memory traces. Below, we present evidence which we feel demonstrates conclusively that the long-term memory traces for this type of learning are formed and stored in the cerebellum.

We and our associates have developed a new approach to the problem of localizing memory traces in the brain, namely the use of methods of reversible inactivation, together with recording of neural activity. Reversible inactivation methods (e.g. using drugs or cooling), *per se*, have existed for some time and have been used very effectively to produce temporary lesions (e.g. Mink and Thach, 1991). What we have done is to apply this method systematically to the major structures and pathways in the cerebellar–brainstem circuit, which we have identified as the essential (necessary and sufficient) circuit for classical conditioning of discrete responses (Figure 12.2), during performance and during acquisition of the CR.

A word about methods of inactivation: infusion of a low dose of muscimol (e.g. 0.7 nmol) over a period of 1–2 min inactivates neuron cell bodies (but not axons) for a period of 2–4 h. It activates $GABA_A$ receptors for this long period of time, thus hyperpolarizing the neurons. Lidocaine acts on sodium channels, thus inactivating both cells and fibers. The duration of action is very brief (a few minutes), so it must be infused continuously. Relatively high doses are necessary and the site of effective action can be very localized. Tetanus toxin (TTX) is a much more effective sodium channel blocker and can yield inactivation for a period of hours with a very low dose infused over a minute or two. It also inactivates both cells and fibers. The exact distribution of muscimol in the brain can be determined by the use of radiolabeled (tritiated) muscimol. It is much more difficult to determine the effective distribution of radiolabeled lidocaine since it must be infused continuously. Finally, reversible cooling, as developed by Lavond and associates (see Clark *et al.*, 1992), can inactivate relatively localized regions of brain tissue for a period up to hours and has the advantage that it can be turned on or off in a matter of seconds. The exact region inactivated cannot be determined but can be estimated computationally and/or with neuronal recording.

As noted above, the diagram of Figure 12.2 shows in highly simplified schematic form the essential memory trace circuit for classical conditioning of discrete responses, based on the lesion, recording and stimulation evidence described above. Interneuron circuits are not shown, only net excitatory or inhibitory actions of projection pathways. Other pathways, known and unknown, may also of course be involved. Many uncertainties still exist, e.g. concerning details of sensory-specific patterns of projection to pontine nuclei and cerebellum (CS pathways), details of red nucleus projections to premotor and motor nuclei (CR pathway) and the possible roles of recurrent circuits.

Several parts of the circuit have been inactivated reversibly for the duration of training (eyeblink conditioning) in naive animals, indicated by shadings labeled a, b, c, d and encircled e in Figure 12.2. The motor nuclei essential for generating the UR and CR (primarily 7th and accessory 6th and adjacent neural tissues; a in Figure 12.2) were inactivated by infusion of muscimol (6 days) or cooling (5 days) during standard tone–airpuff training (Zhang and Lavond, 1991; Thompson *et al.*, 1993; Krupa *et al.*, 1996). The animals showed no CRs and no URs during this inactivation training; indeed, performance was completely abolished. The region of inactivation in the brainstem with muscimol was quite large, including the facial (7th) nucleus, the accessory abducens nucleus and an extensive surrounding region of reticular formation. The motor paralysis on the side of infusion was complete—the external eyelids were flaccid, the left ear hung down and no vibrissae movements occurred—

and lasted at least 3 h, followed by full recovery. [importantly, when the animals were unrestrained, airpuff to the paralyzed (trained) eye caused the animal to jerk its head away, showing that sensory processing of the US occurred]. However, the animals exhibited asymptotic CR performance and normal UR performance from the very beginning of post-inactivation training. Thus, performance of the CR and UR are completely unnecessary for normal learning, and the motor nuclei and adjacent inactivated tissue make no contribution at all to formation of the memory trace—they are completely efferent from the trace.

Inactivation of the magnocellular red nucleus is indicated by b in Figure 12.2. Inactivation by low doses of muscimol for 6 days of training had no effect on the UR but completely prevented expression of the CR (Krupa *et al.*, 1993). Yet animals showed asymptotic learned performance of the CR from the beginning of post-inactivation training. Training during cooling of the magnocellular red nucleus gave identical results—animals learned during cooling, as evidenced in post-inactivation training, but did not express CRs at all during inactivation training (Clark and Lavond, 1993). Consequently, the red nucleus must be efferent from the memory trace.

Inactivation of the dorsal anterior interpositus and overlying cortex (c in Figure 12.2) by low doses of muscimol (6 days), by lidocaine (3 and 6 days) and by cooling (5 days) resulted in no expression of CRs during inactivation training and no evidence of any learning at all having occurred during inactivation training (Clark *et al.*, 1992; Krupa *et al.*, 1993; Nordholm *et al.*, 1993; Hardiman *et al.*, 1996). In subsequent post-inactivation training, animals learned normally as though completely naive; they showed no savings at all relative to non-inactivated control animals. None of the methods of inactivation had any effect at all on performance of the UR on US alone trials. The distribution of [³H]muscimol completely effective in preventing learning in Krupa *et al.* (1993) included the anterior dorsal interpositus and overlying cortex of lobule HVI, a volume approximately 2% of the total volume of the cerebellum. In a more recent study, [³H]muscimol limited to just the anterior interpositus nucleus was also completely effective in preventing learning (Krupa and Thompson, 1997) (see Figure 12.3).

Finally, we infused TTX in the superior cerebellar peduncle (scp) ipsilateral to the critical cerebellar hemisphere before any significant numbers of axons

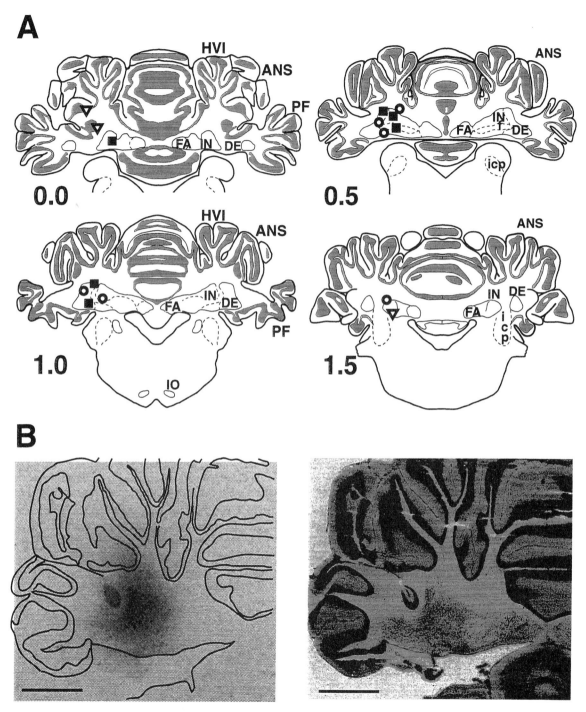

Figure 12.3. Muscimol infusion sites in the cerebellar interpositus nucleus. Effective muscimol infusions completely prevented learning as the subjects were trained for five sessions. (**A**) Cannula locations for each rabbit in coronal sections. ((■) Effective muscimol infusion sites; (O) controls; ((▽) ineffective muscimol infusion sites. ANS, ansiform cortex; DE, dentate nucleus; FA, fastigial nucleus; HVI, hemispheric lobule VI; icp, inferior cerebellar peduncle; IN, interpositus nucleus; IO, inferior olive; PF, paraflocculus. Numbers 0.0–1.5 below and to the left of each section indicate distance (mm) rostral of the lambdoidal suture. (**B**) Maximum extent of infusion, measured by autoradiography following ³H-labeled muscimol infusion. On the left is the auto-radiograph with a superimposed outline drawn from the Nissl-stained section from which it was exposed (right). Diffusion is limited to interpositus and dentate nuclei, with little diffusion into cortex and no evidence of diffusion outside of the cerebellum (from Krupa and Thompson, 1997, with permission).

exited the scp (e in Figure 12.2). This inactivates both descending and ascending efferent projections of the cerebellar hemisphere. The animals exhibited motor symptoms consistent with this effect. TTX infusion in the scp completely prevented expression of the CR (with no effect on the UR) for the 6 days of training. On the seventh day, TTX was not infused and the animals showed asymptotic learned performance of the CR. Control animals were infused with TTX in the scp for 6 days but not trained, and then were trained, and showed normal learning.

Collectively, these data strongly support the hypothesis that the memory trace is formed and stored in a localized region of the cerebellum (anterior interpositus and overlying cortex). Indeed, we can conceive of no rational alternative. Inactivation of this region (c) during training completely prevents learning, but inactivation of the output pathway from the region (d and e) and its necessary (for the CR) efferent target, the red nucleus (b), does not prevent learning at all. In no case do the drug inactivations have any effect at all on performance of the reflex response on US-alone trials. If even a part of the essential memory trace were formed prior to the cerebellum in the essential circuit, then, following cerebellar inactivation training, the animals would have to show savings, and they show none at all. Similarly, if a part of the essential memory trace were formed in the red nucleus or other efferent targets of the interpositus (e.g. brainstem), then, following red nucleus (b), interpositus efferent (d) or scp (e) inactivation training, animals could not show asymptotic CR performance, but they do.

LEARNED ARM MOVEMENTS

William Thach and colleagues at Washington University have investigated the role of the cerebellum in trained arm movements in monkeys. In a task involving learned adaptation of wrist movement to a mechanically induced perturbation, Purkinje cells frequently produced complex spikes following a load change that causes motor error; this complex spike error signal disappeared after readaptation to the new load (Gilbert and Thach, 1977), just as complex spikes evoked by an airpuff US disappear as the CR develops. The same cells displayed a decrease in simple spike activity, again analogous to the changes observed in conditioning. Subsequent studies concluded that cerebellar measures are correlated less

with kinematic parameters of single-jointed movement but rather with smooth execution of learned multijoint movements (Thach *et al.*, 1992).

When glasses containing wedge prisms are placed over a subject's eyes, the subject's visual world is displaced to one side according to the alignment of the prism. When the subject subsequently throws a ball or dart at a target, their aim is off in the same direction, and over the course of 10–30 trials their aim improves until they can once again hit the target (Martin *et al.*, 1996b). When the prism glasses are removed, aim is perturbed in the opposite direction and adaptation begins again ('negative after-effect'). Thach *et al.* (1992) stress that coordination between visual and arm trajectory is a learned skill, and much evidence suggests that corresponding synaptic changes take place in the cerebellum. Prism adaptation is abolished following cerebellar lesions in macaques (Baizer and Glickstein, 1974) and cerebellar disease in humans (Weiner *et al.*, 1983; Martin *et al.*, 1996a).

Keating and Thach (1990) introduced a paradigm similar to prism adaptation and more conducive to an animal study: monkeys were trained to move a lever to align a cursor with a target on a screen. When the experimenter altered the gain of the lever (the ratio of observed cursor movement to lever displacement), the subject had to adapt wrist movements to compensate, over time developing a new 'muscle synergy'. During adaptation, transitory, co-varying changes in both simple and complex spikes were observed; following adaptation, a persistent change in simple spike rates was seen. These changes in Purkinje cell firing rates paralleled those seen in the 1977 study and in a study of adaptation of the vestibulo-ocular reflex (VOR; Watanabe, 1984).

CEREBELLAR DEPENDENCE IN A BUTTON-PRESSING TASK IN MONKEYS

In a series of studies that explored the role of basal ganglia, frontal cortex and cerebellum in skill learning, Okihide Hikosaka's group at Juntendo University trained monkeys in a button-pressing task and observed the effect of brain lesions over the course of learning (for a review, see Hikosaka *et al.*, 1998). Each subject was presented with a 16-button panel (4×4 grid) with another button below these (the 'home' key). When the monkey pressed the home key, two of 16 of the buttons would light simultaneously. The monkey was required to press both keys in the proper sequence (which he could only determine by trial and error). This sequence pair constituted a 'set'; the monkey had to complete five sets (= one 'hyperset') for a fluid reward. A hyperset was repeated until the monkey successfully completed it 10 times. Each repetition of a hyperset is called a trial; usually the subject could obtain a nearly perfect score by trial 10 on the first day (~3 min of training). A given hyperset (i.e. a unique 2×5 sequence) was considered well learned when the monkey made no errors and performance time was nearly minimal (performance time tended to decrease over several days or weeks of training on the same hyperset). Most monkeys over the course of the experiment learned about 20 different hypersets to criterion, with about half the sets learned and tested on the right hand and half on the left.

The effects of muscimol inactivation of supplementary motor area (SMA), pre-SMA, caudate, putamen and cerebellar dentate (DN) on retention of new (randomly generated following the inactivation) and learned hypersets (chosen from those well learned prior to inactivation) were examined in a series of studies. Inactivation of pre-SMA (and, to a lesser extent, SMA) resulted in a significant increase in the number of errors on new hypersets, with negligible change in performance of learned hypersets (Miyashita *et al.*, 1996; Hikosaka *et al.*, 1998). Inactivation of the anterior caudate and putamen impaired recall of new hypersets, while injections in the middle or posterior putamen significantly increased the error count for learned hypersets (Miyachi *et al.*, 1997).

This suggests that different regions of the telencephalon are involved in learning or recalling new versus very well learned motor sequences. Striking results were found when this paradigm was applied to the cerebellum (Lu *et al.*, 1998). Two monkeys were trained until they had learned a repertoire of hypersets (*n* = 21 and 12, respectively), and two recording/injection cannulae were directed into the dentate nucleus (one cannula into each hemisphere). Following injection of muscimol to inactivate the dentate–interpositus, monkeys were tested on both new and very well learned hypersets. In both monkeys, the number of errors significantly increased (more than tripled) for learned hypersets, with no impairment at all on new hypersets. The muscimol effect was limited to the ipsilateral hand. This is in agreement with other cerebellar learning studies and with the anatomical literature indicating that afferent sensory information crosses the midline twice before reaching the cerebellum, as do cerebellar output pathways (see Figure 12.1), so that cerebellar activity in one hemisphere is expected primarily to influence motor behavior on the ipsilateral side. Finally, the effect of the drug was dependent on injection location in the nucleus: of four injection sites in one animal spanning the dorsoventral extent of the DN, and three injection sites in the second animal, the increase in error count was limited to injections in the dorsal region. An increase in movement time was also observed, especially among injections in the ventral dentate. This suggests that 'engrams' corresponding to well-learned movement sequences of this type are stored in the ipsilateral cerebellum, but that initial learning involves other brain structures as well.

Several other behavioral observations provide corroborating evidence that the well-learned hypersets are expressed (and therefore stored) as a motor skill (procedural memory), as distinct from storage of a 2 × 5 sequence alone (declarative memory). Several features distinguish skill learning: while declarative memory can be acquired in a single trial, procedural memory requires many trials to criterion, with gradually improving performance over time, as in this task. Performance speed and timing also improve over time. In classical conditioning, the CR becomes progressively more precisely timed over the course of training, eventually stabilizing such that the peak CR occurs precisely at the onset of the US; this timing is disrupted following cerebellar cortical lesions (Perrett *et al.*, 1993) and in Purkinje cell degeneration (pcd) mice trained in the delay eyeblink task (Chen *et al.*, 1996). Execution time in the 2×5 task decreased over training and continued to improve even after 30 days of training (Hikosaka *et al.*, 1998), and was disrupted following inactivation of the ventral dentate (Lu *et al.*, 1998). Intact monkeys learned their hypersets so well that it became difficult to follow their rapid finger movements recorded on videotape (Hikosaka, 1997). Lastly, learned skilled movements can be recalled for a long time after the conclusion of training; following a 6-month rest period, performance on learned hypersets was 'nearly perfect' (Hikosaka *et al.*, 1998).

These results led these researchers to conclude that different brain regions are involved in the storage and recall of new and well-learned sequences: during early learning, prefrontal cortex, pre-SMA and anterior caudoputamen are critical, while well-learned motor sequences come to be stored in the cerebellum to provide for rapid execution of the sequence as in procedural (skill) learning.

OTHER TYPES OF SKILL LEARNING

There are other types of skill learning, and skilled aspects of learning that appear to involve the cerebellum. Petrosini and Molinari found that hemicerebellectomized rats were impaired in the procedural aspects of maze performance (in terms of restricted spatial search strategies) but not in the declarative aspects, i.e. where the target was located (Petrosini *et al.*, 1996; Molinari *et al.*, 1997a,b; Petrosini *et al.*, 1998). Cerebellectomized rats were also found to be impaired in an open-field search task tested 10 days after initial training. The researchers 'concluded that the cerebellum is not absolutely necessary in the processes that sustain spatial learning but that it is involved in the mechanisms sustaining focused spatial memory and in the cognitive processes of the motor program elaboration and not only in the regulation of the movement being done' (Dahhaoui *et al.*, 1992).

Seitz *et al.* (1990) measured regional blood flow with positron emission tomography (PET; see also Dolan, Chapter 17) while subjects learned a complicated finger sequence of voluntary movements. Motor learning was accompanied by blood flow increases in the cerebellum, decreases in all limbic and paralimbic structures, and striatal decreases that changed to increases as the skill was learned. The authors argue that both cerebellar circuits and striatal circuits are important for the storage of motor skills.

In an unusual skill-learning task, a robot arm was used to provide a programmed set of disturbances (a 'virtual mechanical environment') that human subjects had to learn to counter while holding the robot manipulandum. The results suggested that learning of this task is dependent on corticostriatal circuitry during the early phase of learning, with changes over the course of learning implying an increased dependence on the corticocerebellar loop (Krebs *et al.*, 1998).

While subjects learned a similar tongue robot arm motor task, PET activity was most significant in prefrontal cortex. Six hours after practice and while recalling the learned task, PET activity shifted to premotor and posterior parietal cortices and to cerebellar cortex (Shadmehr and Holcomb, 1997).

Subjects required to learn a visuomotor sequence (implicitly) which contained an embedded sequence that the subjects eventually detected (explicit component) demonstrated an increased rCBF signal in right striatum and cerebellar dentate nucleus (Doyon *et al.*, 1996) following procedural learning of the task. After the subjects detected (made explicit) the embedded sequence, only changes in right mid-ventrolateral frontal cortex were significant, suggesting a transfer from use of the cerebellar-dependent procedural memory to more declarative recall involving frontal cortex. Over the course of learning a task involving complex finger movements, rCBF increases were observed in the cerebellum and striatum (Seitz *et al.*, 1990).

In a variety of motor learning paradigms, the cerebellum has been established as necessary for learning, with neurophysiological measures correlated with changes in learning, in both animals and humans. The common theme among these forms of learning are the spatial and temporal precision of their execution, and the slow development of this skill over practice and the probable role of the cerebellum in long-term storage of these motor memory traces.

MECHANISMS OF MEMORY STORAGE IN THE CEREBELLUM

The localization of memory traces for classical conditioning of discrete responses (learned with aversive USs) to the cerebellum is now sufficiently established that a focus on cerebellar cellular mechanisms of plasticity is warranted. Indeed, since much of the essential circuitry has been identified, this system may provide the first instance in the mammalian brain where the entire circuitry from memory trace to learned behavior, the 'read out' of memory, and the neuronal content of the memory store can be analyzed (Thompson and Krupa, 1994). Similar progress has been made for imprinting in the avian brain (Horn, 1985; see also Horn, Chapter 19).

Many of the Purkinje neurons exhibiting learning-related changes show decreases in simple spike responses in the CS period. This would result in disinhibition of interpositus neurons, consistent with a mechanism of long-term depression (LTD) at the parallel fiber–Purkinje cell synapse. Current evidence suggests that glutamate activation of α-amino-3-hydroxy-5-methyl-4-isoxazole proprionic acid (AMPA) and metabotropic receptors together with increased intracellular calcium (normally by climbing fiber activation) yields the persisting decrease in AMPA receptor function of LTD (see below and Ito and Karachot, 1990; Linden and Connor, 1991, 1995). LTD has been proposed as the mechanism underlying synaptic plasticity in the flocculus that subserves adaptation of the VOR (e.g. Ito, 1989).

Thus, iontophoretic application of L-glutamate in place of parallel fiber stimulation caused a similar depression of glutamate sensitivity. When kynurenate, a glutamate receptor antagonist, was co-applied, the depression did not occur, confirming that glutamate or a glutamate agonist are necessary for LTD induction and expression (Kano *et al.*, 1988). Quisqualate, but not kainate or aspartate, applied with climbing fiber stimulation also leads to LTD, implying that one or both quisqualate subtypes (AMPA and/or mGlu) of glutamate receptor is the receptor involved at the parallel fiber synapse (Kano and Kato, 1988). Linden and Connor (1991) found that application of AMPA instead of quisqualate in conjunction with depolarization was insufficient to induce LTD; likewise, application of a selective mGluR antagonist blocked quisqualate-induced LTD. Therefore, both the AMPA and metabotropic glutamate receptors are necessary for the induction of LTD. This study also concluded that actual depolarization of the Purkinje cell is necessary for induction: voltage-clamped Purkinje cells would not undergo LTD. Inhibitors of protein kinase C (PKC) blocked the induction of LTD, and application of an activator of PKC was sufficient to induce LTD-like responses.

Intracellular calcium is implicated in the chain of events leading from climbing fiber–parallel fiber co-stimulation to LTD. Injection of EGTA (a calcium chelator) into Purkinje dendrites in a cerebellar slice prevented induction of LTD (Sakurai, 1990). Likewise, LTD could not be induced in mouse cerebellar cultures incubated in EGTA (Linden and Connor, 1991).

Recent studies using 'gene knockout' preparations (see also Winder and Kandel, Chapter 10) have strengthened the argument for LTD as a key mechanism of memory storage in cerebellar cortex. Thus, mice that lack the metabotropic glutamate receptor (mGluR1) show marked impairments in cerebellar cortical LTD and eyeblink conditioning (Aiba *et al.*, 1994). They also show generalized motor impairments, i.e. some degree of ataxia, as do the pcd mice (see above). Interestingly, current studies present evidence supporting the view that LTD is more important for learning (eyeblink conditioning) than for motor coordination. Thus, using the protein kinase Cγ (PKCγ) knockout mutant mouse, Kano *et al.* (1995) showed that the Purkinje neurons in adult animals maintained the perinatal condition of more than one climbing fiber per neuron (wild-type adults have only one climbing fiber per Purkinje neuron). Chen *et al.*

(1995) showed that this mutant exhibited normal LTD but impaired motor coordination (due, presumably, to the multiple climbing fiber innervation of Purkinje neurons). In striking contrast, these animals learned the conditioned eyeblink response more rapidly than did the wild-type controls!

Just the opposite result holds for a quite different mutant, namely the glial fibrillary acidic protein (GFAP) knockout mouse (Shibuki *et al.*, 1996) in which the cerebellar cortex appears to be anatomically normal. Cerebellar cortical LTD and eyeblink conditioning are markedly deficient in these animals (their performance is very similar to that of the pcd mice) but they do not show any impairments at all in motor coordination or general motor behavior!

The Shibuki *et al.* (1996) study is also important in another regard. GFAP is not present in neurons, only in glial cells. In the cerebellum, it is normally present in substantial amounts in the Bergmann glia that surround the parallel fiber and climbing fiber–Purkinje neuron dendrite synapses. Although the Bergmann glia appear morphologically normal in the GFAP knockout, they have no GFAP. Thus an abnormality limited to glial cells markedly impairs a form of synaptic plasticity (LTD) and a form of basic associative learning and memory. This may be the first direct evidence for a key role of glia in processes of learning and memory.

Several lines of evidence therefore support the hypothesis that a process of LTD in cerebellar cortex is a mechanism involved in memory storage in classical conditioning of discrete behavioral responses. Similarly, several lines of evidence support such a role for cerebellar cortical LTD in adaptation of the VOR (for detailed discussions, see above and Ito, 1984). However, the fact that some degree of learning occurs in the pcd mouse (see above), a preparation that functionally has a complete cerebellar decortication, argues that some degree of plasticity must occur in the interpositus nucleus. There is just one paper in the literature (Racine *et al.*, 1986) reporting that tetanus of the white matter yields long-term potentiation (LTP) in the interpositus nucleus. Much work remains to be done exploring possible mechanisms of plasticity and memory storage in the cerebellum. The fact that GABA agonists and antagonists infused in the cerebellum have such profound effects on the conditioned response (Mamounas *et al.*, 1987; Krupa *et al.*, 1993; Ramirez *et al.*, 1997) at least raises the possibility that GABAergic processes may be involved in cerebellar memory storage.

ACKNOWLEDGEMENTS

Supported by NSF (IBN-9215069), NIH (AG05142), NIMH (5P01-MH52194), ONR (N00014-95-1-1152) and Sankyo Co., Ltd.

REFERENCES

Aiba, A., Kano, M., Chen, C., Stanton, M.E., Fox, G.D., Herrup, K., Zwingman, T.A. and Tonegawa, S. (1994) Deficient cerebellar long-term depression and impaired motor learning in mGluR1 mutant mice. *Cell*, 79, 377–388.

Aitkin, L.M. and Boyd, J. (1978) Acoustic input to the lateral pontine nuclei. *Hearing Research*, 1, 67–77.

Albus, J.S. (1971) A theory of cerebellar function. *Mathematical Bioscience*, 10, 25–61.

Baizer, J.S. and Glickstein, M. (1974) Proceedings: role of cerebellum in prism adaptation. *Journal of Physiology (London)*, 236, 34P–35P.

Berg, M. and Thompson, R.F. (1995) Neural responses of the cerebellar deep nuclei in the naive and well trained rabbit following NM conditioning. *Society for Neuroscience Abstracts*, 21, 1221.

Berthier, N.E. and Moore, J.W. (1986) Cerebellar Purkinje cell activity related to the classical conditioned nictitating membrane response. *Experimental Brain Research*, 63, 341–350.

Berthier, N.E. and Moore, J.W. (1990) Activity of deep cerebellar nuclear cells during classical conditioning of nictitating membrane extension in rabbits. *Experimental Brain Research*, 83, 44–54.

Blaxton, T.A., Zeffiro, T.A., Gabrieli, J.D., Bookheimer, S.Y., Carrillo, M.C., Theodore, W.H. and Disterhoft, J.F. (1996) Functional mapping of human learning: a positron emission tomography activation study of eyeblink conditioning. *Journal of Neuroscience*, 16, 4032–4040.

Brodal, P. (1978) The corticopontine projection in the rhesus monkey. Origin and principles of organization. *Brain*, 101, 251–283.

Chapman, P.F., Steinmetz, J.E. and Thompson, R.F. (1988) Classical conditioning does not occur when direct stimulation of the red nucleus or cerebellar nuclei is the unconditioned stimulus. *Brain Research*, 442, 97–104.

Chapman, P.F., Steinmetz, J.E., Sears, L.L. and Thompson, R.F. (1990) Effects of lidocaine injection in the interpositus nucleus and red nucleus on conditioned behavioral and neuronal responses. *Brain Research*, 537, 149–156.

Chen, C. and Thompson, R.F. (1995) Temporal specificity of long-term depression in parallel fiber–Purkinje synapses in rat cerebellar slice. *Learning and Memory*, 2, 185–198.

Chen, C., Masanobu, K., Abeliovich, A., Chen, L., Bao, S., Kim, J.J., Hashimoto, K., Thompson, R.F. and Tonegawa, S. (1995) Impaired motor coordination correlates with persistent multiple climbing fiber innervation in PKCγ mutant mice. *Cell*, 83, 1233–1242.

Chen, L., Bao, S., Lockard, J.M., Kim, J.K. and Thompson, R.F. (1996) Impaired classical eyeblink conditioning in cerebellar-lesioned and Purkinje cell degeneration (pcd) mutant mice. *Journal of Neuroscience*, 16, 2829–2838.

Clark, R.E. and Lavond, D.G. (1993) Reversible lesions of the red nucleus during acquisition and retention of a classically conditioned behavior in rabbits. *Behavioral Neuroscience*, 107, 264–270.

Clark, R.E., Zhang, A.A. and Lavond, D.G. (1992) Reversible lesions of the cerebellar interpositus nucleus during acquisition and retention of a classically conditioned behavior. *Behavioral Neuroscience*, 106, 879–888.

Dahhaoui, M., Lannou, J., Stelz, T., Caston, J. and Guastavino, J.M. (1992) Role of the cerebellum in spatial orientation in the rat. *Behavioral and Neural Biology*, 58, 180–189.

Daum, I., Schugens, M.M., Ackermann, H., Lutzenberger, W., Dichgans, J. and Birbaumer, N. (1993) Classical conditioning after cerebellar lesions in humans. *Behavioral Neuroscience*, 107, 748–756.

Donegan, N.H., Foy, M.R. and Thompson, R.F. (1985) Neuronal responses of the rabbit cerebellar cortex during performance of the classically conditioned eyelid response. *Society for Neuroscience Abstracts*, 11, 835.

Doyon, J., Owen, A.M., Petrides, M., Sziklas, V. and Evans, A.C. (1996) Functional anatomy of visuomotor skill learning in human subjects examined with positron emission tomography. *European Journal of Neuroscience*, 8, 637–648.

Du Lac, S., Raymond, J.L., Sejnowski, T.J. and Lisberger, S. (1995) Learning and memory in the vestibulo-ocular reflex. *Annual Review of Neuroscience*, 18, 409–441.

Eccles, J.C. (1977) An instruction–selection theory of learning in the cerebellar cortex. *Brain Research*, 127, 327–352.

Foy, M.R. and Thompson, R.F. (1986) Single unit analysis of Purkinje cell discharge in classically conditioned and untrained rabbits. *Society for Neuroscience Abstracts*, 10, 122.

Foy, M.R., Steinmetz, J.E. and Thompson, R.F. (1984) Single unit analysis of cerebellum during classically conditioned eyelid response. *Society for Neuroscience Abstracts*, 12, 518.

Foy, M.R., Krupa, D.J., Tracy, J. and Thompson, R.F. (1992) Analysis of single unit recordings from cerebellar cortex of classically conditioned rabbits. *Society for Neuroscience Abstracts*, 18, 1215.

Gilbert, P.F. and Thach, W.T. (1977) Purkinje cell activity during motor learning. *Brain Research*, 128, 309–328.

Glickstein, M., Cohen, J.L., Dixon, B., Gibson, A., Hollins, M., Labossiere, E. and Robinson, F. (1980) Corticopontine visual projections in macaque monkeys. *Journal of Comparative Neurology*, 190, 209–229.

Gluck, M.A., Reifsnider, E.S. and Thompson, R.F. (1990) Adaptive signal processing and the cerebellum: models of classical conditioning and VOR adaptation. In: Gluck, M.A. and Rumelhart, D.E. (eds), *Neuroscience and Connectionist Models*. Lawrence Erlbaum Associates, Hillsdale, New Jersey, pp. 131–185.

Goldowitz, D. and Eisenman, L.M. (1992) Genetic mutations affecting murine cerebellar structure and function. In: Driscoll, P. (ed.), *Genetically Defined Animal Models of Neurobehavioral Dysfunctions*. Birkhauser, Boston, pp. 66–88.

Gormezano, I., Kehoe, E.J. and Marshall, B.S. (1983) Twenty years of classical conditioning with the rabbit. *Progress in Psychobiology and Physiological Psychology*, 10, 197–275.

Gould, T.J. and Steinmetz, J.E. (1996) Changes in rabbit cerebellar cortical and interpositus nucleus activity during acquisition, extinction, and backward classical eyelid conditioning. *Neurobiology of Learning and Memory*, 65, 17–34.

Haley, D.A., Thompson, R.F. and Madden, J., IV (1988) Pharmacological analysis of the magnocellular red nucleus during classical conditioning of the rabbit nictitating membrane response. *Brain Research*, 454, 131–139.

Hardiman, M.J., Ramnani, N. and Yeo, C.H. (1996) Reversible inactivations of the cerebellum with muscimol prevent the acquisition and extinction of conditioned nictitating membrane responses in the rabbit. *Experimental Brain Research*, 110, 235–247.

Hesslow, G. and Ivarsson, M. (1994) Suppression of cerebellar Purkinje cells during conditioned responses in ferrets. *NeuroReport*, 5, 649–652.

Hikosaka, O. (1997) Differential roles of the frontal cortex, basal ganglia, and cerebellum in visuo-motor sequence learning. In: *Center for the Neurobiology of Learning and Memory: Annual Fall Conference*: University of California at Irvine.

Hikosaka, O., Miyashita, K., Miyachi, S., Sakai, K. and Lu, X. (1998) Differential roles of the frontal cortex, basal ganglia, and cerebellum in visuomotor sequence learning. *Neurobiology of Learning and Memory*, 70, 137–149.

Horn, G. (1985) *Memory, Imprinting and the Brain*. Clarendon Press, Oxford.

Ito, M. (1984) *The Cerebellum and Neural Control*. Appleton Century-Crofts, New York.

Ito, M. (1989) Long-term depression. *Annual Review of Neuroscience*, 12, 85–102.

Ito, M. (1993) Cerebellar mechanisms of long-term depression. In: Baudry, M., Davis, J.L. and Thompson, R.F. (eds), *Synaptic Plasticity: Molecular and Functional Aspects*. MIT Press, Cambridge, Massachusetts, pp. 117–146.

Ito, M. and Karachot, L. (1990) Messenger mediating long-term desensitization in cerebellar Purkinje cells. *NeuroReport*, 1, 129–132.

Ivkovich, D., Lockard, J.M. and Thompson, R.F. (1993) Interpositus lesion abolition of the eyeblink CR is not due to effects on performance. *Behavioral Neuroscience*, 107, 530–532.

Kano, K. and Kato, M. (1988) Mode of induction of long-term depression at parallel fibre–Purkinje cell synapses in rabbit cerebellar cortex. *Neuroscience Research*, 5, 544–556.

Kano, M., Kato, M. and Chang, H.S. (1988) The glutamate receptor subtype mediating parallel fibre–Purkinje cell transmission in rabbit cerebellar cortex. *Neuroscience Research*, 5, 325–337.

Kano, M., Hashimoto, K., Chen, C., Abeliovich, A., Aiba, A., Kurihara, H., Watanabe, M., Inoue, Y. and Tonegawa, S. (1995) Impaired synapse elimination during cerebellar development in PKCγ mutant mice. *Cell*, 83, 1223–1231.

Keating, J.G. and Thach, W.T. (1990) Cerebellar motor learning: quantitation of movement adaptation and performance in rhesus monkeys and humans implicates cortex as the site of adaptation. *Society for Neuroscience Abstracts*, 16, 762.

Kim, J.J. and Thompson, R.F. (1997) Cerebellar circuits and synaptic mechanisms involved in classical eyeblink conditioning. *Trends in Neurosciences*, 20, 177–181.

Kim, J.J., Clark, R.E. and Thompson, R.F. (1995) Hippocampectomy impairs the memory of recently, but not remotely, acquired trace eyeblink conditioned responses. *Behavioral Neuroscience*, 109, 195–203.

Kim, J.J., Krupa, D.J. and Thompson, R.F. (1998) Inhibitory cerebello-olivary projections mediate the 'blocking' effect in classical conditioning. *Science*, 279, 570–573.

Knowlton, B., and Thompson, R.F. (1988) Microinjections of local anesthetic into the pontine nuclei reduce the amplitude of the classically conditioned eyeblink response. *Physiology and Behavior*, 43, 855–857.

Knowlton, B.J. and Thompson, R.F. (1992) Conditioning using a cerebral cortical conditioned stimulus is dependent on the cerebellum and brain stem circuitry. *Behavioral Neuroscience*, 106, 509–517.

Krebs, H.I., Brashers-Krug, T., Rauch, S.L., Savage, C.R., Hogan, N., Rubin, R.H., Fischman, A.J. and Alpert, N.M. (1998) Robot-aided functional imaging: application to a motor learning study. *Human Brain Mapping*, 6, 59–72.

Krupa, D.J. and Thompson, R.F. (1997) Reversible inactivation of the cerebellar interpositus nucleus completely prevents acquisition of the classically conditioned eyeblink response. *Learning and Memory*, 3, 545–556.

Krupa, D.J., Weiss, C. and Thompson, R.F. (1991) Air puff evoked Purkinje cell complex spike activity is diminished during conditioned responses in eyeblink conditioned rabbits. *Society for Neuroscience Abstracts*, 17, 322.

Krupa, D.J., Thompson, J.K. and Thompson, R.F. (1993) Localization of a memory trace in the mammalian brain. *Science*, 260, 989–991.

Krupa, D.J., Weng, J. and Thompson, R.F. (1996) Inactivation of brainstem motor nuclei blocks expression but not acquisition of the rabbit's classically conditioned eyeblink response. *Behavioral Neuroscience*, 110, 1–9.

Landis, S.C. and Mullen, R.J. (1978) The development and degeneration of Purkinje cells in pcd mutant mice. *Journal of Comparative Neurology*, 177, 125–144.

Lavond, D.G. and Steinmetz, J.E. (1989) Acquisition of classical conditioning without cerebellar cortex. *Behavioral Brain Research*, 33, 113–164.

Lavond, D.G., Steinmetz, J.E., Yokaitis, M.H. and Thompson, R.F. (1987) Reacquisition of classical conditioning after removal of cerebellar cortex. *Experimental Brain Research*, 67, 569–593.

Lavond, D.G., Kim, J J. and Thompson, R.F. (1993) Mammalian brain substrates of aversive classical conditioning. *Annual Review of Psychology*, 44, 317–42.

Lewis, J.L., Lo Turco, J.J. and Solomon, P.R. (1987) Lesions of the middle cerebellar peduncle disrupt acquisition and retention of the rabbit's classically conditioned nictitating membrane response. *Behavioral Neuroscience*, 101, 151–157.

Linden, D.J. and Connor, J.A. (1991) Participation of postsynaptic PKC in cerebellar long-term depression in culture. *Science*, 254, 656–1659.

Linden, D.J. and Connor, J.A. (1995) Long-term synaptic depression. *Annual Review of Neuroscience*, 18, 319–357.

Logan, C.G. (1991) *Cerebellar Cortical Involvement in Excitatory and Inhibitory Classical Conditioning*. Stanford University Press, California.

Logan, C.G. and Grafton, S.T. (1995) Functional anatomy of human eyeblink conditioning determined with regional cerebral glucose metabolism and positron-emission tomography. *Proceedings of the National Academy of Sciences of the United States of America*, 92, 7500–7504.

Lu, X., Hikosaka, O. and Miyachi, S. (1998) Role of monkey cerebellar nuclei in skill for sequential movement. *Journal of Neurophysiology*, 79, 2245–2254.

Lye, R.H., O'Boyle, D.J., Ramsden, R.T. and Schady, W. (1988) Effects of a unilateral cerebellar lesion on the acquisition of eye-blink conditioning in man. *Journal of Physiology (London)*, 403, 58P.

Mamounas, L.A., Thompson, R.F. and Madden, J., IV (1987) Cerebellar GABAergic processes: evidence for critical involvement in a form of simple associative learning in the rabbit. *Proceedings of the National Academy of Sciences of the United States of America*, 84, 2101–2105.

Marr, D. (1969) A theory of cerebellar cortex. *Journal of Physiology*, 202, 437–470.

Martin, T.A., Keating, J.G., Goodkin, H.P., Bastian, A.J. and Thach, W.T. (1996a) Throwing while looking through prisms. I. Focal olivocerebellar lesions impair adaptation. *Brain*, 119, 1183–1198.

Martin, T.A., Keating, J.G., Goodkin, H.P., Bastian, A.J. and Thach, W.T. (1996b) Throwing while looking through prisms. II. Specificity and storage of multiple gaze–throw calibrations. *Brain*, 119, 1199–1211.

Mauk, M.D., Steinmetz, J.E. and Thompson, R.F. (1986) Classical conditioning using stimulation of the inferior olive as the unconditioned stimulus. *Proceedings of the National Academy of Sciences of the United States of America*, 83, 5349–5353.

McCormick, D.A. and Thompson, R.F. (1984a) Cerebellum: essential involvement in the classically conditioned eyelid response. *Science*, 223, 296–299.

McCormick, D.A. and Thompson, R.F. (1984b) Neuronal responses for the rabbit cerebellum during acquisition and performance of a classically conditioned nictitating membrane eyelid response. *Journal of Neuroscience*, 4, 2811–2822.

McCormick, D.A., Clark, G.A., Lavond, D.G. and Thompson, R.F. (1982a) Initial localization of the memory trace for a basic form of learning. *Proceedings of the National Academy of Sciences of the United States of America*, 79, 2731–2742.

McCormick, D.A., Guyer, P.E. and Thompson, R.F. (1982b) Superior cerebellar peduncle lesions selectively abolish the ipsilateral classically conditioned nictitating membrane/eyelid response of the rabbit. *Brain Research*, 244, 347–350.

McCormick, D.A. Steinmetz, J.E. and Thompson, R.F. (1985) Lesions of the inferior olivary complex cause extinction of the classically conditioned eyelid response. *Brain Research*, 359, 120–130.

Mihailoff, G.A. (1993) Cerebellar nuclear projections from the basilar pontine nuclei and nucelus reticularis tegmenti pontis as demonstrated with PHA-L tracing in the rat. *Journal of Comparative Neurology*, 330, 130–146.

Mink, J.W. and Thach, W.T. (1991) Basal ganglia motor control. III. Pallidal ablation: normal reaction time, muscle contraction, and slow movement. *Journal of Neurophysiology*, 65, 330–351.

Mintz, M., Lavond, D.G., Zhang, A.A., Yun, Y. and Thompson, R.F. (1994) Unilateral inferior olive NMDA lesion leads to unilateral deficit in acquisition and retention of eyelid classical conditioning. *Behavioral and Neural Biology*, 61, 218–224.

Miyachi, S., Hikosaka, O., Miyashita, K., Karadi, Z. and Rand, M.K. (1997) Differential roles of monkey striatum in learning of sequential hand movement. *Experimental Brain Research*, 115, 1–5.

Miyashita, K., Sakai, K. and Hikosaka, O. (1996) Effects of SMA and pre-SMA inactivation on learning of sequential movements in monkey. *Society for Neuroscience Abstracts*, 22, 1862.

Molchan, S.E., Sunderland, T., McIntosh, A.R., Herscovitch, P. and Schreurs, B.G. (1994) A functional anatomical study of associative learning in humans. *Proceedings of the National Academy of Sciences of the United States of America*, 91, 8122–8126.

Molinari, M., Grammaldo, L.G. and Petrosini, L. (1997a) Cerebellar contribution to spatial event processing: right/left discrimination abilities in rats. *European Journal of Neuroscience*, 9, 1986–1992.

Molinari, M., Petrosini, L. and Grammaldo, L.G. (1997b) Spatial event processing. *International Review of Neurobiology*, 41, 217–230.

Mower, G., Gibson, A. and Glickstein, M. (1979) Tectopontine pathway in the cat: laminar distribution of cells of origin and visual properties of target cells in dorsolateral pontine nucleus. *Journal of Neurophysiology*, 42, 1–15.

Moyer, J.R., Jr, Deyo, R.A. and Disterhoft, J.F. (1990) Hippocampectomy disrupts trace eyeblink conditioning in rabbits. *Behavioral Neuroscience*, 104, 243–252.

Nelson, B. and Mugnoini, E. (1989) GABAergic innervation of the inferior olivary complex and experimental evidence for its origin. In: Strata, P. (ed), *The Olivocerebellar System in Motor Control*. Springer-Verlag, New York, pp. 86–107.

Nordholm, A.F., Thompson, J.K., Dersarkissian, C. and Thompson, R.F. (1993) Lidocaine infusion in a critical region of cerebellum completely prevents learning of the conditioned eyeblink response. *Behavioral Neuroscience*, 107, 882–886.

Perrett, S.P. and Mauk, M.D. (1995) Extinction of conditioned eyelid responses requires the anterior lobe of cerebellar cortex. *Journal of Neuroscience*, 15, 2074–2080.

Perrett, S.P., Ruiz, B.P. and Mauk, M.D. (1993) Cerebellar cortex lesions disrupt learning-dependent timing of conditioned eyelid responses. *Journal of Neuroscience*, 13, 1708–1718.

Petrosini, L., Molinari, M. and Dell'Anna, M.E. (1996) Cerebellar contribution to spatial event processing: Morris water maze and T-maze. *European Journal of Neuroscience*, 8, 1882–1896.

Petrosini, L., Leggio, M.G. and Molinari, M. (1998) The cerebellum in the spatial problem solving: a co-star or a guest star? *Progress in Neurobiology*, 56, 191–210.

Racine, R.J., Wilson, D.A., Gingell, R. and Sutherland, D. (1986) Long-term potentiation in the interpositus and vestibular nuclei in the rat. *Experimental Brain Research*, 63, 158–162.

Ramirez, O.A., Nordholm, A.F., Gellerman, D., Thompson, J.K. and Thompson, R.F. (1997) The conditioned eyeblink response: a role for the GABA-B receptor. *Pharmacology, Biochemistry and Behavior*, 58, 127–132.

Rosenfield, M.E. and Moore, J.W. (1983) Red nucleus lesions disrupt the classically conditioned nictitating membrane response in rabbit. *Behavioural Brain Research*, 10, 393–398.

Rosenfield, M.D., Dovydaitis, A. and Moore, J.W. (1985) Brachium conjunctivum and rubrobulbar tract: brainstem projections of red nucleus essential for the conditioned nictitating membrane response. *Physiology and Behavior*, 34, 751–759.

Sakurai, M. (1990) Calcium is an intracellular mediator of the climbing fiber in induction of cerebellar long-term depression. *Proceedings of the National Academy of Sciences of the United States of America*, 87, 3383–3385.

Schmahmann, J.D. and Pandya, D.N. (1989) Anatomical investigation of projections to the basis pontis from posterior parietal association corticles in rhesus monkey. *Journal of Comparative Neurology*, 289, 53–73.

Schmahmann, J.D. and Pandya, D.N. (1991) Projections to the basis pontis from the superior temporal sulcus and superior temporal region in the rhesus monkey. *Journal of Comparative Neurology*, 308, 224–248.

Schmahmann, J.D. and Pandya, D.N. (1993) Prelunate, occipitotemporal, and parahippocampal projections to the basis pontis in rhesus monkey. *Journal of Comparative Neurology*, 337, 94–112.

Schreurs, B.G., McIntosh, A.R., Bahro, M., Herscovitch, P., Sunderland, T. and Molchan, S.E. (1997) Lateralization and behavioral correlation of changes in regional cerebral blood flow with classical conditioning of the human eyeblink response. *Journal of Neurophysiology*, 77, 2153–2163.

Schugens, M.M., Egerter, R., Daum, I., Schepelmann, K., Klockgether, T. and Loschmann, P.A. (1997) The NMDA antagonist memantine impairs classical eyeblink conditioning in humans. *Neuroscience Letters*, 224, 57–60.

Sears, L.L. and Steinmetz, J.E. (1991) Dorsal accessory inferior olive activity diminishes during acquisition of the rabbit classically conditioned eyelid response. *Brain Research*, 545, 114–122.

Seitz, R.J., Roland, E., Bohm, C., Greitz, T. and Stone-Elander, S. (1990) Motor learning in man: a positron emission tomographic study. *NeuroReport*, 1, 57–60.

Shadmehr, R. and Holcomb, H.H. (1997) Neural correlates of motor memory consolidation. *Science*, 277, 821–825.

Shibuki, K., Gomi, H., Chen, C., Bao, S., Kim, J.J., Wakatsuki, H., Fujisaki, T., Fujimoto, K., Ikeda, T., Chen, C., Thompson, R.F. and Itohara, S. (1996) Deficient cerebellar long-term depression, impaired eyeblink conditioning and normal motor coordination in GFAP mutant mice. *Neuron*, 16, 587–599.

Shinoda, Y., Suguichi, Y., Futami, T. and Izawa, R. (1992) Axon collaterals of mossy fibers from the pontine nucleus in the cerebellar dentate nucleus. *Journal of Neurophysiology*, 67, 547–560.

Snyder, R.L., Faull, R.L.M. and Mehler, W.R. (1978) A comparative study of the neurons of origin of the spinocerebellar afferents in the rat, cat and squirrel monkey based on the retrograde transport of horseradish peroxidase. *Journal of Comparative Neurology*, 181, 833–852.

Solomon, P.R., Lewis, J.L., LoTurco, J., Steinmetz, J.E. and Thompson, R.F. (1986a) The role of the middle cerebellar peduncle in acquisition and retention of the rabbit's classically conditioned nictitating membrane response. *Bulletin of the Psychonomic Society*, 24, 75–78.

Solomon, P.R., Vander Schaaf, E.R., Thompson, R.F. and Weisz, D.J. (1986b) Hippocampus and trace conditioning of the rabbit's classically conditioned nictitating membrane response. *Behavioral Neuroscience*, 100, 729–744.

Solomon, P.R., Stowe, G.T. and Pendlebury, W.W. (1989) Disrupted eyelid conditioning in a patient with damage to cerebellar afferents. *Behavioral Neuroscience*, 103, 898–902.

Steinmetz, J.E. (1990) Classical nictitating membrane conditioning in rabbits with varying interstimulus intervals and direct activation of cerebellar mossy fibers as the CS. *Behavioral Brain Research*, 38, 97–108.

Steinmetz, J.E. and Sengelaub, D.R. (1992) Possible conditioned stimulus pathway for classical eyelid conditioning in rabbits. *Behavioral and Neural Biology*, 57, 103–115.

Steinmetz, J.E., Rosen, D.J., Chapman, P.F., Lavond, D.G. and Thompson, R.F. (1986) Classical conditioning of the rabbit eyelid response with a mossy-fiber stimulation CS: I. Pontine nuclei and middle cerebellar peduncle stimulation. *Behavioral Neuroscience*, 100, 878–887.

Steinmetz, J.E., Logan, C.G., Rosen, D.J., Thompson, J.K., Lavond, D.G. and Thompson, R.F. (1987) Initial localization of the acoustic conditioned stimulus projection system to the cerebellum essential for classical eyelid conditioning. *Proceedings of the National Academy of Sciences of the United States of America*, 84, 3531–3535.

Steinmetz, J.E., Lavond, D.G. and Thompson, R.F. (1989) Classical conditioning in rabbits using pontine nucleus stimulation as a conditioned stimulus and inferior olive stimulation as an unconditioned stimulus. *Synapse*, 3, 225–233.

Steinmetz, J.E., Lavond, D.G., Ivkovich, D., Logan, C.G. and Thompson, R.F. (1992) Disruption of classical eyelid conditioning after cerebellar lesions: damage to a memory trace system or a simple performance deficit? *Journal of Neuroscience*, 12, 4403–4426.

Swain, R.A., Shinkman, P.G., Nordholm, A.F. and Thompson, R.F. (1992) Cerebellar stimulation as an unconditioned stimulus in classical conditioning. *Behavioral Neuroscience*, 106, 739–750.

Thach, W.T., Goodkin, H.P. and Keating, J.G. (1992) The cerebellum and the adaptive coordination of movement. *Annual Review of Neuroscience*, 15, 403–442.

Thompson, J.K., Lavond, D.G. and Thompson, R.F. (1985) Cerebellar interpositus/dentate nuclei afferents seen with retrograde fluorescent tracers in the rabbit. *Society for Neuroscience Abstracts*, 11, 1112.

Thompson, J.K., Spangler, W.J. and Thompson, R.F. (1991) Differential projections of pontine nuclei to interpositus nucleus and lobule HVI. *Society for Neuroscience Abstracts*, 17, 871.

Thompson, J.K., Krupa, D.J., Weng, J. and Thompson, R.F. (1993) Inactivation of motor nuclei blocks expression but not acquisition of rabbit's classically conditioned eyeblink response. *Society for Neuroscience Abstracts*, 19, 999.

Thompson, R.F. (1989) Role of inferior olive in classical conditioning. In: Strata, P. (ed.), *The Olivocerebellar System in Motor Control*. Springer-Verlag, New York, pp. 347–362.

Thompson, R.F. (1990) Neural mechanisms of classical conditioning in mammals. *Philosophical Transactions of the Royal Society of London, Series B*, 329, 161–170.

Thompson, R.F. and Krupa, D.J. (1994) Organization of memory traces in the mammalian brain. *Annual Review of Neuroscience*, 17, 519–549.

Thompson, R.F., Bao, S., Chen, L., Cipriano, B.D., Grethe, J.S., Kim, J.J., Thompson, J.K., Tracy, J.A., Weninger, M.S. and Krupa, D.J. (1997) Associative learning. *International Review of Neurobiology*, 41, 151–189.

Thompson, R.F., Thompson, J.K., Kim, J.J., Krupa, D.J. and Shinkman, P.G. (1998) The nature of reinforcement in cerebellar learning. *Neurobiology of Learning and Memory*, 70, 150–176.

Timmann, D., Kolb, F.P., Baier, C., Rijntjes, M., Muller, S.P., Diener, H.C. and Weiller, C. (1996) Cerebellar activation during classical conditioning of the human flexion reflex: a PET study. *NeuroReport*, 7, 2056–2060.

Tracy, J. (1995) Brain and behavior correlates in classical conditioning of the rabbit eyeblink response. Unpublished doctoral dissertation, University of Southern California.

Tracy, J., Weiss, C. and Thompson, R.F. (1991) Single unit recordings of somatosensory and auditory evoked responses in the anterior interpositus nucleus in the naive rabbit. *Society of Neuroscience Abstracts*, 17, 322.

Tracy, J.A., Thompson, J.K., Krupa, D.J. and Thompson, R.F. (1998) Evidence of plasticity in the pontocerebellar conditioned stimulus pathway during classical conditioning of the eyeblink response in the rabbit. *Behavioral Neuroscience*, 112, 267–285.

Tusa, R.J. and Ungerleider, L.G. (1988) Fiber pathways of cortical areas mediating smooth pursuit eye movements in monkeys, *Annals of Neurology*, 23, 174–183.

Voneida, T., Christie, D., Boganski, R. and Chopko, B. (1990) Changes in instrumentally and classically conditioned limb-flexion responses following inferior olivary lesions and olivocerebellar tractotomy in the cat. *Journal of Neuroscience*, 10, 3583–3593.

Watanabe, E. (1984) Neuronal events correlated with long-term adaptation of the horizontal vestibulo-ocular reflex in the primate flocculus. *Brain Research*, 297, 169–174.

Weiner, M.J., Hallett, M. and Funkenstein, H.H. (1983) Adaptation to lateral displacement of vision in patients with lesions of the central nervous system. *Neurology*, 33, 766–772.

Woodruff-Pak, D.S. and Jaeger, M.E. (1998) Predictors of eyeblink classical conditioning over the adult age span. *Psychology of Aging*, 13, 193–205.

Woodruff-Pak, D.S. and Thompson, R.F. (1988) Classical conditioning of the eyeblink response in the delay paradigm in adults aged 18–83 years. *Psychology and Aging*, 3, 219–229.

Woodruff-Pak, D.S., Lavond, D.G. and Thompson, R.F. (1985) Trace conditioning: abolished by cerebellar nuclear lesions but not lateral cerebellar cortex aspirations. *Brain Research*, 348, 249–260.

Woodruff-Pak, D.S., Cronholm, J.F. and Sheffield, J.B. (1990) Purkinje cell number related to rate of eyeblink classical conditioning. *NeuroReport*, 1, 165–168.

Yeo, C.H. (1991) Cerebellum and classical conditioning of motor response. *Annals of the New York Academy of Sciences*, 627, 292–304.

Yeo, C.H., Hardiman, M.J. and Glickstein, M. (1985a) Classical conditioning of the nictitating membrane response of the rabbit I. Lesions of the cerebellar nuclei. *Experimental Brain Research*, 60, 87–98.

Yeo, C.H., Hardiman, M.J. and Glickstein, M. (1985b) Classical conditioning of the nictitating membrane response of the rabbit. II. Lesions of the cerebellar cortex. *Experimental Brain Research*, 60, 99–113.

Yeo, C.H., Hardiman, M.J. and Glickstein, M. (1986) Classical conditioning of the nictitating membrane response of the rabbit. IV. Lesions of the inferior olive. *Experimental Brain Research*, 63, 81–92.

Zhang, A.A. and Lavond, D.G. (1991) Effects of reversible lesions of reticular or facial neurons during eyeblink conditioning. *Society for Neuroscience Abstracts*, 17, 869.

13   BRAIN SYSTEMS AND THE REGULATION OF MEMORY CONSOLIDATION

James L. McGaugh, Larry Cahill, Barbara Ferry and Benno Roozendaal

INTRODUCTION

Since the early studies of Lashley (1950), research attempting to understand how memories are stored in the brain has focused, to a considerable extent, on the brain locus (or loci) of memories and the cellular processes essential for creating the neural changes or 'engrams' (Lashley, 1950) that enable lasting memory. The success of Thompson and colleagues (1998; see King and Thompson, Chapter 12) in investigating the neural circuit essential for the formation and maintenance of a conditioned eyelid response has greatly stimulated interest in finding circuits mediating other types of learning. Research on brain systems and memory has also been guided by an interest in discovering the functions of different brain systems in learning and memory (McDonald and White, 1993; Salmon and Butters, 1995; Eichenbaum, 1996; Packard and McGaugh, 1996; Hikosaka et al., 1998). The seminal findings of Milner (1966) that bilateral lesions of medial temporal brain regions significantly disrupt the acquisition of new information stimulated intensive and extensive investigation of the functions of the hippocampal region and the cortex surrounding the hippocampus in explicit or declarative memory (Zola-Morgan et al., 1989; Bussey et al., 1999; Brown, Chapter 11).

Gabriel Horn's extensive and influential research on the neural basis of imprinting examines brain systems and mechanisms involved in the acquisition and retention of the various features of this type of learning in chicks (Horn, 1985, 1998). Horn's findings have identified brain regions in chicks that appear to have functions similar to those of the medial temporal region in rats, monkeys and humans in enabling recognition (i.e. declarative) memory and possibly storing such memory (Horn, 1998). Horn's findings, like those of other investigators, indicate that other forms of memory appear to involve other brain systems (Horn, 1998). Increasing evidence, for example, suggests that the striatum is involved in mediating some types of response or habit learning (Salmon and Butters, 1995; Packard and McGaugh, 1996; Hikosaka et al., 1998) and that the prefrontal cortex is involved in working memory (Fuster, 1995, 1998; Williams and Goldman-Rakic, 1995; Sakurai, 1998).

In drawing conclusions about the roles of different brain systems in learning and memory, the use of the words 'involves' and 'mediates' is usually quite deliberate, simply because the way or ways in which the systems are involved in memory is, in most cases, not as yet fully understood. Of course, any brain system might well have more than one function in learning and memory, and the nature of the functions may involve interactions with other brain systems. It is well established, for example, that lesions of the hippocampal region (and surrounding cortex) impair recognition memory and the consolidation of declarative memory (Zola-Morgan et al., 1989). An implicit assumption of much research investigating long-term potentiation in the hippocampus appears to be that the findings will reveal the cellular processes mediating long-term memory storage in that brain region (see Dudai and Morris, Chapter 9; Winder and Kandel, Chapter 10). However, the findings that lesions of the hippocampus and adjacent regions induced several weeks after learning do not impair retention clearly indicate that this brain region is not the locus of long-term storage of declarative memory (Winocur, 1990; Zola-Morgan and Squire, 1990; Kim and Fanselow, 1992, Squire and Alvarez, 1995). It remains to be determined whether this brain region is the locus of short-term storage or serves some other function(s) in the establishment of long-term memory (Brown, Chapter 11).

Another important lesson learned from Horn's investigations of memory for imprinting is that brain systems interact in creating and maintaining memories (Horn, 1985). It seems highly likely that the hippocampal system interacts with other regions, including the cortex, in forming long-term memories. Interactions among brain systems are also observed in other types of learning. Weinberger (1998) has shown, for example, that the learning of the significance of a particular auditory stimulus involves the action of several subcortical brain systems that influence the functioning of the auditory cortex where the change in the significance appears to be represented. Hikosaka and his colleagues (1998) have demonstrated that the frontal cortex, basal ganglia and cerebellum interact in the learning of motor skills. Clearly, as Horn (1985) has emphasized, such findings indicate that understanding brain mechanisms underlying learning and memory will require detailed knowledge of the functional interactions among brain systems as well as circuitry and cellular plasticity.

EMOTIONAL AROUSAL AND THE REGULATION OF MEMORY CONSOLIDATION

There is now extensive evidence that another system in the medial temporal region, the amygdaloid complex, plays a special role in learning and memory. The amygdala appears to be involved importantly in memory for emotionally arousing experiences. More specifically, the amygdala appears to be part of a system that serves to regulate the strength of explicit/declarative memories in relation to their emotional significance (Cahill and McGaugh, 1998). This chapter summarizes findings of our research investigating the involvement of the amygdala in regulating memory. The basic hypothesis that is suggested by our findings is that emotionally arousing stimulation activates the amygdala, and that amygdala activity regulates the consolidation of long-term explicit memory of events by modulating neuroplasticity in other brain regions (McGaugh *et al.*, 1996; Cahill and McGaugh, 1998).

Adrenal stress hormones also play a critical role. Our findings indicate that hormones released from the adrenal medulla (adrenaline) and adrenal cortex (corticosterone in the rat) activate noradrenergic systems projecting to the amygdala. Additionally, the findings indicate that the amygdala is not critically involved in the retrieval of emotionally influenced explicit memory. This view is based primarily on evidence from our studies examining the involvement of the amygdala in mediating stress hormone and drug influences on memory, as well as findings of studies of the effects of lesions and temporary inactivation of the amygdala or amygdala afferents or efferents. The hypothesis is also supported by recent findings from studies using human subjects (Cahill, 1996).

Our experimental approach is based on the 'consolidation hypothesis' originally proposed by Mueller and Pilzecker a century ago (1900) suggesting that memory traces become consolidated over time. The consolidation hypothesis is supported strongly by clinical as well as experimental findings (McGaugh and Herz, 1972; Weingartner and Parker, 1984). Of particular importance for the issues addressed in this chapter are the early findings that post-training injections of stimulant drugs enhance memory when administered shortly after training (Breen and McGaugh, 1961; McGaugh, 1966, 1968, 1973) and are generally ineffective when administered several hours after learning (McGaugh and Herz, 1972). Such findings indicate that the drugs affect memory by modulating the consolidation of recently acquired information. The use of post-training treatments to alter brain functioning shortly after training has provided an effective technique for distinguishing the effects of treatments on memory from effects of the treatments on the behavior used to make inferences about memory (McGaugh, 1966, 1989a; McGaugh and Herz, 1972; McGaugh, 2000). With the use of post-training treatments, brain functioning is not altered during acquisition or retention testing.

STRESS HORMONE INFLUENCES ON MEMORY CONSOLIDATION

It is well established that hormones of the adrenal medulla and adrenal cortex are released during and immediately after stressful stimulation of the kinds typically used in aversively motivated training tasks (McCarty and Gold, 1981; McGaugh and Gold, 1989). It is also well established that these hormones influence memory consolidation. Early studies focused on the influence of adrenaline on memory consolidation. The basic hypothesis guiding these studies is that if stress hormones regulate memory storage then it should be possible to influence memory by administering hormones post-training. In support of this implication, Gold and van Buskirk (1975) found that post-training injections of adrenaline enhance long-term retention of inhibitory avoidance. As with stimulant drugs, the memory enhancement was greatest when the injections were administered shortly after training. Similar effects have been obtained subsequently with many other types of training tasks (Izquierdo and Diaz, 1983; Sternberg *et al.*, 1985; Introini-Collison and McGaugh, 1986; Liang *et al.*, 1986). These findings strongly support the view that adrenaline enhances memory consolidation.

Stress-released adrenocortical hormones also modulate memory storage (de Kloet, 1991; Bohus, 1994; McEwen and Sapolsky, 1995; Lupien and McEwen, 1997). As with adrenaline, single injections of moderate doses of corticosterone or synthetic glucocorticoids can enhance memory consolidation (Cottrell and Nakajima, 1977; Sandi and Rose, 1994; Roozendaal and McGaugh, 1996a). The memory-modulating effects of glucocorticoids seem to involve selective activation of glucocorticoid receptors, as a blockade of glucocorticoid receptors (but not mineralocorticoid receptors) shortly before or immediately after training impairs memory (Oitzl and de Kloet, 1992; Roozendaal *et al.*, 1996b; Lupien and McEwen, 1997). These findings strongly implicate glucocorticoid receptors in memory storage, and suggest that memory consolidation is also modulated by stress-induced release of endogenous glucocorticoids.

Several findings indicate that catecholamines and glucocorticoids interact in influencing memory storage (Borrell *et al.*, 1983, 1984). We examined glucocorticoid–adrenergic interactions in rats injected with metyrapone, a drug that attenuates the elevation of circulating corticosterone induced by aversive stimulation (Roozendaal *et al.*, 1996a). Rats received systemic injections of metyrapone prior to inhibitory avoidance training, as well as post-training injections of adrenaline, amphetamine or 4-OH amphetamine (a peripherally acting derivative of amphetamine). Amphetamines stimulate the release of adrenaline from the adrenal medulla (Weiner, 1985) and are known to enhance memory in rats as well as human subjects (McGaugh, 1973; Soetens *et al.*, 1993, 1995). Metyrapone blocked the memory-enhancing effects of adrenaline and the amphetamines but did not affect memory when administered alone. Thus, stress-induced release of corticosterone and activation of glucocorticoid receptors appear to be essential in enabling adrenergic modulation of memory consolidation.

AMYGDALA INVOLVEMENT IN STRESS HORMONE INFLUENCES ON MEMORY CONSOLIDATION

Extensive evidence indicates that adrenaline and glucocorticoid effects on memory are mediated by influences involving the amygdala. Our focus on the amygdala as a possible brain site involved in modulating consolidation was guided by evidence that post-training electrical stimulation of the amygdala modulates memory storage. Retention is enhanced by low-intensity stimulation and impaired by high-intensity stimulation (Kesner and Wilburn, 1974; McGaugh and Gold, 1976). These findings indicating that memory storage is enhanced by mild activation of the amygdala suggested the possibility that endogenously induced activation of the amygdala might influence memory storage.

β-Adrenergic influences

The first evidence suggesting that the amygdala is involved in adrenergic effects on memory was provided by the finding that adrenal demedullation and injections of adrenaline alter the memory-modulating effects of electrical stimulation of the amygdala (see Table 13.1). Stimulation that induced retrograde amnesia in control rats enhanced memory in adrenally demedullated rats. In contrast, in adrenally

Table 13.1 Adrenaline modulates the effects of post-training electrical stimulation of the amygdala on consolidation of memory for inhibitory avoidance and active avoidance training

| | Memory on 24 h retention test | |
Treatment[a]	Adrenal intact	Adrenal demedullated
Saline	Impaired	Enhanced
Adrenaline before stimulation	Impaired	Impaired
Adrenaline after stimulation		No effect

[a]Systemic injections were administerd before or after post-training electrical stimulation of the amygdala.
From Liang *et al.* (1985).

demedullated rats given adrenaline prior to electrical stimulation of the amygdala, memory was impaired (Liang *et al.*, 1985). Furthermore, lesions of either the amygdala or the stria terminalis, a major amygdala pathway, block adrenaline effects on memory consolidation (Liang and McGaugh, 1983; Cahill and McGaugh, 1991). These findings strongly suggest that adrenaline modulates amygdala functioning in regulating memory consolidation.

Adrenaline effects on memory for inhibitory avoidance training are also blocked by peripheral administration of the β-adrenergic antagonist propranolol, a drug that readily enters the brain, as well as by sotalol, a β-adrenergic antagonist that does not readily enter the brain (Introini-Collison *et al.*, 1992). Post-training peripheral administration of β-adrenergic agonists that enter the brain, including dipivefrin and clenbuterol, also enhances memory consolidation. The memory enhancement induced by dipivefrin and clenbuterol is blocked by propranolol, but not by sotalol (Introini-Collison *et al.*, 1992). These findings indicate that adrenaline effects on memory storage are initiated by activation of peripheral β-adrenergic receptors but that memory storage is also modulated by activation of β-adrenergic receptors within the brain. There is evidence that β-adrenergic receptors are located on vagal afferents that project to the nucleus of the solitary tract in the brainstem (Schreurs *et al.*, 1986). Furthermore, projections from the nucleus of the solitary tract release noradrenaline within the amygdala (Ricardo and Koh, 1978). These findings suggest that adrenaline effects on memory are mediated at least in part by activation of the nucleus of the solitary tract. In support of this view, we found that inactivation of the nucleus of the solitary tract with infusions of lidocaine blocks adrenaline effects on memory consolidation (Williams and McGaugh, 1993). The findings that in rats, as well as human subjects, memory is enhanced by post-training electrical stimulation of vagal afferents provides additional evidence for the importance of vagal afferents in regulating memory consolidation (Clark *et al.*, 1995, 1999).

The hypothesis that adrenaline effects on memory consolidation involve adrenergic activation within the amygdala suggests that infusions of the β-adrenergic antagonist propranolol administered into the amygdala should block adrenaline effects. Experimental findings are consistent with this hypothesis (Liang *et al.*, 1986). This hypothesis suggests, more generally, that post-training activation of amygdala adrenergic receptors should enhance memory. The findings of

several studies strongly support this implication. Infusions of noradrenaline or the β-adrenergic agonist clenbuterol into the amygdala after inhibitory avoidance training induce dose-dependent enhancement of memory (Liang *et al.*, 1986, 1990, 1995; Introini-Collison *et al.*, 1991, 1996). Furthermore, post-training intra-amygdala infusions of β-adrenergic antagonists block the memory-enhancing effects of noradrenaline and impair retention when administered alone (Liang *et al.*, 1986, 1995). Considered together, these findings provide strong evidence that memory storage is modulated by noradrenergic activation within the amygdala.

A major assumption of this hypothesis is that emotionally arousing training experiences induce the release of noradrenaline in the amygdala. In experiments using *in vivo* microdialysis and high-performance liquid chromatography, we found that footshock stimulation of the kind typically used in inhibitory avoidance training induced noradrenaline release within the amygdala (Galvez *et al.*, 1996). Noradrenaline release in the amygdala induced by footshock stimulation varied directly with the stimulus intensity (Figure 13.1) (Quirarte *et al.*, 1998). Furthermore, hormones and drugs that modulate memory storage influence the release of noradrenaline in the amygdala. Peripheral injections of adrenaline induce the release of noradrenaline (Williams *et al.*, 1998) whereas injections of the opiate antagonist naloxone potentiate noradrenaline release induced by footshock (Quirarte *et al.*, 1998). This latter finding is consistent with evidence that intra-amygdala infusions of β-adrenergic antagonists block naloxone effects on memory storage (McGaugh *et al.*, 1988; Introini-Collison *et al.*, 1989) as well as evidence that opiate agonists inhibit the release of noradrenaline in other regions of the brain (Arbilla and Langer, 1978). Peripheral injections of the GABAergic antagonist picrotoxin also induce noradrenaline release in the amygdala (Hatfield *et al.*, 1999). These findings fit well with previous findings that peripheral or intra-amygdala injections of GABAergic antagonists enhance memory (Brioni and McGaugh, 1988; Brioni *et al.*, 1989).

Glucocorticoid influences

It is well established that activation of adrenal steroid receptors in the hippocampus plays an important role in mediating glucocorticoid influences on memory (Bohus, 1994; McEwen and Sapolsky, 1995). Findings

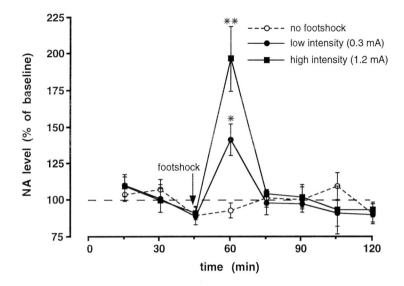

Figure 13.1. Effects of low- and high-intensity footshock on noradrenaline release in the amygdala assessed by *in vivo* microdialysis and HPLC. Noradrenaline levels are expressed as mean (±SEM) of basal levels prior to footshock. *$P <0.05$; **$P <0.01$ as compared with the no footshock group. From Quirarte *et al.* (1998).

from our laboratory indicate that the amygdala is also involved in glucocorticoid effects on memory storage. Lesions of the stria terminalis or amygdala block the memory-enhancing effects of post-training systemic injections of the synthetic glucocorticoid dexamethasone (Roozendaal and McGaugh, 1996a,b). As is discussed below, post-training intra-amygdala infusions of a selective glucocorticoid agonist enhance memory storage and the memory enhancement involves noradrenergic activation in the amygdala. (Roozendaal and McGaugh, 1997a)

Interaction of neuromodulatory systems

As noted above, other neuromodulatory influences on memory, including those of opioid peptidergic and GABAergic systems, involve activation of the amygdala. Systemic injections of opioid peptides and opiates generally impair memory consolidation, and opiate antagonists enhance memory (Izquierdo and Diaz, 1983; McGaugh, 1989b; McGaugh *et al.*, 1993). GABAergic antagonists and agonists enhance and impair retention, respectively (Brioni and McGaugh, 1988; Brioni *et al.*, 1989). Lesions of the amygdala or stria terminalis block opioid peptidergic as well as GABAergic influences on memory storage (McGaugh *et al.*, 1986; Ammassari-Teule *et al.*, 1991). The findings of several experiments indicate that GABAergic influences on memory, like those of adrenaline and glucocorticoids, involve noradrenergic activation in the amygdala. Intra-amygdala infusions of propranolol block opiate and GABAergic influences on

memory (McGaugh *et al.*, 1988; Introini-Collison *et al.*, 1989). Furthermore, in experiments using both inhibitory avoidance and water maze spatial tasks, intra-amygdala infusions of clenbuterol blocked the memory-impairing effects of β-endorphin administered together with clenbuterol. The neuromodulatory interactions found in our experiments are summarized schematically in Figure 13.2. Glucocorticoid influences shown in the figure are discussed below.

Other findings from our laboratory indicate that amygdala influences on memory storage are not restricted to the learning of tasks, such as inhibitory avoidance, that involve the use of aversive stimulation. A series of recent experiments in our laboratory examined the involvement of the amygdala in memory for a change in reward magnitude (CRM). Rats were trained for several days to run in a straight alley for a large reward (10 pellets of food). The reward was then reduced to one pellet and decreases in running speeds were used as an index of memory of the reduced reward. As with memory for other types of training, memory for CRM involves the amygdala. Post-training intra-amygdala infusions of muscimol, lidocaine or propranolol impaired memory for CRM, whereas infusions of the muscarinic cholinergic agonist oxotremorine enhanced memory (Salinas *et al.*, 1993, 1997; Salinas and McGaugh, 1995). Other experiments examined the involvement of the amygdala in memory for an increase in reward. Post-training intra-amygdala infusions of the GABAergic antagonist bicuculline enhanced memory for an increase in reward magnitude (Salinas and McGaugh,

BASOLATERAL AMYGDALA

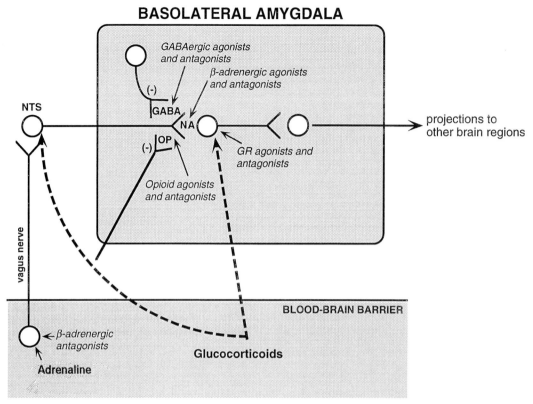

Figure 13.2. Schematic summarizing the interactions of neuromodulatory influences in the basolateral amygdala on memory storage as suggested by the findings of our experiments. (Abbreviations: GR = glucocorticoid receptor; NA = noradrenaline; NTS = nucleus of the solitary tract; OP = opioids).

1996). All of these findings are highly comparable with those obtained with other tasks, including inhibitory avoidance.

Involvement of the basolateral amygdala nucleus

The studies reviewed above investigated the effects of lesions or microinfusions (0.5 or 1.0 μl) affecting the entire amygdaloid complex. However, the findings of many recent studies using much smaller infusion volumes indicate that the basolateral nucleus (BLA) is selectively involved in mediating neuromodulatory influences on memory consolidation (see Table 13.2). Our studies investigating the effects of benzo-diazepines on memory were the first to suggest the selective involvement of the BLA in modulating memory storage. Benzodiazepines are known to impair memory for inhibitory avoidance training through influences on GABAergic mechanisms in the amygdala (Izquierdo *et al.*, 1990a,b). We found that lesions restricted to the BLA blocked the memory-

impairing effects of a benzodiazepine on memory for inhibitory avoidance training, whereas lesions of the central nucleus were ineffective (Tomaz *et al.*, 1992). Additionally, selective infusions of a benzodiazepine or benzodiazepine antagonist into the BLA modulate memory storage (de Souza-Silva and Tomaz, 1995; Da Cunha *et al.*, 1999).

The finding that selective inactivation of the BLA with post-training infusions impairs memory for inhibitory avoidance training provides additional evidence that the BLA is involved in modulating memory consolidation (Parent and McGaugh, 1994). Amygdala noradrenergic influences on memory storage also selectively involve the BLA. Also, as is shown in Figure 13.3, the BLA is involved in modulating memory for spatial training in a water maze (Hatfield and McGaugh, 1999). Post-training infusions of noradrenaline or propranolol administered into the BLA enhanced and impaired memory, respectively.

Other recent findings from our laboratory indicate that α-adrenergic receptors within the BLA are also

Table 13.2 Basolateral amygdala critical to memory modulation

Procedure	Basolateral nucleus	Central nucleus	Reference
Lidocaine infusion post-learning	Modulates memory	No effect	Parent *et al.* (1994)
Infusions of glucocorticoid agonist or antagonist into AC nuclei	Modulates memory	No effect	Roozendaal and McGaugh (1997a)
Lesions of AC nuclei; systemic dexamethasone	Blocks modulation	No effect	Roozendaal and McGaugh (1996a)
Lesions of AC nuclei; adrenalectomy	Blocks modulation	No effect	Roozendaal *et al.* (1996b)
Lesions of AC nuclei; infusion of glucocorticoid agonist or antagonist into hippocampus	Blocks modulation	No effect	Roozendaal and McGaugh (1997b)
Lesions of AC nuclei; systemic diazepam	Blocks modulation	No effect	Tomaz *et al.* (1992)
Infusion of β-blocker into AC nuclei; systemic dexamethasone	Blocks modulation	No effect	Quirarte *et al.* (1997a)
Infusion of noradrenaline into	Modulates memory	No effect	Hatfield and McGaugh (1999)
Infusion of benzodiazepine antagonist into AC nuclei	Modulates memory	No effect	Da Cunha *et al.* (1999)

All lesions are excitotoxic.

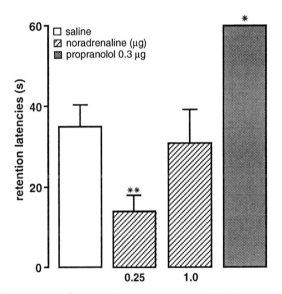

Figure 13.3. Retention latencies (mean ± SEM) for a 24 h water maze spatial task. Effects of immediate post-training infusions of noradrenaline (0.25 or 1.0 μg in 0.2 μl) or the β-adrenergic antagonist propranolol (0.3 μg in 0.2 μl) into the basolateral amygdala. *P <0.05; **P <0.01 as compared with the corresponding saline group. From Hatfield and McGaugh (1999).

involved in consolidation of memory for inhibitory avoidance training (Ferry *et al.*, 1999a). Differential effects are induced by selective activation of α_1- and α_2-adrenergic receptors in the BLA. α_1-Adrenoceptors are located postsynaptically whereas α_2-adrenoceptors are located predominantly presynaptically

and, when activated, inhibit the release of noradrenaline (Starke, 1979). In our experiment, post-training infusions of the selective α_1-adrenergic antagonist prazosin impaired memory. In addition, as is shown in Figure 13.4A, post-training activation of α_1-adrenoceptors by infusing the non-specific α-adrenergic agonist phenylephrine into the BLA together with the selective α_2-adrenoceptor antagonist yohimbine enhanced memory. The α_1-adrenergic influences appear to be mediated by an interaction with β-adrenergic receptors. As shown in Figure 13.4B, infusions of the β-adrenergic antagonist atenolol together with phenylephrine and yohimbine blocked the memory enhancement induced by activation of α_1-adrenoceptors. Other findings (Ferry *et al.*, 1999b) support this hypothesis. The memory-enhancing effects induced by post-training intra-BLA infusions of the β-adrenergic agonist clenbuterol were attenuated (i.e. higher doses were required for enhancement) by concurrent infusions of prazosin (Figure 13.5A). Intra-BLA infusions of the synthetic cAMP analog 8-bromo-cAMP also enhanced retention, and this latter effect was not blocked by prazosin (Figure 13.5B). These findings are consistent with pharmacological evidence suggesting that β-adrenergic receptors modulate memory storage by a direct coupling to adenylate cyclase and that α_1-adrenergic receptors act indirectly by influencing β-adrenergic activation of cAMP (Perkins and Moore, 1973; Pfeuffer, 1977; Ross *et al.*, 1978; Daly *et al.*, 1981).

Glucocorticoid influences on memory storage also selectively involve the BLA. As is shown in Figure

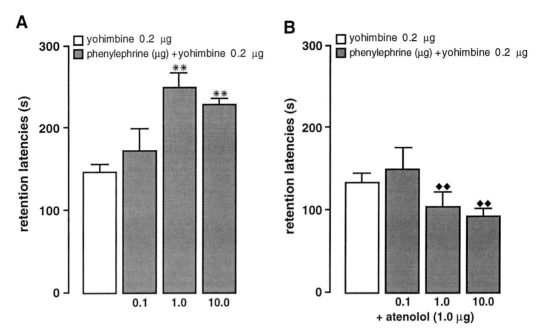

Figure 13.4. Step-through latencies (mean ± SEM) for a 48 h inhibitory avoidance test. Effects of immediate post-training infusions of the non-specific α-adrenergic agonist phenylephrine (0.1–10 μg) + the specific α₂-adrenergic antagonist yohimbine (0.2 μg in 0.2 μl) into the basolateral amygdala alone (**A**) or together with the β₁-adrenergic antagonist atenolol (1.0 μg) (**B**). * *P < 0.01 as compared with the corresponding saline group; ◆◆ P < 0.01 as compared with the corresponding phenylephrine + yohimbine group. From Ferry *et al.* (1999a).

13.6A, lesions of the amygdala restricted selectively to the BLA block the memory-enhancing effects of post-training systemic injections of dexamethasone (Roozendaal and McGaugh, 1996a). Furthermore, as is shown in Figure 13.6B, post-training infusions of the specific glucocorticoid receptor agonist RU 28362 selectively enhance retention when administered into the BLA (Roozendaal and McGaugh, 1997a). In addition to disrupting the memory-modulatory effects of a glucocorticoid in an inhibitory avoidance task, lesions of the BLA also block glucocorticoid effects on memory for water-maze spatial learning (Roozendaal *et al.*, 1996b). These findings indicate that the effects of glucocorticoids on memory storage are mediated, in part, by binding directly to glucocorticoid receptors in the BLA.

Glucocorticoid influences on memory storage also depend critically on β-adrenergic activation within the BLA. As is shown in Figure 13.7, β-adrenergic antagonists infused selectively into the BLA blocked the enhancing effects of post-training systemic dexamethasone on inhibitory avoidance retention (Quirarte *et al.*, 1997a). Additionally, blockade of glucocorticoid receptors in the BLA with a specific antagonist attenuated the dose–response effect of the β-adrenergic agonist clenbuterol infused into the BLA post-training

(Quirarte *et al.*, 1997b). Glucocorticoid receptor activation in the BLA appears to influence the effectiveness of β-adrenergic stimulation in modulating memory consolidation. Some of the effects of systemic glucocorticoids on memory may involve activation of glucocorticoid receptors in the ascending noradrenergic cell groups in the brainstem that have high densities of glucocorticoid receptors (Harfstrand *et al.*, 1986). We recently found that post-training infusions of the glucocorticoid receptor agonist RU 28362 into the nucleus of the solitary tract enhanced memory for inhibitory avoidance training and that the effect was blocked by intra-BLA infusions of the β-adrenergic antagonist atenolol (Roozendaal *et al.*, 1999a). The interaction of both adrenaline and glucocorticoids with noradrenergic mechanisms in the BLA may provide the basis for the interaction of these two stress hormone systems in regulating memory consolidation as described above.

AMYGDALA INTERACTIONS WITH OTHER BRAIN SYSTEMS

Although the findings summarized above strongly support the hypothesis that the BLA is a site for inte-

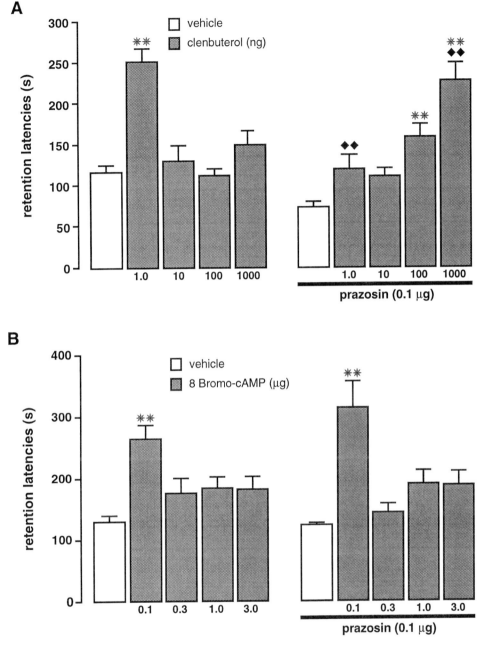

Figure 13.5. Step-through latencies (mean ± SEM) for a 48 h inhibitory avoidance test. Effects of immediate post-training infusions of the α_1-adrenergic antagonist prazosin (0.1 μg in 0.2 μl) into the basolateral amygdala on the dose–response effects of the concurrently administered β-adrenergic agonist clenbuterol (**A**) or the synthetic cAMP analog 8-bromo-cAMP (**B**). ******P <0.01 as compared with the corresponding saline group; ♦♦P <0.01 as compared with the corresponding clenbuterol or 8-bromo-cAMP group. From Ferry *et al.* (1999b).

grating the interactions of neuromodulatory systems influencing memory storage, they do not reveal the brain site(s) at which amygdala activity modulates memory storage. Many findings of experiments using

other methods suggest that the BLA is not a likely locus of neural changes underlying long-term memory for the information acquired in the tasks typically used in our experiments, including inhibitory

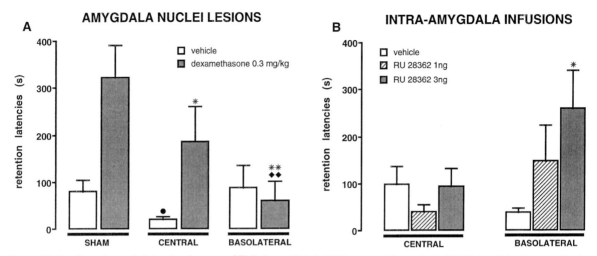

Figure 13.6. Step-through latencies (mean ± SEM) for a 48 h inhibitory avoidance test. (**A**) Rats with sham, or lesions of either the central or basolateral nucleus of the amygdala had been treated with dexamethasone (0.3 mg/kg, subcutaneous) or vehicle immediately after training. (**B**) Rats received post-training infusions of the glucocorticoid receptor agonist RU 28362 (1.0 or 3.0 ng in 0.2 μl) into the central or basolateral nucleus. *P <0.05; **P <0.01 as compared with the corresponding vehicle group; •P <0.05 as compared with the corresponding sham lesion–vehicle group; ••P <0.01 as compared with the corresponding sham lesion–dexamethasone group. From Roozendaal and McGaugh (1996a, 1997a).

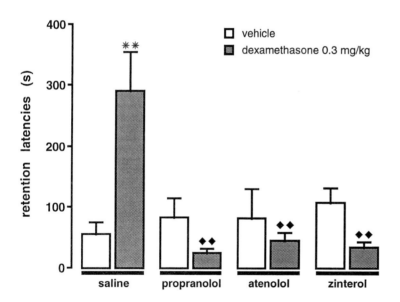

Figure 13.7. Step-through latencies (mean ± SEM) for a 48 h inhibitory avoidance test. Effects of pre-training infusions of either the non-specific β-adrenergic antagonist propranolol (0.5 μg in 0.2 μl), the β_1-adrenergic antagonist atenolol (0.5 μg in 0.2 μl) or the β_2-adrenergic antagonist zinterol (0.5 μg in 0.2 μl) into the basolateral amygdala and immediate post-training injections of dexamethasone (0.3 mg/kg, subcutaneous). **P <0.01 as compared with the corresponding vehicle group; ••P <0.01 as compared with the corresponding vehicle–dexamethasone group. From Quirarte *et al.* (1997a).

avoidance and water-maze spatial tasks. The question of whether the BLA is a locus of memory for other types of fear-based learning also remains an issue of experimental inquiry (Cahill *et al.*, 1999). Lesions of the entire amygdala (Parent *et al.*, 1992, 1994) or BLA (Parent and McGaugh, 1994; Parent *et al.*, 1995) induced a week or longer after training do not block inhibitory avoidance retention performance. Further-

more, large lesions of the amygdaloid complex induced before training typically attenuate but do not block inhibitory avoidance retention performance (Cahill and McGaugh, 1990).

We addressed this issue further in a recent experiment using Pavlovian fear conditioning (Vazdarjanova and McGaugh, 1998). Sham-lesioned and BLA-lesioned rats were first allowed to explore a Y-maze and on the following day received a series of four foot-shocks in one arm of the Y-maze. Additionally, a group of BLA-lesioned controls received no shocks. The next day, each rat was placed in one of the other arms, i.e. an arm where shock was not delivered, and several behavioral measures were assessed for 8 min. The sham-lesioned animals displayed freezing in the arm in which they were placed for approximately 75% of the test period. As a consequence, they moved about the maze very little and spent only about 10% of the time in the other safe arm and almost no time in the shock arm. As was expected, the BLA lesions disrupted freezing behavior. Thus, the critical comparisons are those between the BLA-lesioned rats that had received shock and those that had not received shock. In comparison with BLA-lesioned controls that had not received footshocks, the BLA-lesioned rats that had received shocks (like the sham-lesioned animals that had received shocks) had longer latencies to enter the arm where they had received shock, entered the shock arm less frequently and spent less time there. It is important to note that the BLA-lesioned animals that had received no shock spent equal amounts of time in each of the arms during the 8-min test period. Thus, these findings indicate that the BLA-lesioned animals that received shocks very clearly learned that shock was delivered in one of the three arms of the maze and displayed that knowledge by subsequently avoiding that arm.

Studies of conditioned neuroendocrine responses provide additional evidence that does not support the hypothesis that the amygdala is a long-term site of memory storage. In agreement with findings of others (LeDoux, 1995; Maren and Fanselow, 1996; Vazdarjanova and McGaugh, 1998; Nader and LeDoux, Chapter 14), lesions of the amygdala induced after Pavlovian contextual fear conditioning training significantly attenuated rats' 'freezing' behavior, a somatic response often used as an index of fear. Other findings, however, indicate that lesions of the amygdala induced after fear conditioning do not block conditioned neuroendocrine responses (Roozendaal *et al.*, 1992). Such findings suggest that the memory for the aversive training was not impaired. Moreover, studies using two strains of rats that differ in their preferential behavioral responses to aversive stimulation (mild shock delivered through a probe inserted into the cage) indicated that, in both strains, post-training intra-amygdala infusions of noradrenaline enhanced memory of an aversive stimulation. In the rats that normally dis-

played freezing, the post-training noradrenaline enhanced freezing. In the other rats, the post-training noradrenaline did not enhance freezing but, rather, enhanced other natural defensive responses, i.e. burying and biting of the probe (Roozendaal *et al.*, 1993). Additionally, recent findings indicate that large neurotoxic lesions of the amygdala induced 4 days after rats received a shock delivered through an electrified probe inserted into their cage did not block subsequent retention of the shock experience, as assessed by the latency to contact the probe and number of contacts with the probe (Lehmann, *et al.*, 2000). These findings provide additional evidence that an intact amygdala is not required for the remembrance of danger.

Many of the experiments examining the role of the amygdala in memory have used inhibitory avoidance as the measure of memory. Our own studies have used inhibitory avoidance tasks extensively in such research. Other investigators (e.g. LeDoux, 1995; Maren *et al.*, 1996; Nader and LeDoux, Chapter 14) have suggested that findings based on studies using inhibitory avoidance may differ from those using Pavlovian fear conditioning because inhibitory avoidance and Pavlovian contextual fear conditioning differ procedurally and may have different neural bases. However, it is not at all clear that these two types of training differ in critical ways, and many findings very strongly suggest that they have common bases. For both types of training, learning may occur with only a single training trial in which shock is delivered in a specific place in an apparatus. The critical difference appears not to be behavioral contingency on training but, rather, the way in which memory of the training is assessed. Freezing typically is used as the measure for contextual fear conditioning whereas latency to enter the place where shock was received typically is used as the inhibitory avoidance measure. As 'place' learning is acquired rapidly and response learning typically requires extensive training (e.g. Packard and McGaugh, 1996), it is highly unlikely that inhibitory avoidance is based on the learning of an instrumental response. Just as the learning of contextual fear conditioning based on a single training trial occurs too quickly to be based on instrumental conditioning (Fanselow, 1980), the learning of inhibitory avoidance based on a single training trial also occurs too quickly to be based on learning of an instrumental response. Additionally, post-training treatments affecting the amygdala have comparable effects on memory for inhibitory avoidance training and contextual fear conditioning. For example, recent findings indicate that rats' memory for Pavlovian contextual fear conditioning is impaired by post-training intra-BLA infusions of lidocaine and, equally importantly, enhanced by infusions of oxotremorine (Vazdarjanova and McGaugh, 1999). Comparable findings were obtained previously in studies using inhibitory avoidance training (Parent and McGaugh, 1994; Introini-Collison *et al.*, 1996). These findings very clearly indicate that the BLA has a comparable role in regulating memory storage for fear conditioning and inhibitory avoidance learning, and thus provide additional evidence that the learning resulting from the two types of training is based on the same processes.

Experiments examining the effects of post-training intra-BLA infusions on fear-based learning do not, of course, directly address the issue of whether or not the memory of the shock experience, including the knowledge of *where* the shock was experienced, is located in neural changes within the amygdala. Such experiments very clearly are not designed to address that issue. The findings merely indicate that such post-training treatments modulate, i.e. enhance or impair, such memory and thus provide additional evidence that the two types of training, fear conditioning and inhibitory avoidance, have common neural bases. Other experiments have addressed more explicitly the issue of the locus of the modulatory influences on the consolidation of long-term memory. Extensive evidence suggests that the amygdala regulates memory consolidation occurring in other brain regions. The amygdala projects directly to many brain regions including the striatum, via the stria terminalis. Furthermore, the finding that stimulation of the amygdala induces expression of the proto-oncogene c-*fos* in the dentate gyrus of the dorsal hippocampus and the caudate nucleus indicates that the amygdala is functionally connected with these brain structures (Packard *et al.*, 1995). Substantial evidence from 'double-dissociation' studies indicates that the caudate nucleus and hippocampus are involved in mediating different forms of memory (Packard and McGaugh, 1992, 1996; McDonald and White, 1993). Hippocampal lesions selectively impair water maze spatial learning (swimming to a submerged platform) (Morris *et al.*, 1982; Moser *et al.*, 1993), whereas caudate lesions selectively impair water maze visually cued learning (swimming to a visible platform) (Packard and McGaugh, 1992).

The findings of several studies indicate that the amygdala modulates memory consolidation in both

hippocampal-dependent and caudate nucleus-dependent learning tasks (Packard *et al.*, 1994; Packard and Teather, 1998). Unilateral post-training infusions of amphetamine administered into the dorsal hippocampus immediately after a single training session enhanced memory storage for a spatial, but not for a cued, version of the water maze. In contrast, amphetamine infused into the caudate nucleus after training selectively enhanced memory for a cued task. However, amphetamine injected into the amygdala post-training enhanced memory in both the spatial and the cued versions of the task. Of particular importance was the finding that inactivation of the amygdala prior to the retention test did not block the enhanced retention induced by the intra-amygdala infusions of amphetamine (Packard *et al.*, 1994; Packard and Teather, 1998). The finding that an intact amygdala is not required for the retention of the spatial or cued training clearly indicates that the amygdala is not the locus of the memory of the training.

Recent findings from our laboratory provide additional evidence indicating that the BLA plays a role in enabling the processing of hippocampal-dependent memory consolidation (Roozendaal *et al.*, 1998). Post-training intra-hippocampal administration of a glucocorticoid receptor agonist enhanced retention of inhibitory avoidance training. However, in animals with BLA lesions, the memory enhancement was completely blocked (Roozendaal and McGaugh, 1997b). Additionally, intra-BLA infusions of the β-receptor antagonist atenolol blocked the memory-enhancing effects of the glucocorticoid agonist infused into the hippocampus. (Roozendaal *et al.*, 1999b).

Highly comparable findings have been obtained in studies examining BLA influences on *in vivo* hippocampal long-term potentiation. Selective lesions of the BLA or infusions of a β-adrenergic antagonist into the BLA attenuate the induction of long-term potentiation in the dentate gyrus (Ikegaya *et al.*, 1994, 1995a, 1997). Also, stimulation of the BLA facilitates the induction of long-term potentiation in the dentate gyrus (Ikegaya *et al.*, 1995b). These findings are consistent with those of behavioral studies indicating that modulation of memory storage involves noradrenergic influences in the BLA and that the BLA influences memory by modulating memory storage in other brain structures.

In the studies cited above, the effects of intra-hippocampal infusions of a glucocorticoid receptor agonist on memory consolidation as well as the effects of electrical stimulation of the hippocampus on long-term potentiation were blocked only by treatments affecting the ipsilateral BLA. Thus, the effects are likely to be due to neural connections between the BLA and hippocampus and not to influences mediated by non-specific effects of BLA stimulation. Although the pathway(s) through which the BLA affects hippocampal memory and neuroplasticity are not known, some evidence suggests an involvement of projections from the BLA to the nucleus accumbens via the stria terminalis. The nucleus accumbens also receives a projection from the hippocampus (O'Donnell and Grace, 1995). As discussed above, lesions of the stria terminalis, like lesions of the BLA or large amygdala lesions, block the effects of glucocorticoids and adrenaline on memory consolidation. The finding that lesions of the nucleus accumbens also block the memory-modulating effects of post-training systemic injections of dexamethasone (Setlow *et al.*, 2000) supports the view that the BLA–nucleus accumbens pathway may mediate BLA influences on memory that involve the hippocampus.

As it seems likely that long-term memory is represented ultimately in cortical regions, it will be important to investigate the direct as well as indirect influences of the BLA on cortical activity. Recent findings by Quirk and colleagues (Quirk *et al.*, 1997) provide evidence that a functional connection between the amygdala and cortex may be important for learning. These investigators recorded unit activity in the lateral amygdala and auditory cortex of rats given fear conditioning and extinction, and found that training-induced changes in cell firing in the auditory cortex generally occurred after those seen in the amygdala. Furthermore, during extinction, the amygdala units extinguished relatively rapidly, whereas responses of the cortical units persisted. Such findings are consistent with the hypothesis that the amygdala plays a time-limited role in modulating memory storage processes in the cortex (Cahill and McGaugh, 1998).

INVOLVEMENT OF β-ADRENERGIC ACTIVATION AND THE AMYGDALA IN HUMAN MEMORY

The findings of several studies of memory in human subjects support evidence from animal studies indicating that drugs affecting the noradrenergic system modulate memory storage and that such effects involve the amygdala. As noted above, there is extensive evidence from animal experiments that post-training systemic (or intra-amygdala) adminis-

tration of amphetamine enhances memory storage (McGaugh, 1973; Packard *et al.*, 1994). Comparable results have been obtained in studies with human subjects. Soetens and colleagues (1993, 1995) found that administration of amphetamine to human subjects before or immediately after they learned lists of words enhanced long-term retention of the words. Other recent experiments examined the effects of β-adrenergic antagonists on memory in human subjects. Cahill and colleagues (1994) examined the effect of the β-adrenergic antagonist propranolol on long-term (i.e. 1 week) memory for either an emotionally arousing story or a more emotionally neutral story. Propranolol selectively impaired memory for the arousing portion of the emotionally arousing story. These findings were replicated in a subsequent study (van Stegeren *et al.*, 1998). Additionally, that study found that nadolol, a β-adrenergic antagonist that does not readily cross the blood–brain barrier, did not affect memory. Thus, the impairing effect of propranolol appears to be due to blocking of central β-adrenergic receptors. However, the findings of van Stegeren *et al.* (1998) leave open the possibility that nadolol might well impair memory for more highly emotionally arousing material. In another study, Nielson and Jensen (1994) found that, in elderly subjects, β-adrenergic antagonists blocked the enhanced memory induced by physical arousal (i.e. increased muscle tension).

Amygdala functioning is also implicated in the enhanced memory induced by emotional arousal in humans. In experiments using the same general procedures as used in the experiment by Cahill *et al.* (1994), emotional arousal did not enhance memory in humans with selective, bilateral amygdala lesions (Cahill *et al.*, 1995; Adolphs *et al.*, 1997). In contrast to the memory effects seen in subjects with damaged amygdalae, memory for emotionally arousing material is enhanced in amnesic subjects with intact amygdalae (Hamann *et al.*, 1997ab). The findings of a positron emission tomography (PET) scan study of memory in human subjects provide further evidence that the amygdala is involved in emotionally influenced memory (Cahill *et al.*, 1996). Subjects in this experiment viewed a series of brief, emotionally arousing videos and, in a second session, a series of relatively emotionally neutral videos. Memory of the videos was assessed with a surprise free-recall test 3 weeks later. PET activity (i.e. glucose metabolic rate) of the right amygdala induced by viewing the emotional film clips correlated highly (+0.93) with the number of films recalled on the retention test.

The 'memory modulation' hypothesis of amygdala function predicts amygdala participation in memory formation for emotionally *arousing* events, either positive or negative (Cahill and McGaugh, 1990, 1998). This view is confirmed by another recent PET study (Hamann *et al.*, 1999). Amygdala activity induced by viewing either pleasant or unpleasant emotionally arousing pictures correlated significantly with memory for the pictures 1 month later. Amygdala activity induced while viewing emotionally neutral pictures (including pictures of novel objects) did not correlate with recall. Such findings fit well with the hypothesis that the amygdala functions selectively to influence memory for emotionally arousing experiences (see also Alkire *et al.*, 1998). Interestingly, in the Hamann *et al.* study (1999), hippocampal activity as measured by PET activation also correlated with memory for both types of arousing pictures as well as with memory for pictures of novel objects. Taken together, these findings are consistent with the view that the amygdala modulates hippocampal region functioning in memory (Packard *et al.*, 1994; Cahill and McGaugh, 1998; Packard and Teather, 1998).

Two recent studies using brain functional magnetic resonance imaging (fMRI) techniques to study changes induced by classical fear conditioning in human subjects reported additional evidence indicating the involvement of the amygdala early in conditioning. The findings of LaBar and colleagues (1998) suggested that 'The amygdala, may preferentially signal the detection of affective signals when they are novel, or in the initial stages of learning when their emotional meaning is actively encoded' (LaBar *et al.*, 1998, p. 940). Buchel and colleagues (1998) found habituation in the lateral amygdala nucleus during continued activation of cortical areas. On the basis of these findings, they suggested that, '…with time, mnemonic representations of behaviorally salient contexts are expressed in cortical regions other than medial temporal lobe structures' (Buchel *et al.*, 1998, p. 954; see also Dolan, Chapter 17). Collectively, the findings of studies investigating the involvement of the amygdala in human memory provide additional support for the hypothesis that the amygdala plays a temporally limited role in modulating memory storage occurring elsewhere in the brain (McGaugh *et al.*, 1984, 1996; McGaugh, 1989c; Packard *et al.*, 1995; Cahill and McGaugh, 1998).

CONCLUSIONS

The findings of our studies, like those of Gabriel Horn and his colleagues (1985, 1998), emphasize the importance of understanding the differential roles of neuromodulatory systems and brain systems in orchestrating the storage of information in the brain. An understanding of how the brain enables memory will thus require additional focus on the interactions among these systems as well as the processes by which these systems regulate the cellular machinery underlying memory storage.

ACKNOWLEDGEMENTS

This research was supported by USPHS grants MH12526 (J.L.M.) and MH57508 (L.C.) from the National Institute of Mental Health, and an R.W. and Leona Gerard Family Trust Fellowship (L.C., B.F. and B.R.).

REFERENCES

Adolphs, R., Cahill, L., Schul, R. and Babinsky, R. (1997) Impaired declarative memory for emotional stimuli following bilateral amygdala damage in humans. *Learning and Memory*, 4, 291–300.

Alkire, M.T., Haier, R.J. Fallon, J.F. and Cahill, L.F. (1998) Hippocampal, but not amygdala, activity at encoding correlates with long-term, free recall of nonemotional information. *Proceedings of the National Academy of Sciences of the United States of America*, 95, 14506–14510.

Ammassari-Teule, M., Pavone, F., Castellano, C. and McGaugh, J.L. (1991) Amygdala and dorsal hippocampus lesions block the effects of GABAergic drugs on memory storage. *Brain Research*, 551, 104–109.

Arbilla, S. and Langer, S.Z. (1978) Morphine and beta-endorphin inhibit release of noradrenaline from cerebral cortex but not of dopamine from rat striatum. *Nature*, 271, 559–561.

Bohus, B. (1994) Humoral modulation of memory processes. Physiological significance of brain and peripheral mechanisms. In: Delacour, J. (ed.), *The Memory System of the Brain*. Advanced Series of Neuroscience, Vol. 4. World Scientific, New Jersey, pp. 337–364.

Borrell, J., de Kloet, E.R., Versteeg, D.H.G. and Bohus, B. (1983) Inhibitory avoidance deficit following short-term adrenalectomy in the rat: the role of adrenal catecholamines. *Behavioral and Neural Biology*, 39, 241–258.

Borrell, J., de Kloet, E.R. and Bohus, B. (1984) Corticosterone decreases the efficacy of adrenaline to affect passive avoidance retention of adrenalectomized rats. *Life Sciences*, 34, 99–105.

Breen, R.A. and McGaugh, J.L. (1961) Facilitation of maze learning with posttrial injections of picrotoxin. *Journal of Comparative and Physiological Psychology*, 54, 498–501.

Brioni, J.D. and McGaugh, J.L. (1988) Posttraining administration of GABAergic antagonists enhance retention of aversively motivated tasks. *Psychopharmacology*, 96, 505–510.

Brioni, J.D., Nagahara, A.H. and McGaugh, J.L. (1989) Involvement of the amygdala GABAergic system in the modulation of memory storage. *Brain Research*, 487, 105–112.

Buchel, C., Morris, J., Dolan, R.J. and Friston, K.J. (1998) Brain systems mediating aversive conditioning, an event-related fMRI study. *Neuron*, 20, 947–957.

Bussey, T.J., Muir, J.L. and Aggleton, J.P. (1999) Functionally dissociating aspects of event memory, the effects of combined perirhinal and postrhinal cortex lesions on object and place memory in the rat. *Journal of Neuroscience*, 19, 495–502.

Cahill, L. (1996) The neurobiology of memory for emotional events. Converging evidence from infra-human and human studies. *Cold Spring Harbor Symposia on Quaitative Biology*, 61, 259–264.

Cahill, L. and McGaugh, J.L. (1990) Amygdaloid complex lesions differentially affect retention of tasks using appetitive and aversive reinforcement. *Behavioral Neuroscience*, 104, 532–543.

Cahill, L. and McGaugh, J.L. (1991) NMDA-induced lesions of the amygdaloid complex block the retention enhancing effect of posttraining epinephrine. *Psychobiology*, 19, 206–210.

Cahill, L. and McGaugh, J.L. (1998) Mechanisms of emotional arousal and lasting declarative memory. *Trends in Neurosciences*, 21, 294–299.

Cahill, L., Prins, B., Weber, M. and McGaugh, J.L. (1994) Beta-adrenergic activation and memory for emotional events. *Nature*, 371, 702–704.

Cahill, L., Babinsky, R., Markowitsch, H. and McGaugh, J.L. (1995) The amygdala and emotional memory. *Nature*, 377, 295–296.

Cahill, L., Weinberger, N.M., Roozendaal, B. and McGaugh, J.L. (1999) Is the amygdala a locus of 'conditioned fear'? Some questions and caveats. *Neuron*, 23, 227–228.

Cahill, L., Haier, R.J.F., Alkire, M., Tang, C., Keator, D., Wu, J. and McGaugh, J.L. (1996) Amygdala activity at encoding correlated with long-term, free recall of emotional information. *Proceedings of the National Academy of Sciences of the United States of America*, 93, 8016–8021.

Clark, K.B., Krahl, S.E., Smith, D.C. and Jensen, R.A. (1995) Post-training unilateral vagal stimulation enhances retention performance in the rat. *Neurobiology of Learning and Memory*, 63, 213–216.

Clark, K.B., Naritoku, D.K., Smith, D.C., Browning, R.A. and Jensen, R.A. (1999) Enhanced recognition memory following vagus nerve stimulation in human subjects. *Nature Neuroscience*, 2, 94–98.

Cottrell, G.A. and Nakajima, S. (1977) Effects of corticosteroids in the hippocampus on passive avoidance behavior in the rat. *Pharmacology, Biochemistry and Behavior*, 7, 277–280.

Da Cunha, C., Roozendaal, B., Vazdarjanova, A. and McGaugh, J.L. (1999) Microinfusions of flumazenil into the basolateral but not central nucleus of the amygdala enhance memory consolidation in rats. *Neurobiology of Learning and Memory*, 72, 1–7.

Daly, J.W., Padgett, W., Creveling, C.R., Cantacuzene, D. and Kirk, K.L. (1981) Cyclic AMP-generating systems: regional differences in activation by adrenergic receptors in rat brain. *Journal of Neuroscience*, 1, 49–59.

de Kloet, E.R. (1991) Brain corticosteroid receptor balance and homeostatic control. *Frontiers in Neuroendocrinology*, 12, 95–164.

de Souza-Silva, M.A. and Tomaz, C. (1995) Amnesia after diazepam infusion into basolateral but not central amygdala of *Rattus norvegicus*. *Neuropsychobiology*, 32, 31–36.

Eichenbaum, H. (1996) Is the rodent hippocampus just for space? *Current Opinions in Neurobiology*, 6, 187–195.

Fanselow, M.S. (1980) Conditional and unconditional components of post-shock freezing. *Pavlovian Journal of Biological Science*, 15, 177–182.

Ferry, B., Roozendaal, B. and McGaugh, J.L. (1999a) Involvement of α_1-adrenergic receptors in the basolateral amygdala in modulation of memory storage. *European Journal of Pharmacology*, 372, 9–16.

Ferry, B., Roozendaal, B. and McGaugh, J.L. (1999b) Basolateral amygdala noradrenergic influences on memory storage are mediated by an interaction between β- and α_1-receptors. *Journal of Neuroscience*, 19, 5119–5123.

Fuster, J.M. (1995) *Memory in the Cerebral Cortex. An Empirical Approach to the Neural Networks in the Human and Nonhuman Primate*. MIT Press, Cambridge, Massachusetts.

Fuster, J.M. (1998) Distributed memory for both short and long term. *Neurobiology of Learning and Memory*, 70, 268–274.

Galvez, R., Mesches, M. and McGaugh, J.L. (1996) Norepinephrine release in the amygdala in response to footshock stimulation. *Neurobiology of Learning and Memory*, 66, 253–257.

Gold, P.E. and van Buskirk, R. (1975) Facilitation of time-dependent memory processes with posttrial epinephrine injections. *Behavioral Biology*, 13, 145–153.

Hamann, S.B., Cahill, L., McGaugh, J.L. and Squire, L.R (1997a) Intact enhancement of declarative memory for emotional material in amnesia. *Learning and Memory*, 4, 301–309.

Hamman, S.B., Cahill, L. and Squire, L.R. (1997b) Emotional perception and memory in amnesia. *Neuropsychology* 11, 1–10.

Hamann, S., Ely, T., Grafton, S. and Kilts, C. (1999) Amygdala activity related to enhanced memory for pleasant and aversive stimuli. *Nature Neuroscience*, 2, 289–293.

Harfstrand, A., Fuxe, K., Cintra, A., Agnati, L., Mzini, L., Wikstrom, A.C., Okret, S., Yu, Z.Y., Goldstein, M., Steinbusch, H., Verhofstad, A. and Gustafsson, J.-A. (1986) Glucocorticoid receptor immunoreactivity in monoaminergic neurons of rat brain. *Proceedings of the National Academy of Science of the United States of America*, 83, 9779–9783.

Hatfield, T. and McGaugh, J.L. (1999) Norepinephrine infused into the basolateral amygdala posttraining enhances retention in a spatial water maze task. *Neurobiology of Learning and Memory*, 71, 232–239.

Hatfield, T., Spanis, C. and McGaugh, J.L. (1999) Response of amygdalar norepinephrine to footshock and GABAergic drugs using *in vivo* microdialysis and HPLC. *Brain Research*, 835, 340–345.

Hikosaka, O., Miyashita, K., Miyachi, S., Sakai, K. and Lu, X. (1998) Differential roles of the frontal cortex, basal ganglia and cerebellum in visuomotor sequence learning. *Neurobiology of Learning and Memory*, 70, 137–149.

Horn, G. (1985) *Memory, Imprinting and the Brain*. Clarendon Press, Oxford.

Horn, G. (1998) Visual imprinting and the neural mechanisms of recognition memory. *Trends in Neurosciences*, 21, 300–305.

Ikegaya, Y., Saito, H. and Abe, K. (1994) Attenuated hippocampal long-term potentiation in basolateral amygdala-lesioned rats. *Brain Research*, 656, 157–164.

Ikegaya, Y., Saito, H. and Abe, K. (1995a) Requirement of basolateral amygdala neuron activity for the induction of long-term potentiation in the dentate gyrus *in vivo*. *Brain Research*, 671, 351–354.

Ikegaya, Y., Saito, H. and Abe, K. (1995b) High-frequency stimulation of the basolateral amygdala facilitates the induction of long-term potentiation in the dentate gyrus *in vivo*. *Neuroscience Research*, 22, 203–207.

Ikegaya, Y., Saito, H. Abe, K. and Nakanishi, K. (1997) Amygdala β-noradrenergic influence on hippocampal long-term potentiation *in vivo*. *NeuroReport*, 8, 3143–3146.

Introini-Collison, I.B. and McGaugh, J.L. (1986) Interaction of adrenergic, cholinergic and opioid systems in modulation of memory storage. *Society for Neuroscience Abstracts*, 12, 710.

Introini-Collison, I.B., Nagahara, A.H. and McGaugh, J.L. (1989) Memory-enhancement with intra-amygdala post-training naloxone is blocked by concurrent administration of propranolol. *Brain Research*, 476, 94–101.

Introini-Collison, I., Miyazaki, B. and McGaugh, J.L. (1991) Involvement of the amygdala in the memory-enhancing effects of clenbuterol. *Psychopharmacology*, 104, 541–544.

Introini-Collison, I., Saghafi, D., Novack, G. and McGaugh, J.L. (1992) Memory-enhancing effects of posttraining dipivefrin and epinephrine. Involvement of peripheral and central adrenergic receptors. *Brain Research*, 572, 81–86.

Introini-Collison, I., Dalmaz, C. and McGaugh, J.L. (1996) Amygdala—noradrenergic influences on memory storage involve cholinergic activation. *Neurobiology of Learning and Memory*, 65, 57–64.

Izquierdo, I. and Diaz, R.D. (1983) Effect of ACTH, epinephrine, β-endorphin, naloxone and of the combination of naloxone or β-endorphin with ACTH or epinephrine on memory consolidation. *Psychoneuroendocrinology*, 8, 81–87.

Izquierdo, I., DaCunha, C., Huang, C.H., Walz, R., Wolfman, C. and Medina, J.H. (1990a) Post-training down regulation of memory consolidation by a GABA-A mechanism in the amygdala modulated by endogenous benzodiazepines. *Behavioral and Neural Biology*, 54, 105–109.

Izquierdo, I., DaCunha, C. and Medina, J. (1990b) Endogenous benzodiazepine modulation of memory processes. *Neuroscience and Biobehavioral Reviews*, 14, 419–424.

Kesner, R.P. and Wilburn, M. (1974) A review of electrical stimulation of the brain in the context of learning and retention. *Behavioral Biology*, 10, 259–293.

Kim, J.J. and Fanselow, M.S. (1992) Modality-retrograde amnesia of fear. *Science*, 256, 675–677.

Lashley, K.S. (1950) In search of the engram. *Symposium for Experimental Biology*, 4, 454–482.

LaBar, K.S., Gatenby, J.C., Gore, J.C., LeDoux, J.E. and Phelps, E.A. (1998) Human amygdala activation during conditioned fear acquisition and extinction: a mixed trial fMRI study. *Neuron*, 20, 937–945.

LeDoux, J.E. (1995) Emotion: clues from the brain. *Annual Review of Psychology*, 46, 209–235.

LeDoux, J. (1998) Fear and the brain: where have we been and where are we going. *Biological Psychiatry*, 44, 1229–1238.

Lehmann, H., Treit, D. and Parent, M.B. (2000) Amygdala lesions do not impair shock-probe avoidance retention performance. *Behavioral Neuroscience*, 114, 107–116.

Liang, K.C. and McGaugh, J.L. (1983) Lesions of the stria terminalis attenuate the enhancing effect of posttraining epinephrine on retention of an inhibitory avoidance response. *Behavioural Brain Research*, 9, 49–58.

Liang, K.C., Bennett, C. and McGaugh, J.L. (1985) Peripheral epinephrine modulates the effects of posttraining amygdala stimulation on memory. *Behavioural Brain Research*, 15, 93–100.

Liang, K.C., Juler, R. and McGaugh, J.L. (1986) Modulating effects of posttraining epinephrine on memory: involvement of the amygdala noradrenergic system. *Brain Research*, 368, 125–133.

Liang, K.C., McGaugh, J.L. and Yao, H. (1990) Involvement of amygdala pathways in the influence of posttraining amygdala norepinephrine and peripheral epinephrine on memory storage. *Brain Research*, 508, 225–233.

Liang, K., Chen, L. and Huang, T.-E. (1995) The role of amygdala norepinephrine in memory formation: involvement in the memory enhancing effect of peripheral epinephrine. *Chinese Journal of Physiology*, 38, 81–91.

Lupien, S.J. and McEwen, B.S. (1997) The acute effects of corticosteroids on cognition: integration of animal and human model studies. *Brain Research Review*, 24, 1–27.

Maren, S. and Fanselow, M. (1996) The amygdala and fear conditioning: has the nut been cracked? *Neuron*, 16, 237–240.

Maren, S., Aharonov, G. and Fanselow, M.S. (1996) Retrograde abolition of conditional fear after excitotoxic lesions in the basolateral amygdala of rats: absence of a temporal gradient. *Behavioral Neuroscience*, 110, 718–726.

McCarty, R. and Gold, P.E. (1981) Plasma catecholamines: effects of footshock level and hormonal modulators of memory storage. *Hormones and Behavior*, 15, 168–182.

McDonald,R.J. and White, N.M. (1993) A triple dissociation of memory systems: hippocampus, amygdala and dorsal striatum. *Behavioral Neuroscience*, 107, 3–22.

McEwen, B.S. and Sapolsky, R.M. (1995) Stress and cognitive function, *Current Opinions in Neurobiology*, 5, 205–216.

McGaugh, J.L. (1966) Time-dependent processes in memory storage. *Science*, 153, 1351–1358.

McGaugh, J.L. (1968) Drug facilitation of memory and learning. In: *Psychopharmacology: A Review of Progress*. PHS Publication 1836, US Government Printing Office, Washington, DC, pp. 891–904.

McGaugh, J.L. (1973) Drug facilitation of learning and memory. *Annual Review of Pharmacology*, 13, 229–241.

McGaugh, J.L. (1989a) Dissociating learning and performance. Drug and hormone enhancement of memory storage. *Brain Research Bulletin*, 23, 339–345.

McGaugh, J.L. (1989b) Involvement of hormonal and neuromodulatory systems in the regulation of memory storage. *Annual Review of Neuroscience*, 12, 255–287.

McGaugh, J.L. (1989c) Modulation of memory storage processes. In: Solomon, P.R., Goethels, G.R., Kelly, C.M. and

Stevens, B.R. (eds), *Memory: Interdisciplinary Approaches.* Springer Verlag, New York, pp. 33–64.

McGaugh, J.L. (2000) Memory–a century of consolidation. *Science,* 287, 248–251.

McGaugh, J.L. and Gold, P.E. (1976) Modulation of memory by electrical stimulation of the brain. In: Rosenzweig, M.R. and Bennett, E.L. (eds), *Neural Mechanisms of Learning and Memory.* MIT Press, Cambridge, Massachusetts, pp. 549–560.

McGaugh, J.L. and Gold, P.E. (1989) Hormonal modulation of memory. In: Brush, R.B. and Levine, S. (eds), *Psychoendocrinology.* Academic Press, New York, pp. 305–339.

McGaugh, J.L. and Herz, M.J. (1972) *Memory Consolidation.* Albion, San Francisco.

McGaugh, J.L., Liang, K.C., Bennett, C. and Sternberg, D.B. (1984) Adrenergic influences on memory storage: interaction of peripheral and central systems. In: Lynch, G., McGaugh, J.L. and Weinberger, N.M. (eds), *Neurobiology of Learning and Memory.* The Guilford Press, New York, pp. 313–333.

McGaugh, J.L., Introini-Collison, I.B., Juler, R.G. and Izquierdo, I. (1986) Stria terminalis lesions attenuate the effects of posttraining naloxone and β-endorphin on retention. *Behavioral Neuroscience,* 100, 839–844

McGaugh, J.L., Introini-Collison, I.B. and Nagahara, A.H. (1988) Memory-enhancing effects of posttraining naloxone: involvement of β-noradrenergic influences in the amygdaloid complex. *Brain Research,* 446, 37–49.

McGaugh, J.L., Introini-Collison, I. and Castellano, C. (1993) Involvement of opioid peptides in learning and memory. In: Herz, A., Akil, H. and Simon, E.J. (eds), *Handbook of Experimental Pharmacology, Opioids, Part I and II.* Springer-Verlag, Heidelberg, pp. 419–477.

McGaugh, J.L., Cahill, L. and Roozendaal, B. (1996) Involvement of the amygdala in memory storage: interaction with other brain systems. *Proceedings of the National Academy of Sciences of the United States of America,* 93, 13508–13514.

Milner, B. (1966) Amnesia following operation on the temporal lobes. In: Whitty, C.W.M. and Zangwill, O.L. eds), *Amnesia.* Butterworths, London, pp. 109–133.

Morris, R.G.M., Garrud, P., Rawlins, J.N.P. and O'Keefe, J. (1982) Place navigation impaired in rats with hippocampal lesions. *Nature,* 297, 681–683.

Moser, E., Moser, M.-B. and Andersen, P. (1993) Spatial learning impairment parallels the magnitude of dorsal hippocampal lesions, but is hardly present following ventral lesions. *Journal of Neuroscience,* 13, 3916–3925.

Mueller, G.E. and Pilzecker, A. (1900) Experimentelle Beiträge zur Lehre vom Gedächtniss. *Zeitschrift für Psychologie,* 1, 1–288.

Nielson,K. and Jensen, R. (1994) Beta-adrenergic receptor antagonist antihypertensive medications impair arousal-induced modulation of working memory in elderly humans. *Behavioral and Neural Biology,* 62, 190–200.

O'Donnell, P. and Grace, A.A. (1995) Synaptic interactions among excitatory afferents to nucleus accumbens neurons: hippocampal gating of prefrontal cortical input. *Journal of Neuroscience,* 15, 3622–3639.

Oitzl, M.S. and de Kloet, E.R. (1992) Selective corticosteroid antagonists modulate specific aspects of spacial orientation learning. *Behavioral Neuroscience,* 106, 62–71.

Packard, M.G. and McGaugh, J.L. (1992) Double dissociation of fornix and caudate nucleus lesions on acquisition of two water maze tasks, further evidence for multiple memory systems. *Behavioral Neuroscience,* 106, 439–446.

Packard, M.G. and McGaugh, J.L. (1996) Inactivation of hippocampus or caudate nucleus with lidocaines differentially affects expression of place and response learning. *Neurobiology of Learning and Memory,* 65, 65–72.

Packard, M.G., Cahill, L. and McGaugh, J.L. (1994) Amygdala modulation of hippocampal-dependent and caudate nucleus-dependent memory processes. *Proceedings of the National Academy of Sciences of the United States of America,* 91, 8477–8481.

Packard, M.G., Williams, C., Cahill, L. and McGaugh, J.L. (1995) The anatomy of a memory modulatory system, from periphery to brain. In: Spear, N. Spear, L. and Woodruff, M. (eds), *Neurobehavioral Plasticity, Learning, Development and Response to Brain Insults.* Lawrence Erlbaum Associates, Hillsdale, New Jersey, pp. 149–184.

Packard, M.G. and Teather, L. (1998) Amygdala modulation of multiple memory systems, hippocampus and caudate-putamen. *Neurobiology of Learning and Memory,* 69, 163–203.

Parent, M. and McGaugh, J.L. (1994) Posttraining infusion of lidocaine into the amygdala basolateral complex impairs retention of inhibitory avoidance training. *Brain Research,* 661, 97–103.

Parent, M., Tomaz, C. and McGaugh, J.L. (1992) Increased training in an aversively motivated task attenuates the memory impairing effects of posttraining N-methyl-D-aspartic acid-induced amygdala lesions. *Behavioral Neuroscience,* 106, 791–799.

Parent, M., West, M. and McGaugh, J.L. (1994) Memory of rats with amygdala lesions induced 30 days after foot-shock-motivated escape training reflects degree of original training. *Behavioral Neuroscience,* 6, 1080–1087.

Parent, M., Avila, E. and McGaugh, J.L. (1995) Footshock facilitates the expression of aversively motivated memory in rats given post-training amygdala basolateral complex lesions. *Brain Research,* 676, 235–244.

Perkins, J.P. and Moore, M.M. (1973) Characterization of the adrenergic receptors mediating a rise in cyclic 3',5'-adenosine monophosphate in rat cerebral cortex. *Journal of Pharmacology and Experimental Therapeutics,* 185, 371–378.

Pfeuffer, T. (1977) GTP-binding proteins in membranes and the control of adenylate cyclase activity. *Journal of Biology and Chemistry,* 252, 7224–7234.

Quirarte, G.L., Roozendaal, B. and McGaugh, J.L. (1997a) Glucocorticoid enhancement of memory storage involves noradrenergic activation in the basolateral amygdala. *Proceedings of the National Academy of Sciences of the United States of America,* 94, 14048–14053.

Quirarte, G.L., Roozendaal, B. and McGaugh, J.L. (1997b) Glucocorticoid receptor antagonist infused into the basolateral amygdala inhibits the memory enhancing effects of the noradrenergic agonist infused clenbuterol. *Society for Neuroscience Abstracts,* 1314.

Quirarte, G.L., Galvez, R., Roozendaal, B. and McGaugh, J.L. (1998) Norepinephrine release in the amygdala in response to footshock and opioid peptidergic drugs. *Brain Research,* 808, 134–140.

Quirk, G.J., Armony, J.L. and LeDoux, J.E. (1997) Fear conditioning enhances different temporal components of tone-evoked spike trains in auditory cortex and lateral amygdala. *Neuron*, 19, 613–624.

Ricardo, J. and Koh, E. (1978) Anatomical evidence of direct projections from the nucleus of the solitary tract to the hypothalamus, amygdala and other forebrain structures in the rat. *Brain Research*, 153, 1–26.

Roozendaal, B. and McGaugh, J.L. (1996a) Amygdaloid nuclei lesions differentially affect glucocorticoid-induced memory enhancement in an inhibitory avoidance task. *Neurobiology of Learning and Memory*, 65, 1–8.

Roozendaal, B. and McGaugh, J.L. (1996b) The memory-modulatory effects of glucocorticoids depend on an intact stria terminalis. *Brain Research*, 709, 243–350.

Roozendaal, B. and McGaugh, J.L. (1997a) Glucocorticoid receptor agonist and antagonist administration into the basolateral but not central amygdala modulates memory storage. *Neurobiology of Learning and Memory*, 67, 176–179.

Roozendaal, B. and McGaugh, J.L. (1997b) Basolateral amygdala lesions block the memory-enhancing effect of glucocorticoid administration in the dorsal hippocampus of rats. *European Journal of Neuroscience*, 9, 76–83.

Roozendaal, B., Koolhaas, J.M. and Bohus, B. (1992) Central amygdaloid involvement in neuroendocrine correlates of conditioned stress response. *Journal of Neuroendocrinology*, 4, 483–489.

Roozendaal, B., Koolhaas, J.M. and Bohus, B. (1993) Post-training norepinephrine infusion into the central amygdala differentially enhances later retention in Roman High-Avoidance and Low-Avoidance rats. *Behavioral Neuroscience*, 7, 575–579.

Roozendaal, B., Carmi, O. and McGaugh, J.L. (1996a) Adrenocortical suppression blocks the memory-enhancing effects of amphetamine and epinephrine. *Proceedings of the National Academy of Sciences of the United States of America*, 93, 1429–1433.

Roozendaal, B., Portillo-Marquez, G. and McGaugh, J.L. (1996b) Basolateral amygdala lesions block glucocorticoid-induced modulation of memory for spatial learning. *Behavioral Neuroscience*, 110, 1074–1083.

Roozendaal, B., Sapolsky, R. and McGaugh, J.L. (1998) Basolateral amygdala lesions block the disruptive effects of long-term adrenalectomy on spatial memory. *Neuroscience*, 84, 453–465.

Roozendaal, B., Williams, C.L. and McGaugh, J.L., (1999a) Glucocorticoid receptor activation of noradrenergic neurons within the rat nucleus of the solitary tract facilitates memory consolidation: involvement of the basolateral amygdala. *European Journal of Neuroscience*, 11, 1317–1323.

Roozendaal, B., Nguyen, B.T., Power, A. and McGaugh, J.L. (1999b) Basolateral amygdala noradrenergic influence enables enhancement of memory consolidation induced by hippocampal glucocorticoid receptor activation. *Proceedings of the National Academy of Sciences of the United States of America*, 96, 11642–11647.

Ross, E.M., Howlette, A.C., Ferguson, K.M. and Gilman, A.G. (1978) Reconstitution of hormone-sensitive adenylate cyclase activity with resolved components of the enzyme. *Journal of Biological Chemistry*. 253, 6401–6412.

Sakurai, Y. (1998) Cell assembly coding in several memory processes. *Neurobiology of Learning and Memory*, 70, 212–225.

Salinas, J. and McGaugh, J.L. (1995) Muscimol induces retrograde amnesia for changes in reward magnitude. *Neurobiology of Learning and Memory*, 63, 277–285.

Salinas, J. and McGaugh, J.L. (1996) The amygdala modulates memory for changes in reward magnitude, involvement of the amygdaloid GABAergic system. *Behavioural Brain Research*, 80, 87–98.

Salinas, J., Packard, M.G. and McGaugh, J.L. (1993) Amygdala modulates memory for changes in reward magnitude, reversible post-training inactivation with lidocaine attenuates the response to a reduction reward. *Behavioural Brain Research*, 59, 153–159.

Salinas, J., Introini-Collison, I.B., Dalmaz, C. and McGaugh, J.L. (1997) Posttraining intra-amygdala infusion of oxotremorine and propranolol modulate storage of memory for reduction in reward magnitude. *Neurobiology of Learning and Memory*, 68, 51–59.

Salmon, D.P. and Butters, N. (1995) Neurobiology of skill and habit learning. *Current Opinions in Neurobiology*, 5, 184–190.

Sandi, C. and Rose, S.P.R. (1994) Corticosterone enhances long-term retention in one day-old chicks trained in a week passive avoidance learning paradigm. *Brain Research*, 647, 106–112.

Schreurs, J., Seelig, T. and Schulman, H. (1986) β_2-Adrenergic receptors on peripheral nerves. *Journal of Neurochemistry*, 46, 294–296.

Setlow, B., Roozendaal, B. and McGaugh, J.L. (2000) Involvement of a basolateral amygdala complex–nucleus accumbens pathway in glucocorticoid-induced modulation of memory storage. *European Journal of Neuroscience*, 12, 367–375.

Soetens, E., D'Hooge, R. and Hueting, J.E. (1993) Amphetamine enhances human-memory consolidation. *Neuroscience Letters*, 161, 9–12.

Soetens, E., Casaer, S., D'Hooge, R. and Hueting, J.E. (1995) Effect of amphetamine on long-term retention of verbal material. *Psychopharmacology*, 119, 155–162.

Squire, L.R. and Alvarez, P. (1995) Retrograde amnesia and memory consolidation: a neurobiological perspective. *Current Opinions in Neurobiology*, 5, 169–177.

Starke, K. (1979) Presynaptic regulation of catecholamines release in the centrla nervous system. In: Paton, D.M. (ed.), *The Release of Catecholamines from Adrenergic Neurons*. Pergamon Press, New York, pp. 143–183.

Sternberg, D.B., Isaacs, K., Gold, P.E. and McGaugh, J.L. (1985) Epinephrine facilitation of appetitive learning: attenuation with adrenergic receptor antagonists. *Behavioral and Neural Biology*, 44, 447–453.

Thompson, R.F., Thompson, J.K., Kim, J.J., Krupa, D.J. and Shinkman, P.G. (1998) The nature of reinforcement in cerebellar learning. *Neurobiology of Learning and Memory*, 70, 150–176.

Tomaz, C., Dickinson-Anson, H. and McGaugh, J.L. (1992) Basolateral amygdala lesions block diazepam-induced anterograde amnesia in an inhibitory avoidance task. *Proceedings of the National Academy of Sciences of the United States of America*, 89, 3615–3619.

van Stegeren, A.H., Everaerd, W., Cahill, L., McGaugh, J.L. and Gooren, L.J.G. (1998) Memory for emotional events, differential effects of centrally versus peripherally acting beta-blocking agents. *Psychopharmacology*, 138, 305–310.

Vazdarjanova, A. and McGaugh, J.L. (1998) Basolateral amygdala is not a critical locus for memory of contextual fear conditioning. *Proceedings of the National Academy of Sciences of the United States of America*, 95, 15003–1507.

Vazdarjanova, A. and McGaugh, J.L. (1999) Basolateral amygdala is involved in modulating consolidation of memory for classical fear conditioning. *Journal of Neuroscience*, 19, 6615–6622.

Weinberger, N.M. (1998) Physiological memory in primary auditory cortex: characteristics and mechanisms. *Neurobiology of Learning and Memory*, 70, 226–251.

Weiner, N. (1985) Norepinephrine, epinephrine and the sympathomimetic amines. In: Gilman, A.G., Goodman, L.S., Rall, T.W. and Murad, F. (eds), *The Pharmacological Basis of Therapeutics*. Macmillan Publishing Company, New York, pp. 145–180.

Weingartner, H. and Parker, E.S. (1984) *Memory Consolidation*. Lawrence Erlbaum Associates, Hillsdale, New Jersey.

Williams, C.L. and McGaugh, J.L. (1993) Reversible lesions of the nucleus of the solitary tract attenuate the memory-modulating effects of posttraining epinephrine. *Behavioral Neuroscience*, 107, 1–8.

Williams, C.L., Men, D., Clayton, E.C. and Gold, P.E. (1998) Norepinephrine release in the amygdala following systemic injection of epinephrine or escapable footshock: contribution of the nucleus of the solitary tract. *Behavioral Neuroscience*, 112, 1414–1422.

Williams, G.V. and Goldman-Rakic, P.S. (1995) Modulation of memory fields by dopamine D1 receptors in prefrontal cortex. *Nature*, 376, 572–575.

Winocur, G. (1990) Anterograde and retrograde amnesia in rats with dorsal hippocampal or dorsomedial thalamic lesions. *Behavioural Brain Research*, 38, 145–154.

Zola-Morgan, S. and Squire, L.R. (1990) The primate hippocampal formation: evidence for a time-limited role in memory storage. *Science*, 250, 288–290.

Zola-Morgan, S., Squire, L.R., Amaral, D.G. and Suzuki, W.A. (1989) Lesions of perirhinal and parahippocampal cortex that spare the amygdala and hippocampal formation produce severe memory impairment. *Journal of Neuroscience*, 9, 4355–4370.

14 HOW THE BRAIN LEARNS ABOUT DANGER

Karim Nader and Joseph LeDoux

INTRODUCTION

Life is dangerous. Most animals live on both sides of the food chain and, to stay alive for even a day, it is essential that they be able to identify efficiently things that are likely to cause them harm. This is the job of the brain's fear system. The fear system is wired by evolution to respond to some stimuli, such as those that signal the presence of predators or other perennial sources of danger to the individual. For example, the very first time that a rat is exposed to a cat, even an anesthetized one, it crouches or freezes (Blanchard and Blanchard, 1971), a typical fear or defense response in rats (Bolles and Fanselow, 1980; Marks, 1987). However, not all dangers are hard-wired. Many of the things that cause harm have to be learned about. This is especially true in the lives of contemporary humans, who are seldom attacked by blood-thirsty beasts, but who nevertheless face threats of various kinds, including threats to personal or family well-being and social status. We can even learn to fear things that are harmless.

The manner in which the fear system learns about danger and stores the results for future reference has been studied extensively in recent years using a behavioral task called classical fear conditioning. In this chapter, we will briefly describe the view of how the fear system works that has emerged from fear-conditioning studies conducted over the past two decades, and then go on to consider some newer issues and controversies that have developed regarding the organization and functioning of this system.

WHAT IS FEAR CONDITIONING?

'Fear conditioning' can be used to refer to both a behavioral procedure that an experimenter employs and a process that occurs in the brain. The behavioral procedure is a tool for engaging the process, but, as noted above, the process is also engaged naturally

whenever an animal encounters danger. When we use artificial fear-conditioning tasks involving stimuli that an animal seldom encounters naturally, we nevertheless are tapping into the system that the brain normally uses to learn about dangerous stimuli.

In a typical fear-conditioning experiment, a relatively neutral stimulus, which does not elicit fear responses, can come to do so if it occurs prior to some painful or otherwise noxious event. In most fear-conditioning studies, footshock is used as the unconditional stimulus (US) that modifies the way in which the neutral conditional stimulus (CS), often a tone, is reacted to. A single pairing of the CS and US is often sufficient to allow the tone to acquire the capacity to elicit a full spectrum of defensive responses, including behavioral reactions such as crouching and changes in body physiology (Figure 14.1; Fanselow and Bolles, 1979; LeDoux, 1996).

Most studies use a variant called forward conditioning, where the onset of the US follows the onset of the CS. With this procedure, the CS reliably comes to elicit defensive responses. In contrast, when US occurs prior to CS onset, so-called backward conditioning, the likelihood of the CS eliciting defense responses is lower, and the responses, when they occur, are weaker. Thus, the fear system is most sensitive to cues that predict future dangerous events. However, through independent tests, it can be shown that even when behavioral responses are not expressed explicitly to the CS after backward conditioning, the association between the CS and US is present (e.g. Matzel et al., 1988).

ORGANIZATION OF THE FEAR-CONDITIONING SYSTEM

Studies over the past two decades from several different laboratories using different species, different kinds of stimuli as CSs and measuring different conditioned responses have led to a common conclusion:

A

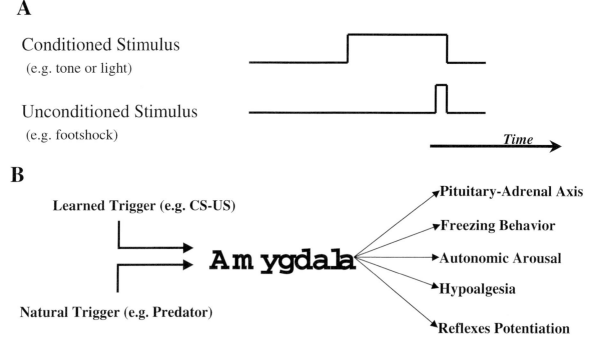

Figure 14.1. (**A**) The fear-conditioning paradigm entails presenting a neutral CS which co-terminates with footshock. (**B**) Natural and learned triggers (such as a CS that had been paired with footshock) require the integrity of a structure called the amygdala in order to engage defensive responses. Note that both triggers elicit similar spectra of behaviors.

the amygdala is a key structure in the neural system underlying fear conditioning (Kapp *et al.*, 1992; Davis *et al.*, 1994; LeDoux, 1996; Maren and Fanselow, 1996). Positioned along neural paths in such a way as to link sensory systems processing the CS and the motor systems controlling the conditioned fear responses, the amygdala is the centerpiece of the fear system. Much has been learned about how the amygdala performs the sensory–learning–motor linkages that constitute fear conditioning.

Most studies of the neural basis of fear conditioning have utilized an auditory stimulus as a CS. Auditory information reaches the amygdala via two pathways. One goes from the auditory thalamus directly to the amygdala, while the other goes from the auditory thalamus to the auditory cortex and then to the amygdala (LeDoux *et al.*, 1990b; Turner and Herkenham, 1991; Mascagni *et al.*, 1993; Romanski and LeDoux, 1993) These pathways converge onto single cells in the lateral nucleus of the amygdala (LA) (Li *et al.*, 1996). While each pathway can mediate conditioning in the absence of the other (Romanski and LeDoux, 1992), they are not equivalent. Information transmitted to LA via the direct pathway arrives in the amygdala sooner, though with less fidelity than,

information from the cortex (see LeDoux *et al.*, 1986; LeDoux, 1996). The thalamo-amygdala pathway therefore allows for rapid but possibly inappropriate responses to environmental events, while the cortico-amygdala pathway allows for more accurate stimulus evaluation but at the expense of time.

What naturally emerges from the 'quick and dirty' structural relationship of the thalamo-amygdala pathway is a 'better safe than sorry' defensive strategy. Because the first information to get to the amygdala is coarse, it is likely that some otherwise neutral stimuli that resemble either a natural or conditioned trigger in some physical dimension might engage the fear system. In the case of such false alarms, information from the cortex possibly can correct the evaluation and turn the fear system off (LeDoux, 1986, 1996). If the direct pathway from the thalamus to LA has diagnosed the situation correctly, the fear system will have already begun to engage the defensive responses.

The shorter response time of the direct pathway may mean the difference between life and death in situations where rapid responses are useful, as, for example, when a predator or other danger suddenly appears. Nevertheless, there are also obvious advantages to integrating the quick and dirty information with cortical input. At the same time, it is conceivable that integration between the two routes may also fail to occur. In some people, for example, it may be the case that for constitutional or experiential reasons the two pathways are uncoupled such that the information attended to by the cortex fails to coincide with the trigger features that activate the amygdala by way of the thalamus. In such a situation, one would have fear reactions for reasons that are poorly understood. That this is all too common is suggested by the fact that fear and anxiety are the leading causes of visits to mental health professionals each year.

The basic requirement for conditioning, at the cellular level, is the convergence of information about the CS and US onto single cells. It is thus significant that such convergence occurs in LA and that the responses of cells in LA to the CS are modified following associative pairing with the US (Romanski *et al.*, 1993; Quirk *et al.*, 1995, 1997b). Plasticity also occurs in LA in the form of long-term potentiation (LTP), a popular model of how memories are formed at the synaptic level (see Kandel, 1989; Lynch *et al.*, 1991; Bliss and Collingridge, 1993; see also Dudai and Morris, Chapter 9; Winder and Kandel, Chapter 10). LTP has been induced in both the thalamic (Clugnet *et al.*,

1990; Rogan and LeDoux, 1995; Weisskopf and LeDoux, 1998) and cortical (Chapman *et al.*, 1990; Huang and Kandel, 1998) inputs to LA. That LTP in these pathways may explain or contribute to memory formation is suggested by studies showing that synaptic responses elicited by the CS in LA are changed similarly by fear conditioning and LTP induction (McKernan and Shinnick-Gallagher, 1997; Rogan *et al.*, 1997).

The LA is the emotional baggage check in reverse. You do not drop off, you pick up. In order for the learning to be expressed, information needs to get from LA to the central nucleus (CE), which is the output nucleus for conditioned fear responses of all types, including species-typical defensive behaviors (freezing), autonomic nervous system responses (blood pressure and heart rate), neuroendocrine responses (stress hormones) and others (see Davis, 1994; LeDoux, 1996; Maren and Fanselow, 1996). Information processed in LA reaches the CE either via a direct route or via projections to the basal (B) and accessory basal (AB) nuclei (see Pitkänen *et al.*, 1997). Lesions of the CE block the expression of all fear responses, while lesions of brainstem areas to which CE projects selectively block individual responses (see

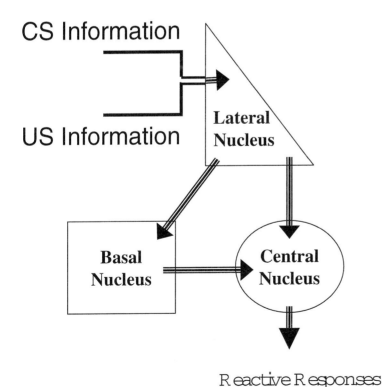

Figure 14.2. The standard model of the amygdala pathways mediating fear conditioning. Learning is thought to involve the lateral nucleus (LA). Information then goes to the central nucleus (CE) either directly or indirectly via the basal nucleus (B). The output of the CE engages defensive responses.

Davis, 1994; LeDoux, 1996; Maren and Fanselow, 1996) (Figure 14.2).

The pathways mediating information about the US still have not been delineated clearly. Recently, however, it has been suggested that there are two independent US pathways, analogous to the pathways transmitting CS information (Shi and Davis, 1998). One pathway is thought to project from the posterior thalamic complex, which sends information concerning footshock directly to the amygdala. The second pathway is believed to project from the thalamus to the posterior insular cortex and then to the amygdala (Shi and Davis, 1998). If this is correct, then the neural organization of CS and US pathways would closely mirror each other. However, this conclusion must wait for further evidence, especially since there are other routes by which US information can reach the amygdala. There are direct projections to CE from pain pathways originating in the spinal cord (Cliffer *et al.*, 1991), as well as from pathways making intermediate synaptic stops in the parabrachial nucleus (Bernard and Besson, 1990). While it is generally believed that conditioning involves plasticity in the LA nucleus rather than the CE, recent studies show that CE projects to the LA and B nuclei (Pitkänen *et al.*, 1997), suggesting that unconditioned stimulus information could reach these areas by way of CE. Thus, the essential US pathway for plasticity in the lateral amygdala is not known.

The view of fear conditioning that has emerged is one of a serially organized, but somewhat redundant neural system. It is serially organized because information necessarily must go through distinct, interconnected nodes within the system, such as the projections from auditory areas to LA and from LA to CE. It is redundant in the sense that at several hierarchical levels there are indirect and direct ways that information can travel from one place to the next, such as the thalamo-amygdala and thalamo-cortico-amygdala routes to LA, and the direct projection from LA to CE versus the indirect projection from LA to B and AB, and from these to CE.

ISSUES AND CONTROVERSIES REGARDING THE NEURAL BASIS OF FEAR CONDITIONING

Sufficiency of thalamic sensory transmission to mediate conditioning

Although the thalamic and cortical pathway can each mediate conditioning when the other is removed before training (Romanski and LeDoux, 1992), lesions of corti-cal areas after training disrupt the expression of fear responses (Campeau and Davis, 1995; Corodimas and LeDoux, 1995). Campeau and Davis argued from these data that the CS normally reaches the amygdala by way of the cortex during training. Thus, when lesions are made after training, the thalamic pathway cannot elicit the memory because it did not learn. In contradiction to this interpretation, however, are the findings that post-training auditory cortex lesions block differential conditioned autonomic responses (Jarrell *et al.*, 1987). Interestingly, the lesions did not result in a decreased responding to the CS that predicted shock; rather, the animal responded as much to the non-reinforced CS (CS–) as to the reinforced CS (CS+). Thus if, as Campeau and Davis (1995) have suggested, animals acquire fear conditioning using the cortical pathway, then there should have been no responding to either CS+ or CS–. The findings are consistent with the view that posits (i) that the direct thalamic projections to the amygdala can mediate fear learning and (ii) that the direct pathway does not represent auditory information with great accuracy and, therefore, animals are not able to differentiate the CS– from the CS+. Other interpretations are also possible. The lesion, which involved the perirhinal cortex, also interfered with context memory, suggesting that information flow into or out of the hippocampus regarding context may have been affected (Corodimas and LeDoux, 1995; see also Brown, Chapter 11; Buckley and Gaffan, Chapter 17). Since the strength of conditioned responses elicited by a CS can be modulated by context, the lesions may have affected the relationship between CS and context (Bouton, 1994). Finally, it is also possible that the memory of the CS is in part stored by way of interactions between the amygdala and cortex.

It will be difficult to disentangle these issues using lesion studies, which can only infer function from dysfunction. Physiological recordings, on the other hand, allow the direct assessment of function and may shed some light on issues regarding the role of thalamic versus cortical CS routes to the amygdala. In one such study, unit activity was recorded in the LA and auditory association cortex during fear conditioning (Quirk *et al.*, 1997a). The earliest responses elicited by the CS developed later in the auditory cortex than in LA. This suggests that the LA uses thalamic rather than cortical sensory information during conditioning, at least for the conditioning of the earliest responses. Further support comes from a recent functional imaging study in humans showing that during fear conditioning to visual stimuli, activity increases in the amygdala co-varied with the visual thalamus but not with the visual cortex (Morris *et al.*, 1999).

Together, these findings strongly suggest that the thalamic pathway is likely to contribute to conditioning. This conclusion does not rule out a role for the cortical pathway, but instead suggests that both are likely to contribute to fear learning.

Does the amygdala learn or does it just modulate?

One of the most heated controversies at present is centered around the question of learning versus modulation. While these are not necessarily mutually exclusive options, they have become so in a version of modulation proposed by McGaugh and colleagues (Cahill and McGaugh, 1998; Vazdarjanova and McGaugh, 1998; Cahill *et al.*, 1999; see also McGaugh *et al.*, Chapter 13). According to their theory, the amygdala mainly modulates learning and memory processes occurring in other brain systems. We begin by addressing the least controversial aspect of this work, i.e. the role of the amygdala in the modulation of the memory for tasks other than fear conditioning. We then turn to the question of whether the amygdala modulates fear learning. Finally, we consider whether the amygdala is involved in learning at all.

Modulation of tasks other than fear conditioning

The modulation hypothesis stems in part from the fact that in humans, explicit or declarative memories of emotionally charged experiences are more vivid and enduring than memories of neutral events (e.g. Christianson, 1989), and in part from studies in experimental animals over many years showing that systemic or intra-amygdala injection of pharmacological agents immediately after training can alter the strength of memories (McGaugh *et al.*, 1992, 1995; Cahill and McGaugh, 1998).

The clearest results come from studies involving tasks which are themselves not dependent on the amygdala. Spatial learning in mazes is perhaps the best example. Thus, injection of certain drugs into 'basolateral amygdala' (a term that refers to the lateral and basal nuclei collectively) immediately after learning, but not immediately before testing, can increase or decrease the strength of the memory formed (e.g. Packard *et al.*, 1994). The basic idea is that during the task some emotional event causes the release of chemicals both within the brain and from peripheral organs (such as the adrenal gland) that activate the amygdala and in turn modulate memory consolidation in other learning systems. Because the amygdala is not directly required for learning, its removal does

not prevent memory formation. At the same time, because the amygdala is involved in modulation, its removal does prevent the acquisition or expression of various learned behaviors.

Modulation of inhibitory avoidance

The task that has been used most extensively to study amygdala modulation of memory is inhibitory avoidance. In this task, a rat is placed in one part of a chamber and is then punished (shocked) for leaving that location. Subsequently, the rat is removed from the chamber and at some later time is returned to the original (unpunished) location in the chamber. If it takes a longer time to leave the unpunished location, an aversive memory is said to have been established. As with the maze studies, manipulations of the amygdala immediately after training can influence the strength of the memory formed. Unlike the maze studies, though, damage to the amygdala sometimes affects the baseline learning of inhibitory avoidance.

Numerous studies have demonstrated an effect of amygdala lesions on the acquisition and performance of passive avoidance tasks, of which inhibitory avoidance is one example (Ursin, 1965; Cahill and McGaugh, 1990; Parent *et al.*, 1992, 1994; Takashina *et al.*, 1995; Bermudez-Rattoni *et al.*, 1997; Oakes and Coover, 1997). In some cases, however, the effects are partial.

In order to understand the confusing nature of amygdala lesion effects on passive avoidance conditioning, it is necessary to ask what is being learned in this task. First of all, inhibitory avoidance is operationally an instrumental learning task, one in which the behavior is controlled by its consequences (stepping into the opposite environment is punished by shock, so the probability of performing this behavior is decreased). This is essentially a habit-learning task, and such tasks are in general known to depend on the striatum (Mishkin *et al.*, 1984; McDonald and White, 1993). At the same time, because of the use of shock, the animal is also undergoing Pavlovian fear conditioning to the local cues where the shock occurs. As we have seen, amygdala damage disrupts Pavlovian fear conditioning and, therefore, we might expect some effects on inhibitory avoidance as well. However, depending on the circumstances, the Pavlovian conditioning that occurs in passive avoidance may or may not be a part of the strategy an animal uses to solve inhibitory avoidance. The fact that striatal lesions alone can disrupt learning suggests that passive avoidance can be completely independent of the Pavlovian processes that are believed to occur through the amygdala (e.g. Prado-Alcala *et al.*, 1975; Rothman and Glick, 1976).

On the other hand, even in cases where the amygdala is required for inhibitory conditioning, it is possible that Pavlovian processes involving the amygdala can modulate memory conditionally. Shock presentation leads to Pavlovian conditioning to local cues (Fanselow, 1980). The presence of these cues in the time after shock elicits many of the neurochemical changes posited as being critical for memory modulation, such as increased peripheral and central corticosterone, changes in peripheral adrenaline levels and changes in amygdala noradrenaline levels (e.g. Tsuda *et al.*, 1986; Weyers *et al.*, 1989; Pitman *et al.*, 1995). Although the extent to which memory modulation is a conditioned versus unconditioned phenomenon has not been addressed explicitly, the fact that conditioned cues elicit the neurochemical changes that underlie modulation suggests that conditioned cues probably play an important role in memory modulation. If so, the amygdala is likely to be required to recognize situations in which the modulators should be released. Modulation, thus, is secondary to conditioning.

Does the amygdala modulate Pavlovian fear conditioning?

On the basis of inhibitory avoidance learning studies, proponents of the modulation hypothesis have argued that the amygdala modulates fear memory, and in particular the memory of fear conditioning (Vazdarjanova and McGaugh, 1998). However, as we have suggested, inhibitory avoidance measures instrumental responses as opposed to Pavlovian fear conditioning. If we want to determine whether the amygdala modulates the memory of Pavlovian fear conditioning we should measure the Pavlovian response in a task that is not contaminated by instrumental response learning.

One of the main ways to determine whether learning and memory are modulated by the amygdala is to turn the amygdala off immediately after learning has taken place. This is typically done by infusing either a local anesthetic or the γ-aminobutyric acid (GABA) agonist muscimol into the amygdala (Helmstetter and Bellgowan, 1994; Muller *et al.*, 1997; Vazdarjanova and McGaugh, 1999). Recently, Vazdarjanova and McGaugh (1999) have demonstrated that post-training infusions of lidocaine, an anesthetic, block the acquisition of freezing behavior

in a Pavlovian task where the US was not contingent on the animal performing a response. This would seem to be strong evidence for the amygdala acting as a modulator, even for fear-conditioned responses. However, the use of lidocaine compromises the strength of their interpretation. Lidocaine has been shown to inhibit cAMP production in various tissue types including neural tissue (Roux *et al.*, 1989; Onozuka *et al.*, 1993). This second messenger cascade is the leading putative molecular pathway mediating memory consolidation (Dudai *et al.*, 1976; Kandel, 1989). Thus, given lidocaine's ability to interact with the molecular pathways mediating memory consolidation, the post-training findings with lidocaine can easily be reinterpreted as supporting the contention that memory is being consolidated in the amygdala itself! When muscimol, an agonist at the ionotropic $GABA_A$ receptor is used, a very different pattern of results emerge. Now, pre- but not post-training infusions of muscimol inhibit the acquisition of freezing behavior (Wilensky *et al.*, 1998). Furthermore, the post-training doses that had no effect on the consolidation of freezing behavior impaired the consolidation of inhibitory avoidance (Wilensky, Schafe and LeDoux, personal communications). These findings tell us two things. First, the amygdala has to be active during CS–US presentations but not afterwards in order for learning to occur. Secondly, the evidence so far favors the view that the amygdala does not modulate itself.

The case for the amygdala being involved in learning and memory is made stronger by recent findings demonstrating that intra-amygdala manipulations of the intracellular cascades thought to underlie memory consolidation impair freezing behavior. Specifically, post-training intra-amygdala infusions of inhibitors of protein synthesis and proteins that are activated by cAMP, such as protein kinase A (PKA), inhibit the consolidation of fear conditioning (Nadel *et al.*, 1999). Together with the above-mentioned data, we know that amygdala activity is necessary during the CS–US presentation and not afterwards. In order for learning to occur, intracellular messengers such as PKA are required to engage the genetic machinery to produce new proteins.

Evidence that learning takes place in the amygdala

Throughout, we have mentioned various pieces of evidence suggesting that the amygdala does indeed learn. Here we will summarize the main points.

(i) Damage to the LA or LA and B together prior to (e.g. LeDoux *et al.*, 1990a), immediately after (Campeau and Davis, 1995) or long after (Kim and Davis, 1993; Maren *et al.*, 1996a) training prevents the expression of the memory of Pavlovian fear conditioning. (ii) Pharmacological manipulation of the amygdala during learning prevents learning, but the same treatment immediately after training has no effect (Maren *et al.*, 1996b; Wilensky *et al.*, 1998; see above). (iii) Neural activity changes in the amygdala as fear responses are acquired both in animals (Quirk *et al.*, 1995, 1997a) and in humans (LaBar *et al.*, 1998; Morris *et al.*, 1999). (iv) Manipulations of intra-amygdala intracellular molecular pathways that are involved in memory consolidation affect consolidation of fear conditioning (Nadel *et al.*, 1999).

In contrast to the wealth of positive evidence implicating the amygdala, and specifically the LA and B, in Pavlovian fear conditioning, there are two studies reporting 'negative' results (Selden *et al.*, 1991; Vazdarjanova and McGaugh, 1998). In neither case was the standard conditioning procedure used. Specifically, fear conditioning was measured as a variant of place learning. Both studies reported that following lesions of the LA and B, animals preferred a location that had not been paired with footshock over one that had been paired.

For example, in the study by Vazdarjanova and McGaugh (1998), animals were shocked in one of three arms of a Y-maze. Amygdala-lesioned animals demonstrated no freezing when placed in the shocked arm (consistent with a deficit in fear conditioning) but they also showed significant avoidance of the place where the shock occurred (suggesting that fear learning had occurred). However, closer analysis of the data revealed that the unlesioned control animals did not spend equivalent amounts of time in the two non-shocked arms. In fact, the amount of time spent in one of the safe or unshocked arms was closer to the amount of time they spent in the shocked arm than to the amount of time spent in the other unshocked arm. With this kind of inconsistency in the baseline measure, it is impossible to draw conclusions on the basis of this task.

In the study by Selden *et al.* (1991), lesions of the LA and B had no effect on the acquisition of place aversions to environments paired with footshock. There were two independent variables, one was the lesion and the other was the delay between the CS and US. Short and long traces were used to vary the amount of conditioning to a CS versus context, respectively.

Amygdala-lesioned animals demonstrated similar preferences for the safe side as sham animals at both trace intervals. At face value, this is clear evidence that amygdala-lesioned animals can form and express a Pavlovian fear association. However, in the short trace interval groups, the amount of time spent on the safe side after conditioning was almost identical to the baseline amount of time spent in that environment prior to training. Thus, the simplest explanation of the short trace data is that little conditioning occurred to the context. Therefore, there is nothing there for the amygdala lesions to affect. The data from the long trace groups are slightly stronger. There is an increase in the amount of time spent in the safe environment of about 25 s (out of 300 s) for both lesion and control groups. However, there are no data demonstrating how unpaired controls would have performed. Thus, the small increase in time on the safe side, and the lack of an unpaired control group, begs the question of whether there is any conditioned place aversion to be blocked at all.

Methodological problems with these two lesion studies weaken their ability to overthrow the vast literature (based on lesions, pharmacological manipulations and physiological recordings) pointing to an essential role of the amygdala in Pavlovian fear conditioning.

Short- versus long-term amygdala contributions to fear memory

Above, we argued that the amygdala is involved in learning. One argument put forth against the learning position is that some studies have found that neural activity changes are most obvious during early training trials, after which activity appears to return to the lower pre-training level (e.g. Quirk *et al.*, 1995; LaBar *et al.*, 1998), suggesting a time-limited modulatory role of the amygdala in conditioning (Cahill and McGaugh, 1998). While some cells do indeed exhibit this behavior, not all do. In fact, with the collection of additional data, it now seems that cells that continue to fire at the higher conditioned rate are just as common, if not more so, than cells that reset (Repa *et al.*, 1999).

However, let us put the new data aside for now and just consider whether the observation that some cells reset is indeed rock solid evidence for the modulatory and against the encoding view of amygdala contributions to fear learning. For the sake of argument, let us say that all cells in LA that condition reset during late training. Would this argue against a critical role for LA in learning? Not necessarily. Two other interpretations are possible.

Prominent learning theories, for example, predict that the amount of learning occurring at any time is a direct function of the difference in what the animal experiences and what the CS predicts (e.g. Rescorla and Wagner, 1972; Pearce and Hall, 1980). With extended training, the CS comes to predict US occurrence accurately; therefore, little new learning takes place. If the CS–US contingency is changed by withholding the US, then a discrepancy once again exists between what is expected and experienced, and additional learning should occur during extinction. This is exactly what the studies found. Activity increased in early training, when the CS–US relationship was being learned about, decreased once the relationship was learned and then increased again when the US was withheld during extinction.

Alternatively, it is possible that during learning, information is encoded by the rate of firing of individual cells, but once learning has occurred an assembly of cells is formed (Hebb, 1949) and the memory is encoded not by firing rate but by the linkage between the cells. That such linkages occur is suggested by the finding that the cross-correlation of spike timing between pairs of LA cells increases during training (Quirk *et al.*, 1995). Spike timing can remain correlated even when spike rate (activity) is no longer changed by the occurrence of the CS, as during extinction (Quirk *et al.*, 1995, 1997). This suggests that the amygdala may shift from a rate to a time code to store the effects of training as learning proceeds. The resetting of cells would, in this case, not indicate an absence of involvement in learning but instead would reflect the shift in coding.

These two alternative explanations are admittedly *post hoc*. They were not experimental predictions, though they can now be predictions for new experiments. The modulatory hypothesis cannot explain the resetting of the cells. Specifically, the cells stop responding in spite of the fact that the stimuli that elicit modulation, the US and environmental cues conditioned to it, continue to occur.

Action versus reaction

So far we have been dealing with fear reactions, responses that occur automatically in the face of danger. However, in addition to being fear reactors, we also often take action when we encounter danger. Reactions are programmed, stereotyped responses

that occur in more or less the same way in all members of a species. Actions, however, are highly individualistic, and can vary considerably. In the case of fear, the main emotional action is avoidance, i.e. the willful or habitual control of behavior in such a way as to prevent harm from occurring.

The variability of emotional actions is readily illustrated by the different ways in which you can avoid a threatening situation that you anticipate. For example, if while walking down the street you see someone threatening, you can cross the street, back track, take a taxi or do any of a number of things to reduce the chances that you will encounter the person. In the laboratory, this process can be operationalized using avoidance conditioning tasks. One such task is inhibitory avoidance, which was described above. As noted, we suggest that this is an instrumental learning task. The subject learns to do something that prevents the harmful or threatening stimulus from occurring. In the case of passive avoidance, withholding responses (i.e. staying put) achieves the goal, whereas in active avoidance some specific response is required (i.e. crossing to the other side of the chamber).

Many studies of the brain mechanisms of avoidance learning have been performed (Goddard, 1964; Grossman *et al.*, 1975; Sarter and Markowitsch, 1985; McGaugh *et al.*, 1995). Unfortunately, these have led to confusing and contradictory results. The flexibility that characterizes emotional action is also a curse on the study of avoidance. That is to say, just as avoidance can be achieved in many ways when one encounters danger, many different kinds of task arrangements can be used to study avoidance. The tasks vary in terms of the stimuli that signal the danger to be avoided and the kind of responses that will be successful in achieving avoidance. Also, since different processing and motor control demands are made on the subject when the stimuli and responses differ, the brain will perform these different tasks in different ways. This no doubt accounts, at least in part, for why avoidance studies have led to a less consistent picture of the brain mechanisms of emotion than studies of conditioned fear, where the responses that are expressed are selected by evolution rather than by the experimenter.

For these reasons, we recently have chosen to begin studying the neural basis of fear action using a task that builds directly upon the simple fear conditioning task we have used extensively. Specifically, we modified a task developed by Neal Miller (1948), and popularized by McAllister and McAllister (1971), to study fear responses. This task is called the escape from fear paradigm. Rats were first given tone–shock pairings in a standard fear-conditioning chamber. They were placed in a new apparatus in which the tone CS could be presented. No shocks were delivered. When the tone came on, the rats initially exhibited freezing. Once freezing extinguished a little, they began to move somewhat, which led to the cessation of the tone. With time, they learned that the tone would cease as soon as they crossed to the other side of the chamber. In other words, in the presence of a stimulus that predicted harm (shock), they learned to take an action that would remove the warning stimulus and end the threat it predicted. Eventually, the response was performed as soon as the rat was placed in the chamber. The action, in other words, became a habit.

The beauty of this avoidance task is that it is controlled by the same stimulus that controls conditioned fear reactions. Since the LA is the region through which auditory inputs reach the amygdala, we predicted that the LA would be involved in the actions performed in the presence of the tone as well as the reactions elicited by the tone. The key question we were interested in was whether the CE would also be involved. As noted above, the CE is required for automatic fear reactions because of its connections with brainstem areas involved in the control of these stereotyped responses.

Indeed, we found that damage to the LA and B together interfered with the learning of the active responses, whereas lesions of CE had no effect. Additional studies showed that damage restricted to B had the same detrimental effect as damage involving both LA and B. Given that the tone CS is most likely to come into the amygdala by way of LA, we concluded that the LA projection to B mediates the learning of emotional actions provoked by a tone just as the LA projection to CE mediates the emotional reactions elicited by the same stimulus. Given that B projects to the striatum, which is known to be involved in instrumental learning (Mishkin *et al.*, 1984; White, 1997), it would seem that the LA–B–striatum connection might be an important circuit for emotional action/habit learning (Figure 14.3).

Single or multiple emotional learning systems

Findings reported by Killcross *et al.* (1997) support the conclusion that distinct components of the fear system mediate active and reactive responses. In contrast to our findings suggesting that the learning mediating both types of responses is occurring in the LA, Killcross *et al.* found that the reactive and active systems were mediated by two independent learning systems. In their elegant study designed to measure both conditioned fear and active avoidance, the authors found that damage to the LA and B interfered with the avoidance of a lever that sometimes led to shock, an active response, but had no effect on the suppression of an ongoing response, a reflexive fear response. Lesions of the CE produced the opposite pattern of results: they blocked suppression of ongoing behavior but had no effect on avoidance of a lever that led to shock. Based on these findings, the authors concluded that two independent emotional learning systems existed within the amygdala. One mediated by the LA and B mediating active responses to emotional cues and the second which mediated the reflexive fear responses such as suppression and freezing.

Although the models are consistent with regard to positing separate mechanisms mediating active and reactive responses, they differ in whether a single or two independent emotional learning systems exits. One reason for the discrepant findings may be the fact that animals were highly overtrained in the Killcross *et al.* study. In a typical fear-conditioning study, rats will receive 2–10 CS–US pairings. In the Killcross *et al.* study, the animals received 120 pairings. Thus, the use of small numbers of pairings may have missed a second fear learning system that comes online only after extensive overtraining. Speaking against this possibility, however, are the findings that overtraining does not rescue either freezing behavior or suppression in rats with LA and B lesions (Maren, 1998; Sun *et al.*, 1999).

The amygdala and appetitive conditioning

One of the reasons for focusing our research on fear, to the exclusion of other emotions, is to facilitate the description of the underlying circuitry for this emotion. Once this has been done, multiple comparisons can be made between emotional systems in the brain. One such comparison is whether appetitive and aversive Pavlovian conditioning are mediated by the same or distinct neural systems. Before we can embark on such comparisons, we need to determine first the appetitive equivalent of freezing: the species-typical response to positive stimuli. For example, should we compare the data from aversive Pavlovian conditioning with the results of studies that have examined approach behavior, 'US-related' behaviors or orientation responses to name a few possibilities? If freezing

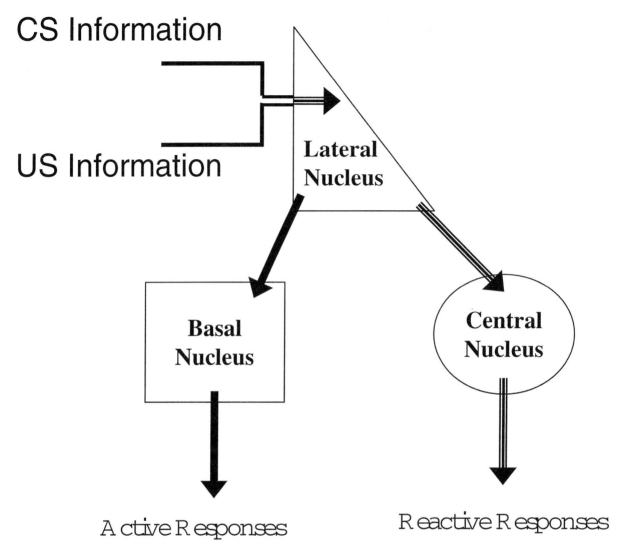

Figure 14.3. A revised model of fear conditioning. There is a new hierarchical level in its organization. First, learning involves the LA. Secondly, information travels to the B and CE carrying qualitatively different information. Information being projected to the B mediates the conditioned reinforcing properties acquired by the CS. Thus, the output of this system leads to the acquisition of 'active responses'. This is in contrast to information being transmitted to the CE which mediates the hard-wired 'reactive responses' such as freezing, etc.

is evolution's hard-wired answer for evading detection by a predator, then what is the analogous hard-wired behavior for situations that predict something beneficial? Correct identification of the appetitive response is likely to be the single most important variable that will determine how successful our comparisons will be.

Conditioned orientation behaviors, which are dependent on the CE of the amygdala, can be ruled out (Gallagher *et al.*, 1990). This is because they are acquired with either appetitive or aversive USs

(Holland, 1977, 1979). Thus, these responses are not specific to a particular emotion.

Approach is an attractive candidate intuitively. It makes sense that signals predicting food should automatically engage mechanisms that mediate approach behavior. Animals approach a place previously paired with food or where they received injections of rewarding drugs. Paradigms of this sort have implicated the amygdala in mediating conditioned place preferences (e.g. amygdala lesions block place preferences for environments paired with traditional reinforcers such as food which elicit approach responses (Everitt *et al.*, 1991; Hiroi and White, 1991; Brown and Fibiger, 1993; McDonald and White, 1993; White and McDonald, 1993). The most notable finding from these studies is that lesions confined to the LA block the acquisition and expression of these place preferences (Hiroi and White, 1991; White and McDonald, 1993). Therefore, approach behavior requires the integrity of the LA, as does freezing. The similarity ends there, however, as the CE is not necessary for this behavior (Hiroi and White, 1991). Thus, if we assume approach to be the appetitive equivalent of freezing, then we can conclude that the mechanisms mediating appetitive and aversive Pavlovian conditioning overlap (the LA is necessary for both) but are distinct (the CE is necessary for freezing but not approach). It should be noted that at this stage it remains unclear whether approach is a reactive or active response to cues predicting something rewarding.

Another possible response that may represent the hard-wired conditioned appetitive responses is what has been called US-like responses (Holland, 1977). If the US is food, the responses include standing motionless in front of the food cup and head jerking (Holland, 1977). Neither the LA and B nor the CE mediate the acquisition of these responses (Gallagher *et al.*, 1990; Hatfield *et al.*, 1996). However, the mechanisms mediating conditioned appetitive active responses and which support the acquisition of second-order conditioning of these responses are mediated by the LA and B (Hatfield *et al.*, 1996). Thus, if the US-like responses discussed above represent the appetitive equivalent of feeding, then we come to a different conclusion: specifically, that appetitive and aversive Pavlovian conditioning are mediated by distinct neural systems in the brain.

It should be obvious to the reader at this point that a comparison of the mechanisms mediating appetitive and aversive conditioning will not be a trivial exercise. Its success will tell us a great deal about how the brain has evolved to learn about biologically significant stimuli in the environment. As we hope is apparent, the results of the comparison will change drastically depending on what appetitive response we consider to be evolution's hard-wired solution to being in the presence of cues that predict something beneficial.

CONCLUSIONS

Our knowledge of the fear system continues to grow exponentially. Studies at different levels of analyses are delineating the biological mechanisms mediating fear at the behavioral, physiological, cellular and molecular levels. Regardless of the data supporting the hypothesis, it is important occasionally to stop and ask whether our initial hypothesis, that the amygdala mediates learning, is correct. As we have argued, alternative interpretations of amygdala function which reinterpret the amygdala's role in fear conditioning as modulatory in nature are lacking. This interpretation can be ruled out on a number of grounds. It is likely that the amygdala is involved in both modulation and learning. Furthermore, we are at a point where it is valuable to compare the organization of the fear system with the organization of other emotions.

REFERENCES

Bermudez-Rattoni, F., Introini-Collison, I., Coleman-Mesches, K. and McGaugh, J.L. (1997) Insular cortex and amygdala lesions induced after aversive training impair retention: effects of degree of training. *Neurobiology of Learning and Memory*, 67, 57–63.

Bernard, J.F. and Besson, J.M. (1990) The spino (trigemino)pontoamygdaloid pathway: electrophysiological evidence for an involvement in pain processes. *Journal of Neurophysiology*, 63, 473–489.

Blanchard, R.J. and Blanchard, D.C. (1971) Defensive reactions in the albino rat. *Learning and Motivation*, 2, 351–362.

Bliss, T.V.P. and Collingridge, G.L. (1993) A synaptic model of memory: long-term potentiation in the hippocampus. *Nature*, 361, 31–39.

Bolles, R.C. and Fanselow, M.S. (1980) A perceptual–defensive–recuperative model of fear and pain. *Behavioral and Brain Sciences*, 3, 291–323.

Bouton, M.E. (1994) Conditioning, remembering and forgetting. *Journal of Experimental Psychology: Animal Behavior Processes*, 20, 219–231.

Brown, E.E. and Fibiger, H.C. (1993) Differential effects of excitotoxic lesions of the amygdala on cocaine-induced conditioned locomotion and conditioned place preference. *Psychopharmacology (Berlin)*, 113, 123–30.

Cahill, L. and McGaugh, J.L. (1990) Amygdaloid complex lesions differentially affect retention of tasks using appetitive and aversive reinforcement. *Behavioral Neuroscience*, 104, 532–543.

Cahill, L. and McGaugh, J.L. (1998) Mechanisms of emotional arousal and lasting declarative memory. *Trends in Neurosciences*, 21, 294–9.

Cahill, L., Weinberger, N.M., Roozendaal, B. and McGaugh, J.L. (1999) Is the amygdala a locus of 'conditioned fear'? Some questions and caveats. *Neuron*, 23, 227–228.

Campeau, S. and Davis, M. (1995) Involvement of subcortical and cortical afferents to the lateral nucleus of the amygdala in fear conditioning measured with fear-potentiated startle in rats trained concurrently with auditory and visual conditioned stimuli. *Journal of Neuroscience*, 15, 2312–2327.

Chapman, P.F., Kairiss, E.W., Keenan, C.L. and Brown, T.H. (1990) Long-term synaptic potentiation in the amygdala. *Synapse*, 6, 271–278.

Christianson, S.-A. (1989) Flashbulb memories: special, but not so special. *Memory and Cognition*, 17, 435–443.

Cliffer, K.D., Burstein, R. and Giesler, G.J. (1991) Distributions of spinothalamic, spinohypothalamic and spinotelencephalic fibers revealed by anterograde transport of PHA-L in rats. *Journal of Neuroscience*, 11, 852–868.

Clugnet, M.C., LeDoux, J.E. and Morrison, S.F. (1990) Unit responses evoked in the amygdala and striatum by electrical stimulation of the medial geniculate body. *Journal of Neuroscience*, 10, 1055–1061.

Corodimas, K.P. and LeDoux, J.E. (1995) Disruptive effects of posttraining perihinal cortex lesions on conditioned fear: contributions of contextual cues. *Behavioral Neuroscience*, 109, 613–619.

Davis, M., Falls, W.A., Campeau, S. and Kim, M. (1994) Fear potentiated startle: a neural and pharmacological analysis. *Behavioural Brain Research*, 58, 175–198.

Dudai, Y., Jan, Y.N., Byers, D., Quinn, W.G. and Benzer, S. (1976) Dunce, a mutant of *Drosophila* deficient in learning. *Proceedings of the National Academy of Sciences of the United States of America*, 73, 1684–1688.

Everitt, B.J., Morris, K.A., O'Brien, A. and Robbins, T.W. (1991) The basolateral amygdala–ventral striatal system and conditioned place preference: further evidence of limbic–striatal interactions underlying reward-related processes. *Neuroscience*, 42, 1–18.

Fanselow, M.S. (1980) Conditional and unconditional components of post-shock freezing. *Pavlovian Journal of Biological Science*, 15, 177–182.

Fanselow, M.S. and Bolles, R.C. (1979) Naloxone and shock-elicited freezing in the rat. *Journal of Comparative and Physiological Psychology*, 93, 736–744.

Gallagher, M., Graham, P.W. and Holland, P.C. (1990) The amygdala central nucleus and appetitive Pavlovian conditioning: lesions impair one class of conditioned behavior. *Journal of Neuroscience*, 105, 1906–1911.

Goddard, G. (1964) Functions of the amygdala. *Psychological Review*, 62, 89–109.

Grossman, S.P., Grossman, L. and Walsh, L. (1975) Functional organization of the rat amygdala with respect to avoidance behavior. *Journal of Comparative and Physiological Psychology*, 88, 829–50.

Hatfield, T., Han, J.-S., Conley, M., Gallagher, M. and Holland, P. (1996) Neurotoxic lesions of basolateral, but not central, amygdala interfere with Pavlovian second-order conditioning and reinforcer devaluation effects. *Journal of Neuroscience*, 16, 5256–5265.

Hebb, D.O. (1949) *The Organization of Behavior*. John Wiley & Sons, New York.

Helmstetter, F.J. and Bellgowan, P.S. (1994) Effects of muscimol applied to the basolateral amygdala on acquisition and expression of contextual fear conditioning in rats. *Behavioral Neuroscience*, 108, 1005–1009.

Hiroi, N. and White, N.M. (1991) The lateral nucleus of the amygdala mediates expression of the amphetamine-produced conditioned place preference. *Journal of Neuroscience*, 11, 2107–2116.

Holland, P.C. (1977) Conditioned stimulus as a determinant of the form of the Pavlovian conditioned response. *Journal of Experimental Psychology: Animal Behavior Processes*, 3, 77–104.

Holland, P.C. (1979) The effects of qualitative and quantitative variation in the US on individual components of Pavlovian appetitive conditioned behavior in rats. *Animal Learning and Behavior*, 17, 424–432.

Huang, Y.Y. and Kandel, E.R. (1998) Postsynaptic induction and PKA-dependent expression of LTP in the lateral amygdala. *Neuron*, 21, 169–178.

Jarrell, T.W., Gentile, C.G., Romanski, L.M., McCabe, P.M. and Schneiderman, N. (1987) Involvement of cortical and thalamic auditory regions in retention of differential bradycardia conditioning to acoustic conditioned stimuli in rabbits. *Brain Research*, 412, 285–294.

Kandel, E.R. (1989) Genes, nerve cells and the remembrance of things past. *Journal of Neuropsychiatry*, 103–125.

Kapp, B.S., Whalen, P.J., Supple, W.F. and Pascoe, J.P. (1992) Amygdaloid contributions to conditioned arousal and sensory information processing. In: Aggleton, J.P. (ed.), *The Amygdala: Neurobiological Aspects of Emotion, Memory and Mental Dysfunction*. Wiley-Liss, New York, pp. 229–254.

Killcross, S., Robbins, T.W. and Everitt, B.J. (1997) Different types of fear-conditioned behavior mediated by separate nuclei within amygdala. *Nature*, 388, 377–380.

Kim, M. and Davis, M. (1993) Lack of a temporal gradient of retrograde amnesia in rats with amygdala lesions assessed with the fear-potentiated startle paradigm. *Behavioral Neuroscience*, 107, 1088–1092.

LaBar, K.S., Gatenby, J.C., Gore, J.C., LeDoux, J.E. and Phelps, E.A. (1998) Human amygdala activation during conditioned fear acquisition and extinction: a mixed-trial fMRI study. *Neuron*, 20, 937–945.

LeDoux, J.E. (1986) Sensory systems and emotion. *Integrative Psychiatry*, 4, 237–248.

LeDoux, J.E. (1996) *The Emotional Brain*. Simon and Schuster, New York.

LeDoux, J.E., Morrison, S.F. and Reis, D.J. (1986) The geniculo-amygdala projection: electrophysiological characteristics of cells in a fear conditioning pathway. *Society for Neuroscience Abstracts*, 12, 748.

LeDoux, J.E., Cicchetti, P., Xagoraris, A. and Romanski, L.M. (1990a) The lateral amygdaloid nucleus: sensory interface of the amygdala in fear conditioning. *Journal of Neuroscience*, 10, 1062–1069.

LeDoux, J.E., Farb, C.F. and Ruggiero, D.A. (1990b) Topographic organization of neurons in the acoustic thalamus that project to the amygdala. *Journal of Neuroscience*, 10, 1043–1054.

Li, X.F., Stutzmann, G.E. and LeDoux, J.L. (1996) Convergent but temporally separated inputs to lateral amygdala neurons from the auditory thalamus and auditory cortex use different postsynaptic receptors: *in vivo* intracellular and extracellular recordings in fear conditioning pathways. *Learning and Memory*, 3, 229–242.

Lynch, G., Larson, J., Staubli, U. and Granger, R. (1991) Variants of synaptic potentiation and different types of memory operations in hippocampus and related structures. In: Squire, L.R., Weinberger, N.M., Lynch, G. and McGaugh, J.L. (eds), *Memory: Organization and Locus of Change*. Oxford University Press, New York, pp. 330–363.

Maren, S. (1998) Overtraining does not mitigate contextual fear conditioning deficits produced by neurotoxic lesions of the basolateral amygdala. *Journal of Neuroscience*, 18, 3088–3097.

Maren, S. and Fanselow, M.S. (1996) The amygdala and fear conditioning: has the nut been cracked? *Neuron*, 16, 237–240.

Maren, S., Aharonov, G. and Fanselow, M.S. (1996a) Retrograde abolition of conditional fear after excitotoxic lesions in the basolateral amygdala of rats. *Behavioral Neuroscience*, 110, 718–726.

Maren, S., Aharonov, G., Stote, D.L. and Fanselow, M.S. (1996b) N-Methyl-D-aspartate receptors in the basolateral amygdala are required for both acquisition and expression of the conditional fear in rats. *Behavioral Neuroscience*, 110, 1365–1374.

Marks, I. (1987) The development of normal fear: a review. *Journal of Child Psychological Psychiatry*, 28, 667–697.

Mascagni, F., McDonald, A.J. and Coleman, J.R. (1993) Corticoamygdaloid and corticocortical projections of the rat temporal cortex: a *Phaseolus vulgaris* leucoagglutinin study. *Neuroscience*, 57, 697–715.

Matzel, L.D., Held, F.P. and Miller, R.R. (1988) Information and expression of simultaneous and backward associations: implications for contiguity theory. *Learning and Motivation* 19, 317–344.

McAllister, W.R. and McAllister, D.E. (1971) Behavioral measurement of conditioned fear. In: Brush, F.R. (ed.), *Aversive Conditioning and Learning*. Academic Press, New York, pp. 105–179.

McDonald, R.J. and White, N.M. (1993) A triple dissociation of memory systems: hippocampus, amygdala and dorsal striatum. *Behavioral Neuroscience*, 107, 3–22.

McGaugh, J.L., Introini-Collison, I.B., Cahill, L., Kim, M. and Liang, K.C. (1992) Involvement of the amygdala in neuromodulatory influences on memory storage. In: Aggleton, J.P. (eds), *The Amygdala: Neurobiological Aspects of Emotion, Memory and Mental Dysfunction*. Wiley-Liss, New York, pp. 431–451.

McGaugh, J.L., Mesches, M.H., Cahill, L., Parent, M.B., Coleman-Mesches, K. and Salinas, J.A. (1995) Involvement of the amygdala in the regulation of memory storage. In: McGaugh, J.L., Bermudez-Rattoni, F. and Prado-Alcala, R.A. (eds), *Plasticity in the Central Nervous System*. Lawrence Erlbaum Associates, Mahwah, New Jersey, pp. 18–39.

McKernan, M.G. and Shinnick-Gallagher, P. (1997) conditioning induces a lasting potentiation of synaptic currents *in vitro*. *Nature*, 390, 607–611.

Miller, N.E. (1948) Studies of fear as an acquirable drive: I. Fear as motivation and fear reduction as reinforcement in the learning of new responses. *Journal of Experimental Psychology*, 38, 89–101.

Mishkin, M., Malamut, B. and Bachevalier, J. (1984) Memories and habits: two neural systems. In: McGaugh, J.L., Lynch, G. and Weinberger, N.M. (eds), *The Neurobiology of Learning and Memory*. Guilford Press, New York, pp. 65–77.

Morris, J.S., Ohman, A. and Dolan, R.J. (1999) A subcortical pathway to the right amygdala mediating 'unseen' fear. *Proceedings of the National Academy of Sciences of the United States of America*, 96, 1680–1685.

Muller, J., Corodimas, K.P., Fridel, Z. and LeDoux, J.E. (1997) Functional inactivation of the lateral and basal nuclei of the amygdala by muscimol infusion prevents fear conditioning to an explicit CS and to contextual stimuli. *Behavioral Neuroscience*, 111, 683–691.

Nadel, N.V., Schafe, G.E., Harris, A., Sullivan, G.M. and LeDoux, J.E. (1999) Immediate post-training injection of inhibitors of protein synthesis and PKA activity in the lateral and basal amygdala, but not the hippocampus, interferes with memory consolidation for contextual and auditory fear conditioning. *Society for Neuroscience Abstracts*, 25, 1618.

Oakes, M.E. and Coover, G.D. (1997) Effects of small amygdala lesions on fear, but not aggression, in the rat. *Physiology and Behavior*, 61, 45–55.

Onozuka, M., Watanabe, K., Imai, S., Nagasaki, S. and Yamamoto, T. (1993) Lidocaine suppresses the sodium current in Euhadra neurons which is mediated by cAMP-dependent protein phosphorylation. *Brain Research*, 628, 335–9.

Packard, M.G., Cahill, L. and McGaugh, J.L. (1994) Amygdala modulation of hippocampal-dependent and caudate nucleus-dependent memory processes. *Proceedings of the National Academy of Sciences of the United States of America*, 91, 8477–8481.

Parent, M.B., Tomaz, C. and McGaugh, J.L. (1992) Increased training in an aversively motivated task attenuates the memory-impairing effects of posttraining N-methyl-D-aspartate-induced amygdala lesions. *Behavioral Neuroscience*, 106, 789–798.

Parent, M.B., West, M. and McGaugh, J.L. (1994) Memory of rats with amygdala lesions induced 30 days after foot-shock-motivated escape training reflects degree of original training. *Behavioral Neuroscience*, 108, 1080–1087.

Pearce, J.M. and Hall, G. (1980) A model of Pavlovian conditioning: variations in effectiveness of conditioned but not unconditioned stimuli. *Psychological Review*, 87, 332–352.

Pitkänen, A., Savander, V. and LeDoux, J.L. (1997) Organization of intra-amygdaloid circuitries: an emerging framework for understanding functions of the amygdala. *Trends in Neurosciences*, 20, 517–523.

Pitman, D.L., Natelson, B.H., Ottenweller, J.E., McCarty, R., Pritzel, T. and Tapp, W.N. (1995) Effects of exposure to stressors of varying predictability on adrenal function in rats. *Behavioral Neuroscience*, 109, 767–76.

Prado-Alcala, R.A., Grinberg, Z.J., Arditti, Z.L., Garcia, M.M., Prieto, H.G. and Brust-Carmona, H. (1975) Learning deficits produced by chronic and reversible lesions of the corpus striatum in rats. *Physiology and Behavior*, 15, 283–7.

Quirk, G.J., Repa, J.C. and LeDoux, J.E. (1995) Fear conditioning enhances short-latency auditory responses of lateral amygdala neurons: parallel recordings in the freely behaving rat. *Neuron*, 15, 1029–1039.

Quirk, G.J., Armony, J.L. and LeDoux, J.E. (1997a) Fear conditioning enhances different temporal components of toned-evoked spike trains in auditory cortex and lateral amygdala. *Neuron*, 19, 613–624.

Quirk, G.J., Armony, J.L., Repa, J.C., Li, X.-F. and LeDoux, J.E. (1997b) Emotional memory: a search for sites of plasticity. *Cold Spring Harbor Symposia on Quantitative Biology*, 61, 247–257.

Repa, J.C., Muller, J., Aspergis, J. and LeDoux, J.E. (1999) Single unit plasticity in the lateral amygdala: relationship to behavioral learning during fear conditioning. *Learning and Memory Meeting Abstracts*, 67.

Rescorla, R.A. and Wagner, A.R. (1972) A theory of Pavlovian conditioning: variations in the effectiveness of reinforcement and nonreinforcement. In: Black, A.A. and Prokasy, W.F. (eds), *Classical Conditioning II: Current Research and Theory*. Appleton-Centry-Crofts, New York, pp. 64–99.

Rogan, M.T. and LeDoux, J.E. (1995) LTP is accompanied by commensurate enhancement of auditory-evoked responses in a fear conditioning circuit. *Neuron*, 15, 127–136.

Rogan, M., Staubli, U. and LeDoux, J. (1997) Fear conditioning induces associative long-term potentiation in the amygdala. *Nature*, 390, 604–607.

Romanski, L.M. and LeDoux, J.E. (1992) Equipotentiality of thalamo-amygdala and thalamo-cortico-amygdala projections as auditory conditioned stimulus pathways. *Journal of Neuroscience*, 12, 4501–4509.

Romanski, L.M. and LeDoux, J.E. (1993) Information cascade from primary auditory cortex to the amygdala: corticocortical and corticoamygdaloid projections of temporal cortex in the rat. *Cerebral Cortex*, 3, 515–532.

Romanski, L.M., LeDoux, J.E., Clugnet, M.C. and Bordi, F. (1993) Somatosensory and auditory convergence in the lateral nucleus of the amygdala. *Behavioral Neuroscience*, 107, 444–450.

Rothman, A.H. and Glick, S.D. (1976) Differential effects of unilateral and bilateral caudate lesions on side preference and passive avoidance behavior in rats. *Brain Research*, 118, 361–9.

Roux, S., Escoubet, B., Friedlander, G., Le Grimellec, C., Bertrand, I. and Amiel, C. (1989) Effects of lidocaine on sarcolemmal fluidity and cellular cAMP in rat cardiomyocytes. *American Journal of Physiology*, 256, H422–H427.

Sarter, M.F. and Markowitsch, H.J. (1985) Involvement of the amygdala in learning and memory: a critical review, with emphasis on anatomical relations. *Behavioral Neuroscience*, 99, 342–380.

Selden, N.R., Everit, B.J., Jarrard, L.E. and Robbins, T.W. (1991) Complementary roles for the amygdala and hippocampus in aversive conditioning to explicit and contextual cues. *Neuroscience*, 42, 335–350.

Shi, C. and Davis, M. (1998) Pain pathways involved in fear conditioning measured with fear potentiated startle: lesion studies. *Journal of Neuroscience*, 19, 420–430.

Sun, P., Nader, K. and LeDoux, J.E. (1999) The basolateral amygdala is required for auditory conditioned suppression even in animals that are overtrained. *Society for Neuroscience Abstracts*, 25, 1618.

Takashina, K., Saito, H. and Nishiyama, N. (1995) Preferential impairment of avoidance performances in amygdala-lesioned mice. *Japanese Journal of Pharmacology*, 67, 107–15.

Tsuda, A., Tanaka, M., Ida, Y., Tsujimaru, S., Ushijima, I. and Nagasaki, N. (1986) Effects of preshock experience on enhancement of rat brain noradrenaline turnover induced by psychological stress. *Pharmacology Biochemistry and Behavior*, 24, 115–119.

Turner, B. and Herkenham, M. (1991) Thalamoamygdaloid projections in the rat: a test of the amygdala's role in sensory processing. *Journal of Comparative Neurology*, 313, 295–325.

Ursin, H. (1965) Effect of amygdaloid lesions on avoidance behavior and visual discrimination in cats. *Experimental Neurology*, 11, 298–317.

Vazdarjanova, A. and McGaugh, J.L. (1998) Basolateral amygdala is not critical for cognitive memory of contextual fear conditioning. *Proceedings of the National Academy of Sciences of the United States of America*, 95, 15003–15007.

Vazdarjanova, A. and McGaugh, J.L. (1999) Basolateral amygdala is involved in modulating consolidation of memory for classical fear conditioning. *Journal of Neuroscience*, 19, 6615–22.

Weisskopf, M.G. and LeDoux, J.E. (1998) NMDA-independent LTP at cortical and thalamic input synapses to the lateral amygdala. *Society for Neuroscience Abstracts*, 24 1914.

Weyers, P., Bower, D.B. and Vogel, W.H. (1989) Relationships of plasma catecholamines to open-field behavior after inescapable shock. *Neuropsychobiology*, 22, 108–16.

White, N.M. (1997) Mnemonic functions of the basal ganglia. *Current Opinions in Neurobiology*, 7, 164–9.

White, N.M. and McDonald, R.J. (1993) Acquisition of a spatial conditioned place preference is impaired by amygdala lesions and improved by fornix lesions. *Behavioural Brain Research*, 55, 269–281.

Wilensky, A.E., Schafe, G.E. and LeDoux, J.E. (1998) Immediate post-training infusion of muscimol into the amygdala does not interfere with fear conditioning. *Society for Neuroscience Abstracts*, 24, 1684.

15 MODELS OF MEMORY: THE CASE OF IMPRINTING

Patrick Bateson

INTRODUCTION

As the result of relatively brief exposure to an object early in life, many birds and mammals will form strong and exclusive social attachments to that object. This process is known as 'filial imprinting' since the object to which the young animal has become attached is treated as though it were a parent. Some of the characteristics of imprinting are due to the naive animal searching for and responding selectively to particular stimuli. Before imprinting takes place, the young bird has clear preferences for the type of stimuli which it subsequently will learn about. It also has already developed a repertoire of motor activities that facilitate the learning process and maintain proximity to the object of its attachment. Learning takes place at a biologically appropriate time in the life cycle and few would doubt that the whole process has been adapted during evolution for the kin recognition function which it currently serves under natural conditions.

The image conjured up by the term is vivid and simple. At a certain stage, the wax of the young animal's brain is soft and it receives the imprint of the first conspicuous thing which the animal encounters. The German term *Prägung* (translated as 'imprinting') was first used by (Heinroth, 1911), although Spalding (1873) had used a similar metaphor, namely 'stamping in'. Lorenz (1935), who did so much to make the phenomenon famous, liked the image because it suggests, as he believed to be the case, an instantaneous, irreversible process. It also led to strong claims that imprinting is quite different from associative learning (Hess, 1973). As more evidence became available, the claims were disputed and the term was held to be misleading (Bateson, 1966; Sluckin, 1972). Nevertheless, 'imprinting' has been retained in the literature by advocates and critics alike. [Confusingly, 'imprinting' has also been used for a quite different process oper-

ating at the genomic level. The influence of one gene on another may be determined not by the dominance of the gene itself but by the sex of the parent from which it comes (Constancia *et al.*, 1998).]

Leaving on one side the matter of whether or not the terminology is appropriate, what happens as a young animal learns the characteristics of its parent? To understand imprinting properly from a behavioral standpoint, it is not necessary to know how genes are switched on and off or any of the other intricate mechanisms of cellular machinery, interesting though such details might be. Instead, what is required is a good understanding of how the various neural subprocesses involved in learning are activated in development and how they fit together. Such an understanding can be enhanced by theoretical models that are built on plausible biological assumptions.

Early experience can also have long-lasting effects on sexual preferences, but the conditions are different from those in which the first attachments are formed. Long-term retention of sexual preferences is found in the face of considerable sexual experience with other objects (Immelmann, 1972). However, the final hook-up between the representation of the imprinting object stored in early life and the output system controlling sexual behavior probably does not occur until much later than the original storage of the representation (Hutchison and Bateson, 1982; Bischof and Clayton, 1991; Kruit and Meeuwissen, 1991; Oetting *et al.*, 1995). As Bischof (1997) has argued, the parallels between 'sexual imprinting' and song learning in birds are striking.

Filial imprinting with a novel and conspicuous object usually occurs most readily at a particular stage of development (Bolhuis, 1991). The range of objects that motivate and elicit social behavior is restricted by the animal's experience. When the young bird becomes familiar with one object, the likelihood of it withdrawing from dissimilar conspicuous objects increases. The first preferences to be formed are likely to be the ones that last, within certain constraints such as the age of the animal at its first exposure and the length of that exposure (Cherfas and Scott, 1981; Immelmann and Suomi, 1981; Bolhuis *et al.*, 1990; Cook, 1993). When a bird is well imprinted, it can be exposed to another object. At first the bird withdraws, showing every sign of great alarm. By degrees, this alarm habituates. Sometimes the bird starts to direct social behavior towards the new object and may become attached to it. However, if it has been well imprinted with the first object, it does not express any social behavior towards the second object—it is tame but unattached.

The so-called sensitive period seems to be brought to an end by the formation of a social attachment (Bateson, 1987). However, even dark-reared chicks eventually are less easy to imprint than they were at first, which may suggest that the ending of the sensitive period may not be entirely experience dependent (Parsons and Rogers, 1997).

FACTORS INFLUENCING IMPRINTING

Many factors have relatively short-term effects on responsiveness. For example, Polt and Hess (1966) found that domestic chicks given 2 h of social experience with siblings beforehand followed a moving object more strongly than isolated birds (Lickliter and Gottlieb, 1985, 1988). Stimulation in other modalities, when presented concurrently with visual stimuli, can have a powerful motivating effect. Gottlieb (1971) found that, in domestic chicks and mallard ducklings, the sounds most effective in eliciting pursuit of a moving visual stimulus are conspecific maternal calls. Furthermore, young birds learn the characteristics of auditory stimuli played to them shortly after hatching (Gottlieb, 1988). In forming a social attachment under natural conditions, auditory signals are important in guiding the process. Also ten Cate (1989) has found that in Japanese quail, the posture of a live adult female has a powerful motivating effect on the response to her by the chicks.

At one time, movement was regarded as essential in 'releasing' the following response of domestic chicks and domestic ducklings and hence in initiating the imprinting process. However, the effectiveness of the many visual stimuli used in the imprinting situation depends on properties such as their size and shape, as well as on the angle they subtend and the

intensity and wavelength of light they reflect. Moreover, the rates at which these variables change are also important—hence the undoubted effectiveness of movement and flicker.

The bird clearly responds to a pattern of stimulation, and characterization of the most effective stimulus must be cast in terms of compounds. Gilbert Gottlieb and his colleagues (Johnston and Gottlieb, 1981; Lickliter and Gottlieb, 1985) argued that the conditions under which imprinting is studied in the laboratory are so impoverished and artificial that the results can give a seriously misleading view of what happens in the wild. However, it does not follow that experimental analysis is, therefore, useless or that different neural systems are studied in laboratory and natural conditions. A car that is filled with low-octane fuel and runs badly does not become another car on that account. Nevertheless, the well-known sensitive period curves for chicks and ducklings, with their peaks within the first day after hatching, probably are misleading. Most processing and storage of information about the mother probably takes place at least a day later under natural conditions. Anyhow, the work on predispositions has been focused increasingly on stimulus features found in the natural world. Strong evidence suggests that head and neck features are particularly attractive to domestic chicks (Horn and McCabe, 1984; Johnson and Horn, 1988).

The discovery of the head and neck detector was important because it suggested a dissociation of the analysis subsystem required for imprinting from that involved in the recognition learning. Under laboratory conditions, the necessary feature detectors take longer to develop than do those driven by flashing lights and movement (Horn and McCabe, 1984; Bolhuis *et al.*, 1985, 1989; Johnson *et al.*, 1985). The dissociation, which had been anticipated (Bateson, 1981), was confirmed by the analysis that led to the identification of a specific region of the brain concerned with storing a representation of imprinting objects.

IDENTIFICATION OF A NEURAL SITE FOR IMPRINTING

An array of different neurobiological techniques have implicated the intermediate and medial part of the hyperstriatum ventrale (IMHV) on both sides of the brain as being sites of a neural representation of the imprinting object (Horn and Johnson, 1989; Horn, 1991, 1998). When evidence is open to a variety of interpretations, greater confidence in a particular explanation may be achieved by tackling the problem from a number of different angles. Each piece of evidence obtained by the different approaches may be ambiguous, but the ambiguities are different in each case. When the whole body of evidence is considered, therefore, much greater confidence may be placed on a particular meaning. An analogy is trying to locate on a map the position of a visible mountain top. One compass bearing is usually not enough. Two bearings from different angles provide a much better fix, and three bearings give the most reliable position for the top.

An important component of the triangulation procedure was to exploit the asymptotic character of learning: a phase of rapid change is followed by one of much slower change. Therefore, animals that are at the rapid phase will be likely to show greater activity in brain sites that are specifically involved in learning than those that have moved onto the slower phase, even though many other aspects of the animals' experience and activity are matched. Animals may be prepared in advance by under-training them or over-training them on the task in question. This technique was exploited successfully when identifying the role of IMHV as a site for the neural representation of the imprinting object in imprinting (Bateson *et al.*, 1973; Horn *et al.*, 1979).

Chicks that have had both left and right IMHV removed surgically are unable to imprint and, if bilateral lesions are placed immediately after imprinting, the birds show no recognition of the imprinting object (see Horn, 1985). Nevertheless, these lesioned chicks will show a preference for a stimulus that has a head and neck feature over one that does not, thereby dissociating the analysis component of the imprinting process from the recognition component. The lesioning experiments also dissociated recognition learning from learning involving external reward. Chicks will learn a visual discrimination rewarded with heat after bilateral removal of IMHV (Cipolla-Neto *et al.*, 1982; Honey *et al.*, 1995). They will also learn to press a pedal rewarded by the view of an imprinting stimulus even though they do not go on to learn the characteristics of that stimulus (Johnson and Horn, 1986).

Many of the detailed cellular and molecular events occurring in IMHV are beginning to be worked out, and the connections between IMHV and other structures have been described (Horn, 1998). However, the links between imprinting and other learning processes occurring in parallel with it are still poorly understood.

DIFFERENT LEARNING RULES

The effects of lesions placed in IMHV are consistent with the view that imprinting might be separated from rewarded learning on functional grounds. Many of the transactions between animals and their environments involve elements of both perceptual learning, occurring without external reward, and elements of event-relating learning which does depend on external reward (or punishment). These components of an overall change in behavior may be seen as subprocesses that normally are used in conjunction, but may depend on different rules (Bateson, 1990; Hollis *et al.*, 1991).

When characterizing classical conditioning, Dickinson (1980) used a definition which relates to the utility of the learning process. The learning process serves to uncover the causal structure of the environment. The jobs of learning to predict and to control the environment are not the same as that of learning to categorize it. At the physiological level, similar if not identical mechanisms *may* be used to achieve these different jobs. At the behavioral level, however, different design rules would be plausible. Detecting causal structure may require classification, but establishing a classification does not involve an association of cause with effect.

In uncovering causality, detecting order usually is crucial. If the supposed cause follows an event, then the necessary contingency is likely to be missing. By contrast, when establishing a category, temporal contiguity may be important, but the order in which the features occur is not. Undoubtedly, under some experimental arrangements, a backward contingency may be extracted in classical conditioning. This raises two possibilities: the regularity of an association might allow the computation of a causal link even when the 'cause' appears to follow the 'effect'; alternatively, when backward conditioning does not occur, the impact of a biologically significant event might distract the subject's attention from events that follow.

The thrust of some theoretical approaches has been to explain perceptual learning and event-relating learning processes in the same terms (McLaren *et al.*, 1989). Also the well-tried methodologies, which were developed from the study of conditioning, have been applied to imprinting itself (Abercombie and James, 1961; Zolman, 1982; Bolhuis *et al.*, 1990; de Vos and

Bolhuis, 1990; van Kampen and de Vos, 1995). Since neither the theory nor the experimental evidence has decisively suggested a unitary mechanism, it is worth examining the case for learning processes that are governed by different rules.

In the real world, a complicated object often presents a substantially different set of features from one view than it does from another. In many circumstances, an animal would benefit from treating these different sets as though they were equivalent (Bateson, 1973). Consider the problem facing the bird which has to gather information about the front, side and back views of its mother. All these views are physically distinct and they may also take on different appearances when viewed at different distances. Information from two separate arrays of features may be combined into a single representation when the two arrays occur in the same context or within a short time of each other (Bateson and Chantrey, 1972).

Chantrey (1974) exposed chicks to two separate imprinting stimuli. He varied the time between the onset of presentation of one imprinting object and the onset of presentation of another and subsequently required domestic chicks to discriminate between the two familiar objects in order to receive a food reward. If the objects were presented five or more minutes apart, the birds learnt to discriminate between the two objects more quickly than those in the control group that had not been exposed to these two objects. However, when the two objects were presented 30 s or less apart, the imprinted birds took longer than the control group to learn the discrimination.

Circumstances are likely to arise when elements of a compound stimulus presented in rapid succession are processed separately. Indeed, Stewart *et al.* (1977) were only able to obtain a classification-together effect when they replicated Chantrey's experimental conditions exactly. When they used less salient features than color, or presented the stimuli in different places, they did not get the effect which, they argued, was fragile. Nevertheless, the point remains that when the elements of a compound are treated by an animal as part of a whole, the order of presentation does not matter. The fragility of the effect will be considered later.

Honey *et al.* (1993), using a different technique from that of Chantrey, double-imprinted chicks and then required them to discriminate between the two imprinting stimuli in order to receive a heat reward if they approached one of them but not the other. In the imprinting regime, the birds were either given alternate exposures with a mean inter-exposure interval of 14 s,

the mixed condition, or they were exposed to periodic exposures to one stimulus and then after a gap of 2 h to periodic exposures to the other, the separate condition. The pattern of imprinting was otherwise the same and the total exposure to the two stimuli was identical in the two conditions. The birds imprinted in the mixed condition took significantly longer to learn the heat-rewarded visual discrimination than the chicks exposed to the separate condition. The explanation is that, when stimuli are presented in alternation close together in time, they are classified together; if, subsequently, the birds are required to learn the discrimination, they first have to disaggregate the two representations before they are able to master the task.

A MODEL OF IMPRINTING

In order to understand more fully the classification-together effect, it is helpful to have a model of what might be happening. One such model was developed by Bateson and Horn (1994). The first step in the model simulates detection of features in a stimulus presented to a young bird. Aspects of the stimulus which the bird is predisposed to find attractive are picked out at this stage. The second step involves comparison between what has already been experienced and the current input. Before imprinting has taken place, no comparison is involved. Once it has occurred, recognition of what is familiar and what is novel is crucial. Finally, the third stage involves control of the various motor patterns involved in executing filial behavior. The behavioral scaffolding for the imprinting process is provided by a direct link between the analysis and executive systems.

A simplified version of the architecture of the Bateson and Horn (1994) model is shown in Figure 15.1. All modules in the analysis system initially are linked to all modules in the recognition system which, in their turn, are linked to all modules in the executive system, only one of which is shown here. Initial strengths of links are indicated by the thickness of the lines. All modules in the analysis system are also linked at maximum strength directly through a by-pass to the module in the executive system that controls filial behavior (such as approach and following). The starting condition is shown first (Figure 15.1a). The strengths of linkages between modules after the model has been exposed to a stimulus that activated analysis module A1 is shown next (Figure 15.1b). The spontaneous excitability in the recognition module,

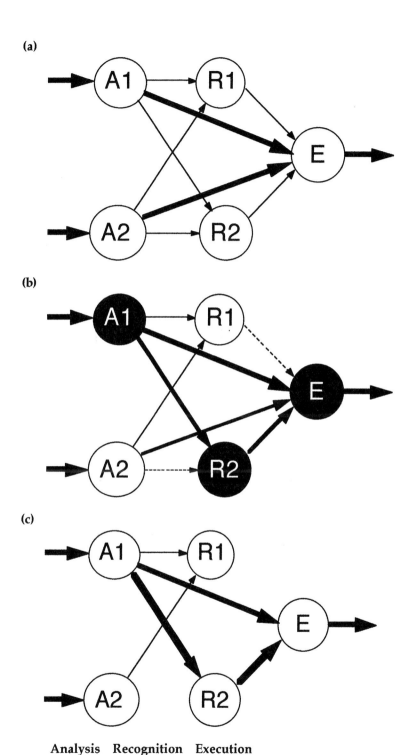

(a)

(b)

(c)

Analysis   Recognition   Execution

Figure 15.1. Simplified architecture of Bateson and Horn's (1994) model for imprinting. All modules in the analysis system are linked initially to all modules in the recognition system which, in their turn, are linked to all modules in the executive system, only one of which is shown here. Initial strengths of links are indicated by the thickness of the lines. All modules in the analysis system are also linked at maximum strength directly through a bypass to the module in the executive system that controls filial behavior (such as approach and following). The starting condition is shown in (a). In (b) the strengths of linkages between modules after the model has been exposed to a stimulus that activated analysis module, A1. The spontaneous excitability in the recognition module, R2, happened to be higher than that in R1 at the time that the input from A1 arrived; activity in R1 was inhibited. The strengthening rule is that modules are active conjointly. The weakening rule is that the upstream module is inactive when the downstream module is active. The completed process is shown in (c).

R2, happened to be higher than that in R1 at the time that the input from A1 arrived and the activity in R1 was inhibited. The strengthening rule is that modules are active conjointly (from Hebb, 1949). The weakening rule is that the upstream module is inactive when the downstream module is active (from Stent, 1973). The completed process is shown in Figure 15.1c.

The three functions separate conveniently into three layers, found in many neural net models (e.g. Mitchison, 1989; Davalo and Naïm, 1991; Levine, 1991). However, the model involves no correction by 'backpropagation' and in that sense is 'unsupervised' (see McClelland, 1989); it requires few components in each layer to operate in a powerful way and, as a consequence, is fast. A convenient feature of its simplicity is that the nature of its behavior is easily understood; this simplicity is particularly valuable when the model behaves in surprising ways in the course of varying parameter values. Despite its simplicity, the subprocesses are plausible in neural terms and the characteristics of the whole system resemble those of an intact animal.

The model can perform a classification-together process readily by retaining the excitability of the recognition modules for a finite period after they had been activated. If a second set of features are presented in alternation with the first, the level of residual excitation in the recognition modules is critical in determining whether the two stimuli are represented subsequently in the same module. The degree of overlap in features between the two stimuli is also critical. If the overlap is high, the probability of the two stimuli sharing a recognition module is also high, even when residual excitation from previous stimulation is zero. Conversely, when the overlap of features is low, the probability of sharing the same recognition module is low, even with maximum levels of residual excitation.

The model also provides a ready explanation for some new empirical evidence (Bolhuis and Honey, 1994, 1998; Honey and Bolhuis, 1997). When the maternal call of the domestic hen accompanies the presentation of a visual stimulus, the domestic chick is more responsive and develops a stronger preference for the visual stimulus. However, if the auditory stimulus is played in the absence of the visual stimulus before presentation of the compound stimulus, the preference for the visual stimulus is weaker. From the standpoint of animal learning, an even more striking result is that if the auditory stimulus is played on its own after the compound stimulus, the preference for the visual stimulus is also weaker than when the post-compound exposure is omitted. Somewhat similar results have been obtained in other contexts (e.g. Dwyer *et al.*, 1998) and have been referred to as 'retrospective revaluation'. In terms of the Bateson and Horn model, the playing of the auditory stimulus on its own weakens the link between the analysis modules processing the features of the visual system and the recognition system. This is because the downstream modules are active when the upstream modules are inactive.

The strengthening and weakening aspects of imprinting have been explored further by Griffiths (1998). Chicks were exposed for 120 min to a moving red triangle. Half of them were then exposed for a further 180 min to a moving purple circle, at the end of which their preference for the red triangle was compared with that for the purple circle or with that for a novel stimulus which was a moving blue cylinder. These preferences were compared with those of the remaining chicks which were not given a second period of exposure with the purple circle (see Figure 15.2). In terms of the Bateson and Horn model, the reduction in the preference for the red triangle after exposure to the purple circle is due to both a strengthening between the analysis modules processing the purple circle and the recognition system and a weakening between the analysis modules processing the red triangle and the recognition system. The extent of weakening alone may be obtained by comparing the birds given a choice between the red triangle and the blue cylinder after no further exposure or after exposure to the purple circle for 180 min.

Not too much should be made of the calculation of the strengthening to weakening ratio because it is difficult to allow for generalization and for the inevitable non-linearities in the underlying processes. However, throwing caution to the winds, a ratio of 4.3:1 for strengthening to weakening is obtained from the Griffiths data, which is close to the Bateson and Horn guess of 4:1. Other neural net models of perceptual learning might be able to cope well with these data (e.g. McLaren *et al.*, 1989; O'Reilly and Johnson, 1994). Their interest lies in showing how a model generates an experiment which then allows parameter values in that model to be estimated.

OPTIMAL TIME INTERVALS

Despite some of the successes of the Bateson and Horn model, it did lead to an interesting failure. In

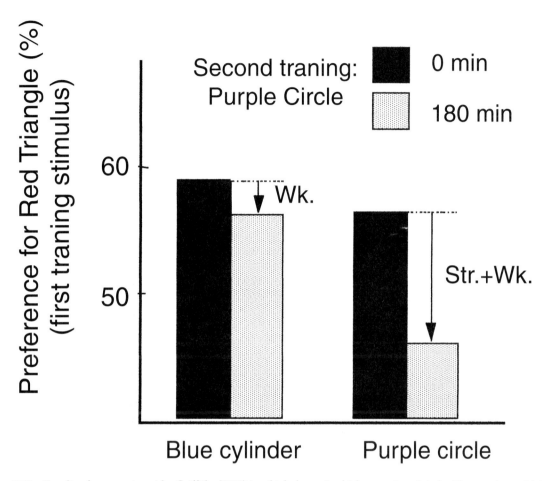

Figure 15.2. Results of an experiment by Griffiths (1998) in which domestic chicks were imprinted with a moving red triangle for 120 min. One group was given no further imprinting while the other was imprinted with a moving purple circle for a further 180 min. At the end of imprinting, chicks were either given a choice between the red triangle and a novel blue cylinder or between the red triangle and the purple circle. In the first test, reduction in the preference for the red triangle as the result of imprinting with the purple circle is attributed to a weakening of the control by the red triangle. In the second test, the reduction is attributed to both the weakening of control by the red cylinder and the strengthening of the control by the purple circle.

the mixed–separate design which was used to replicate the Chantrey result, a mixed presentation of a purple circle and a red triangle during imprinting led to significantly poorer performance than a separate presentation in the heat-rewarded visual discrimination between the purple circle and red triangle (Honey *et al.*, 1993). However, the result was inverted when the strong purple feature was shared by the stimuli and the stimuli were a purple circle and a purple triangle. Now the mixed presentation gave a

significantly better performance than the separate presentation (Honey *et al.*, 1994).

The combined results are summarized in Figure 15.3. The Bateson and Horn model had anticipated that two stimuli sharing a highly attractive feature would be more likely to be represented in the same recognition module, particularly after prolonged exposure to one of the stimuli. This is because a strong link from the analysis module responding to the high stimulus value feature, established during

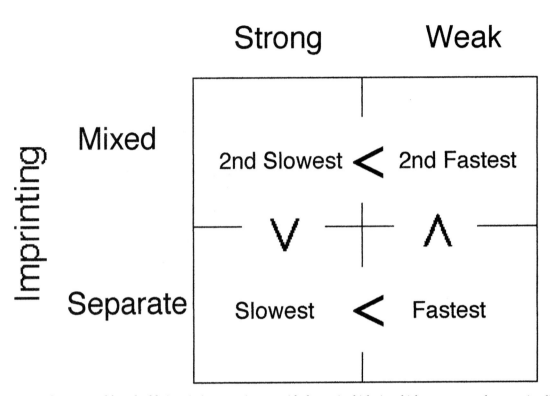

Figure 15.3. Summary of four double imprinting experiments with domestic chicks in which exposure to the two stimuli was either 'mixed' or 'separate' and the stimuli shared either a strongly attractive feature in common (color) or relatively weak features (such as the pattern of movement). After imprinting, the chicks were required to discriminate between the stimuli with which they had been imprinted. The chicks given the separate imprinting condition in which the shared features of the stimuli were relatively weak learned the discrimination most quickly. The chicks which had been given the separate condition in which the stimuli shared a strong feature learned the discrimination most slowly.

exposure to the first stimulus, increases the likelihood that the recognition module responding most strongly to the first stimulus will also respond most strongly to the second stimulus. However, the effect of the mixed condition using a purple circle and a purple triangle was not readily explained by the Bateson and Horn model.

The Honey *et al.* (1994) experiment was repeated with two naturalistic stimuli, a side view of a jungle fowl and a back view of a jungle fowl. This time a control was included which had not been imprinted with the two stimuli. Once again, in discrimination learning, the mixed presentation gave rise to significantly better performance than the separate presentation, which was, if anything, marginally worse than not having had experience with either stimulus (Honey and Bateson, 1996).

The Bateson and Horn model can be modified to cope with these results when an additional feature is added. Supposing that some habituation occurs in the analysis modules, then the shared features of the stimuli will habituate more than the non-shared features. As a result, in the mixed condition, the non-shared features will stand out more relative to each other than in the separate condition. This effect has to be superimposed on some residual activity in the recognition system. If such residual activity was set to decay more rapidly than the dishabituation of analysis modules, the revised model simulated the empirical data. As the time between the presentations of the two imprinting stimuli was increased, the likelihood of them being classified together started high, then declined and then rose again.

It is an empirical matter whether decay of the inferred residual activity and recovery of inferred habituation have different time courses. Therefore, a further experiment was carried out. The interval between presentation was either a mean of 14 s or a mean of 28 s. The results of this experiment showed that doubling the time interval led to an improved performance in discrimination learning (Honey and Bateson, 1996). This supported the notion that residual activity declines more rapidly than the effects of habituation decay, leading to a lowered probability of classification together. The probability then climbs again as the powerful shared feature detector dishabituates and, when reactivated, pulls the representations of the two stimuli together.

How general are these results? If they represent a universal feature of perceptual learning, the prediction is a strong one. Perceptual learning will be improved if the stimuli which are to be discriminated between are presented fairly close together in time, but the gap between them must not be too short. An optimal time interval between presentations is called for.

LINKS BETWEEN IMPRINTING AND REWARDED LEARNING

The possibility of transfer of training after imprinting means that the neural system underlying recognition learning is connected with the one underlying rewarded learning in the intact animal. Chicks show a strong preference for the imprinting object immediately after imprinting. In contrast, when transfer of training in heat-rewarded discrimination learning is tested immediately after imprinting, the rate of learning the discrimination is unaffected by imprinting. However, if discrimination learning between a purple circle and a red triangle is delayed by 6 h, then imprinting does affect the rate of learning, with those given the mixed condition learning significantly more slowly than those that were imprinted in the separate condition (Honey *et al.*, 1995). While the memory required for recognition is formed quickly, the memory sustaining transfer of training is not.

Lesion studies suggest that another representation of the imprinting stimulus (known as S′) is consolidated in another region of the brain about 6 h after imprinting (McCabe, 1991). The formation or the use of this representation can be prevented by placing a lesion in the right IMHV soon after imprinting. If the lesion is delayed for more than 6 h, the imprinted chicks retain their preference. Moreover, the representation may be used in the heat-rewarded discrimination learning task (Honey *et al.*, 1995). The lateralization of the processes involved in forming the second store is of great interest because of the strong evidence accumulated over many years that many processes involved in the visual control of behavior are lateralized (Andrew, 1991; Vallortigara and Andrew, 1991, 1994). The dynamics of changes taking place after imprinting have certain similarities to what happens when humans learn about faces since the left prefrontal cortex is activated during encoding new memories for faces, whereas the right prefrontal cortex is activated during later recognition of those faces (Haxby *et al.*, 1996). In view of the transfer of training studies with IMHV-lesioned chicks (Honey *et al.*, 1995), the second store formed after imprinting might provide a point of contact between imprinting and rewarded learning.

Why are the two independent memory systems needed? Possibly because the associative process dependent on external reward requires different rules from the simple recognition process involved in imprinting. Why should the systems be linked? The biological advantages of using the same information in a variety of contexts can be great. In the case of the young bird, the mother's actions may prove extremely important in predicting where and when it can find crucial resources for itself. While the mother gives signals such as the food call which the chicks respond to without learning, all the chicks hear this and they are in competition with each other. Therefore, capacity for transfer of training is likely to benefit the individual possessing such a mechanism.

CONCLUSION

Imprinting is an example of tightly constrained learning. Paradoxically, its general interest lies in its particularity. The predispositions to respond to particular features and give particular responses to the stimulus are central in the case of imprinting. Mechanisms that change as a result of experience are obviously dependent on mechanisms that have developed before imprinting has taken place. Moreover, the mechanisms that existed before imprinting has occurred are sometimes changed by the experience and sometimes not. In other examples of learning with different functions and involved in different motivational systems, the interdependence is less obvious, but present nonetheless.

Perhaps the most important conclusion from the behavioral work is the need to think of a given phenomenon in terms of a series of subprocesses. These subprocesses were referred to as 'modules' by Bateson and Horn (1994). Clearly such usage can cause confusion since 'module' is a word that has come to have as many meanings as 'instinct'. As with instinct, belief in the validity of one meaning does not imply belief in the validity of other meanings. For example, many believe that the subsystems involved in imprinting have evolved as the result of a Darwinian process of evolution (which is one meaning of module). It does not follow from such a belief that the subsystems are 'hard-wired' and do not change in the course of individual development (which is another meaning of module). Nor does it follow that the subsystems are dedicated to one function (which is yet another meaning).

Despite the ambiguities, the concept of a modular subsystem goes some way toward reconciling alternative perspectives on the mechanisms of learning. On the one hand, differences in the ways in which animals learn may be explained in terms of variation in the perceptual and motivational mechanisms used in the various contexts in which learning occurs. Looked at as a whole, the properties of the entire system are different, which would then have allowed for the evolution of differences in function. In other words, whole learning systems may have different uses. Nonetheless, the subsystems used in one learning context may also be used in another. The subsystems involved in storage of a representation of the external world may operate in the same way. However, the study of imprinting suggests that representations of causality and representations of perceptual categories are achieved in different ways.

The work on imprinting has focused on the analysis of the features of the stimuli that start off the formation of the social attachment, the establishment of a representation of that combination of features and the linking of such a representation to the system controlling social behavior. The common denominator with a great many other learning processes is creating a representation of the object to which the animal has been exposed. Representations must be formed during exploration, latent learning and, indeed, virtually every transaction that a complicated animal has with its environment. The inference is, though, that different subprocesses have different underlying rules for plastic change. Contiguity of the various elements is likely to be important in forming a category, whereas contingency is crucial in learning dependent on external reward.

Inferences about the subprocesses involved in an overall transaction with the environment currently are being examined at the neural level. The behavioral theories undoubtedly make assumptions about the nervous system, and these assumptions may prove to be false. As the neural understanding grows, the enquiry has to return to the behavioral level so that the parts may be reassembled and, if necessary, new behavioral experiments may be done. The return flow of ideas from lower to higher levels of analysis seems a much more attractive and plausible picture of collaboration between disciplines than that of relentless reductionism in which the behavioral people hand a problem to the neural people who, having done their stuff, hand it on to the molecular people.

SUMMARY

The timing of imprinting, the features that most readily trigger learning and the motor systems that are linked to representations stored as a result of learning are all specific to the functional context of forming a social attachment to one or both parents. The underlying neural mechanisms might be the same as those involved in other learning processes. Nevertheless, it is worth asking whether the rules involved in learning about the causal structure of the environment are different from those used in perceptual learning (of which imprinting is a special case). Time plays a different role in classical or instrumental conditioning from that which it does in perceptual learning. The order in which different events are experienced may matter a lot when one event causes the other. However, the order does not matter at all when the experiences are different views of the same object. Some behavioral and physiological evidence from studies of imprinting in chicks suggests that these two broad functions are served by different subprocesses but that the subprocesses are, nevertheless, in touch with each other.

ACKNOWLEDGEMENTS

Gabriel Horn and I have collaborated for more than 30 years. His friendship and working with him have provided me with some of the most enjoyable aspects of my scientific life. It is a pleasure to dedicate this chapter to him. I am grateful to Johan Bolhuis for the care with which he read an earlier version of this chapter.

REFERENCES

Abercombie, B. and James, H. (1961) The stability of the domestic chick's response to visual flicker. *Animal Behaviour*, 9, 205–212.

Andrew, R.J. (1991) *Neural and Behavioural Plasticity*. Oxford University Press, New York.

Bateson, P.P.G. (1966) The characteristics and context of imprinting. *Biological Reviews*, 41, 177–220.

Bateson, P.P.G. (1973) Internal influences on early learning in birds. In: Hinde, R.A. and Stevenson-Hinde, J. (eds), *Constraints on Learning: Limitations and Predispositions*. Academic Press, London, pp. 101–116.

Bateson, P. (1981) Control of sensitivity to the environment during development. In: Immelmann, K., Barlow, G.W., Petrinovich, L. and Main, M. (eds), *Behavioral Development*. Cambridge University Press, Cambridge, pp. 432–453.

Bateson, P. (1987) Imprinting as a process of competitive exclusion. In: Rauschecker, J.P. and Marler, P. (eds), *Imprinting and Cortical Plasticity*. Wiley, New York, pp. 151–168.

Bateson, P. (1990) Is imprinting such a special case? *Philosophical Transactions of the Royal Society London, Series B*, 329, 125–131.

Bateson, P.P.G. and Chantrey, D.F. (1972) Discrimination learning: retardation in monkeys and chicks previously exposed to both stimuli. *Nature*, 237, 173–174.

Bateson, P. and Horn, G. (1994) Imprinting and recognition memory—a neural-net model. *Animal Behaviour*, 48, 695–715.

Bateson, P.P.G., Rose, S.P.R. and Horn, G. (1973) Imprinting: lasting effects on uracil incorporation into chick brain. *Science*, 181, 576–578.

Bischof, H.J. (1997) Song learning, filial imprinting and sexual imprinting: three variations of a common theme? *Biomedical Research, Tokyo*, 18, 133–146.

Bischof, H.J. and Clayton, N. (1991) Stabilization of sexual preferences by sexual experience. *Behaviour*, 118, 144–155.

Bolhuis, J.J. (1991) Mechanisms of avian imprinting: a review. *Biological Reviews*, 66, 303–345.

Bolhuis, J.J. and Honey, R.C. (1994) Within-event learning during filial imprinting. *Journal of Experimental Psychology: Animal Behavior Processes*, 20, 240–248.

Bolhuis, J.J. and Honey, R.C. (1998) Imprinting, learning and development: from behaviour to brain and back. *Trends in Neurosciences*, 21, 306–311.

Bolhuis, J.J., Johnson, M.H. and Horn, G. (1985) Effects of early experience on the development of filial preferences in the domestic chick. *Developmental Psychobiology*, 18, 299–308.

Bolhuis, J.J., Johnson, M.H. and Horn, G. (1989) Interacting mechanisms during the formation of filial preferences: the development of a predisposition does not prevent learn-

ing. *Journal of Experimental Psychology: Animal Behavior Processes*, 15, 376–382.

Bolhuis, J.J., de Vos, G.J. and Kruijt, J.P. (1990) Filial imprinting and associative learning. *Quarterly Journal of Experimental Psychology*, 42B, 313–329.

Chantrey, D.F. (1974) Stimulus preexposure and discrimination learning by domestic chicks: effect of varying interstimulus time. *Journal of Comparative and Physiological Psychology*, 87, 517–525.

Cherfas, J.J. and Scott, A.M. (1981) Impermanent reversal of filial imprinting. *Animal Behaviour*, 29, 301.

Cipolla-Neto, J., Horn, G. and McCabe, B.J. (1982) Hemispheric asymmetry and imprinting: the effect of sequential lesions to the hyperstriatum ventrale. *Experimental Brain Research*, 48, 22–27.

Constancia, M., Pickard, B., Kelsey, G. and Reik, W. (1998) Imprinting mechanisms. *Genome Research*, 8, 881–900.

Cook, S.E. (1993) Retention of primary preferences after secondary filial imprinting. *Animal Behaviour*, 46, 405–407.

Davalo, E. and Naïm, P. (1991) *Neural Networks*. Macmillan, London.

de Vos, G.J. and Bolhuis, J.J. (1990) An investigation into blocking of filial imprinting in the chick during exposure to a compound stimulus. *Quarterly Journal of Experimental Psychology*, 42B, 289–312.

Dickinson, A. (1980) *Contemporary Animal Learning Theory*. Cambridge University Press, Cambridge.

Dwyer, D.M., Mackintosh, N.J. and Boakes, R.A. (1998) Simultaneous activation of the representations of absent cues results in the formation of an excitatory association between them. *Journal of Experimental Psychology: Animal Behavior Processes*, 24, 163–171.

Gottlieb, G. (1971) *Development of Species Identification in Birds*. University of Chicago Press, Chicago.

Gottlieb, G. (1988) Development of species identification in ducklings: XV Individual auditory recognition. *Developmental Psychobiology*, 21, 509–522.

Griffiths, D.P. (1998) The dynamics of stimulus representation during filial imprinting: behavioural analysis and modelling. Unpublished PhD Dissertation, University of Cambridge.

Haxby, J.V., Ungerleider, L.G., Horwitz, B., Maisog, J.M., Rapoport, S.I. and Grady, C.L. (1996) Face encoding and recognition in the human brain. *Proceedings of the National Academy of Sciences of the United States of America*, 93, 922–927.

Hebb, D.O. (1949) *Organization of Behavior*. Wiley, New York.

Heinroth, O. (1911) Beiträge zur Biologie, namentlich Ethologie und Psychologie der Anatiden. *Verhandlung der 5 Internationale Ornithologie Congressus*, 589–702.

Hess, E.H. (1973) *Imprinting*. Van Nostrand Reinhold, New York.

Hollis, K.L., ten Cate, C. and Bateson, P. (1991) Stimulus representation: a subprocess of imprinting and conditioning. *Journal of Comparative Psychology*, 105, 307–317.

Honey, R.C. and Bateson, P. (1996) Stimulus comparison and perceptual-learning—further evidence and evaluation from an imprinting procedure. *Quarterly Journal of Experimental Psychology*, 49B, 259–269.

Honey, R.C. and Bolhuis, J.J. (1997) Imprinting, conditioning and within-event learning. *Quarterly Journal of Experimental Psychology*, 50B, 97–110.

Honey, R.C., Horn, G. and Bateson, P. (1993) Perceptual-learning during filial imprinting—evidence from transfer of training studies. *Quarterly Journal of Experimental Psychology*, 46B, 253–269.

Honey, R.C., Bateson, P. and Horn, G. (1994) The role of stimulus comparison in perceptual learning: an investigation with the domestic chick. *Quarterly Journal of Experimental Psychology*, 47B, 83–103.

Honey, R.C., Horn, G., Bateson, P. and Walpole, M. (1995) Functionally distinct memories for imprinting stimuli: behavioral and neural dissociations. *Behavioral Neuroscience*, 109, 689–698.

Horn, G. (1985) *Memory, Imprinting and the Brain*. Clarendon Press, Oxford.

Horn, G. (1991) Cerebral function and behaviour investigated through a study of filial imprinting. In: Bateson, P. (ed.), *The Development and Integration of Behaviour*. Cambridge University Press, Cambridge, pp. 121–148.

Horn, G. (1998) Visual imprinting and the neural mechanisms of recognition memory. *Trends in Neurosciences*, 21, 300–305.

Horn, G. and Johnson, M.H. (1989) Memory systems in the chick: dissociations and neuronal analysis. *Neuropsychologia*, 27, 1–22.

Horn, G. and McCabe, B.J. (1984) Predispositions and preferences. Effects on imprinting of lesions to the chick brain. *Animal Behaviour*, 32, 288–292.

Horn, G., McCabe, B.J. and Bateson, P.P.G. (1979) An autoradiographic study of the chick brain after imprinting. *Brain Research*, 168, 361–373.

Hutchison, R.E. and Bateson, P. (1982) Sexual imprinting in male Japanese quail: the effects of castration at hatching. *Developmental Psychobiology*, 15, 471–477.

Immelmann, K. (1972) Sexual and other long-term aspects of imprinting in birds and other species. *Advances in the Study of Behavior*, 4, 147–174.

Immelmann, K. and Suomi, S.J. (1981) Sensitive phases in development. In: Immelmann, K., Barlow, G.W., Petrinovich, L. and Main, M. (eds), *Behavioral Development*. Cambridge University Press, Cambridge, pp. 395–431.

Johnson, M.H., Bolhuis, J. and Horn, G. (1985) Interaction between acquired preferences and developing predispositions in an imprinting situation. *Animal Behaviour*, 33, 1000–1006.

Johnson, M.H. and Horn, G. (1986) Dissociation between recognition memory and associative learning by a restricted lesion to the chick forebrain. *Neuropsychologia*, 24, 329–340.

Johnson, M.H. and Horn, G. (1988) Development of filial preferences in dark-reared chicks. *Animal Behaviour*, 36, 675–683.

Johnston, T.D. and Gottlieb, G. (1981) Development of visual species identification in ducklings: what is the role of imprinting? *Animal Behaviour*, 29, 1082–1099.

Kruijt, J.P. and Meeuwissen, G.B. (1991) Sexual preferences of male zebra finches: effects of early and adult experince. *Animal Behaviour*, 42, 91–102.

Levine, D.S. (1991) *Introduction to Neural and Cognitive Modeling*. Erlbaum, Hillsdale, New Jersey.

Lickliter, R. and Gottlieb, G. (1985) Social interaction with siblings is necessary for the visual imprinting of species-specific maternal preference in ducklings. *Journal of Comparative Psychology*, 99, 371–379.

Lickliter, R. and Gottlieb, G. (1988) Social specificity: interaction with own species is necessary to foster species-specific maternal preference in ducklings. *Developmental Psychobiology*, 21, 311–321.

Lorenz, K. (1935) Der Kumpan in der Umwelt des Vogels. *Journal für Ornithologie*, 83, 137–213, 289–413.

McCabe, B.J. (1991) Hemispheric asymmetry of learning-induced changes. In: Andrew, R.J. (ed.), *Neural and Behavioural Plasticity*. Oxford University Press, New York, pp. 262–276.

McClelland, J.L. (1989) Parallel distributed processing: implications for cognition and development. In: Morris, R.G.M. (ed.), *Parallel Distributed Processing: Implications for Psychology and Neurobiology*. Oxford University Press, New York, pp. 8–45.

McLaren, I.P.L., Kaye, H. and Mackintosh, N.J. (1989) An associative theory of the representation of stimuli: application to perceptual learning and latent inhibition. In: Morris, R.G.M. (ed.), *Parallel Distributed Processing: Implications for Psychology and Neurobiology*. Oxford University Press, New York, pp. 102–130.

Mitchison, G. (1989) Learning algorithms and networks of neurons. In: Durbin, R., Miall, C. and Mitchison, G. (eds), *The Computing Neuron*. Addison-Wesley, Wokingham, UK, pp. 35–53.

O'Reilly, R.C. and Johnson, M.H. (1994) Object recognition and sensitive periods—a computational analysis of visual imprinting. *Neural Computation*, 6, 357–389.

Oetting, S., Pröve, E. and Bischof, H.J. (1995) Sexual imprinting as a 2-stage process—mechanisms of information-storage and stabilization. *Animal Behaviour*, 50, 393–403.

Parsons, C.H. and Rogers, L.J. (1997) Pharmacological extension of the sensitive period for imprinting in *Gallus domesticus*. *Physiology and Behavior*, 62, 1303–1310.

Polt, J.M. and Hess, E.H. (1966) Effects of social experience on the following response in chicks. *Journal of Comparative Physiology and Psychology*, 61, 268–270.

Sluckin, W. (1972) *Imprinting and Early Learning*, 2nd edn. Methuen, London.

Spalding, D.A. (1873) Instinct with original observations on young animals. *Macmillan's Magazine*, 27, 282–293.

Stent, G.S. (1973) A physiological mechanism for Hebb's postulate of learning. *Proceedings of the National Academy of Sciences of the United States of America*, 70, 997–1001.

Stewart, D.J., Capretta, P.J., Cooper, A.J. and Littlefield, V.M. (1977) Learning in domestic chicks after exposure to both discriminanda. *Journal of Comparative and Physiological Psychology*, 91, 1095–1109.

ten Cate, C. (1989) Stimulus movement, hen behavior and filial imprinting in japanese quail (*Coturnix coturnix japonica*). *Ethology*, 82, 287–306.

Vallortigara, G. and Andrew, R.J. (1991) Lateralization of response by chicks to change in a model partner. *Animal Behaviour*, 41, 187–194.

Vallortigara, G. and Andrew, R.J. (1994) Differential involvement of right and left-hemisphere in individual recognition in the domestic chick. *Behavioural Processes*, 33, 41–57.

van Kampen, H.S. and de Vos, G.J. (1995) A study of blocking and overshadowing in filial imprinting. *Quarterly Journal of Experimental Psychology*, 48B, 346–356.

Zolman, J.F. (1982) Ontogeny of learning. In: Bateson, P.P.G. and Klopfer, P.H. (eds), *Perspectives in Ethology. Vol. 5. Ontogeny*. Plenum Press, New York, pp. 275–323.

16 THE HIPPOCAMPUS, PERIRHINAL CORTEX AND MEMORY IN THE MONKEY

Mark J. Buckley and David Gaffan

INTRODUCTION

New insights into the neuropsychology of primate learning and memory were precipitated in 1953 by the patient H.M. who underwent surgical bilateral resection of the medial temporal lobe for the relief of intractable epilepsy (Scoville and Milner, 1957; Milner, 1958). It was found that the operation had the desired effect of alleviating his seizures but had also left H.M. with a severe and selective memory impairment in that H.M. was unable to retrieve and store new information about stimuli and events; however, his perceptual and intellectual abilities were unchanged. Although H.M. and similar patients demonstrate rapid and complete memory loss for most events, they remain capable of learning motor and cognitive procedures and skills at a normal rate and can exhibit intact perceptual priming (see also Weiskrantz, Chapter 17). However, these patients are unable to report what it is that they have learnt and manifest little or no awareness of the context in which such learning occurred (Cohen and Squire, 1980). It appears that in amnesic patients, the memory system that stores specific facts, episodes or events is adversely affected, whereas the system that stores procedures or rules is unaffected. A similar dichotomy of memory systems has been proposed in non-human primates (Mishkin *et al.*, 1984). Stored information about specific events or facts has been termed representational, declarative or explicit memory, and stored information about rules is known as procedural, nondeclarative or implicit memory. Thus, representational memory is used when future actions are planned and for the association of the *what, where and when* of events, and forming representational memories allows organisms to identify and attach meanings to objects in their environment.

The demonstration that memory was a distinct cerebral function dissociable from other perceptual and cognitive abilities led to attempts to develop an animal model of human amnesia in the monkey. The aim of this model was to identify which structures and connections within the medial temporal lobe were important for declarative memory. Early research initially led to the idea that the hippocampus and amygdala together were the medial temporal lobe structures critical for declarative memory. With subsequent research, this hypothesis was later revised and there was a shift in emphasis away from the hippocampus and toward the importance of the role of the underlying cortical areas, in particular the perirhinal cortex, in mediating such memory (see also Brown, Chapter 11). After an overview of the research which contributed to this shift in emphasis, we will proceed to argue that yet further clarification and revision of the present model is required in the light of more recent findings.

THE 'COMBINED AMYGDALA AND HIPPOCAMPUS DAMAGE' HYPOTHESIS

Early studies (Orbach *et al.*, 1960; Correll and Scoville, 1965a,b, 1967) provided little evidence that lesions of medial temporal lobe structures in the monkey, designed to replicate the lesions that H.M. had received, impaired stimulus memory to the extent of the amnesia demonstrated in H.M. These early studies often used delayed non-matching to sample (DNMS) and delayed matching to sample tasks (DMS) with only small numbers of stimulus objects. These recognition memory tasks consist of two stages. In the sample presentation stage, the subject is confronted with a single sample object overlying a central well of a three-well test tray in a Wisconsin General Test Apparatus (WGTA). The monkey must displace this object in order to obtain the food reward that is located in the well underneath the object. In the choice stage, after a delay of 10 s, the subject is presented with the sample and a non-sample object positioned over the two lateral wells of the test tray. In DNMS, the monkey can obtain another food reward by displacing the non-sample (i.e. non-matching) object, whereas in DMS the monkey can obtain another food reward by displacing the sample (i.e. matching) object.

Subsequent research also employed these tasks, together with certain modifications, to reveal important new evidence which has led to progress in the development of an animal model of amnesia. One modification was the use of much larger stimulus sets (Gaffan, 1974; Mishkin and Delacour, 1975). The intention behind this modification was to have (or to approximate to the state of having) trial-unique stimuli whereby novel objects would be presented on each choice trial. This modification was considered to be more appropriate for several reasons. It was thought that memories could be made to be more powerful by avoiding interference effects between different sample presentations of the same object. It was also considered to provide a more direct measure of stimulus recognition as the subject was now in effect asked the question 'which of these two objects have you seen before?' Furthermore with the adoption of trial-unique stimuli, the recognition memory task become more similar to the tasks traditionally used to assess human memory. A second modification was the addition of manipulations designed to tax memory further (Gaffan, 1974). These modifications have been termed performance tests. For instance, after the subject had relearned the basic task with 10 s delay, a performance test would then be given in which each sample object is required to be remembered for a longer period of time (e.g. by increasing the delays between the sample presentation and choice stage from 10 s to 30, 60 and 120 s), and subsequently the subject would be required to remember longer lists of sample objects (e.g. three, then five then 10 objects) before the choice stage commenced.

Using both of these modifications to the recognition memory task, Mishkin (1978) found that monkeys with combined amygdala and hippocampus lesions could relearn the non-matching rule and perform the DNMS task with short delays (~10 s) but were impaired with long delays (≥60 s), whereas monkeys

with either amygdala ablations alone or hippocampus ablations alone, like the controls, performed the task well at all delays tested (up to 3.5 min). Mishkin concluded that damage to both the amygdala and hippocampus was necessary for the recognition memory impairment and, likewise, damage to both structures was responsible for the global anterograde amnesia in H.M. Several subsequent studies followed which examined the effects of combined as well as separate damage to the amygdala and hippocampus, and these too appeared to substantiate Mishkin's conclusion and further strengthen the 'combined amygdala and hippocampus damage' hypothesis (Zola-Morgan *et al.*, 1982; Murray and Mishkin, 1984; Saunders *et al.*, 1984; Zola-Morgan and Squire, 1984, 1986; Bachevalier *et al.*, 1985).

However, this hypothesis was challenged with the accumulation of several contradictory findings which showed that severe recognition memory impairments could be found in animals with either the amygdala (Mahut *et al.*, 1982; Zola-Morgan and Squire, 1986) or the hippocampus (Murray and Mishkin, 1986) still intact. Resolving these contradictions required a more careful anatomical analysis as little weight had been given to the possibility that the damage sustained to cortical regions surrounding the amygdala and hippocampus might actually underlie the behavioral deficits previously ascribed to combined hippocampal and amygdala damage. Proceeding in this direction, subsequent research lead to the development of the 'rhinal cortex' hypothesis.

THE 'RHINAL CORTEX' HYPOTHESIS

The perirhinal and entorhinal cortex together can be called, for brevity, the rhinal cortex (See Figure 16.1). The perirhinal cortex lies in the anterior medial part of the inferior temporal gyrus; it is made up of Brodmann's areas 35 and 36 and is situated in the lateral bank of the rhinal sulcus and in the cortex laterally adjacent to it, although the recognized extent of the perirhinal cortex differs slightly between species and across investigators (Brodmann, 1909; Amaral *et al.*, 1987; Insausti *et al.*, 1987; see also Brown, Chapter 11). Indeed, although the inferior temporal gyrus previously was thought to be composed of cortex designated as TE (von Bonin and Bailey, 1947) or area 20 (Brodmann, 1909), it now appears on connectional grounds that the lateral boundary of perirhinal cortex (Brodmann's areas 35 and 36) may be located more

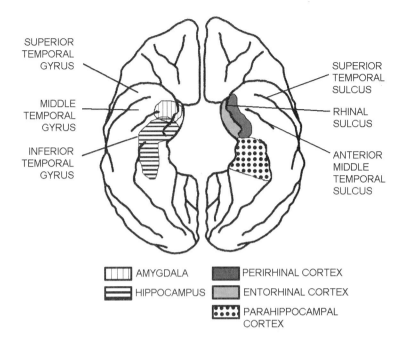

SUPERIOR
TEMPORAL
GYRUS

MIDDLE
TEMPORAL
GYRUS

INFERIOR
TEMPORAL
GYRUS

SUPERIOR
TEMPORAL
SULCUS

RHINAL
SULCUS

ANTERIOR
MIDDLE
TEMPORAL
SULCUS

AMYGDALA
HIPPOCAMPUS
PARAHIPPOCAMPAL
CORTEX

PERIRHINAL CORTEX
ENTORHINAL CORTEX

Figure 16.1. Schematic diagram of the ventral view of a rhesus monkey brain: the approximate locations of the hippocampus and amygdala within the medial temporal lobe are indicated on the left. The approximate extent of the perirhinal, entorhinal and parahippocampal cortices are indicated on the right. The major gyri and sulci are labeled on the left and right, respectively.

laterally than previously believed (Amaral *et al.*, 1987; Insausti *et al.*, 1987; Suzuki *et al.*, 1993). The entorhinal cortex (Brodmann's area 28) is situated medial to the rhinal sulcus, including the medial bank of the sulcus. It is defined uniquely by its robust layer II projection to the molecular layer of the dentate gyrus (Witter *et al.*, 1989) and includes the areas designated as prorhinal and entorhinal cortices by Van Hoesen and Pandya (1975a).

Whereas the anterior parts of the rhinal cortex underlie the amygdala, the posterior parts of the rhinal cortex underlie the hippocampus. Therefore, during amygdala removals, approximately the anterior half of the entorhinal cortex is also removed, in addition to some piriform and periamygdaloid cortex, whereas with hippocampal removals, approximately the posterior half of the entorhinal cortex is removed in addition to the cortex of the parahippocampal gyrus. Thus, only the combined amygdala and hippocampus removals included the entire entorhinal cortex. Further, as perirhinal efferent fibers course in a sheet immediately lateral to the amygdala (see Murray, 1992), there was also the possibility of extensive damage to critical efferents projecting outside of the temporal lobe. The possibility remained that damage to the cortex underlying the amygdala and hippocampus was responsible for the severe memory

deficits that followed combined ablation of the amygdala and hippocampus.

Initially it was found that lesions of the perirhinal and parahippocampal cortex that spared the amygdala and hippocampal formation produced a severe deficit in recognition memory (Zola-Morgan *et al.*, 1989). Although these findings were taken to support the idea that the underlying cortex was critical for recognition memory, these studies remained inconclusive in this regard as branches of the posterior cerebral artery are necessarily severed during the course of making parahippocampal cortex lesions. Thus these behavioral deficits may have been due entirely or in part to interruption of the blood supply to inferotemporal cortex visual area TE which, unlike the perirhinal cortex, receives its blood supply predominantly from the posterior cerebral artery (see Gaffan and Lim, 1991). Confirmation of the 'rhinal cortex' hypothesis was, however, provided by the demonstration that removal of the entorhinal and perirhinal cortex alone, without damage to the amygdala or hippocampus, produced a severe deficit in recognition memory (Murray *et al.*, 1989; Meunier *et al.*, 1993). These studies proved to be consistent with an earlier study (Horel *et al.*, 1987) which showed that a severe impairment in DNMS followed either ablation or reversible cooling lesions of the inferior temporal gyrus, which includes a large portion of the perirhinal cortex. In addition, combined lesions of the amygdala and hippocampus made with the excitotoxin ibotenic acid in order to spare the rhinal cortex failed to produce an impairment on DNMS with delay intervals ranging from 10 s to 3.5 min (O'Boyle *et al.*, 1993; see Murray and Mishkin, 1998). Therefore, damage to the cortex underlying the amygdala and hippocampus was shown to be both necessary and sufficient to produce severe impairment in recognition memory, whereas combined amygdala and hippocampal damage, sparing the underlying cortex, was shown to be neither necessary nor sufficient to produce the impairment.

The mnemonic contributions of the cortical fields underlying the amygdala and hippocampus were examined in greater detail, and, of the perirhinal cortex, entorhinal cortex and parahippocampal cortex, the perirhinal cortex was implicated as the area most important for visual recognition memory. Combined lesions of the perirhinal and entorhinal cortex were found to produce an impairment greater than that which followed lesions of either structure alone and which approaches the size of the impairment that followed large medial temporal lobe lesions; thus, both the perirhinal and entorhinal cortex contribute to recognition memory (Meunier *et al.*, 1993). However, whereas lesions of the perirhinal cortex alone were found to lead to large impairments in recognition memory (Meunier *et al.*, 1993), lesions of the entorhinal cortex alone have only been shown to lead to mild or transient impairments (Meunier *et al.*, 1993; Leonard *et al.*, 1995), and lesions restricted to the parahippocampal cortex alone were shown to produce little or no impairment (Ramus *et al.*, 1994). The aim of more recent studies discussed below has been to elucidate further the particular role played by the perirhinal cortex in vision and memory.

IS THE PERIRHINAL CORTEX PART OF THE INFEROTEMPORAL CORTEX VISUAL SYSTEM?

The inferior temporal cortex consists of the middle temporal gyrus dorsally and the inferior temporal gyrus ventrally, which largely correspond to Brodmann's areas 21 and 20, respectively (Brodmann, 1905). The anterior portions of both the middle and inferior temporal gyrii were considered to be part of a single division in *Macaca mulatta* and were labeled TE

by von Bonin and Bailey (1947) who also identified a more caudal area adjacent to TE which they labeled TEO. These areas have been established to be the visual part of the temporal lobe.

Being located in the anterior medial part of the inferior temporal gyrus, the perirhinal cortex may be viewed as merely a functional component of, or continuation of, the inferior temporal cortex visual system and therefore considered to be a cortical area primarily involved in object perception rather than stimulus memory. Indeed, the most prominent inputs to the perirhinal cortex (64%) are from the laterally adjacent unimodal visual areas TE and TEO (Suzuki and Amaral, 1994a). Despite these prominent visual inputs, the perirhinal cortex also receives inputs from polymodal association cortices including the parahippocampal cortex (25%), dorsal superior temporal sulcus (6%), orbitofrontal cortex (2%) and cingulate cortex (<1%), and from unimodal areas including somatosensory insular cortex (2%) and auditory superior temporal gyrus (<1%). While this pattern of inputs is not consistent with a purely visual perceptual role for the perirhinal cortex, it is still consistent with the view that the perirhinal cortex might have a higher order polymodal role in object perception, associating together perceptual information about objects arising from different stimulus modalities.

However, a recent study by Buckley *et al.* (1997) showed that bilateral perirhinal cortex ablation produced impairments in DNMS but not in color discrimination, whereas bilateral ablation of the middle temporal gyrus, a part of visual area TE, produced the opposite pattern of results and impaired color discrimination but not DNMS. This, the first study to demonstrate a functional double dissociation between the perirhinal cortex and cortex within TE, supports the hypothesis that the perirhinal cortex is a functionally distinct cortical area which should not therefore be considered to be just a part or continuation of the inferotemporal cortex perceptual system.

IS THE PERIRHINAL CORTEX PART OF THE LIMBIC MEMORY SYSTEM?

The perirhinal cortex is characterized by robust interconnections with limbic system structures which are thought to be crucial for memory. The perirhinal cortex is strongly interconnected with the hippocampal formation via the entorhinal cortex. Approximately 40% of the direct input to the entorhinal cortex, terminating in its anterior and lateral regions, is provided by the perirhinal cortex, and there are also strong return projections from these same regions back to the perirhinal cortex (Insausti *et al.*, 1987; Suzuki and Amaral, 1994b; Suzuki, 1996). Accordingly, another prevailing view is that the perirhinal cortex is involved exclusively in memory and is just one constituent part of the temporal lobe memory system.

Squire and Zola-Morgan (1991) proposed that the hippocampal formation, entorhinal cortex and anatomically related perirhinal and parahippocampal cortices constitute a single functional memory system in the temporal lobe and that the gradation of memory impairments after temporal lobe damage simply reflected the amount of total damage to structures in this system. However, there is now evidence for multiple memory systems in the primate temporal lobe. Gaffan (1994a) showed that on a test of DMS with complex naturalistic scenes, monkeys with bilateral perirhinal cortex ablation were far more severely impaired than monkeys with transection of the fornix, the main output of the hippocampus. Conversely, the monkeys with fornix transection were impaired on a test of simple spatial discrimination learning while monkeys with perirhinal cortex damage remained unimpaired. Thus the role of the perirhinal cortex can be doubly dissociated from that of the fornix. Furthermore, using tests of acquisition of systematic food preference, it was shown that the role of both the perirhinal cortex and the fornix can be dissociated from that of the amygdala. Together, these experiments indicate that the limbic system is comprised of multiple functionally distinct components and that the argument for a single functional system was incorrect.

As the perirhinal cortex has been functionally doubly dissociated on the one hand from structures considered to constitute the limbic memory system and on the other hand from structures considered to constitute the inferotemporal visual system, then the perirhinal cortex may be better viewed as a functionally distinct cortical area which is specialized exclusively for neither perception nor memory. The fact that the perirhinal cortex interacts heavily with both the inferotemporal cortex (IT) and limbic system structures suggests that the role of the perirhinal cortex is closely related to both perception and memory. The following section addresses in greater detail what the particular role of this functionally distinct cortical area may be.

THE ROLE OF THE PERIRHINAL CORTEX IN THE MONKEY

Several selective rhinal and perirhinal lesion studies have been performed to investigate what the particular role of these cortical areas might be. What initially appeared to be quite opposing findings from different laboratories, with different interpretations provided accordingly, can now be attributed largely to differences in detail of the behavioral tasks employed and the experimental methodologies used. DMS and DNMS tasks as described earlier have been widely used to test recognition memory, whereas discrimination learning tasks, either with single problems or several problems tested concurrently, have been used to test associative learning.

The basic form of the discrimination learning task is as follows. Monkeys are presented with a pair of objects, either real objects over food wells in a WGTA, computer-generated stimuli or digitized photographs of objects upon a touchscreen, and they have to learn by trial and error which object is baited. In single trial discrimination learning, each pair of objects is presented repeatedly until that problem is learnt to criterion, whereas in concurrent discrimination learning each of a number of pairs of objects are presented one after another until the whole set of problems has been learnt to criterion. In either version, all the stimulus objects are equally familiar to the monkey whether baited or not; therefore, unlike DMS and DNMS, this task cannot be solved by recognition memory alone; instead the monkey has to learn and remember particular associations between individual stimuli and reward.

The memory versus habit debate

Both recognition memory tasks and associative memory tasks have been used extensively but, as the recognition memory tasks appeared to be much more sensitive to temporal lobe damage, the consensus emerged that this type of task was more appropriate to be used as the basis for the development of an animal model of human amnesia. Monkeys with large aspiration lesions of the medial temporal lobe, including the amygdala and hippocampus and parts of the ventral temporal cortex, could learn without impairment a list of concurrent discrimination problems, with 24 h intervals between subsequent sessions in which each of the problems in the set were tested, yet were severely impaired in DNMS (Malamut *et al.*,

1984; Overman *et al.*, 1990). These studies provided the main behavioral evidence supporting Mishkin's popular hypothesis that memories and habits relied upon separate brain systems, with memory thought to be supported by limbic system structures and habit learning (concurrent discrimination learning over long intertrial intervals) supported by interaction of the neocortex and the striatum (Malamut *et al.*, 1984; Mishkin and Petri, 1984). Impairments in new postoperative discrimination learning were either absent as in the above experiments or remained ambiguous. For instance, both Gaffan and Murray (1992) and Eacott *et al.* (1994) found significant impairments in DMS but not in concurrent discrimination learning with 24 h intertrial intervals after rhinal damage. Similarly, not withstanding the problems interpreting damage to the perirhinal cortex combined with parahippocampal aspiration lesions, Zola-Morgan and colleagues found consistent impairments in recognition memory whereas concurrent discrimination learning was sometimes impaired (Zola-Morgan *et al.*, 1989) and sometimes unimpaired (Zola-Morgan *et al.*, 1993).

More recent studies in our laboratory have resolved these ambiguities in concurrent discrimination learning and have challenged the idea that memories and habits are supported by different brain systems. In a series of studies, we showed that bilateral perirhinal cortex ablation does in fact produce new postoperative concurrent discrimination learning impairments when the basic concurrent discrimination learning task is manipulated in a variety of ways. We showed that increasing the number of distracting stimuli that were presented together with the rewarded object in each trial leads to impairments in concurrent discrimination learning (Buckley and Gaffan, 1997). We showed that increasing the number of problems that had to be learnt concurrently also leads to impairments in the task (Buckley and Gaffan, 1997). We also showed that impairments in new postoperative concurrent discrimination learning could be revealed even with set sizes as small as 10 if the views of the objects are changed between trials (Buckley and Gaffan, 1998a). We concluded that the magnitude of impairment in new postoperative concurrent discrimination learning is sensitive to the demands placed by the task upon the ability of monkeys to identify multiple individual objects, and accordingly the lack of impairments in all the concurrent discrimination learning studies described above simply reflects a lack of such demand by the consistent use of relatively few

problems. This pattern of results is also mirrored in recognition memory, as Eacott *et al.* (1994) demonstrated that DMS was impaired after rhinal damage when large object sets were used but not when small object sets were used. As both recognition memory and associative learning have been shown to be impaired similarly under appropriate conditions, the initial observed contrasts in the magnitude of impairment upon each task following damage to these structures can be considered to be merely an artifact of the level of demands placed by the task upon object identification. Furthermore, it has been argued that the cortico-striatal pathway which was proposed to support habit learning is also capable of supporting normal memory (see Gaffan, 1996a). Thus the basis for the above-proposed distinction between short-term memory and long-term habit has been eroded.

In spite of these arguments, some authors still maintain that spared concurrent discrimination learning performance under certain conditions after perirhinal cortex damage implies that concurrent discrimination learning must be a task which can be learnt by habit formation as well as by declarative memory (see Buffalo *et al.*, 1998b). These authors propose that the habit formation process is based outside of the perirhinal cortex in neighboring visual cortical area TE, whereas the perirhinal cortex, in contrast, functions exclusively in declarative memory processes. This view does not easily accommodate the finding of an impairment on both simultaneous and zero-second delay conditions in DMS, where the demands upon memory are minimal or absent, respectively, following rhinal cortex ablation (Eacott *et al.*, 1994). Nor does this easily accommodate the finding of a large impairment following perirhinal cortex ablation in reacquisition of discriminations that were overlearnt preoperatively (Easton and Gaffan, 2000) which, according to the view outlined above, should be classified as 'habits'.

The perirhinal cortex has a role in perception as well as in memory

Further grounds to reject the above argument were provided by the demonstration that the perirhinal cortex also plays a role in perception as well as in memory. Buckley and Gaffan (1998b) showed that performance on a concurrent discrimination learn task was impaired again when 10 familiar problems that had been learnt to criterion were re-tested using slightly different views of the objects that had not been seen before. This manipulation to the task was designed to manipulate the demands placed upon object identification while leaving the demands placed upon memory unchanged. In light of this, we (Buckley *et al.*, 1998, 2000) investigated the perceptual role of the perirhinal cortex in greater detail in a series of 'oddity' tasks. In these perceptual tasks, the subjects have to touch one of six stimuli presented upon a touchscreen to indicate which stimulus is the odd stimulus in the display. For example, in the basic version of the task, five identical patterned stimuli are presented together with one different patterned stimulus. We subsequently varied the nature of the stimulus material to investigate whether there would be any selective perceptual impairments to certain kinds of stimuli. We found that bilateral perirhinal cortex ablation impaired perceptual oddity judgements when the odd stimulus was one view of an object presented together with five different views of a second object. Performance was unimpaired when the odd stimulus was one view of an object presented together with five identical views of a second object. Whereas the latter task can be solved by simple pattern discrimination, this is not the case in the former version as none of the stimuli are identical and judging oddity would be aided by the ability to attain a somewhat view-invariant concept of the individual objects. Furthermore, performance became increasingly poor as problem difficulty increased, which again is likely to reflect the greater involvement of the perirhinal cortex as the demands placed by the task upon object identification are increased. In contrast, performance on color, shape and size oddity were all found to be unimpaired even at very high levels of difficulty. These are tasks which would be very sensitive to the effects of TE damage as they involve discriminating between simple perceptual features. For instance, Buckley *et al.* (1997) demonstrated that ablation of the middle temporal gyrus part of TE severely impairs color discrimination. Thus, the lack of impairment on color, shape and size oddity in the present studies implies that the impairments in object oddity cannot be ascribed to inadvertent damage to area TE. This argument, as made by Buffalo *et al.* (1998b), is in any case refuted by the fact that the monkeys with perirhinal lesions in our studies had either no damage to TE or had only very slight non-bilateral damage. Further studies using the oddity paradigm showed that face oddity (both human and monkey faces) and scene oddity judgements were also impaired, which is further consistent with the idea that the perirhinal

cortex is necessary when the task requires animate or inanimate object identity to be processed and not simply when tasks are perceptually hard *per se*. Faces, for example, are made up of the same set of similar features arranged in a similar spatial relationship in each face and, as such, faces are more easily discriminated on the basis of their being whole 'objects' than on the basis of their individual features alone, and for this reason the processing of face identity is likely to be sensitive to perirhinal cortex damage. Likewise, visual processing of scenes requires multiple objects to be distinguished from the background, which may explain why we found that scene oddity was also sensitive to perirhinal cortex damage. All these findings show that the role of the perirhinal cortex in the monkey is clearly not restricted to memory but that it is also involved in perception. This provides further grounds for rejecting the contrast made between the perirhinal cortex and TE on the basis of their proposed roles in declarative memory and habit learning, respectively.

What is the functional specialization of the perirhinal cortex?

The dual role of the perirhinal cortex in perception and memory reflects the specialization of the anatomical connections of the perirhinal cortex to other structures, which places the perirhinal cortex in an ideal position to process object identity. This has somewhat blurred the traditional distinction that has been made between structures involved exclusively in memory on the one hand and those involved exclusively in perception on the other. However, it is intuitive to think that a brain structure such as the perirhinal cortex which is highly specialized for processing object identity should be able to contribute to both object perception and object memory. Furthermore, there is mounting evidence that the same is also true for other structures. Evidence that memory retrieval is organized retinotopically (Gaffan and Hornak, 1997a) implies that the function of retinotopic early visual areas, usually thought of as being perceptual in function, may be to maintain a representation of the visual world based on both retinal input and memory. Conversely, it remains to be tested to what extent impairments in perceiving scenes or object–place configurations, in addition to impairments in memory, may follow damage to the hippocampal system. The suggestion that the cortical plasticity that underlies perceptual learning and memory is not fundamentally different also supports this general erosion of a potentially misleading perception versus memory distinction (Gaffan, 1996b). We have suggested previously (Gaffan, 1996b; Buckley and Gaffan, 1998c) that the specializations of memory systems are conferred by the specialization of their anatomical connections to other structures rather than by any specialization in specific memory processes. So, whereas the perirhinal cortex owes its specialization in object identity processing to the prominent cortical inputs it receives from visual areas TE and TEO in addition to information from other sensory modalities from diverse unimodal and polymodal association cortices, the hippocampus owes its specialization in contributing to episodic, whole-scene or spatial memory to the fact that it receives multiple inputs from higher order polymodal cortical areas.

Buckley and Gaffan (1998c) provided experimental evidence in support of the above suggestion by showing that perirhinal cortex ablation disrupts configural learning. Configural learning is a task which cannot be solved by associating individual features alone with reward, rather, it can only be solved by associating specific 'combinations' of features with reward. This further refutes the idea proposed by Sutherland and Rudy (1989) that the hippocampus is the site of one such specialized memory process, namely the configural association system. It also illustrates that the information processed by a particular area, in this case the perirhinal cortex, can be put to a variety of uses as required, in this case memory for stimulus configurations. Furthermore, the disruption of configural learning is consistent with the proposed role for the perirhinal cortex in processing object identity, as real objects consist of configural arrangements of spatially continuous features. Object recognition therefore requires analysis of the configural arrangement of these features. Thus the role of the perirhinal cortex in discriminating visual configural cues is closely related to the general role of the perirhinal cortex in identifying individual objects.

The earlier argument that the functional specialization of memory structures is conferred by the pattern of anatomical inputs can now be extended further and strengthened by considering that the use of the information processed in any particular area need not be restricted to a single process such as memory and instead can contribute to both perception and memory. This may explain why experimental findings have led to diverse roles for the hippocampus being proposed in the past, as the particular information

processed by the hippocampus may be used to contribute to a range of processes such as episodic memory, whole-scene memory, spatial memory and perception too, as required. What the particular nature of the information processed by the hippocampus might be is discussed in a later section.

Independent electrophysiological, functional anatomical and neural network modeling evidence also provides support for a role for the perirhinal cortex in processing object information. Visual processing in the inferior temporal cortex is organized non-retinotopically. Electrophysiological studies have shown that cells in TE respond best to moderately complex features rather than whole objects, and these cells have been shown to be organized in a columnar manner with nearby cells within a column responding to similar features and cells in different columns responding to quite different features (for a review, see Tanaka, 1996). Saleem and Tanaka (1996) indicated that sites in the perirhinal cortex may receive convergent inputs from multiple widely distributed sites in the ventral part of anterior TE. This suggests that different moderately complex features of objects represented by distant columns in TE could be associated together in the perirhinal cortex to represent whole objects.

In addition to the prominent inputs from unimodal visual areas TEO and TE, the perirhinal cortex also receives projections from other diverse unimodal and polymodal areas of association cortex (Suzuki and Amaral, 1994a). Therefore, unlike unimodal association cortices, the perirhinal cortex is in a position to associate together information about individual stimuli from different modalities. This is consistent with the proposed specialized role for the perirhinal cortex in processing coherent polymodal concepts of multiple individual objects (Buckley and Gaffan, 1998b,c).

Further, electrophysiological evidence consistent with the proposed role for the perirhinal cortex in processing information about objects was provided initially by Brown *et al.* (1987) who demonstrated that neurons in the anterior inferior temporal cortex and perirhinal cortex showed recognition-related responses. They found cells in these areas which responded more strongly to the first than to subsequent presentations of unfamiliar stimuli. Fahy *et al.* (1993) went on to show that some neurons demonstrate an equal decrement on stimulus repetition regardless of the relative familiarity of the stimuli; these were termed 'recency neurons' as they signal that a stimulus has been seen recently but do not signal the relative familiarity of the stimulus. In contrast, certain neurons were found to respond more strongly to unfamiliar stimuli than to familiar stimuli but do not change their response when a stimulus is shown a second time after a short interval. Such neurons were termed 'familiarity neurons' as they signal the relative familiarity of a stimulus but not whether it has been seen recently. Several further studies have investigated similar declining responses which have been described alternatively as 'adaptive filtering' (Li *et al.*, 1993; Miller *et al.*, 1993) or 'stimulus-specific adaptation' (Sobotko and Ringo, 1993, 1994; Ringo, 1996). It was proposed that these decremental responses might constitute the neural basis of object recognition memory which on the face of it appears to support a role for the anterior inferior temporal cortex and perirhinal cortex in mnemonic processesing.

However, the above interpretation has been called into question by Miller and Desimone (1993) who showed that monkeys tested on a serial DMS task while under the influence of systemically administrated scopolamine, a cholinergic muscarinic receptor blocker, showed a behavioral impairment even though the repetition suppression of perirhinal neuronal activity remained entirely normal. Tang *et al.* (1997) ruled out the possibility that the drug-induced dissociation between memory scores and neuronal activity acted entirely outside the perirhinal cortex. They showed that stimulus recognition could be interrupted by injecting scopolamine directly into the perirhinal cortex but not by injection into neighboring TE or into the dentate gyrus. Thus scopolamine must disrupt some other critical mechanism within the perirhinal cortex itself. The stimulus-specific response decrements themselves have been found in a range of behavioral tasks and have also been found with the presentation of visual stimuli in the absence of any behavioral requirement. This, together with the fact that a majority of cells in the perirhinal cortex that have been recorded from show stimulus selectivity without showing decremental responses, suggests that a more parsimonious account of the relationship between these neuronal responses and behavior would be to consider that a range of neuronal mechanisms in the perirhinal cortex can contribute to a range of behaviors. Recognition memory itself, for instance, requires both stimulus identification as well as judgements about prior occurrence. Thus the evidence from electrophysiology is also consistent with the idea that the perirhinal cortex is specialized for processing information about objects, and that it is not an area which is functionally specialized either for purely mnemonic or purely perceptual processes.

Higuchi and Miyashita (1996) showed that ibotenic acid lesions of the rhinal cortex disrupt the association together of information about paired visual stimuli stored in TE. There is also evidence that a small proportion of cells in TE store view-invariant information about objects (Booth and Rolls, 1998). It is possible, therefore, that the perirhinal cortex may associate together various features of objects, including information from different views, and direct the storage of these associations into respective areas of unimodal association cortex. It is unlikely that multimodal invariant information about each and every individual object experienced by the monkey is actually stored in the animal's perirhinal cortex itself as the perirhinal cortex in the monkey is relatively small in area compared with visual association cortex. Further behavioral evidence that the perirhinal cortex at least maintains the association between information stored elsewhere is that damage to the perirhinal or rhinal cortex typically produces more severe retrograde memory deficits than deficits in new associative learning (Gaffan and Murray, 1992; Buckley and Gaffan, 1997; Thornton *et al.*, 1997). After perirhinal cortex damage, although new visual object associative learning is impaired (Buckley and Gaffan, 1997, 1998a,b), new concurrent visual discrimination problems do eventually proceed to be learnt to a normal level, and in the absence of the perirhinal cortex this new learning may be supported by area TE. It is notable that in the absence of the perirhinal cortex, while concurrent discrimination tasks with small numbers of objects are unimpaired, those involving discriminations between larger number of objects, those which involve objects to be identified across different views or those which require objects to be discriminated from complex backgrounds are impaired (Buckley and Gaffan, 1997, 1998a,b). Thus it would appear that TE is well capable of supporting, even in the absence of perirhinal cortex, discrimination learning between moderately complex features of objects but is less capable of supporting those tasks which require a greater degree of object discrimination as opposed to feature discrimination in order to be solved. These latter tasks are ones in which the specialized function of the perirhinal cortex is likely to be recruited to a greater extent in order to facilitate performance in the intact brain.

Assuming the perirhinal cortex to be the final stage of visual processing in the inferotemporal cortex, Saksida and Bussey (1998) used a neural network model of IT function to examine the effects of lesions to the part of their model, the 'feature conjunction layer', corresponding to the perirhinal cortex. They found that lesions to the 'perirhinal cortex' in their model replicated several of the effects of lesions to the perirhinal cortex in experimental animals in a range of learning paradigms. Firstly, lesioning the 'perirhinal cortex' of their network reproduced stimulus set size effects similar to those observed following lesions of the perirhinal cortex in monkeys upon concurrent discrimination learning tasks (Buckley and Gaffan, 1997). Secondly, lesioning the 'perirhinal cortex' of their model also had a devastating effect on the acquisition of a biconditional discrimination task despite a small set size which reproduces the configural learning impairments that have been shown to exist in monkeys with perirhinal cortex ablation (Buckley and Gaffan, 1998c). Thirdly, lesioning the 'perirhinal cortex' of their network produced an impairment on retention but not upon acquisition when the set size was small, but when the set size was larger an impairment in new learning emerged which again replicates the findings from perirhinal cortex ablation studies in monkeys (Gaffan and Murray, 1992; Eacott *et al.*, 1994; Buckley and Gaffan, 1997; Thornton *et al.*, 1997). The authors explain this differential effect upon new acquisition and new learning in their model as being due to simple properties intrinsic to their model. They argue that that under normal circumstances, simple small set size discriminations can be solved either by using representations of the features of the stimulus or conjunctions of those features, and that normal animals will use both as the learning is distributed across these two types of representation. However, when the perirhinal cortex is lesioned following acquisition of the discrimination, a major contributor to the associative connections leading to the response is removed. The result is an impairment in the performance of the discrimination relative to the intact animal. If, however, the lesioned animal is then presented with a new simple small set size discrimination, all of the learning can be accomplished using the feature representation alone and there will be no difference between the lesioned and the intact animal in their ability to solve the discrimination.

To conclude this section, representations of objects are likely to be stored in a diffuse manner throughout diverse unimodal and polymodal cortical areas. We have argued that each of these different areas are likely to have roles in both perception and memory and have argued that each area will be specialized to process particular aspects of stimuli depending upon the specific patterns of anatomical projections to that area. Thus, while many different brain areas will be involved in processing the different aspects of any individual stimulus, the areas which will be most crucial for performance on any particular perceptual or memory task will be those areas specialized for processing the type of information best manipulated in order to solve that task. Thus the perirhinal cortex is most likely to be crucial in tasks which require the manipulation of representations of configural associations between multiple complex features from one or more sensory modalities, or, in short, when task performance requires the processing of concepts of objects.

WHAT ARE THE ROLES OF ANALOGOUS MEDIAL TEMPORAL LOBE CORTICAL AREAS IN THE HUMAN BRAIN?

Information regarding the cytoarchitecture and precise borders of the perirhinal cortex in the human brain is relatively scarce. Insausti *et al.* (1994) observed close similarities in humans between Brodmann's area 38, the rostrally situated medial temporal cortex or temporal polar cortex, and Brodmann's areas 35 and 36, the ventrally situated cortex lining the banks of the collateral sulcus (Insausti *et al.*, 1994). They concluded that the perirhinal cortex in humans extends from the temporal pole to the level of the uncus, mostly hidden in both banks of the collateral sulcus, and three main portions of the perirhinal cortex were distinguished: a medial portion that surrounds the entirety of the entorhinal cortex, a lateral portion bordering the inferotemporal cortex and a rostral portion up to the temporal pole (see Amaral and Insausti, 1990).

Buffalo *et al.* (1998a) reported that two amnesic patients (E.P and G.T.) with extensive bilateral medial temporal lobe damage including the hippocampal formation, the amygdaloid complex, perirhinal cortex and parahippocampal cortices (and, in the case of G.T., the inferior, middle and superior temporal gyri were also damaged) were impaired at visual recognition tasks over long delays but not short delays, which was thought to be indicative of an impairment in memory. In the task, their subjects were presented with four visual stimuli in turn and, after a delay, were asked whether or not a subsequent stimulus was the same as any of the previously presented stimuli. They argued that as these patients had damage which included the perirhinal cortex, and as they found no impairment at short delays, then the perirhinal cortex in humans is not involved in perception. However, this cannot be taken to be conclusive as the stimuli chosen which had to be recognized were complex colored fractals and not objects. Although these stimuli were chosen because they cannot be verbalized easily, as we argued earlier the visual processing of stimuli such as these which can be discriminated on the basis of simple features are more likely to recruit the function of TE and TEO than the perirhinal cortex. Thus it is likely that E.P and G.T. did not show signs of perceptual impairments because the areas most involved in processing these colored fractal stimuli were spared. As Buffalo *et al.* (1998a) argued, the reason that G.T. was spared any perceptual impairments given his extra damage may have been due to the lateral temporal lobe area involved in processing moderately complex visual features being situated more posteriorly and ventrally in humans than in the monkey (Sergent *et al.*, 1992; Haxby *et al.*, 1994; Ungerleider and Haxby, 1994).

Similarly, humans may also show perceptual deficits following damage to the perirhinal cortex but, as in monkeys, the deficits will be subtle and may only be revealed in perceptual tasks which primarily tax object identity judgements and at the same time cannot be solved readily on the basis of simple or complex feature discrimination. The same pattern of impairments may be found in memory tasks. Studies which have contributed to defining animal models of human amnesia have for the large part concentrated upon visual memory. It is no surprise then that the visual association areas of the temporal lobe have long been thought to be important in memory function. However, the memory deficits in human amnesia are not generally thought of as being limited largely to deficits in visual memory. Damage to the anterior lateral inferotemporal cortex in humans has instead been associated with selective deficits in semantic memory termed semantic dementia. Hodges *et al.* (1992) reported five such cases of patients with focal atrophy largely in the left temporal region deemed to show a relatively pure breakdown of semantic knowledge. These patients showed a striking loss of vocabulary, particularly affecting nouns, which leads to difficulty in remembering the names of people, places and things and produces severe impairments in gener-

ating exemplars from semantic categories. The patients were also profoundly impaired in a battery of semantic tests designed to assess input to and output from semantic memory via different modalities. Semantic dementia patients have also shown deficits in fundamental aspects of knowledge about living and man-made things such as impairments in the use of real household items and impairments in recognizing people from sight, sound or descriptions. In contrast, syntax and phonology of language were relatively preserved, arithmetic skills, visuospatial skills and digit span were normal, and personal autobiographical memory was unimpaired. Some of the deficits in semantic dementia patients are closely related to language, and as such may not be mirrored in animal studies. However, as many of the deficits can be related to a lack of understanding of 'items' or 'things', in this light they may be seen to be analogous in some ways to the perceptual and memory impairments in monkeys ascribed to deficits in processing information about objects following perirhinal cortex damage.

In humans, the semantic dementia syndrome can follow extensive temporal neocortical damage limited initially to the language dominant hemisphere. By contrast, monkeys show much less functional lateralization, and unilateral perirhinal cortex ablations in monkeys do not result in significant impairments. Warrington (1985) suggested that agnosic patients with right hemisphere damage (including some patients with right temporal lobectomy in addition to patients with right parietal or right posterior lesions) showed what she termed apperceptive agnosia characterized by the inability adequately to organize a coherent visual percept, whereas patients with left temporal lobe damage showed what she termed associative agnosia in which a coherent visual percept could be experienced but it was stripped of meaning. Patients with apperceptive agnosia were impaired on tasks such as matching objects in different views, whereas patients with associative agnosia were impaired on tasks such as matching the function of different objects. We have seen that monkeys with bilateral perirhinal cortex ablation are impaired on analogous tasks of both kinds. They are impaired at identifying objects presented in new unfamiliar views (Buckley and Gaffan, 1998) and at learning knowledge about objects in associative learning tasks, respectively (Buckley and Gaffan, 1997, 1998a,b). If one considers the deficits which follow perirhinal cortex ablation in the monkey to be more akin to agnosia than amnesia, then this at least raises the possibility that, despite there being less evidence for such functional lateralization in the monkey brain, the apperceptive and associative roles of the perirhinal cortex may well be lateralized to a much greater extent in the human brain. This would be consistent with a greater degree of focal atrophy in the left temporal regions in human semantic dementia patients and would be consistent with the language-related semantic impairments shown by these patients.

Patients with dementia of Alzheimer type are also impaired characteristically on tasks dependent upon semantic memory including object naming, generation of definitions for spoken words, word–picture and picture–picture matching and the generation of exemplars on category fluency tests (Hodges *et al.*, 1992). Additionally, these patients show severe impairments in episodic memory and eventually show impairments in many cognitive domains. Alzheimer's disease is characterized neuropathologically by a loss of neurons and the appearance of neuritic plaques and neurofibrillary tangles. As the perirhinal cortex has been identified as one of the most vulnerable and earliest sites of the neuropathological changes in Alzheimer's disease (Braak and Braak, 1985; Bowen *et al.*, 1989; Van Hoesen *et al.*, 1991; Arnold *et al.*, 1994), it is possible that this cell loss may account for the semantic memory impairments shown by these patients. Van Hoesen *et al.* (1991) found that the entorhinal and surrounding cortical areas showed atrophy and shrinkage in Alzheimer's disease.

WHAT IS THE CAUSE OF DENSE AMNESIA?

Earlier in this chapter, we argued that damage to the hippocampus alone, or in combination with the amygdala, does not in itself lead to dense amnesia. We subsequently argued that perirhinal cortex damage produces some kinds of memory impairments but that the pattern of impairments are more like agnosia than amnesia. Thus the functional impairments after perirhinal cortex damage likewise do not amount to dense amnesia either. So how may dense amnesia be explained?

Horel (1978) suggested that the deficit in H.M. produced by Scoville's surgery was due to damage of the temporal lobe white matter referred to as the temporal stem due to its thick stem-like appearance with branches extending into the gyri of the temporal lobe

as viewed in coronal cross-sections. The temporal stem covers the dorsal and lateral aspect of the inferior horn of the lateral ventricle and amygdala and is clearly visible in both humans and monkeys. Horel and Misantone (1976) provided initial evidence for the temporal stem hypothesis; they used a frontal approach intended to resemble the frontal approach used by Scoville and transected the temporal stem in monkeys and produced an impairment in learning and retention of visual discriminations. However, Zola-Morgan *et al.* (1982) subsequently found that monkeys with temporal stem section performed normally on DNMS but were impaired on visual discriminations, whereas monkeys with conjoint amygdala and hippocampal damage showed the opposite pattern of results. At the time, they concluded that this double dissociation implied that the two tasks involved fundamentally different processing requirements and hence were mediated by different brain structures. This appeared to provide evidence in favor of the then popular combined amygdala and hippocampus model of amnesia, and at the same time appeared to disprove Horel's temporal stem hypothesis; it also further bolstered the idea that DNMS was more appropriate than discrimination learning as a task to measure the kind of abilities lost in amnesic patients such as H.M. However, as Zola-Morgan *et al.*'s transections spared the anterior 15 mm of the temporal stem, the output of the anterior extreme of temporal cortex may have been left intact. Thus the part of the temporal stem damaged in limbic lesions that included the anterior hippocampus and amygdala would have been spared and, as the anterior part of the inferotemporal cortex and temporal pole, which include the perirhinal cortex, have been shown to be important for DNMS performance, then the contribution of this part of the temporal stem could indeed be critical for normal memory performance. Cirillo *et al.* (1989) tested this hypothesis by sectioning the anterior extreme of the temporal stem in monkeys and then assessing their performance on tests of learning and memory. They found that the anterior temporal stem section produced a large deficit upon DMS at all delays, whereas re-acquisition and new learning of visual discriminations were not impaired reliably. These impairments differed from those found by Zola-Morgan *et al.* (1982) in that in the latter case the recognition memory impairments were only found at long delays. A delay-dependent deficit may seem to be in greater accord with a memory impairment and with the human data in which short-term memory span is relatively unimpaired. However, this is not necessarily the case as H.M. has been shown to have a deficit even with a zero-second delay in DMS with ellipses (Sidman *et al.*, 1968). Furthermore, unlike Cirillo *et al.* (1989), Zola-Morgan *et al.* (1982) only trained their monkeys postoperatively starting with an 8 s delay and then trained to criterion using progressively longer delays. Thus their delay-dependent deficit may simply be an artifact of this training procedure whereby the monkeys received more practice at the shorter delays prior to testing at longer delays which would be expected to lead to better performance at shorter delays relative to longer delays. In conclusion, Cirillo *et al.* (1989) demonstrated that damage to the temporal lobe white matter in monkeys is sufficient to disrupt a task claimed to measure a form of memory lost in human amnesia. Although the impairments after anterior temporal stem section do not on their own amount to dense amnesia, they may, like damage to the perirhinal cortex, contribute to some of the symptoms found in the human amnesic syndrome.

The impairments after temporal stem section may be due to deafferentation of limbic structures. Additionally, temporal stem section would also disrupt the flow of information between temporal cortical areas and frontal areas involved in memory. It is possible that frontal cortex may exert an influence upon inferior temporal cortex via modulation through subcortical structures such as the hypothalamus or basal forebrain. Indeed afferent connections from frontal cortex to the hypothalamus (Ongur *et al.*, 1998) and to the basal forebrain have been found (Russchen *et al.*, 1985; Irle and Markowitsch, 1986), as have projections from both of these structures to the inferior temporal cortex (Webster *et al.*, 1993). The connections from the basal forebrain to the inferior temporal cortex in the macaque have been observed in retrograde tracing studies to course through the anterior temporal stem and amygdala (Kitt *et al.*, 1987; Seldon *et al.*, 1998). Thus fibers between the inferior temporal cortex and these subcortical structures would be disrupted by lesions in the anterior temporal stem and amygdala. Gaffan and colleagues (Gaffan *et al.*, 1998) found that various combinations of anterior temporal stem section with amygdalectomy and fornix transection in monkeys led to a range of impairments in various tasks including DMS, concurrent visual discrimination learning and object-in-place learning. However, complete disconnection of the basal forebrain from inferior temporal cortex by section of the anterior temporal stem, amygdala and fornix together led to severe impairments in new learning in all of the above tasks. Thus they argued that isolating the basal forebrain from inferior temporal cortex in these ways produced dense amnesia by preventing communication between the inferior temporal cortex and the particular subcortical and frontal structures where interaction by these routes is necessary in particular memory tasks. Subsequent disconnection studies were used to specify further which particular basal forebrain structures may be important in frontal lobe-mediated influence upon inferior temporal cortex via the temporal stem. Interaction between the lateral hypothalamus and the inferior temporal cortex in particular has been shown to be important for concurrent visual discrimination learning, object recognition memory and object-in-place learning (Easton and Gaffan, 1997, 2000; Parker *et al.*, 2000). As the impairments in these tasks were found to be as severe after disconnection of the lateral hypothalamus from either the inferior temporal cortex or the frontal lobe as after section of the temporal stem and amygdala, then this further supports the idea that the subcortically mediated interaction between the frontal lobe and the inferior temporal lobe, via fibers running through the anterior temporal stem and amygdala, are important for performance of these memory tasks.

We suggest, therefore, that dense amnesia is not caused by damage to the hippocampus, amygdala, perirhinal cortex, anterior temporal stem, basal forebrain or frontal lobes alone, but rather by preventing interaction between a number of these structures together typically due to a combination of damage to cortical structures, subcortical structures and white matter, and thereby interrupting multiple interactions mediating a range of memory processes. Future research may be able to specify in greater detail which particular interactions between specific structures are critical for performance of each of the different types of memory tasks so far employed.

Corkin *et al.* (1997) recently conducted magnetic resonance imaging (MRI) studies in an attempt to specify precisely the extent of the bilateral resection in H.M. and to document any other brain abnormalities. According to these MRI studies, the lesion was bilaterally symmetrical and included the medial temporal polar cortex, most of the amygdaloid complex, most or all of the entorhinal cortex and approximately half of the rostrocaudal extent of the intraventricular portion of the hippocampal formation (dentate gyrus, hippocampus and subicular complex). Although the caudal portions (~2 cm) of the hippocampus body were intact, they appeared atrophic bilaterally. The collateral sulcus was visible throughout much of the temporal lobe, indicating that portions of the ventral perirhinal cortex, located on the banks of the sulcus, were spared; in particular, the resection appears to have included rostral levels while leaving caudal portions intact. The parahippocampal cortex (areas TF and TH) was largely intact as was the temporal stem, although the subcortical white matter associated with the most anterior portions of the superior, middle and inferior temporal gyri may have been compromised by the resection. Outside of the temporal lobes, additional damage included marked atrophy of the cerebellum and shrinkage of the mammillary bodies.

As we have argued above, the dense amnesia produced in H.M. as a result of the surgical damage is unlikely to be ascribed to damage to any one structure alone but is likely to be due to interruption of the exchange of information between different areas of the brain involved in memory via a variety of routes each involved to a greater or lesser extent in a range of mnemonic processes. Thus the damage to the perirhinal cortex and temporal polar regions in H.M. obviously will preclude the frontal lobes from receiving, or influencing the processing of, information processed in those specialist areas, which we have argued is particularly likely to be information about object concepts. Furthermore, even the areas of visual cortex which remain intact are unable to interact normally with the portions of the hippocampus which remain intact as the major route of interaction with the hippocampus, of visual information together with information from other higher order sensory cortices, namely the entorhinal cortex, was completely damaged. As the white matter comprising the most anterior portion of the temporal stem was observed to be damaged in H.M., then there will be some disruption of the subcortically mediated interactions between the inferior temporal and frontal lobe which course through the temporal stem. The subcortically mediated interactions between the inferior temporal and frontal lobe which course through the amygdala, on the other hand, will certainly have been severely disrupted due to damage to most of the amygdaloid complex in H.M. Although cholinergic innervation of the hippocampus from the basal forebrain may be intact, its function is likely to be impaired as normal processing in the hippocampus is likely to be precluded due to extensive hippocampal damage and atrophy of the remaining portions. Even if the remaining portions of the hippocampus retain any processing capability, the information cannot interact at all with other structures via the entorhinal cortex and amygdala which are both absent, and any interaction via the intact fornix or remaining portions of intact temporal stem, for example with the frontal lobes via the basal forebrain, will be abnormal.

Clearly there are a host of contributing factors to H.M.'s dense amnesia. Similarly, alternative combinations of factors may also lead to dense amnesia in other patients with differing extents of damage to these and related structures involved in visual learning and memory. Nevertheless, we now possess a greater appreciation of the distinct functional roles of many of these structures which has allowed our present animal model of human amnesia to progress far beyond the early idea that the medial temporal lobe structures merely comprise a single functional system whereby greater damage leads to more severe memory impairments (Squire and Zola-Morgan, 1991).

WHERE DOES THIS LEAVE OUR UNDERSTANDING OF THE ROLE OF THE HIPPOCAMPUS?

Initially, the role of the hippocampus together with the amygdala was considered to be central to animal models of human amnesia. Earlier in this chapter, we outlined how there was then a shift in emphasis away from the hippocampus and toward the underlying cortical areas, especially the perirhinal cortex. We then reviewed more recent evidence which suggests that the perirhinal cortex contributes to both memory and perception. We subsequently argued that the impairments after perirhinal cortex damage may be more akin to agnosia than amnesia, but in any case they do not by themselves amount to dense amnesia. Finally, in the light of evidence from lesion studies, temporal stem section and disconnection experiments considered together, we suggested an etiology of dense amnesia. In the light of all this, where does our understanding of the particular role of the hippocampus now lie?

First, it should be noted that the role of the hippocampus in humans cannot be inferred directly even from those amnesic patients with anoxic damage limited to the fields of the hippocampus as there is evidence that the extent of functional damage after anoxia in animals can extend beyond the region of neuronal cell loss (see Bachevalier and Meunier, 1996;

Gaffan, 1997). Neither can the role of the hippo-campus in monkeys be inferred directly from the behavioral impairments in monkeys with bilateral hippocampal aspiration lesions, as in the course of making these lesions the posterior cerebral artery necessarily is severed and there is, therefore, the possibility of impaired function of adjacent non-hippocampal tissue in area TE which can occur even in the absence of any observable infarcts in TE (Gaffan and Lim, 1991). Experiments in monkeys using selec-tive neurotoxic lesions of the hippocampus recently have begun to be performed (Murray and Mishkin, 1998) but, as argued above, these cannot be compared directly with any human patients with similar restricted damage. Instead the function of the hippo-campus in both monkeys and humans has largely been inferred from damage to the fornix which is the major source of efferent fibers from the hippocampus.

Humans and monkeys both show impairments in memory for complex scenes following fornix damage. Patients with fornix section are impaired at remem-bering photographs of complex scenes (Gaffan *et al.*, 1991) and monkeys with fornix section are impaired in both recognition memory with photographs (Gaffan, 1977) and discrimination learning between still cinema frames (Gaffan, 1992). Thus it was argued that memory for complex scenes may form the basis of episodic memory. According to this view, patients with fornix transection do not possess the ability to reconstruct the scene in which an event occurred in order to retrieve the target information easily. In this way, whole-scene memory was thought to help dif-ferentiate between memories of similar events in that a memory for the scene could protect episodic memo-ries from interference. However, it follows from this that deficits in whole-scene memory may also lead to impairments in tasks that do not overtly test or require scene memory. For instance, although visual object discrimination learning is unimpaired in monkeys with fornix transection when they are restricted to the WGTA, monkeys with fornix tran-section are impaired when they are trained and tested in different environments (Gaffan, 1992). Thus, only when the setting in which the problems are set varies can any memory for the background scene be used to protect memories from confusion and thereby provide an advantage to having an intact fornix. Object recog-nition memory tasks are also not overtly spatial tasks, yet they too are impaired in monkeys with fornix transection. In this case, the impairments may be due to the insensitivity to the different spatial positions of

objects between sample and retention tests which may lead to an impairment in differentiating between the two types of trial. This too is consistent with the idea that it is the processing of the spatial organization of complex scenes which is impaired following fornix transection. Furthermore, monkeys are also impaired in some object–place memory tasks after fornix tran-section even when presented in a constant scene (Gaffan and Harrison, 1989a,b; Gaffan *et al.*, 1984).

The function of the human and monkey hippocam-pus appeared for a long time to be quite different. According to this view, patients were supposed to have dense amnesia following fornix or hippocampus damage, whereas monkeys were supposed to have spared object memory and only show impairments in spatial tasks. However, these differences have now been resolved somewhat. First, monkeys with fornix damage, like patients, have also now been shown be impaired in a range of tasks which are not overly spatial as described above. Secondly, amnesic patients with fornix damage have been shown to be un-impaired in the Warrington recognition memory test for faces (Warrington, 1984; McMackin *et al.*, 1995) which is a task set in a single place. This is analogous to the lack of impairment shown in monkeys with fornix section upon certain tasks when they are set in unchanging backgrounds. Thus the pattern of impair-ments following fornix transection in humans and monkeys are empirically similar.

Thus it appears that the hippocampus of the human and monkey brain has a common function which is to contribute towards processing spatial relationships of objects and memory for object–place configurations which, when interrupted, leads to widespread effects upon episodic memory. However, the nature of the spatial information entering into these object–place configurations and the location of the memories them-selves are as yet unclear. There is strong evidence from ablation studies that the hippocampus of the rat processes 'idiothetic' spatial information (Whishaw *et al.*, 1997; Whishaw and Maaswinkel, 1998). Idio-thetic information is an estimate of animals' current environmental position derived from 'path integra-tion'. Path integration is the process of keeping track of the animal's own movements in space in reference to a known starting or reference point, integrating signals of the animal's locomotor movements over time. Idiothetic information contrasts with allothetic information which is knowledge about the animal's current location derived from exteroceptive input such as the relationship between currently visible landmarks. The idiothetic hypothesis of hippocampal function in the rat is also strongly supported by a weight of electrophysiological evidence (Golob and Taube, 1999).

Gaffan and Eacott (1997) trained rats in a Y-maze on a concurrent discrimination learning task with scenes and objects. However, they found that, unlike monkeys, fornix-transected rats were not impaired with spatially complex scenes relative to objects, nor were the rats impaired in encoding position as revealed by subsequent transfer tests. This is in contrast to fornix-transected monkeys which are impaired with spatially complex scenes relative to objects and are impaired in encoding spatial location as revealed, for example, by an object-in-place memory task (Gaffan, 1994b) and as predicted by the complex scene-learning hypothesis outlined above. However, one difference between the tasks as presented to monkeys in a fixed single touchscreen apparatus and the tasks as presented to rats in the Y-maze is the degree of idiothetic constancy associated with the correct stimuli. In scene memory tasks with monkeys, the reward is always in the same location relative to the environment, while in the rat's Y-maze the position of the scene can vary between the different arms. So whereas the monkeys can learn to associate a specific spatial position in their environment with the correct stimulus, the rats cannot.

In light of evidence such as this, Gaffan (1998) recently proposed an idiothetic role for the hippocampus in primates too. According to this hypothesis, the primate hippocampus provides idiothetic information about the environmental location of body parts, the main function of which is to become configured with object identity information provided by temporal lobe cortex outside of the hippocampus such as the perirhinal cortex which we showed to be involved in object identification (Buckley and Gaffan, 1998c; Buckley *et al.*, 2000) and which is known to interact with the fornix in object-in-place memory (Gaffan and Parker, 1996). The idiothetic hypothesis applied to primates assumes that idiothetic information is available for specific body parts such as the eyes and hand as well as for the body as a whole, because fornix transection has been seen to impair some tasks in which only the monkey's hands and eyes and not its whole body move through space. This extension of the idiothetic hypothesis to apply to primates is intuitively attractive, since although rats largely explore their environment by moving around in it, primates can also explore their environment visually and tactually

to a far greater extent while remaining in the same location. Recent electrophysiological evidence from monkeys shows that the hippocampus contains spatial view cells (Robertson *et al.*, 1998) which signal which part of the environment the animal is looking at independently of the animal's location within the environment itself. This is consistent with the idiothetic hypothesis of hippocampal function in monkeys and not consistent with an earlier hypothesis that the hippocampus provides a 'snapshot' type of encoding of the spatial relationships between objects in the scene as witnessed from the observer's point of view (see Gaffan, 1994b). Furthermore there is no fundamental difference between 'objects' and 'scenes' according to the idiothetic hypothesis as the presence of either type of stimulus can enter into a configuration with the idiothetic signal for that location. Thus the idiothetic hypothesis can explain fornix-dependent knowledge of both object-within-a-background and place-within-a-background which is consistent with the findings that both types of task are impaired after fornix transection in the monkey (Gaffan, 1994b) and is also consistent with the fact that impairments in both monkeys and humans after fornix damage are not limited to overtly spatial tasks.

The idiothetic hypothesis is of particular value as it has the potential to provide a common explanation for the underlying role of the hippocampus in rats, monkeys and humans. In this light, the role of the hippocampus can be seen to provide idiothetic spatial information to a broader based temporal lobe memory system. However, the role of the hippocampus need not be limited to contributing toward memory. Idiothetic information may also be useful to build up a representation of a scene, and in this way the hippocampus may also be thought of as contributing towards perception of scenes or episodic events which, as we discussed earlier, if found to be true would further erode the traditional, and potentially misleading, distinction often made as to whether particular structures are involved exclusively in either perception or memory.

REFERENCES

Amaral, D.G. and Insausti, R. (1990) The hippocampal formation. In: Paxinos, G. (ed.), *The Human Nervous System*. Academic Press, San Diego, pp. 711–755.

Amaral, D.G., Insausti, R. and Cowan, W.M. (1987) The entorhinal cortex of the monkey. I. Cytoarchitectonic organization. *Journal of Comparative Neurology*, 230, 465–496.

Arnold, S.E., Hyman, B.T. and Van Hoesen, G.W. (1991) Neuropathologic changes of the temporal pole in Alzheimer's disease and Pick's disease. *Archives of Neurology*, 51, 145–150.

Bachevalier, J. and Meunier, M. (1996) Cerebral ischemia: are the memory deficits associated with hippocampal cell loss? *Hippocampus*, 6, 553–560.

Bachevalier, J., Parkinson, J.K. and Mishkin, M. (1985) Visual recognition in monkeys: effects of separate vs combined transection of fornix and amygdalofugal pathways. *Experimental Brain Research*, 57, 554–561.

Booth, M.C.A. and Rolls, E.T. (1998) View-invariant representations of familiar objects by neurons in the inferior temporal visual cortex. *Cerebral Cortex*, 8, 510–523.

Bowen, D.M., Najlerahim, E., Procter, A.W., Francis, P.T. and Murphy, E. (1989) Circumscribed changes of the cerebral cortex in neuropsychiatric disorders of later life. *Proceedings of the National Academy of Sciences of the United States of America*, 86, 9504–9508.

Braak, H. and Braak, E. (1985) On areas of transition between entorhinal allocortex and temporary isocortex in the human brain. Normal morphology and lamina-specific pathology in Alzheimer's disease. *Acta Neuropathologica*, 68, 325–332.

Brodmann, K. (1905) Beiträge zur histologischen lokalisation der Grosshirnrinde. Dritte Mitteilung: die Rindenfelder der niederen Affen. *Journal für Psychologie und Neurologie*, 4, 177–226.

Brodmann, K. (ed.) (1909) *Vergleichende Lokalisationslehre der Grosshirnrinde in ihren Prinzipien dargestellt auf Grund des zellenbaus*. Barth, Leipzig.

Brown, M.W., Wilson, F.A.W. and Riches, I.P. (1987) Neuronal evidence that inferotemporal cortex is more important than hippocampus in certain processes underlying recognition memory. *Brain Research*, 409, 158–162.

Buckley, M.J. and Gaffan, D. (1997) Impairment of visual object-discrimination learning after perirhinal cortex ablation. *Behavioral Neuroscience*, 111, 467–475.

Buckley, M.J. and Gaffan, D. (1998a) Learning and transfer of object–reward associations and the role of the perirhinal cortex. *Behavioral Neuroscience*, 112, 15–23.

Buckley, M.J. and Gaffan, D. (1998b) Perirhinal cortex ablation impairs visual object identification. *Journal of Neuroscience*, 18, 2268–2275.

Buckley, M.J. and Gaffan, D. (1998c) Perirhinal cortex ablation impairs configural learning and paired-associate learning equally. *Neuropsychologia*, 36, 535–546.

Buckley, M.J., Gaffan, D. and Murray, E.A. (1997) A functional double-dissociation between two inferior temporal cortical areas: perirhinal cortex vs middle temporal gyrus. *Journal of Neurophysiology*, 77, 587–598.

Buckley, M.J., Booth, M.C.A., Rolls, E.T. and Gaffan, D. (1998) Selective visual–perceptual deficits following perirhinal cortex ablation in the macaque. *Society for Neuroscience Abstracts*, 24, 18.

Buffalo, E.A., Reber, P.J. and Squire, L.R. (1998a) The human perirhinal cortex and recognition memory. *Hippocampus*, 8, 330–339.

Buffalo, E.A., Stefanacci, L., Squire, L.R. and Zola, S.M. (1998b) A reexamination of the concurrent discrimination learning task: the importance of anterior inferotemporal cortex, area TE. *Behavioral Neuroscience*, 112, 3–14.

Cirillo, R.A., Horel, J.A. and George, P.J. (1989) Lesions of the anterior temporal stem and the performance of delayed match-to-sample and visual discriminations in monkeys. *Behavioural Brain Research*, 34, 55–69.

Cohen, N.J. and Squire, L.R. (1980) Preserved learning and retention of pattern-analysing skill in amnesia: dissociation of knowing how and knowing that. *Science*, 210, 207–210.

Corkin, S., Amaral, D.G., Gonzalez, R.G., Johnson, K.A. and Hyman, B. (1997) H.M.'s medial temporal lobe lesion: findings from magnetic resonance imaging. *Journal of Neuroscience*, 17, 3964–3979.

Correll, R.E. and Scoville, W.B. (1965a) Effects of medial temporal lesions on visual discrimination performance. *Journal of Comparative Physiology*, 60, 175–181.

Correll, R.E. and Scoville, W.B. (1965b) Performance of delayed match following lesions of medial temporal lobe structures. *Journal of Comparative and Physiological Psychology*, 60, 360–367.

Correll, R.E. and Scoville, W.B. (1967) Significance of delay in the performance of monkeys with medial temporal lobe resections. *Experimental Brain Research*, 4, 85–96.

Eacott, M.J., Gaffan, D. and Murray, E.A. (1994) Preserved recognition memory for small sets and impaired stimulus identification for large sets following rhinal cortex ablation in monkeys. *European Journal of Neuroscience*, 6, 1466–1478.

Easton, A. and Gaffan, D. (2000). Crossed unilateral lesions of the medial forebrain bundle and either inferior temporal cortex or frontal cortex impair object-reward association learning in rhesus monkeys. *Neuropsychologia* (in press).

Easton, A. and Gaffan, D. (2000) Comparison of perirhinal cortex ablation and crossed unilateral lesions of medial forebrain bundle from inferior temporal cortex in the rhesus monkey. *Behavioral Neuroscience* (in press).

Fahy, F.L., Riches, I.P. and Brown, M.W. (1993) Neuronal activity related to visual recognition memory: long-term memory and the encoding of recency and familiarity information in the primate anterior and medial inferior temporal and rhinal cortex. *Experimental Brain Research*, 96, 457–472.

Gaffan, D. (1974) Recognition impaired and association intact in the memory of monkeys after transection of the fornix. *Journal of Comparative and Physiological Psychology*, 86, 1100–1109.

Gaffan, D. (1977) Monkey's recognition memory impairment for complex pictures and the effect of fornix transection. *Quarterly Journal of Experimental Psychology*, 29, 505–514.

Gaffan, D. (1992) Amnesia for complex naturalistic scenes and for objects following fornix transection in the monkey. *European Journal of Neuroscience*, 4, 381–388.

Gaffan, D. (1994a) Dissociated effects of perirhinal cortex ablation, fornix transection and amygdalectomy: evidence for multiple memory systems in the primate temporal lobe. *Experimental Brain Research*, 99, 411–422.

Gaffan, D. (1994b) Scene-specific memory for objects: a model of episodic memory impairment in monkeys with fornix transection. *Journal of Cognitive Neuroscience*, 6, 305–320.

Gaffan, D. (1996a) Memory, action and the corpus striatum: current developments in the memory–habit distinction. *Seminars in the Neurosciences*, 8, 33–38.

Gaffan, D. (1996b) Associative and perceptual learning and the concept of memory systems. *Cognitive Brain Research*, 5, 69–80.

Gaffan, D. (1997) Episodic and semantic memory and the role of the not-hippocampus. *Trends in Cognitive Sciences*, 1, 246–248.

Gaffan, D. (1998) Idiothetic input into object–place configuration as the contribution to memory of the monkey and human hippocampus: a review. *Experimental Brain Research*, 123, 201–209.

Gaffan, D. and Harrison, S. (1989a) A comparison of the effects of fornix transection and sulcus principalis ablation upon spatial learning by monkeys. *Behavioural Brain Research*, 31, 207–220.

Gaffan, D. and Harrison, S. (1989b) Place memory and scene memory: effects of fornix transection in the monkey. *Experimental Brain Research*, 74, 202–212.

Gaffan, D. and Hornak, J. (1997) Visual neglect in the monkey: representation and disconnection. *Brain*, 120, 1647–1652.

Gaffan, D. and Lim, C. (1991) Hippocampus and the blood supply to TE: parahippocampal pial section impairs visual discrimination learning in monkeys. *Experimental Brain Research*, 87, 227–231.

Gaffan, D. and Murray, E.A. (1992) Monkeys (*Macaca fascicularis*) with rhinal cortex ablations succeed in object discrimination learning despite double sample presentations. *Behavioral Neuroscience*, 106, 30–38.

Gaffan, D. and Parker, A. (1996) Interaction of perirhinal cortex with the fornix-fimbria: memory for objects and 'object-in-place' memory. *Journal of Neuroscience*, 16, 5864–5869.

Gaffan, D., Saunders, R.C., Gaffan, E.A., Harrison, S., Shields, C. and Owen, M.J. (1984) Effects of fornix transection upon associative memory in monkeys: role of the hippocampus in learned action. *Quarterly Journal of Experimental Psychology*, 36B, 173–221.

Gaffan, D., Easton, A. and Parker, A. (1998) Dense amnesia in macaques after section of anterior temporal stem, amygdala and fornix. *Society for Neuroscience Abstracts*, 24, 18.

Gaffan, E.A., Gaffan, D. and Hodges, J.R. (1991) Amnesia following damage to the left fornix and to other sites: a comparative study. *Brain*, 114, 1297–1313.

Gaffan, E.A. and Eacott, M.J. (1997) Spatial memory impairment in rats with fornix transection is not accompanied by a simple encoding deficit for directions of objects in visual space. *Behavioral Neuroscience*, 111, 937–954.

Golob, E.J. and Taube, J.S. (1999) Head direction cells in rats with hippocampal or overlying neocortical lesions: evidence for impaired angular path integration. *Journal of Neuroscience*, 19, 7198–7211.

Haxby, J.V., Horwitz, B., Ungerleider, L.G., Maisog, J.M., Pietrini, P. and Gradby, C.L. (1994) The functional organization of human extrastriate cortex: a PET-rCBF study of selective attention to faces and locations. *Journal of Neuroscience*, 14, 6336–6353.

Higuchi, S. and Miyashita, Y. (1996) Formation of mnemonic neuronal responses to visual paired associates in inferotemporal cortex is impaired by perirhinal and entorhinal lesions. *Proceedings of the National Academy of Sciences of the United States of America*, 93, 739–743.

Hodges, J.R., Patterson, K., Oxbury, S. and Funnell, E. (1992) Semantic dementia: progressive fluent aphasia with temporal lobe atrophy. *Brain*, 115, 1783–1806.

Horel, J.A. (1978) The neuroanatomy of amnesia: a critique of the hippocampal memory hypothesis. *Brain*, 101, 403–445.

Horel, J.A. and Misantone, L.J. (1976) Visual discrimination impaired by cutting temporal lobe connections. *Science*, 193, 336–338.

Horel, J.A., Pytoko-Joiner, D.E., Voytko, M.L. and Salsbury, K. (1987) The performance of visual tasks while segments of the inferotemporal cortex are suppressed by cold. *Behavioural Brain Research*, 23, 29–42.

Insausti, R., Amaral, D.G. and Cowan, W.M. (1987) The entorhinal cortex of the monkey. II. Cortical afferents. *Journal of Comparative Neurology*, 264, 356–395.

Insausti, R., Salinas, A., Sanz, E., Insaust, A., Sobreviela, T. and Gonzalo, L.M. (1994) The human perirhinal cortex. Architecture in controls and in Alzheimer's disease. *Society for Neuroscience Abstracts*, 20, 359.

Irle, E. and Markowitsch, H.J. (1986) Afferent connections of the substantia innominata/basal nucleus of Meynert in carnivores and primates. *Journal für Hirnforschung*, 27, 343–367.

Kitt, C.A., Mitchell, S.J., DeLong, M.R., Wainer, B.H. and Price, D.L. (1987) Fiber pathways of basal forebrain cholinergic neurons in monkeys. *Brain Research*, 406, 192–206.

Leonard, B.W., Amaral, D.G., Squire, L.R. and Zola-Morgan, S. (1995) Transient memory impairment in monkeys with bilateral lesions of the entorhinal cortex. *Journal of Neuroscience*, 15, 5637–5659.

Li, L., Miller, E.K. and Desimone, R. (1994) The representation of stimulus familiarity in anterior inferior temporal cortex. *Journal of Neurophysiology*, 69, 1918–1929.

Mahut, H., Zola-Morgan, S. and Moss, M. (1982) Hippocampal resections impair associative learning and recognition memory in the monkey. *Journal of Neuroscience*, 2, 1214–1229.

Malamut, B.L., Saunders, R.C. and Mishkin, M. (1984) Monkeys with combined amygdalo-hippocampal lesions succeed in object discrimination learning despite 24-hour intertrial intervals. *Behavioral Neuroscience*, 98, 759–769.

McMackin, D., Cockburn, J., Anslow, P. and Gaffan, D. (1995) Correlation of fornix damage with memory impairment in six cases of colid cyst removal. *Acta Neurochirurgica*, 135, 12–18.

Meunier, M., Bachevalier, J. and Mishkin, M. (1993) Effects on visual recognition of combined and separate ablations of the entorhinal and perirhinal cortex in rhesus monkeys. *Journal of Neuroscience*, 13, 5418–5432.

Miller, E.K. and Desimone, R. (1993) Scopolamine affects short-term memory but not inferior temporal neurons. *Neuroreport*, 4, 81–84.

Miller, E.K., Li, L. and Desimone, R. (1993) Activity of neurons in anterior inferior temporal cortex during a short-term memory task. *Journal of Neuroscience*, 13, 1460–1478.

Milner, B. (1958) Psychological defects produced by temporal lobe excision. *Research Publications of the Association for Nervous and Mental Disease*, 36, 244–257.

Mishkin, M. (1992) A memory system in the monkey. *Philosophical Transactions of the Royal Society of London, Series B*, 298, 85–95.

Mishkin, M. and Delacour, J. (1975) An analysis of short-term visual memory in the monkey. *Journal of Experimental Psychology: Animal Behavior Processes*, 1, 326–334.

Mishkin, M. and Petri, H.L. (1984) Some implications for the analysis of learning and retention. In: Squire, L.R. and Butters, N. (eds), *Neuropsychology of Memory*. Guildford Press, New York, pp. 287–296.

Mishkin, M., Malamut, B.L. and Bachevalier, J. (1984) Memories and habits: two neural systems. In: Lynch, G., McGaugh, J.L. and Weinberger, N.M. (eds), *Neurobiology of Learning and Memory*. Guilford Press, New York, pp. 65–77.

Murray, E.A. (1992) Medial temporal lobe structures contributing to recognition memory: The amygdaloid complex versus the rhinal cortex. In: Aggleton, J.P. (ed.), *The Amygdala: Neurobiological Aspects of Emotion, Memory and Mental Dysfunction*. Wiley-Liss, New York, pp. 453–470.

Murray, E.A. and Mishkin, M. (1984) Severe tactual as well as visual memory deficits follow combined removal of the amygdala and hippocampus in monkeys. *Journal of Neuro-science*, 4, 2565–2580.

Murray, E.A. and Mishkin, M. (1986) Visual recognition in monkeys following rhinal cortical ablations combined with either amygdalectomy or hippocampectomy. *Journal of Neuroscience*, 13, 3681–3691.

Murray, E.A. and Mishkin, M. (1998) Object recognition and location memory in monkeys with excitotoxic lesions of the amygdala and hippocampus. *Journal of Neuroscience*, 18, 6568–6582.

Murray, E.A., Bachevalier, J. and Mishkin, M. (1989) Effects of rhinal cortical lesions on visual recognition memory in rhesus monkeys. *Society for Neuroscience Abstracts*, 15, 342.

O'Boyle, V.J., Murray, E.A. and Mishkin, M. (1993) Effects of excitotoxic amygdalo-hippocampal lesions on visual recognition in rhesus monkeys. *Society for Neuroscience Abstracts*, 19, 438.

Ongur, D., An, X. and Price, J.L. (1998) Prefrontal cortical projections to the hypothalamus in macaque monkeys. *Journal of Comparative Neurology*, 401, 480–505.

Orbach, J., Milner, B. and Rasmussen (1960) Learning and retention in monkeys after amygdala–hippocampus resection. *Archives of Neurology*, 3, 1214–1229.

Overman, W.H., Ormsby, G. and Mishkin, M. (1990) Picture recognition vs. picture discrimination learning in monkeys with medial temporal removals. *Experimental Brain Research*, 79, 18–24.

Parker, A., Easton, A. and Gaffan, D. (2000). Crossed uni-lateral lesions of medial forebrain bundle and either inferior temporal or frontal cortex impair object recognition memory in rhesus monkeys. *Society for Neuroscience Abstracts* (in press).

Ramus, S.J., Zola-Morgan, S. and Squire, L.R. (1994) Effects of lesions of perirhinal cortex or parahippocampal cortex on memory in monkeys. *Society for Neuroscience Abstracts*, 20, 1074.

Ringo, J.L. (1996) Stimulus specific adaptation in inferior temporal neurons during visual discrimination. *Journal of Neurophysiology*, 58, 1292–1306.

Robertson, R.G., Rolls, E.T. and Georges-Francois, P. (1998) Spatial view cells in the primate hippocampus: effects of removal of view details. *Journal of Neurophysiology*, 79, 1145–1156.

Russchen, F.T., Amaral, D.G. and Price, J.L. (1985) The afferent connections of the substantia innominata in the monkey, *Macaca fascicularis. Journal of Comparative Neurology*, 242, 1–27.

Saksida, L.M. and Bussey, T.J. (1998) Toward a neural network model of visual object identification in primate inferotemporal cortex. *Society for Neuroscience Abstracts*, 24, 1906.

Saleem, K.S. and Tanaka, K. (1996) Divergent projections from the anterior inferotemporal area TE to the perirhinal and entorhinal cortices in the macaque monkey. *Journal of Neuroscience*, 16, 4757–4775.

Saunders, R.C., Murray, E.A. and Mishkin, M. (1984) Further evidence that amygdala and hippocampus contribute equally to recognition memory. *Neuropsychologia*, 22, 785–796.

Scoville, W.B. and Milner, B. (1957) Loss of recent memory after bilateral hippocampal lesions. *Journal of Neurology, Neurosurgery and Psychiatry*, 20, 11–21.

Seldon, N.R., Gitelman, D.R. and Salamon-Murayama, N. (1998) Trajectories of cholinergic pathways within the cerebral hemispheres of the human brain. *Brain*, 121, 2249–2257.

Sergent, J., Ohta, S. and Macdonald, B. (1992) Functional neuroanatomy of face and object processing. *Brain*, 115, 15–36.

Sidman, M., Stoddard, L.T. and Mohr, J.P. (1968) Some additional quantitative observations of intermediate memory in a patient with bilateral hippocampal lesions. *Neuro-psychologia*, 6, 245–254.

Sobotka, S. and Ringo, J.L. (1993) Investigations of long-term recognition and association memory in unit responses from inferotemporal cortex. *Experimental Brain Research*, 96, 28–38.

Sobotka, S. and Ringo, J.L. (1994) Stimulus specific adaptation in excited but not in inhibited cells in inferotemporal cortex of macaque. *Brain Research*, 646, 95–99.

Squire, L.R. and Zola-Morgan, S. (1991) The medial temporal lobe memory system. *Science*, 253, 1380–1386.

Sutherland, R.J. and Rudy, J.W. (1989) Configural association theory: the role of the hippocampal formation in learning, memory and amnesia. *Psychobiology*, 8, 3–12.

Suzuki, W.A. (1996) Neuroanatomy of the monkey ento-rhinal, perirhinal and parahippocampal cortices: organization of cortical inputs and interconnections with amygdala and striatum. *Seminars in the Neurosciences*, 8, 3–12.

Suzuki, W.A. and Amaral, D.G. (1994a) Perirhinal and parahippocampal cortices of the macaque monkey: cortical afferents. *Journal of Comparative Neurology*, 350, 497–533.

Suzuki, W.A. and Amaral, D.G. (1994b) Topographical organization of the reciprocal connections between monkey entorhinal cortex and the perirhinal and parahippocampal cortices. *Journal of Neuroscience*, 14, 1856–1877.

Suzuki, W.A., Zola-Morgan, S., Squire, L.R. and Amaral, D.G. (1993) Lesions of the perirhinal and parahippocampal cortices in the monkey produce long-lasting memory impairment in the visual and tactual modalities. *Journal of Neuroscience*, 13, 2430–2451.

Tanaka, K. (1996) Inferotemporal cortex and object vision. *Annual Review of Neuroscience*, 19, 109–139.

Tang, Y., Mishkin, M. and Aigner, T.G. (1997) Effects of muscarinic blockade in perirhinal cortex during visual recognition. *Proceedings of the National Academy of Sciences of the United States of America*, 94, 12667–12669.

Thornton, J.A., Rothblat, L.A. and Murray, E.A. (1997) Rhinal cortex removal produces amnesia for preoperatively learned discrimination problems but fails to disrupt postoperative acquisition and retention in rhesus monkeys. *Journal of Neuroscience*, 17, 8536–8549.

Ungerleider, L.G. and Haxby, J.V. (1994) 'What' and 'where' in the human brain. *Current Opinions in Neurobiology*, 4, 157–165.

Van Hoesen, G.W., Pandya, D.N. and Butters, N. (1975) Some connections of the entorhinal area (area 28) and the perirhinal (area 35) cortices of the rhesus monkey. II. Frontal lobe afferents. *Brain Research*, 95, 25–38.

Van Hoesen, G.W., Hyman, B.T. and Damasio, A.R. (1991) Entorhinal cortex pathology in Alzheimer's disease. *Hippocampus*, 1, 1–8.

von Bonin, G. and Bailey, P. (eds) (1947) *The Neocortex of Macaca mulatta*. University of Illinois Press, Urbana, Illinois.

Warrington, E.K. (1984) *Recognition Memory Test*. NFER-Nelson, Windsor, UK.

Warrington, E.K. (1985) Agnosia: the impairment of object recognition. In: Fredericks, J.A.M. (ed.), *Handbook of Clinical Neurology*. Elsevier Science, Amsterdam, pp. 333–349.

Webster, M.J., Bachevalier, J. and Ungerleider, L.G. (1993) Subcortical connections of inferior temporal areas TE and TEO in macaque monkeys. *Journal of Comparative Neurology*, 335, 73–91.

Whishaw, I.Q. and Maaswinkel, H. (1998) Rats with fimbria-fornix lesions are impaired in path integration: a role for the hippocampus in 'sense of direction'. *Journal of Neuroscience*, 18, 3050–3058.

Whishaw, I.Q., McKenna, J.E. and Maaswinkel, H. (1997) Hippocampal lesions and path integration. *Current Opinion in Neurobiology*, 7, 228–234.

Witter, M.P., Van Hoesen, G.W. and Amaral, D.G. (1989) Topographical organization of the entorhinal cortex projection to the dentate gyrus of the monkey. *Journal of Neuroscience*, 9, 216–228.

Zola-Morgan, S. and Squire, L.R. (1984) Preserved learning in monkeys with medial temporal lesions: sparing of motor and cognitive skills. *Journal of Neuroscience*, 4, 1071–1085.

Zola-Morgan, S. and Squire, L.R. (1986) Memory impairment in monkeys following lesions limited to the hippocampus. *Behavioral Neuroscience*, 100, 155–160.

Zola-Morgan, S., Squire, L.R. and Mishkin, M. (1982) The neuroanatomy of amnesia: amygdalo-hippocampus versus temporal stem. *Science*, 218, 1137–339.

Zola-Morgan, S., Squire, L.R., Amaral, D.G. and Suzuki, W.A. (1989) Lesions of perirhinal and parahippocampal cortex that spare the amygdala and hippocampal formation produce severe memory impairment. *Journal of Neuroscience*, 9, 4335–4370.

Zola-Morgan, S., Squire, L.R., Clower, R.P. and Rempel, N.L. (1993) Damage to the perirhinal cortex exacerbates memory impairment following lesions to the hippocampal formation. *Journal of Neuroscience*, 13, 251–265.

17 FUNCTIONAL NEUROIMAGING AND MEMORY SYSTEMS

Raymond J. Dolan

INTRODUCTION

Psychologists have long assumed that there is more than one type of learning and memory (Tolman, 1949). A corollary of this perspective is the idea that different forms of learning and memory are implemented within independent neural substrates. In this chapter, I address brain mechanisms involved in human memory and learning from a functional neuroimaging perspective. It is clearly impossible to do justice to the entire diversity of memory systems within the constraints of a single chapter. Consequently, I will restrict myself to a consideration of two types of learning: perceptual priming and associative learning.

What is meant by learning and memory may seem self-evident, but it is surprisingly difficult to find agreed definitions. Here the term learning refers to experience-dependent generation of internal representations or experience-dependent modifications of these representations. Learning in this sense is a generic property of the brain. It should be distinguished from neural plasticity, a presumed physical substrate of learning. Memory, as opposed to learning, refers to the retention of these experience-dependent representations as stable traces over time (Dudai, 1989). This latter view of memory closely accords with what many now view as the arcane notion of an engram.

Learning and memory have been subjected to scientific analysis at many different levels of organization that extend from the cellular to the behavioral level. From a psychological perspective, the term memory embodies several distinct abilities. These abilities, reflecting prior experience of an organism, are expressed through a variety of means including improved motor skill, enhanced perceptual fluency or increased factual or personal autobiographical knowledge about the world. However, only certain forms of memory are available to conscious awareness, of which the latter are the prime examples. How the disparate psychological abilities that constitute memory are reflected in the functioning of the human brain and whether they reflect distinct or unique mechanisms is a major research theme in the biological sciences.

The focus of the present discussion is on a systems level analysis of learning and memory in the human brain using functional neuroimaging techniques. As outlined, I focus on two distinct types of learning, priming and associative learning. Both are conceived as expressions of implicit memory reflecting the fact that this type of learning can occur without concurrent awareness of what is being learned (see Weiskrantz, Chapter 18). This is in contrast to more explicit forms of memory where awareness of what is being learned is a critical component.

BRAIN MECHANISMS OF ASSOCIATIVE LEARNING

Associative learning is a type of learning driven primarily by changes in expectations about whether future events involve rewards or punishment. This anticipatory capacity is of crucial adaptive significance in that it provides a fundamental basis for selection between different courses of future action based upon past experience within similar environments. One of the best characterized forms of associative learning is what is termed classical conditioning. In standard conditioning paradigms, a sensory cue (the conditioned stimulus or CS) comes to predict reward or punishment. For this type of learning to occur, the cue (CS) must consistently precede the reward (the unconditioned stimulus or US, which usually is a motivationally relevant stimulus) in order for a predictive association to develop. In a standard paradigm, known as delay conditioning, the US onset precedes CS offset. With repeated parings of a CS and US, the CS comes to elicit a response previously expressed to the US alone. This CS-elicited response is the behavioral signature of learning.

As already suggested, the basic mechanism that drives this type of learning is a change in the behavioral relevance of a stimulus. Take a simple example of an airpuff delivered to the eye (an aversive US) which will, without prior experience, elicit a defensive eyeblink response. If an unrelated sensory stimulus (CS), such as a tone, is presented repeatedly just prior to the onset of the airpuff, it comes to predict its occurrence. Consequently, following repeated pairings, the tone will on its own elicit an eyeblink response (see also King and Thompson, Chapter 12). It is in this sense that classical conditioning is conceived of as a form of associative learning in that it essentially involves linkage between a neutral stimulus and a stimulus with high intrinsic emotional or behavioral significance. Unlike explicit forms of learning, this type of learning can occur without any awareness of the relationship between the CS and US (Weiskrantz and Warrington, 1979; see Weiskrantz, Chapter 18).

A traditional view of conditioning emphasized its passive and reflex-like mode of operation. This conceptualization has been revised by more complex models where the critical component is seen to be the predictive power of a stimulus. The essential cognitive nature of conditioning derives from the fact that the ability of a CS to elicit a learnt behavioral response depends upon establishing an association between representations of the CS and US. Consequently, altering the value of a US representation is reflected in spontaneous changes in responses to the CS when it subsequently is presented alone (Holland, 1990; Stanhope, 1992).

LEARNING ABOUT BEHAVIORAL RELEVANCE

The mechanisms for acquisition of associative learning have been studied extensively in animals under a variety of experimental paradigms. A great source of interest is the degree to which human data accord with those acquired in animals. To study this type of learning satisfactorily with functional neuroimaging techniques has become technically feasible only recently. In general, there are two principle types of

functional neuroimaging techniques that are used in studying cognition, positron emission tomography (PET) and functional magnetic resonance imaging (fMRI). Both techniques essentially index changes in local perfusion that occur as a consequence of increased neural activity. The main limitations of PET, apart from the fact that is involves administration of a radiotracer, is its poor temporal resolution which at best is of the order of 30 s. This means that study designs involve blocked presentation of stimuli across this temporal window. fMRI, on the other had, has a greatly enhanced temporal resolution and, with the use of event-related designs, where changes in perfusion are measured in response to the occurrence of isolated events, it is possible to measure differential activity to events occurring every 2 s. This technique also has superior antomical resolution capabilites with respect to PET, and in current applications it is possible to resolve activations that are separated by as little as 5 mm.

The optimal conditions for studying associative learning require the use of mixed-trial paradigms where sensory stimuli that predict the occurrence (CS+) or absence (CS–) of reward or punishment can be presented in an interleaved and random manner. Thus, to address how classical conditioned behavioral responses are acquired needed the advent of event-related fMRI (Buckner *et al.*, 1996; Josephs *et al.*, 1997). This technique resembles event-related potentials in electrophysiology where stimuli pertaining to distinct experimental conditions are presented repeatedly, and randomly, over time. This type of stimulus presentation allows sampling of multiple similar event types which can then be averaged (to improve signal to noise) and compared.

In an aversive classical conditioning study, my colleagues and I used this approach to condition subjects to human faces using a partial reinforcement strategy. In this paradigm, two distinct faces were paired with an aversive event (white noise 10% above threshold, the US) and became the CS+, while two other faces were never paired with the noise and became the CS–. Note that using a partial reinforcement schedule meant that only half the presentations of the CS+ faces were paired with noise. The noise followed the 3 s presentation time of the face and lasted 500 ms. On-line skin conductance responses (SCRs) were obtained simultaneously and provided independent evidence that learning took place. Using this approach, it is possible to compare evoked hemodynamic responses (an index of neural activity) elicited by a CS+ in the absence of noise with responses evoked by the CS– (faces never paired with noises).

Four different event types can be characterized, three of which were time locked to the onset of the presentation of the face; the remaining response was time locked to the onset of the tone, coinciding with the offset of the visual stimulus. The three visual events were subdivided into (i) CS–; (ii) CS+ paired; and (iii) CS+ unpaired face stimuli. The critical comparison in this experiment was that between the unpaired CS+ evoked responses and those evoked by the CS– during conditioning. This comparison revealed differential activation of the anterior cingulate gyrus and bilateral anterior insula for the CS+ condition (Büchel *et al.*, 1998). This analysis assumes that neural responses to the CS+ and CS– do not vary with time and, consequently, isolates systems where there are time-invariant neural responses during conditioning. Such a profile would be in keeping with an output system response in so far as the continued reinforcement of the CS+ over the entire time course of the study would be expected to be associated with an ongoing adaptive behavioral output.

A region where animal studies would predict a response with this type of associative learning is the amygdala (see McGaugh *et al.*, Chapter 13; Nader and LeDoux, Chapter 14). As already noted, such a response was not seen in the categorical comparison of the CS+ and CS–. Bear in mind that this comparison assumes a response profile in neural populations mediating learning that is equivalent across time. There are compelling reasons to suggest that this assumption would not lead to the best characterization of the neural systems involved in associative learning. In particular, animal studies and intracranial recording from human subjects have shown rapid adaptation in neuronal response in the amygdala during conditioning (Fried *et al.*, 1997; Quirk *et al.*, 1997). Consequently, using a statistical model that allows for adaptation in neural response over time, in effect modeling for a time by condition interaction, a distinct profile of neural response was characterized. An initial increase in response to the CS+ and a subsequent decrease over time was highly significant for bilateral amygdalae (see Figure 17.1).

The time-limited role of the amygdala in associative learning that we identified relates to a number of key theoretical issues. Most notably, Pearce and Hall (1980) proposed a distinction between two kinds of attentional processing of CSs; automatic processing responsible for CSs and controlled 'attentional' processing of CSs which determines the extent of new learning. Specifically, this model suggests that controlled processing of a CS is reduced whenever the CS

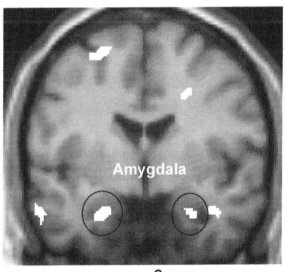

y = -3 mm

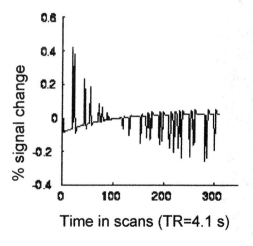

Figure 17.1. (**A**) A coronal MRI slice of a canonical brain on which has been superimposed the area of significant activation in a time by condition contrast of CS+ and CS– faces. The area highlighted corresponds to the left amygdala. This time by condition interaction is illustrated further in (**B**) where the neural response in the amygdala with repeated presentation of a CS+ is seen to diminish with time.

predicts its consequences. In early stages of learning, a CS can elicit considerable controlled processing because it is a relatively poor predictor of the US. Consequently, early CS–US pairings result in substantial learning. However, as learning is acquired, the CS is a better predictor of the US and, in this model, it becomes less able to engender new learning. Note that the automatic processing of the CS is unaltered and, consequently, it continues to elicit a CR.

Extending this theoretical model to our physiological data, a striking parallel is evident between the time-limited role of the amygdala and the proposed temporally modulated 'attentional' processing of the CS associated with enhanced learning. This would suggest that the amygdala is critical in associative learning, and that it initiates the neurobiological changes associated with learning but that these changes are expressed elsewhere in the brain (see McGaugh *et al.*, Chapter 13). Indeed, there is considerable neurobiological evidence from animal studies for this suggestion of a neuromodulatory role for the amygdala (Edeline and Weinberger, 1991; Packard *et al.*, 1994; Weinberger, 1995; McGaugh *et al.*, 1996). Responses in other regions associated with conditioning, such as the cingulate, did not vary across time, and this pattern would conform to a conceptualization that these regions mediate learnt behaviorial responses. More specifically, activation in the cingulate may reflect neural processes related to rapid formation and maintenance of stimulus–response associations.

Unconscious learning of emotional responses

We have already referred to a distinction between explicit and implicit forms of memory. Note that the former refers to a type of memory associated with the ability consciously to report the contingencies of the learning situation, while the latter refers to a type of memory that is independent of reportablility. In the previous section, we described a learning experiment where learning takes place in a context where subjects subsequently could report contingencies between a CS and a US. Thus, even though this type of associative learning frequently is assumed to be implicit, it is clear that in the type of experimental paradigm we describe, process purity, meaning that learning is driven by one process alone, is extremely unlikely.

Behaviorally, it can be shown that associative learning can take place even when subjects' awareness of the contingencies between a CS and a US is non-existent. In other words, associative learning, using delay conditioning paradigms, does not require awareness of stimulus contingencies, unlike a closely associated form of learning, trace conditioning, where explicit awareness seems to be necessary (Clark and Squire, 1998). The independence of associative learning from memory that depends on an ability to report prior occurrence is underlined by studies of patients with hippocampal damage. These patients can acquire reliable SCRs to CSs but cannot discriminate consciously between stimuli paired with an aversive US when these stimuli are presented post-learning (Bechara *et al.*, 1995). Conversely, patients with selective amygdala damage, but intact hippocampi, no longer acquire conditioned SCRs, but show intact declarative knowledge concerning stimulus associations (Bechara *et al.*, 1995; LaBar and LeDoux, 1996).

One approach to studying mechanisms of associative learning without awareness in neurologically intact individuals is to use backward masking techniques. The data that relate directly on this issue include evidence that neurologically intact subjects make discriminatory SCRs to aversively conditioned stimuli that have been backwardly masked to prevent conscious awareness of their occurrence (Esteves *et al.*, 1994; Parra *et al.*, 1997). In a study within our laboratory, we presented volunteer subjects pictures of two angry faces, one of which (prior to test) was paired (CS+) and the other unpaired (CS–) with a US consisting of a 100 dB white noise burst. The target faces were then presented sequentially but masked by a neutral face, without the US, while neural activity was measured by PET.

The critical manipulation was to prevent subjects' awareness of the angry target faces (CS+ and CS–) by backwardly masking with neutral faces under a condition where the task requirement was for subjects to report the occurrence of an angry face. The responses of the subjects in the explicit task indicated that they were unable to detect the target masked faces. In the masked condition, none of the angry faces were reported, whereas the detection rate of the unmasked angry faces was 100%. Mean SCRs were significantly greater for CS+ than CS– faces ($P < 0.001$), both for masked (mean CS + SCR = 0.605 μS; mean CS – SCR = 0.473 μS) and unmasked (mean CS+ SCR = 0.748 μS; mean CS– SCR = 0.426 μS) presentations (see Figure 17.2A). [Note that microSiemans (μS) is a standard unit for indexing SCRs.]

The critical question in this experiment was whether a differential neural response in the amyg-

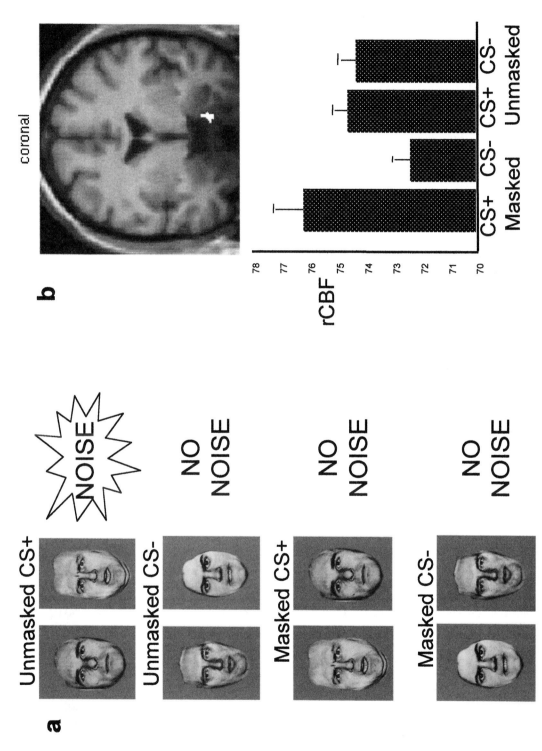

Figure 17.2. (A) The basic design of the study involving presentation of target stimuli (an angry face which may be a CS+ or a CS–) under masked (by an neutral face) or unmasked conditions. (B) The differential response in the right amygdala in the contrast of a masked CS+ and masked CS– angry face.

dala would characterize a situation where subjects showed evidence of differential SCRs but could not report awareness of the target stimuli that had acquired behavioral value through associative learning. Contrasting neural responses associated with masked CS+ and CS– conditions revealed a significant enhanced response in the right amygdala specific to presentation of the masked CS+ faces (see Figure 17.2B).

It is important to recall that the only difference between the CS+ and CS– conditions was the subjects' prior associative experience of a temporal association between the CS+ faces and an aversive noise. During scanning, the CS+ and CS– conditions involved identical physical stimuli, i.e. angry faces, and the same explicit task. Consequently, the neural response expressed must reflect engagement of systems that discriminate between stimuli on the basis of their behavioral significance or predictive ability.

On the basis of these findings, we suggest that neural processing in the human amygdala is involved in the behavioral expression of previously learnt emotionally relevant stimulus associations. Furthermore, this behavioral expression is independent of conscious reportability. These neuroimaging findings therefore complement data from animal and human lesion studies (LeDoux, 1993; Esteves *et al.*, 1994; Bechara *et al.*, 1995; LaBar *et al.*, 1995; LaBar and LeDoux, 1996; Parra *et al.*, 1997). Critically, the differential amygdala response during masked presentations, when subjects were unable to report the occurrence of the target stimuli, indicates that the amygdala can mediate consequences of associative learning in the absence of conscious (reportable) awareness of the presence of the eliciting stimulus.

A common thread through these studies is the idea that the amygdala is involved in assigning emotional value or significance to events through associative learning. In the illustrated examples, the common value in the stimuli, following learning, is that they signal or predict future danger. Given the salience of fear as an emotion, it is conceivable that activation of the amygdala is a mechanism by which autonomic and associative, including mnemonic, processes that are pertinent to marshalling adaptive responses, both prepared and planned, to the current or future context are triggered rapidly. The amygdala in this regard may be required to link visual or other sensory signals of danger to central representations that constitute the concept of fear (Adolphs *et al.*, 1995).

PRIMING

By contrast with associative learning, priming is a facilitation of recognition or production of a stimulus by prior exposure to a stimulus with which the recognized item has a relationship of physical similarity or associated meaning (see also Brown, Chapter 11; Weiskrantz, Chapter 18). Two broad types of priming are recognized, modality-specific perceptual priming and an amodal conceptual priming (Blaxton, 1989). The focus here is solely on the former. As outlined, priming, like associative learning, is an example of implicit memory that usually is studied by indirect tasks that do not engage intentional memory retrieval mechanisms. It has long been recognized that this type of learning is preserved in amnesic patients (Milner *et al.*, 1968; Warrington and Weiskrantz, 1974). For example, perceptual identification of degraded line drawings of familiar objects improves in amnesic patients if they previously had seen the intact drawing even though their explicit memory for the drawing is impaired. However, it is important to note that improved performance does not match that of normals, suggesting that the latter group may also use explicit memory to enhance performance on these types of tasks. At the very least, this implies that in everyday life psychologically distinct forms of memory rarely operate in isolation.

The effect of priming on perceptual processing can be demonstrated using degraded or fragmented stimuli. As shown in Figure 17.3, a naive viewing of degraded stimuli is associated with a low likelihood of an associated perception. However, following priming with the full gray-scale image, a perception can be elicited automatically and effortlessly. This perceptual priming can persist for as long as several weeks (Ramachandran, 1994). A critical question is where and how this rapid perceptual learning is expressed in the human brain? One influential proposal is that perceptual priming is mediated by a retuning of perceptual input modules in posterior neocortex, specifically inferior temporal cortex (Miller *et al.*, 1991).

One experimental approach adopted by my colleagues and I to identify brain mechanisms involved in perceptual priming involved showing subjects two-tone images prior to, and following, exposure to a uniquely associated gray-scale image, as already illustrated. The two-tone binarized images were derived from either real objects or faces. Exposure to uniquely associated gray-scale images, in a learning phase,

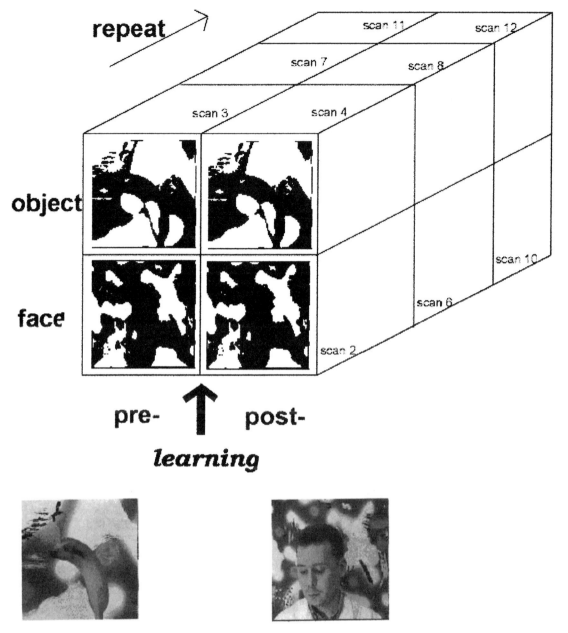

Figure 17.3. The critical experimental manipulation. Binarized images of faces or objects were presented to subjects either before or after exposure to their non-degraded versions. As a control, we used a similar manipulation but the interposed non-degraded stimuli did not correspond to the degraded versions so no priming could take place. Prior to priming, degraded images do not lead to a perception, while post-priming there is a high probability of a perception of a face or object.

increased the likelihood that subjects would see the whole object or face during a subsequent presentation of its two-tone version. The design of the experiment involved four conditions: two-tone images of objects before and after exposure to the associated gray-scale images of the objects; and two-tone images of faces before and after exposure to the associated gray-scale images of the faces (see Figure 17.3). In addition, there were matched control conditions involving repetition of two-tone images of either category without priming. The question of interest in the experiment was the neural events that ensue when priming leads to a change in perceptual experience. A general hypothesis was that this form of learning would modulate activation in extrastriate visual cortex within regions specifically associated with object and face processing (Gross *et al.*, 1979; Moran and Desimone, 1985; Baylis and Rolls, 1987).

We first identified category-specific activations by directly comparing face with object conditions (combining the pre- and post-learning scans, i.e. main effects). Activations in the right superior temporal region extending into the right inferior temporal region were identified in association with the face conditions. Activations in the left inferior temporal region were identified in association with the object conditions. The occurrence of selective activations, due to learning, were determined subsequently by a direct comparison of pre- and post-learning activations for objects and faces, respectively. Control for order of stimulus presentation was effected by the separate non-primed presentation of identical stimuli (i.e. category-specific interactions). This analysis was constrained to areas that revealed main effects during object or face presentation. Category-specific learning effects, involving augmentations of activations, were found within these inferior temporal regions located in the right fusiform gyrus for faces and left fusiform gyrus for objects (Dolan *et al.*, 1997). Note that this region of fusiform gyrus is in the inferior temporal cortex caudal to perirhinal cortex (for a consideration of the function of this region, see Brown, Chapter 11; Buckley and Gaffan, Chapter 16). This region has also been referred to as the fusiform face area (FFA) though whether its role is exclusive to face processing is unresolved (for a fuller discussion, see also Johnson and Bolhuis, Chapter 4).

These data demonstrate that priming-facilitated perception of faces in degraded stimuli is associated with an enhanced neural response in regions of inferior temporal cortex. Note that these enhanced neural responses are associated with a vivid visual perception. This effect was most striking for the enhanced perception of a face where the maximal effect was observed in the right fusiform gyrus. Selective activation of right fusiform gyrus during face perception has been reported previously in functional imaging studies (Haxby *et al.*, 1994; Clark *et al.*, 1996; Courtney *et al.*, 1996). Likewise, left inferior temporal cortex and nearby occipital regions play a role in pattern and object recognition (Gross, 1972; Desimone and Gross,

1979; Ungerleider and Mishkin, 1982; Tanaka *et al.*, 1991; Malach *et al.*, 1995). However, our findings specifically address the brain areas activated when learning facilitates perception of faces and objects. The perception-related activations in fusiform regions, particularly on the right, may reflect learning-related retuning of neural activity similar to that seen in monkeys (Sakia and Miyashita, 1994, 1995; Tovee *et al.*, 1996). Single unit recordings demonstrate that memory and attention can tune responses of inferior temporal cortex to repeated encounters with stimuli (Gross *et al.*, 1979; Moran and Desimone, 1985; Baylis and Rolls, 1987).

The results of our initial study seem at odds with the general finding of a decreased neural response associated with repetition priming (Schacter and Buckner, 1998). One possibility is that our priming-related activation is associated with an enhanced perception of either objects or faces in response to representation of the primed stimuli. In our next experiment, we sought to replicate this basic finding using an experimental design that did not involve stimulus repetition and where priming led to an enhanced perception in one condition but no change of perception in the other condition.

Priming for known and unknown faces

For this study, we used 40 famous faces comprising well-known individuals such as politicians and movie stars and 40 unknown faces matched for sex, image size and age. Priming effects were addressed by determining whether there were differential neural responses to faces arising when a particular face, that had appeared in one block, reappeared in a later block, but now with the reverse contrast polarity (in simple terms, as a positive or a negative).

This type of experimental manipulation arises out of a psychological observation that previous experience with a positive face facilitates subsequent identification of its negative. Note that this phenomenon only applies for known faces and, consequently, primed non-famous negatives provide an ideal matched control group in so far as they rule out mere repetition of low-level features (spatial frequencies and edges) shared by positives and their negatives. In a related behavioral study, we confirmed this type of priming effect arising out of prior exposure to famous positives upon the subsequent recognition of their negatives. Famous positives were recognized more often than famous negatives when unprimed (69%

Seeing the positive of a famous face ....

... primes the recognition of its negative

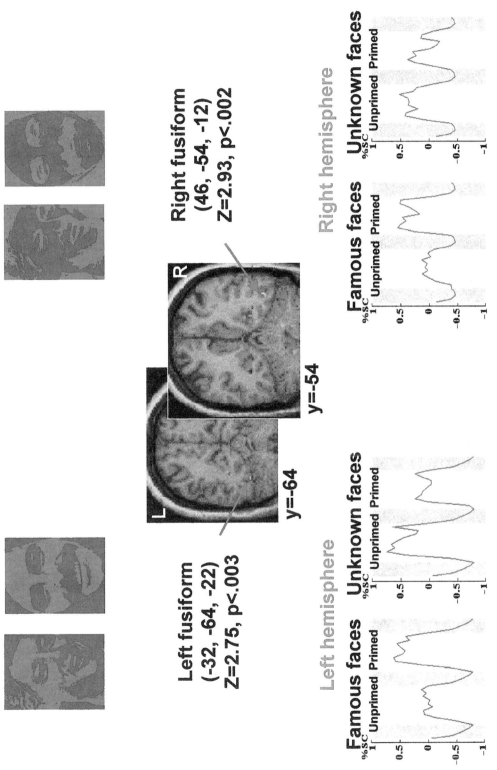

Left fusiform
(-32, -64, -22)
Z=2.75, p<.003

Right fusiform
(46, -54, -12)
Z=2.93, p<.002

y=-64

y=-54

Left hemisphere

Right hemisphere

Famous faces
%SC
Unprimed Primed
1
0.5
0
-0.5
-1

Unknown faces
%SC
Unprimed Primed
1
0.5
0
-0.5
-1

Famous faces
%SC
Unprimed Primed
1
0.5
0
-0.5
-1

Unknown faces
%SC
Unprimed Primed
1
0.5
0
-0.5
-1

Figure 17.4. The coronal sections of the MRI scan are superimposed with areas where there is a priming-related response in left and right fusiform cortex. The lower graphs plot the time course of mean corrected signal change for primed and unprimed known and unknown faces. Note that only with priming of famous negatives is there enhanced recogntion and a parallel enhacement of activity in right fusiform cortex.

versus 17%, P <0.0001); previous recognition of famous positives significantly increased the rate of subsequent recognition for their negatives (45% after priming versus 17% unprimed, P <0.001)].

The basic prediction was that following a 'priming' manipulation, where the corresponding positive is shown shortly beforehand (and which boosts recognition of famous negatives), primed negatives of known faces would induce a stronger neural response than negatives of non-primed known faces. Furthermore, since unknown faces cannot yield identification even in positive form, the predicted increase in neural responses for primed negatives (i.e. those previously seen in positive) versus unprimed negatives would not be seen for unknown faces (see Figure 17.4).

Accordingly, we looked for changes in neural response in the famous face blocks for a simple effect showing greater activation for primed negatives (previously seen as positive) than unprimed negatives (not previously seen in postive form) of known faces. Our data revealed bilateral fusiform activations for primed famous negatives (compared with unprimed famous negatives). The right hemisphere activation peaked at the lateral border of the fusiform gyrus, and extended into mid-fusiform gyrus. The left hemisphere activation peaked more posteriorly in the fusiform. Thus, the very same negatives of famous faces produced more fusiform activation when they had been seen previously as positives and subsequently were more identifiable.

To demonstrate that this effect was associated specifically with priming-related recognition, we carried out a similar analysis with data for unknown faces. No priming-related increase was identified in this analysis. A significant interaction between primed versus unprimed, and famous versus unknown negative faces, was found for the activated regions, indicating that previous exposure to positives of famous negatives led to increased activation solely for those negatives. Strikingly, we found that such previous exposure had the opposite effect for unknown faces, leading to reduced activation.

This priming effect with famous faces on their negatives can be interpreted broadly as evidence that a face-responsive fusiform region is functionally related to recognition processes. This finding recapitulates our previous finding in which recognition in binarized images of faces was facilitated by prior exposure to the full gray-scale version (Dolan *et al.*, 1997). In this instance, we found increased fusiform responses to the very same negative famous face stim-

ulus, depending on whether this stimulus was identified or not (i.e. when primed versus unprimed, respectively). The qualitative difference between the priming effects for known versus unknown faces confirms that the priming effect for famous negatives was indeed due specifically to an influence on their recognition, rather than merely repetition of low-level features; recall that the latter was associated with a decrease in neural response.

These and other findings suggest two physiologically distinct priming effects that are also associated with two psychologically distinct forms of priming. In one form of priming, repeating a stimulus merely increases the fluency (or speed) with which the same information is extracted, but is not associated with any change in what is perceived. This repetition priming, leading to perceptual fluency, is associated consistently with an attenuated neural response (Squire *et al.*, 1992; Dolan *et al.*, 1997; Schacter and Buckner, 1998). By contrast, the second form of priming, illustrated in both our studies of face priming, has the additional effect of changing what is actually perceived in the primed stimulus. Recall that in the previous study a degraded or ambiguous stimulus becomes recognizable for the first time after priming by its corresponding full gray-scale image (Dolan *et al.*, 1997). One other previous study has observed increased activation with priming which also involved ambiguous stimuli whose perception changed when primed (Schacter *et al.*, 1995).

The two forms of perceptual priming we propose can be considered manifestations of implicit memory and they would appear to share common psychological features. These features include an obligatory mechanism for their elicitation involving repeated exposure to identical or structurally similar perceptual inputs. Additionally, one assumes that there is an informational encapsulation constraint on this form of memory in so far as its influence does not generalize to other cognitive domains. However, one type of priming leads to an altered conscious perception without an associated change in the sensory input, and this form of priming is associated with enhanced neural activity.

CONCLUSIONS

The focus of this chapter has been the application of functional neuroimaging to understanding human memory systems. Two examples of implicit memory, associative memory and perceptual priming, were considered. In both examples, functional neuro-imaging can be seen to have provided novel data that have enhanced, and indeed challenged, our existing understanding of the neural mechanisms mediating these distinct forms of memory. In the case of associative learning using aversive conditioning, a crucial role for the amygdala has been highlighted. While this might be predicted from animal and lesion data, the functional neuroimaging experiments indicate that its role in this form of learning is time limited. Furthermore, its role in the expression of associative learning is independent of explicit awareness of the eliciting stimulus. In the case of perceptual priming, functional neuroimaging data indicate that there are two distinct mechanisms involved. One mechanism is associated with an augmented neural response while the other is associated with an attenuated neural response. Phenomenologically, these distinct mechanisms are mirrored by an enhanced perceptual experience on the one hand and an absence of perceptual change on the other.

REFERENCES

Adolphs, R., Tranel, D., Damasio, H. and Damasio, A.R. (1995) Fear and the human amygdala. *Journal of Neuro-science*, 15, 5879–5891.

Baylis, G.C. and Rolls, E.T. (1987) Responses of neurones in the inferior temporal cortex in short term and serial recognition memory tasks. *Experimental Brain Research*, 65, 614–622.

Bechara, A., Tranel, D., Damasio, H., Adolphs, R., Rockland, C. and Damasio, A.R. (1995) Double dissociation of conditioning and declarative knowledge relative to the amygdala and hippocampus in humans. *Science*, 269, 1115–1118.

Blaxton, T.A. (1989) Investigating dissociations among memory measures in memory-impaired subjects: evidence for a processing account of memory. *Journal of Experimental Psychology: Learning, Memory and Cognition*, 15, 657–668.

Büchel, C., Morris, J., Dolan, R.J. and Friston, K.J. (1998) Brain systems mediating aversive conditioning: an event related fMRI study. *Neuron*, 20, 947–957.

Buckner, R.L., Bandettini, P.A., Ocraven, K.M., Savoy, R.L., Petersen, S.E., Raichle, M.E. and Rosen, B.R. (1996) Detection of cortical activation during averaged single trials of a cognitive task using functional magnetic-resonance-imaging. *Proceedings of the National Academy of Science of the United States of America*, 93, 14878–14883.

Clark, R.E. and Squire, L.R. (1998) Classical conditioning and brain systems: the role of awareness. *Science*, 280, 77–81.

Clark, V.P., Keil, K., Maisog, Ma.J., Courtney, S., Ungerleider, L.G. and Haxby, J.V. (1996) Functional magnetic resonance imaging of human visual cortex during face matching: a comparison with positron emission tomography. *Neuro-image*, 4, 1–15.

Courtney, S.M., Ungerleider, L.G., Keil, K. and Haxby, J.V. (1996) Object and spatial visual working memory activate separate neural systems in human cortex. *Cerebral Cortex*, 6, 39–49.

Desimone, R. and Gross, C.G. (1979) Visual areas in the temporal lobe of the macaque. *Brain Research*, 178, 363–380.

Dolan, R.J., Fink, G.R., Rolls, E., Booth, M., Holmes, A., Frackowiak, R.S.J. and Friston, K.J. (1997) How the brain learns to see objects and faces in an impoverished context. *Nature*, 389, 596–599.

Dudai, Y. (1989) *The Neurobiology of Memory*. Oxford University Press, Oxford.

Edeline, J.-M. and Weinberger, N.M. (1991) Thalamic short term plasticity in the auditory system: associative retuning of receptive fields in the ventral medial geniculate body. *Behavioral Neuroscience*, 105, 618–639.

Esteves, F., Dimberg, U. and Ohman, A. (1994) Automatically elicited fear: conditioned skin conductance responses to masked facial expressions. *Cognition and Emotion*, 9, 99–108.

Fried, I., Macdonald, K.A. and Wilson, C.L. (1997) Single neuron activity in hippocampus and amygdala during recognition of faces and objects. *Neuron*, 18, 875–887.

Gross, C.G., Bender, D.B. and Gerstein, G.L. (1979) Activity of inferior temporal neurons in behaving monkey. *Neuropsychologia*, 17, 215–229.

Gross, G.C. (1972) Visual functions of the inferotemporal cortex. In: Jung, B.R. (ed.), *Handbook of Sensory Physiology*. Springer, Berlin, pp. 451–482.

Haxby, J., Horwitz, B., Ungerleider, L.G., Maisog, J.M., Pietrini, P. and Grady, C.L. (1994) The functional organisation of human extrastriate cortex: a PET-rCBF study of selective attention to faces and locations. *Journal of Neuro-science*, 14, 6336–6353.

Holland, P.C. (1990) Event representation in Pavlovian conditioning: image and action. *Cognition*, 37, 105–131.

Josephs, O., Turner, R. and Friston, K. (1997) Event-related fMRI. *Human Brain Mapping*, 5, 243–248.

LaBar, K.S. and LeDoux, J.E. (1996) Partial disruption of fear conditioning in rat with unilateral amygdala damage—correspondence with unilateral temporal lobe damage in humans. *Behavioral Neuroscience*, 110, 991–997.

LaBar, K.S., LeDoux, J.E., Spencer, D.D. and Phelps, E.A. (1995) Impaired fear conditioning following unilateral temporal lobectomy. *Journal of Neuroscience*, 15, 6846–6855.

LeDoux, J.E. (1993) Emotional memory systems in the brain. *Behavioural Brain Research*, 58, 69–79.

Malach, R., Reppas, J.B., Benson, R.R., Kwong, K.K., Jiang, H., Kennedy, W.A., Ledden, P.J., Brady, T.J., Rosen, B.R. and Tootell, R.B.H. (1995) Object-related activity revealed by functional magnetic resonance imaging in human occipital cortex. *Proceedings of the National Academy of Sciences of the United States of America*, 92, 8135–8139.

McGaugh, J.L., Cahill, L. and Roozendaal, B. (1996) Involvement of the amygdala in memory stroage: interaction with other brain systems. *Proceedings of the National Academy of Sciences of the United States of America*, 93, 13508–13514.

Miller, E.K., Li, L. and Desimone, R. (1991) A neural mechanism for working and recognition memory in inferior temporal cortex. *Science*, 254, 1377–1379.

Milner, B., Corkin, S. and Teuber, H.L. (1968) Further analysis of the hippocampal amnesic syndrome: fourteen year follow-up study of H.M. *Neuropsychologia*, 6, 215–234.

Moran, J. and Desimone, R. (1985) Selective attention gates visual processing in the extrastriate cortex. *Science*, 229, 782–784.

Packard, M.G., Cahill, L. and McGaugh, J.L. (1994) Amygdala modulation of hippocampal-dependent and caudate nucleus-dependent memory processes. *Proceedings of the National Academy of Sciences of the United States of America*, 91, 8477–8481.

Parra, C., Esteves, F., Flykt, A. and Ohman, A. (1997) Pavlovian conditioning to social stimuli: backward masking and dissociation of implicit and explicit cognitive processes. *European Psychologist*, 2, 106–117.

Pearce, J.M. and Hall, G. (1980) A model for Pavlovian learning: variations in the effectiveness of conditioned but not of unconditioned stimuli. *Psychological Review*, 82, 532–552.

Quirk, G.J., Armony, J.L. and LeDoux, J.E. (1997) Fear conditioning enhances different temporal components of tone-evoked spike trains in auditory cortex and lateral amygdala. *Neuron*, 19, 613–624.

Ramachandran, V.S. (1994). 2-D or not 2-D that is the question. In: Gregory R.L. and Harris, J. (eds), *The Artful Eye*. Oxford University Press, Oxford, pp. 249–267.

Sakai, K. and Miyashita, Y. (1995) Neural organisation for the long-term memory of paired associates. *Nature*, 354, 152–155.

Sakia, K. and Miyashita, Y. (1994) Neuronal tuning to learned complex forms in vision. *NeuroReport*, 5, 829–832.

Schacter, D.L. and Buckner, R.L. (1998) Priming and the brain. *Neuron*, 20, 185–195.

Schacter, D.L., Reiman, E., Uecker, A., Polster, M.R., Yun, L.S. and Cooper, L.A. (1995) Brain regions associated with retrieval of structurally coherent visual information. *Nature*, 376, 587–590.

Squire, L.R., Ojemann, J.G., Miezin, F.M., Petersen, S.E., Videen, T.O. and Raichle, M.E. (1992) Activation of the hippocampus in normal humans: a functional anatomical study of memory. *Proceedings of the National Academy of Sciences of the United States of America*, 89, 1837–1841.

Stanhope, K.J. (1992) The representation of the reinforcer and force of the pigeon's keypeck in first- and second-order conditioning. *Quarterly Journal of Experimental Psychology*, 44B, 137–158.

Tanaka, K., Saito, H., Fukada, Y. and Moriya, M. (1991) Coding visual images of objects in the inferotemporal cortex of the macaque monkey. *Journal of Neuroscience*, 6, 134–144.

Tolman, E.C. (1949) There is more than one kind of learning. *Psychological Bulletin*, 56, 144–155.

Tovee, M.J., Rolls, E.T. and Ramachandran, V.S. (1996) Visual learning in neurons of the primate temporal visual cortex. *NeuroReport*, 7, 2757–2760.

Ungerleider, L.G. and Mishkin, M. (1982) Two cortical visual systems. In: Goodale, M.A. and Mansfield, R.J.Q. (eds), *Analysis of Behaviour*. MIT Press, Cambridge, Massachusetts, pp. 549–586.

Warrington, E.K. and Weiskrantz, L. (1974) The effect of prior learning on subsequent retention in amnesic patients. *Neuropsychologia*, 12, 419–428.

Weinberger, N.M. (1995) Retuning the brain by fear conditioning. In: Gazzaniga, M. (ed.), *The Cognitive Neurosciences*. MIT Press, Cambridge, Massachusetts, pp. 1071–1090.

Weiskrantz, L. and Warrington, E.K. (1979) Conditioning in amnesic patients. *Neuropsychologia*, 17, 187–194.

18　TO HAVE BUT NOT TO HOLD

Lawrence Weiskrantz

INTRODUCTION

I am honored to be able to contribute to this volume dedicated to my old friend and colleague, Gabriel Horn, whose work has been original, insightful and seminal. What a marvellous idea it was to recognize the enormous potential for using imprinting as a paradigm with which to uncover the neural mechanisms of initial learning, and then to proceed so skilfully to the uncovering itself. Even though his own imprinting on Cambridge has been so difficult for him to overcome, I have had the good fortune to have crossed paths with him not only there, but at various other places. There was a time, which he will remember well from our earlier days at Cambridge, when the psychological effects of brain damage were rejected by theorists as curious but unfortunate perturbations, no more helpful than fragments of Humpty Dumpty for recreating the original. It gradually has become realized by neuropsychologists and cognitive scientists alike that such brain-damaged patients can be a source of highly privileged knowledge yielding fascinating, illuminating insights. They can tell us what capacities can be disturbed in relative isolation from others, which anatomical systems of the brain are important for their processing and, in conjunction with modern imaging methods, can reveal the functioning of both the normal and the damaged living brain. Beyond that, they offer a special route to the study of consciousness. It turns out, surprisingly, that in virtually all of the major cognitive categories that are disturbed by brain damage, there can be remarkably preserved functioning without the patients themselves being aware of this.

It took quite a long time for such phenomena with patients to be recognized even in neuropsychology—they were deeply disbelieved. When first encountered, they call to mind an exchange between Alice and the Queen in *Through the Looking Glass*.

Said Alice plaintively, 'One cannot believe impossible things.'

'I dare say you haven't had much practice,' said the Queen. 'When I was your age, I always did it for half an hour a day. Why, sometimes, I've believed as many as six impossible things before breakfast.'

I shall describe at least six such things—breakfast is optional.

There is no shortage of reviews and studies in each of the areas of interest, and here I wish only to give an indication, a flavor, of the type of evidence that exists for residual so-called implicit processing.

PERFORMANCE WITHOUT AWARENESS: AMNESIA

The best and most thoroughly studied example of this 'performance without awareness' is the severe memory disorder known as the amnesic syndrome, for which experimentally proven evidence of residual function after damage emerged some 30 years ago (Corkin, 1968; Warrington and Weiskrantz, 1968). However, the evidence was so counterintuitive in nature that it inevitably led to resistance among researchers during the ensuing 5–10 years, although ironically the study of residual memory function is now something of an industry.

Amnesic syndrome patients are grossly impaired in remembering recent experiences even after an interval as short as a minute. If the person with whom they have been conversing leaves the room and then returns a minute or two later, the patient does not recognize him; the patient cannot recall a story or information related a short time earlier. The patients do not necessarily have an impairment of short-term memory, for example in reciting back strings of digits, nor do they necessarily have any perceptual or intellectual impairments, but they have grave difficulty in acquiring and holding new information ('anterograde amnesia'). Memory for events from before the onset of the injury or brain disease also is typically affected ('retrograde amnesia'), especially for those events that occurred a few years before the brain damage. Older *knowledge* can be retained—the patients retain their vocabulary and acquired language skills, they know who they are, they may know where they went to school, although in some of the severe and densely amnesic cases patients may be vague even about such early knowledge, e.g. how many children they have, or whether their spouse is alive or dead. The striking aspect of the amnesic syndrome is that it can be relatively pure and in isolation from other cognitive, motor and perceptual difficulties.

The disorder is severely crippling, and such patients typically need constant custodial care. Yet—and here is the surprise—there is good evidence of storage of experiences. Indeed, some of the anecdotal evidence for this is more than a 100 years old. Korsakoff (Delay and Brion, 1969) describes an amnesic patient who openly exhibited fear of a shock apparatus—justifiably, as he had been shocked by it! However, he denied having seen the apparatus nor was there any overt acknowledgement of the shocking experience as such. Another anecdote, told by Claparède, is now often cited: he described the amnesic subject whose hand was stuck with a pin by Claparède (1911) during a neurological examination, and who thereafter vigorously withdrew her hand whenever she saw him. On questioning, she denied having any idea of why she did so. Claparède persisted relentlessly with his questioning and, she would say 'it is just an idea that came into my mind'. Eventually, after much pressing, she said, 'well, you never know who might have a pin in his hand!'

More experimentally robust evidence was reported in the 1950s of the famous patient, H.M., who became and still remains severely amnesic after bilateral surgery to structures in the medial portions of his temporal lobes for the relief of intractable epilepsy (Scoville and Milner, 1957). Because the hippocampus was included in the surgery, it tended to capture most of the interpretative attention, although the lesion also included other structures which have turned out to be important (see Brown, Chapter 11; Buckley and Gaffan, Chapter 16). In any event, it soon became apparent that H.M. was able to learn various perceptual and motor skills, such as mastering the path of a pursuit rotor in which one must learn to keep a stylus on a narrow track on a moving drum. He was also able to learn mirror drawing, i.e. learning to copy from the reversed image of a pattern seen in a mirror (Corkin, 1968). He was able to retain such skills excel-

lently from session to session. However, he demonstrated *no* awareness of having remembered the experimental situations nor could he recognize them; he claimed he had never seen them before (Corkin, 1968). That type of demonstration of excellent acquisition and retention of perceptual motor skills for H.M. and other amnesic subjects, without explicit recognition or recall, has been confirmed in a variety of situations by various authors (e.g. Brooks and Baddeley, 1976; Schacter, 1992).

If you recall the Claparède anecdote, in which the amnesic lady pulled her hand away from the doctor who prodded her hand with a sharp pin, this is of course an example of avoidance conditioning. It is possible to put avoidance conditioning under direct study, although not using such punitive measures, with repeated trials of a light or a sound occurring just before a puff of air to the eye—which generates a kind of conditioned bracing of the eyelids. Results with this procedure work very well with amnesic patients; they acquire and retain eyelid conditioning very well, but acknowledge no memory of this (for control subjects) highly memorable procedure (Weiskrantz and Warrington, 1979).

The examples of perceptual motor skill learning and possibly even of classical conditioning did not stretch credulity unduly because such skills can become more or less automatic, devoid of cognition. Indeed, it was argued originally that the hippocampus and its anatomical cousins need not be concerned with such servile perceptual or motor matters. However, counterintuitive results were much more pressing when it was shown that amnesic subjects could also retain information about verbal material, but again without recognition. The use of verbal material also allowed direct quantitative comparisons to be made between retention of the words using various indirect tests of retention, on the one hand, and explicit recognition of the words, on the other.

The demonstration depended on showing the patients lists of pictures or words and, after an interval of some minutes, testing for recognition in a standard yes/no test, i.e. asking them to say whether they did or did not *recognize* having seen the previously exposed words or pictures (together with new items that had not been exposed). Not surprisingly, the patients performed at the level of chance. However, when asked to 'guess' the *identity* of pictures or words from difficult fragmented drawings, they were much better able to do so for those items to which they had been exposed. For example, if they had first been exposed to drawings of complete words or objects, they were much better able to 'guess' the identity of their fragmented, degraded versions (Warrington and Weiskrantz, 1968).

Another way of demonstrating this phenomenon was to present just some of the letters of the previously exposed word, for example the initial pair or triplet of letters (Weiskrantz and Warrington, 1970). The patients showed enhanced ability for finding the correct words to which they had been exposed earlier compared with control items to which they had not been exposed. This is a procedure that is called priming—the facilitation of retention induced by previous exposure. The demonstration of retention by amnesic patients has been confirmed repeatedly, and retention intervals can be as long as several months: in H.M., successful retention was reported for an interval of 4 months (Milner *et al.*, 1968).

It has turned out that such patients, in fact, can learn a variety of novel types of tasks and information, such as new words, new meanings and new rules (McAndrews *et al.*, 1987; Knowlton *et al.*, 1992). Learning of novel pictures and diagrams has also been demonstrated by Schacter *et al.* (1991) and Gabrieli *et al.* (1990). There also has been intense interest in discovering which brain structures are necessary for explicit as well as for implicit memory. At this stage, however, my object is to record the fact that amnesic patients can store and access information when tested indirectly, but for which they have no acknowledged experience of a memory.

An early response by some memory researchers to the reports of positive memory retention by subjects who could not 'remember' was that they might be just like normal people but with 'weak' memory. This was a natural interpretation of the evidence at hand. However, when dissociations started to appear for other specific forms of memory disorders that were different from the amnesic syndrome, it gradually became clear that there are a number of different memory systems in the brain operating in parallel, although of course normally in interaction with each other. For example, it was found that lesions well removed from the medial temporal lobes, in the basal ganglia, produced loss of 'skills', such as learning a pursuit rotor route, or riding a bicycle, and yet another lesion far removed from the temporal lobe (in the cerebellum) could interfere selectively with conditioned eyelid responses, in neither case causing any loss of 'recognition'. Yet other subjects had brain damage elsewhere that caused them to lose the meanings of words, but without

behaving like amnesic subjects, i.e. they could remember having been shown a word before, and that on that occasion they also did not know its *meaning*! Other brain-damaged subjects could have very impoverished short-term memory—being able to repeat back only one or two digits from a list—and yet were otherwise normal for remembering events and recognizing facts. They could remember that they could only repeat back two digits when tested the day before! (see reviews by Weiskrantz, 1987, 1990b). The research of Horn and his colleagues on chicks demonstrates, with physiological underpinnings as well, the clear dissociation between different memory systems (Horn, 1985, 1990, 1998, Chapter 19).

Such sets of double and multiple dissociations thus demonstrated that 'memory' is not a term to be used as a singular concept; amnesia is not just weak normal memory. The brain apparently has a variety of systems that deal with types of material according to their different demands and, at the very least, has a variety of independent processing modes. Depending on the situation and the material to be stored (or not to be stored) or recovered, different processes will be entailed, with different time constants and different matching operations. However, that is another story; the point is that there is excellent capacity for acquisition and retention of material by amnesic patients.

OTHER EXAMPLES: THE BROAD SPECTRUM

Other examples of residual function following brain damage have now been found across virtually the whole spectrum of neuropsychological defects. *Unilateral neglect* is associated with lesions of the parietal lobe in humans, typically the right parietal lobe, resulting from stroke or other causes. The patients behave as though the left half of their visual (and sometimes also their tactile) world is missing. If shown a picture of a butterfly and asked to copy it, they draw only its right half. This striking syndrome is the subject of quite intense experimental research and attracts a number of theories. Even though the subjects neglect the left half of their visual world, it can be shown in some cases that 'missing' information is being processed by the brain. In an experiment by John Marshall and Peter Halligan (1988), such a subject was shown two pictures of houses that were identical on their right halves, but different on the left. In one picture, a fire was projecting vigorously from the chimney on the left side of the picture, and in the other no fire was shown. Because the subject neglected the left halves of the pictures, she repeatedly judged them as being identical and scored at chance in discriminating between them. However, when asked which house she would prefer to live in she retorted that it was a silly question, because they were the *same*, but nevertheless she reliably chose the house not on fire. Edoardo Bisiach (1992) has carried out some variations on this theme. Other studies have asked whether an 'unseen' stimulus in the neglected left field can 'prime' a response by the subject to a stimulus in the right half-field. Thus, Ladavas *et al.* (1993) have shown that a word presented in the right visual field was processed more quickly when the word was preceded by a brief presentation of an associated word in the 'neglected' left field. When the subject was actually forced to respond directly to the word on the left, for example by reading it aloud, he was not able to do so—it was genuinely 'neglected'. A similar demonstration was made by Berti and Rizzolatti (1992) using pictures of animals and fruit in the left neglected field as primes for pictures in the right which their patients had to classify as quickly as possible, either as animals or fruit, by pressing the appropriate key. The unseen picture shown on the left generated faster reaction times when it matched the category of the picture on the right. Thus material, both pictorial and verbal, of which the subject has no awareness in the left visual field, and to which he or she cannot respond explicitly, nevertheless gets processed. The subject may not 'know' it, but some part of the brain does.

There is a type of memory disorder that is socially awkward for the patient, but intriguing to the scientist. *Prosopagnosia* is an impairment in the ability to recognize and identify familiar faces. The problem is not one of knowing that a face is a face, i.e. it is not a perceptual difficulty, but one of facial *memory*. The condition is associated with damage to the inferior, posterior temporal lobe, especially in the right hemisphere. The condition can be so severe that patients do not recognize the faces of members of their own family. However, it has been demonstrated clearly that the autonomic nervous system can tell the difference between familiar and unfamiliar faces. In one study, Bauer (1984) measured the skin conductance responses (SCRs) of prosopagnosic patients when they were asked to read names when shown an individual face of a famous person or a family member. Some names were correct matches for the

face, others were not. When the correct name was read, SCR responses were much larger than those to the incorrect names. Tranel and Damasio (1985) carried out a similar study in which patients were required to pick out familiar from unfamiliar faces. They scored at chance but, notwithstanding, their SCRs were reliably larger for the familiar faces than for the unfamiliar faces. Thus the patients do not 'know' the faces, but some part of their autonomic nervous system obviously does.

It is not only the autonomic system that can respond differentially to familiar faces in the absence of explicit recognition by the patient. Andy Young and his colleagues (e.g. Young *et al.*, 1990; Young and De Haan, 1992) have demonstrated intact processing of familiar faces. Thus a patient showed faster matching of familiar faces than of unfamiliar faces even though he was at chance when asked to select familiar from unfamiliar ones. It was also shown that recognition of target *names* of familiar people was helped by priming them with a picture of a face that the subject does not recognize, and also that a patient learns the 'true' pairings of faces and names more rapidly than 'incorrect' pairings.

Even for that uniquely human cognitive achievement, the skilled use of language, when severely disturbed by brain damage, evidence exists of residual processing of which subjects remain unaware. One example comes from patients who cannot read whole words, although they can painfully extract the word by reading it 'letter by letter'. This form of *acquired dyslexia* is associated with damage to the left occipital lobe. In a study by Shallice and Saffran, (1986), one such patient was tested with written words that he could not identify—he could neither read them aloud nor report their meanings. Nevertheless, he performed reliably above chance on a lexical decision task, when asked to guess the difference between real words and nonsense words. Moreover, he could correctly categorize words at above chance levels according to their meanings, using forced-choice responding to one of two alternatives. He could say, for example, whether the written name of a country belonged inside or outside Europe, whether the name of a person was that of an author or politician, or whether the name of an object was living or non-living. All this, despite his not being able to read or identify the word aloud or explicitly give its meaning.

An even more striking outcome emerges from studies of patients with severe loss of linguistic comprehension and production, *aphasia* (Frederici, 1982;

Linebarger *et al.*, 1983). An informative study that tackled both grammatical and semantic aspects of comprehension in a severely impaired patient is that by Tyler (1988, 1992). She presented the subject with sentences that were degraded either semantically or syntactically. The subject succeeded in being able to follow the instruction to respond as quickly as possible whenever a particular target word was uttered. It is known that normal subjects are slower to respond to the target word when it is in a degraded context than when in a normal sentence. Even though Tyler's aphasic patient was severely impaired in his ability to judge whether a sentence was highly anomalous or normal, his pattern of reaction times to target words in a degraded context showed the same pattern of slowing as is characteristic of normal control subjects. By this means, it was demonstrated that the patient retained an intact capacity to respond to both the semantic and grammatical structure of the sentences. However, he could not use such a capacity, either in his comprehension or in his use of speech. Tyler distinguishes between the 'on-line' use of linguistic information, which was preserved in her patient, and its exploitation 'off-line'. The subject could 'develop the appropriate representations of an utterance; his problem lies in being unable to gain access to them for the purpose of making explicit decisions about them.'

In all of the examples so far, there has been, in some sense, a retained capacity in the absence of an acknowledged awareness—either of the information content itself or of the knowledge of the residual existence of the capacity. However, there is a more subtle way in which *subparts* of perception can be shown to behave similarly, such that patients can be said not to perceive in one sense, but to perceive very well in another. In evidence garnered impressively by Milner and Goodale (1995), patients are described who are 'agnosic' for judging the shape of objects, or cannot even tell different orientations of lines apart. Yet such a patient might be able, without difficulty, when forced to *act*, to slot cards into a 'mail box' the orientation of which is set to various different angles. Milner and Goodale describe a lovely experiment in which it was demonstrated that the patient still had the capacity for the orientation of a stimulus to make itself 'seen' indirectly by showing that orientation could control a color after-effect (the 'McCulloch After-Effect'), even though the subject could not discriminate different orientations as such.

Another example of a fractionation of perception without awareness has been analyzed in some detail by Heywood *et al.* (1991). They studied a patient suffering from '*achromatopsia*—the loss of perceived color, caused by brain damage to the ventral and posterior temporo-occipital region. Their subject, like other achromatopsic patients, saw the world only in shades of gray, devoid of color (although he had possessed normal color vision prior to the brain damage). However, he demonstrated an excellent capacity for 'color discrimination' even though he could not *see* color under the very same conditions in which he discriminated. Heywood *et al.* showed clearly that the information *must* have arisen from intact color processing mechanisms, even though the subject had lost the color 'qualia'. Thus, he could identify shapes arising out of chromatic information, or the orientation of lines in a grating, even though they were matched with the luminance of the background. The information had to arise from color mechanisms, and yet the subject saw no colors whatsoever, only shades of gray.

Another neuropsychological patient (L.M.) has attracted much attention because she has apparently lost the ability to see movement, at least within wide limits of speed (Zihl *et al.*, 1983). She describes a moving bus, for example, as advancing in a series of discrete 'stills'. The spout of tea emerging from a teapot is seen as a solid curved cylinder. Nevertheless, Peter McLeod and his co-workers find that she catches a ball thrown straight at her with skill, or at least as one would expect of a normal middle-aged woman! She also has no difficulty in identifying the 'natural' movements of 'Johansson' figures, which are films of persons moving in the dark with small lamps fixed at the ankle, knee, hip, elbow and shoulder joints. They were filmed walking, running, jumping, crawling, etc. Normal persons can recognize and name these different 'biological' movements. So can L.M. (McLeod *et al.*, 1996).

Perhaps the most celebrated and dramatic evidence of function without awareness has come from the study of commissurotimized patients, colloquially known as '*split-brain*' patients. Because epileptic electrical outbursts in the brain tend to spread from one cerebral hemisphere to another (and, in fact, thereafter to become autonomous), surgeons have cut the massive connections between the hemispheres, the corpus callosum, in an effort to contain the electrical conflagration. Thus, at least at the cortical level, the two hemispheres are rendered independent, although the lower connecting structures of the midbrain still remain intact.

What Sperry and co-workers found, as is well known, was that when they projected visual stimuli to the left, 'speaking' hemisphere, of split-brain sub-jects (by flashing it on the right visual hemifield), they reported seeing the stimuli quite normally and could identify them. However, when they were projected to the 'silent, non-speaking' right hemisphere (via the left visual hemifield), the subjects *said* they saw nothing at all. Nevertheless, they could be shown, by indirect means, to have identified the 'unseen' visual events. For example, they correctly retrieved with their left hand (which is controlled by the right hemisphere) the object that had been shown to the right hemisphere, even though it was reported as not 'seen' by the subject. Numerous other experiments have demon-strated dramatically how information that reached the 'silent' hemisphere could be processed even though the subject denied seeing it at all (Sperry, 1974).

To summarize, neuropsychology has exposed a large variety of examples in which, in some sense, awareness is disconnected from a capacity to discrim-inate or to remember or to attend or to read or to speak. They are no longer surprising. The Queen has educated Alice. Of course, there is nothing surprising in our performing without awareness—it could even be said that most of our bodily activity is uncon-scious, and that many of our interactions with the outside world are carried on 'automatically' and, in a sense, thoughtlessly. Who is aware of the delicate bodily adjustments that continuously are being made when we maintain our balance, or play tennis or what have you. What is surprising about these examples from neuropsychology is that in all these cases the patients are unaware in precisely the situations in which we would normally expect someone to be very much aware.

BLINDSIGHT

I have left to the end the most dramatic and most counterintuitive, and perhaps still the most controver-sial, of all such examples—where Alice still remains a bit skeptical about thinking impossible thoughts: it is the residual function that can be demonstrated after damage to the *visual cortex*, a condition that has been dubbed *blindsight*. The story actually starts with animal research, some of it more than a century old, and the underlying neuroanatomy of the visual sys-tem. The major target of the eye lies in the occipital lobe (after a relay via the thalamus), in the 'striate cortex' ('V1'). However, while this so-called geniculo-striate pathway is the largest one from the eye des-

tined for targets in the brain, it is not the only pathway. There are at least nine other pathways from the retina to targets in the brain that remain open after blockade or damage to the primary visual cortex (Cowey and Stoerig, 1991). We still do not know whether these are parallel and *potentially independent* (but normally interacting) systems, each with a spe-cialized function and, if so, what these functions might be. It is possible to speculate, for example, that the pathway terminating in the suprachiasmatic nucleus of the hypothalamus is specialized for the control of the diurnal sleep/wakefulness cycle by light, given that lesions in that structure interfere with that cycle—it might be a center that is involved criti-cally in the generation of jet lag. The important point is that, in the absence of striate cortex, there are a number of routes over which information from the eye can reach and be processed at various stages in the brain. Retinal information can reach subcortical areas directly via the collicular and tectal routes, as well as via the accessory optic tract. Also cortical areas, including the temporal lobes, can be reached via thalamic routes, the pulvinar and the lateral geniculate nucleus as well as from midbrain projec-tions. Beyond that, information can reach large regions of the other, intact hemisphere, including its striate cortex, via brain commissures at both the sub-cortical and cortical levels. One such alternative route has been identified directly by Rodman and col-leagues (1989) for neurons in area MT, a region of cortex in the monkey in which cells respond espe-cially to visual moving stimuli and their direction of movement. In the absence of striate cortex, cells in MT still fire normally although the numbers doing so are reduced. It was demonstrated that the critical route sustaining the responses acts via the superior collicu-lus, and thence via the pulvinar to MT (Gross, 1991). Thus, given this state of affairs, it is perhaps not sur-prising that monkeys can still carry out visual dis-criminations even in the absence of V1. Their ability is altered in some important ways (see below), but it is still quite impressive. One of the main demonstrations came from years of observation by Nicholas Humphrey (1970, 1974; Humphrey and Weiskrantz, 1967) of a monkey 'Helen' who had bilateral lesions of V1. She could locate and retrieve visual objects, even quite small specks of dust, and avoid obstacles with considerable ease. The evidence is quite similar to that reported more than 100 years ago by Luciani in 1884. The vision of monkeys without V1 allows the animal to discriminate a difference in orientation in the frontal plane of about 8°, to have a visual acuity better than that of the normal cat, for example, and to reach out correctly for even very briefly presented stimuli.

The paradox is that human patients in whom the striate cortex is damaged say that they are blind in that part of the visual field that maps onto the damaged V1. (Typically, such patients have damage only to one hemisphere and, therefore, are blind in only one-half of the visual fields of both eyes. Of course, with damage to both V1s, they would be blind across the whole of the visual field, but fortunately for the patients, and unfortunately for science, such cases are very rare.) William James summarized the contemporary wisdom of his time in 1890, which has remained as current wisdom until quite recently: 'The literature is tedious *ad libitum*..... The occipital lobes are indispensable for vision in man. Hemiopic disturbance comes from lesion of either one of them, and total blindness, sensorial as well as psychic, from destruction of both' (1980, p. 47). Given that it was known even in James' times that monkeys without visual cortex could still make visual discriminations, a thesis emerged that visual function in people becomes 'encephalized', that visual cortex may be less essential in monkeys but, because of an upward evolutionary 'migration' of function from older midbrain structures to cortex, it becomes essential in humans. This is a strange view in many ways—what happens to the millions of cells that lost their jobs at the level of the midbrain as a result of this upward evolution (cf. Weiskrantz, 1961)?

The detailed anatomy of the visual pathways appears very similar in monkey and humans, and so why are the human patients apparently unable to make use of the parallel visual pathways from the retina that remain after damage to the occipital cortex and to V1? Why are they are blind? Or are they *really* blind? The answer to the question gradually emerged when such patients were tested in the way that one is forced to test animals. One cannot, alas, ask an animal to describe what it sees, or to read a list of letters on an eye chart. One must provide it with a choice of alternatives, and reward it for choosing one or the other. Or one trains the animal to retrieve a reward at one or another position at which one places a cue. In short, you do not ask the animal directly about what it 'sees', but only test what it can discriminate.

The first clue about residual vision in people with visual cortex damage came from a study at MIT in 1973 (Pöppel *et al.*, 1973) in which brain-damaged US war veterans were asked simply to move their eyes to the position of a briefly presented spot of light shone into their blind fields. The position of the light was varied from trial to trial in a random order. As they could not 'see', the subjects thought the instruction odd, but it emerged that, in fact, they did move their eyes to the correct position of where the light had been more often than expected by chance. The effect was not strong, but it was statistically reliable. The 'unseen' light was having some control over the subjects' visual responses.

Soon afterwards a patient, D.B., was seen at the National Hospital in London; he had a visual field defect caused by surgical removal of a small nonmalignant tumor that had invaded V1. He was studied by Elizabeth Warrington, other colleagues and myself, and given a variety of tests that extended, in fact, over some 10 years (Weiskrantz *et al.*, 1974; Weiskrantz, 1986, 1998). The MIT results on eye gaze were confirmed, but, in addition, a range of 'monkeytype' tests were administered in which D.B. had either to reach out to locate a stimulus, or to guess which of two alternative stimuli had been projected into his blind hemifield. In the latter case, he was told what the two choices were before the random trials in the blind half-field were administered. The result was that D.B. could succeed in a variety of discriminations by 'guess-work' in his blind field, even though he said he did not 'see' the stimuli. He could, for example, discriminate whether a circular patch of lines was oriented in one or another direction, or whether a stimulus was moving or stationary. His visual acuity could be measured by varying the spacing of a grating. His ability to locate the position of stimuli in his blind field was not absolutely normal, but remarkably good. In fact, his ability matched that of a monkey without V1 reasonably well.

After these tests, the subject was questioned as to how well he thought had done. In many cases he said he was just guessing, and thought he was not performing better than chance. When he was shown his results (which never took place until the end of testing sessions, which typically lasted 2 or 3 days) in the early days he expressed open astonishment. There were conditions under which D.B. did have *some* kind of awareness, and this has turned out to be of interest in its own right, i.e. with some stimuli, especially those with very rapid movement or sudden onset, he 'knew' that something had moved in his blind field, even though he did not 'see' them as such. However, he could discriminate other stimuli without any awareness of them. The phenomenon, in a passing moment as a response to an urgent request for a seminar title, was dubbed 'blindsight', and the term has stuck. The contrast between 'aware' and 'unaware' modes, as we shall see, turned out to be useful.

The results on the studies of D.B. were among the first to be documented. Other subjects have been tested by a number of researchers. As in the early days of memory research, much work depended, and still depends, on sessions lasting several days or even longer. One of the subjects in this category, still being tested in several different research centers throughout the world, is G.Y., about whom I will say more in due course. The question of just what proportion of patients with occipital damage show 'blindsight', and in what form, is a taxing one, not yet satisfactorily studied. Taken together, subjects with V1 damage have been reported who are able, in their 'blind' hemifields, to detect the presence of stimuli, to locate them in space, to discriminate direction of movement of a spot of light, to discriminate the orientation of lines, to be able to judge whether stimuli in the blind field 'match' or 'mismatch' those in the intact field, to detect chromatic signals (Brent *et al.*, 1094) and to discriminate between different wavelengths of light, i.e. to tell colors apart. Recently the reports have extended also to the semantic biasing by words in the blind field, and to the appropriate adjustments of the hand for grasping differently shaped objects in the blind field (Marcel, 1998).

The discrimination of 'color' presses credulity to the limit, because in those tests—which by their nature were very time consuming and lasted for several days—the subjects uniformly and consistently denied seeing color at all, and yet reliably discriminated above chance between wavelengths, even those falling relatively closely together (Stoerig and Cowey, 1991, 1992). Moreover, the fine-grained features of the spectral sensitivity curves of these subjects (carried out, again, by forced-choice guessing) suggested that wavelength opponency, i.e. color contrast, was intact. The subjects seem to be able to respond to the stimuli that would normally generate the philosophers' favorite species of 'qualia', namely colors, but in the absence of the very 'qualia' themselves! This is, in principle, no more striking or mysterious than being able to discriminate or identify any kind of visual event in the absence of awareness.

It is not only in the visual mode that examples of 'unaware' discrimination capacity have been reported. There are reports of 'blind touch' and also a report of 'deaf hearing.' The first case of 'blind touch' (Paillard

et al., 1983) was closely similar to the early accounts of blindsight. The patient had a severe right tactile anesthesia caused by a left parietal lobe lesion. She did not respond to touch on her right arm, even with 'the strongest pressure'. However, when asked to point (blindfolded) to where she was touched with the pressure instrument, she was able to point, afterwards 'to her own considerable surprise', to the approximate locus of the stimulus, The patient's comment was 'but I do not understand that! You put something here. I don't feel anything and I go there with my finger... How does that happen?' Again in parallel with some blindsight phenomena, she did react positively to a moving tactile stimulus and could judge its direction. A similar recent case has been described more recently by Rossetti and his colleagues in Lyon (Rossetti *et al.*, 1995, 1996), who have invented the splendid oxymoron, 'numbsense'.

Returning to blindsight, that the gap between monkey and man should be narrowed was no surprise to us, but the manner in which it happened *was* surprising and deeply counterintuitive—to us and everyone else. How could anyone discriminate visually events they could not 'see'? A number of possible objections and alternatives were raised for what seemed such a puzzling outcome, as is the healthy response in science. Perhaps, it was suggested, light could spread from the blind half-field into the intact half-field. Or perhaps the effect was purely quantitative—after all, the total output retina is reduced; blindsight vision may be just weakened normal vision. With weak visual stimuli we can all sometimes respond above chance even when we say we do not see. Or perhaps blindsight subjects just became more cautious about admitting that they had a visual experience even though they did. Or perhaps there were small rogue bits of V1 still lurking in the damaged areas of the brain that were responsible for the residual capacity.

These are important issues. There are good reasons and good evidence, much of it of course rather technical, to discount all such explanations of blindsight, although this is not the place to discuss them; detailed accounts can be found elsewhere (Weiskrantz, 1996; Azzopardi and Cowey, 1997; Kentridge *et al.*, 1997; Weiskrantz, 1997, 1998; Weiskrantz *et al.*, 1998).

There is one particular feature of blindsight research that is especially demanding: it is the very strangeness of the question the researcher asks a subject in such a study. For example, 'tell me whether the stimulus which you could not see at all occurred in the first or second of two successive time intervals'. Such questions do not favor easy cooperation or credibility. Indeed, some subjects refuse to play such a strange game, and some experimenters no doubt find it awkward to ask these strange questions and may well indicate shared, even bemused, skepticism when doing so.

INDIRECT APPROACHES

There are interesting possible solutions to the dilemma of having to talk to potential blindsight patients about something they find ineffable. In almost all other cognitive neuropsychological syndromes, a residual 'implicit' capacity can sometimes be found that co-exists with a severe 'explicit' deficit. In most syndromes, the demonstration of residual implicit capacities is made indirectly by using an alternative method of testing which creates no operational or phenomenal conflict for the subject. Thus, amnesic subjects show good priming or conditioning even though the same material does not yield an acknowledged memory of the retained information: the indirect test can be carried out independently of the recognition or recall tests. In aphasia, reaction times to 'target' words in particular semantic or syntactic contexts can be used to demonstrate the integrity of semantics and syntax capacities which the subject cannot use in normal communication. Similar examples exist in other syndromes. In the case of blindsight, however, where residual visual capacity is found, a conflict does arise: a 'guess' or a 'reach' is required for a stimulus that the subject would normally expect to be unable to detect or discriminate because it is unseen. There is incredulity.

Therefore, indirect methods of testing for residual visual processing have been developed that allow firm inferences to be drawn about its characteristics without forcing an instrumental response to an unseen stimulus (Torjussen, 1976, 1978; Marzi *et al.*, 1986; cf. Weiskrantz, 1990a). For example, responses to stimuli in the intact hemifield can be shown to be influenced by stimuli in the blind hemifield, as with visual completion or by visual summation between the two hemifields. Of the various indirect methods, pupillometry, offers a special opportunity because the pupil is surprisingly sensitive to spatial and temporal parameters of visual stimuli in a quantitatively precise way. Barbur and his colleagues have shown that, among other parameters, the pupil constricts

sensitively to movement, to color, and to contrast and spatial frequency of a grating, and that the acuity estimated by pupillometry correlates closely with that determined by conventional psychophysical methods in normal subjects (Barbur, 1995; Barbur and Forsyth, 1986; Barbur and Thomson, 1987; Barbur *et al.*, 1992, 1994b). Such pupillary measurements can be obtained in the absence of verbal interchange about the effective visual stimuli. Therefore, obviously, the method is available not only for testing normal visual fields, but for the blind fields of patients, for animals, for human infants, indeed in any situation where verbal interchange is impossible or is to be avoided.

Therefore, we have measured the profile of the pupillary response in monkeys with unilateral removal of striate cortex, as well as in a human subject, G.Y., in whom there also is unilateral damage to striate cortex (Weiskrantz *et al.*, 1998). We measured the pupillary responses to projected gratings of various spacings and wavelengths into their blind and their intact hemifields, with fixation monitored and controlled. The results were very clear. The human subject and the monkeys showed the same profile. Its peak was at approximately 1 cycle/° (Figure 18.1), and the resulting visual acuity was also approximately the same, about 7 or 8 cycles/°, reduced from that of the normal field by approximately the same amount (~2 octaves).

Now, you might say, just a reflex. What does this tell us about discrimination which the subject has to carry out in a forced-choice task? There is classical published material available for such a task (Pasik and Pasik, 1982) for monkeys without V1. As regards the human subject, it happens that Barbur, Harlow and myself (1994a) had already carried out a discrimination task for gratings with the same human subject a few years earlier. The closeness of the fit between the pupillometry and psychophysical results is striking (see Figure 18.1). The results support the conclusion that visual processing at this early stage in the visual system is comparable in the two species, and this can be shown without the torturous business of requesting the subjects to report about stimuli he or she cannot see. The results also identify a narrowly tuned spatial visual channel that remains intact in the absence of V1.

The impetus for blindsight research actually started with results from monkeys with striate cortex lesions, and it is now possible to complete the circle. We now know, from the ingenious and instructive experiments of Cowey and Stoerig (1995, 1997), that the monkey

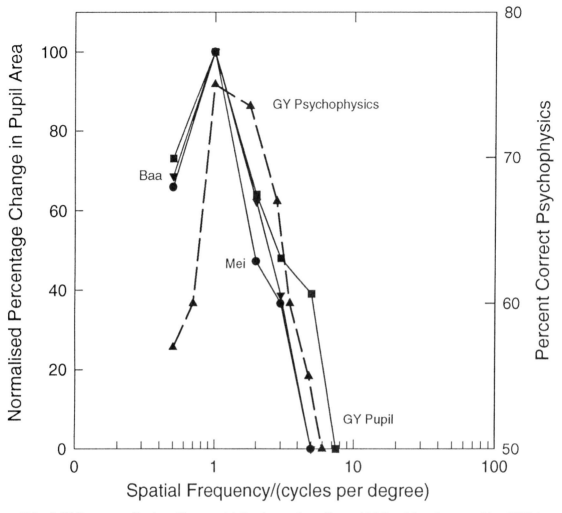

Figure 18.1.   Solid lines: normalized pupillary constriction for monkeys (Baa and Mei) and for a human subject (G.Y.) for gratings as a function of spatial frequency (80% contrast) projected to the affected hemifields. Peak responses have been set to 100 (scale on left). Dashed line: G.Y.'s percentage correct responses (scale on right) for psychophysical tests of grating detection, for 75% contrast, from Barbur *et al.* (1994a). (Reprinted with permission from Weiskrantz *et al.*, 1998.)

with a unilateral lesion of striate cortex also has blindsight in the sense that it treats visual stimuli in the affected half-field as *non-visual* events. Cowey and Stoerig put the matter to monkeys as follows: they first demonstrated that they could respond exquisitely well to visual stimuli in their blind half-fields. So much we have known for a long time, but it was necessary to confirm it for these animals. They then went on to teach the monkeys to make a judgement about visual events, using their intact half-fields. In brief, the monkeys were trained to discriminate between a light and a non-light—a 'blank'—randomly presented in their intact fields. They had to reach for a

light target when it occurred, but press a neutral panel when no light occurred, both in response to an auditory warning signal. That is a very easy task for the monkey. Now the question was, how would the monkeys treat a light stimulus presented to their *'blind'* field? The answer was clear, and was robustly stable. The monkeys judged such a stimulus to be a non-light, a 'blank'. Cowey and Stoerig have pressed the monkeys harder, in still unpublished work, by making the light in the blind field much brighter, by having it flicker, or move. The result is the same. The monkey treats the stimulus in the same way as the human blindsight subject would do for a stimulus in his or her blind field. One had to go 'off-line' to demonstrate it in both species; one had to obtain a parallel judgement about the discriminative events independently of the discrimination itself.

IMAGING AND AWARENESS

Let me remind you where we are. We have seen that there are syndromes caused by brain damage in which good performance occurs in the absence of acknowledged awareness, and so we might be able to compare brain states when a subject is aware or when he or she is unaware but performing well. Of the various syndromes, blindsight offers certain definite advantages over the others. First, we know the anatomy of the various visual pathways in fine detail, starting with the cells of origin of the optic nerve in the retina, and proceeding to various cortical targets, as well as their electrophysiological properties at various stages. Secondly, the typical blindsight subject is blind in only one visual half field, and so one can compare the residual function in the blind field with the normal function of the intact field, using the subject as his or her own control.

However, as it happens, with blindsight, we can do even better than that: we can compare discrimination *with* and *without* awareness within the *blind field* itself, and compare both of them with the intact normal half-field, all within the same subject (Weiskrantz *et al.*, 1995). As mentioned above, some stimuli presented to the blindsight field give rise to a 'feeling' or an 'awareness' or 'knowing' that an event has taken place, even though the subject does not 'see' as such. Such evocative stimuli are typically those with rapid temporal or spatial transients. However, one can damp these transient signals and remove the 'awareness' and, under the right conditions, discriminative performance can still be very good. In relating performance to awareness, of course, one must have a method of assessing awareness. For this purpose, in addition to the standard discrimination keys (e.g. first or second temporal interval?), we introduced 'commentary keys' on which the subject indicates his awareness of the event (e.g. yes, no or degree of?) in each trial (Weiskrantz *et al.*, 1995). The matter and the methods have been discussed in detail elsewhere (Weiskrantz, 1997).

Note one implication that follows: one can obtain good and matched performance in the blind field either with or without awareness. The subject had no

visual image in either condition, but in one condition he had awareness, a 'knowing', and in the other none. Also, in his normal half-field, of course, he had both awareness and vision. Thus the opportunity arose for colleagues at City University and at the Institute of Psychiatry in London and myself to carry out brain imaging of those two modes—good performance either with or without awareness with this same subject (Sahraie *et al.*, 1997). I will not go into the technical details of the movement discrimination situation, which had to be altered to fit into the confines of the functional magnetic resonance imaging (fMRI) magnet, nor of the details of the imaging itself (see also Dolan, Chapter 17). The details and the results have been published.

We did not quite know what to expect—it was a fishing expedition. The answer is that we did find that some brain regions increased their activity when, and only when, G.Y. was in the aware mode—and this was the case whether the stimulus was in the intact half-field or moving quickly in the blind half-field. These regions were situated in the dorsal prefrontal cortex, especially area 46. However, in the unaware mode, and only in that mode, other structures were activated, and these were in the midbrain, the older target of a pathway from the retina, and especially in the superior colliculus (see also Stein *et al.*, Chapter 3). Posterior visual areas were common to both modes, as was the activation of structures such as the cingulate cortex.

However, the main overall result was not a 'consciousness center', as it were, secreting sensory awareness like a gland, but a shift in the detailed pattern of activity from dorsolateral cortical in the awareness mode, to medial cortical and subcortical in the unawareness mode. It is important to point out how dependent imaging results are on statistical assumptions and where one sets the thresholds. In fact, there is a huge constellation of changes, and one has to decide how much of a change is a change. We set our criteria at a very conservative level, and required changes to be of a certain minimal value, as well as requiring a minimal cluster size of areas of activation. However, even on our very conservative assumptions, the list is long. Nevertheless, some structures came to light, so to speak, *only* in the awareness mode, and other *only* in the unawareness mode.

What to make of this result of the shift to the subcortex, and especially the midbrain? On the neuroscientific side, we succeeded in becoming wise after the event. Animal evidence had already suggested, some years ago, in fact, that the superior colliculus has a special role in mediating visual capacity after removal of visual cortex. If a monkey is given lots of practice carrying out visual discrimination in its blind half-field, it gradually improves and the field defect actually shrinks. Robert Wurtz and colleagues at NIH (Mohler and Wurtz, 1977) showed that the superior colliculus plays a crucial role in this improvement in monkeys. The defect returns to being static and apparently absolutely blind if the superior colliculus is removed after the training. It can be removed with impunity if the striate cortex is intact. Human subjects, as it happens, also show improvement in the sensitivity of their blind fields with practice (Zihl and von Cramon, 1985; Kerkhoff *et al.*, 1994; Kasten and Sabel, 1995).

It also turns out, in a further imaging study with G.Y. by our group, that the midbrain structure, the superior colliculus, is also activated by color, perhaps an even more surprising finding, and its activation is correlated both with psychophysical ratings and with the response of the pupil (Barbur *et al.*, 1998). G.Y., or any blindsight subject, has never reported an experience of color in the blind field, and yet, for example, he can reliably detect a red stimulus against a white background, independently of its contrast, and even when matched in luminance to the background. The superior colliculus lights up with the red stimulus in the blind field, but not when it falls in the intact field.

What do we make of the dorsolateral frontal activation, area 46, which was found to be activated uniquely in the aware mode, both for the blind half-field and for the intact half-field? This part of the brain is seemingly a long way from the visual cortex—as the crow flies, so to speak—and is usually not thought to be specialized for visual stimuli. However, Malcolm Young (1992, 1993) has shown, in an anatomical analysis, how visual pathways leaving the visual cortex, via both the dorsal and ventral pathways, converge so strikingly in just this region.

We know that visual association areas, and indeed many other regions of cortex, can be and are activated in the absence of striate cortex. However, while such activation may be *necessary* for awareness, is it *sufficient*? Here animal experiment provides a striking answer in the negative. Long ago Roger Sperry (Sperry *et al.*, 1960), and his then student Michael Gazzaniga (1966), asked whether vision was possible when all visual cortices were left intact, but all non-visual cortex was removed. More recently, Nakamara and Mishkin (1980, 1986; Nakamara *et al.*, 1986) have pursued the same question quite intensively. Without going into the

details, the clear answer is that the animal fails to respond to visual stimuli behaviorally when all visual cortices—generously defined—are intact, but non-visual cortex is removed. This is the case even though the neurons in striate cortex are shown to be responding normally to visual events. Therefore, the visual cortices may be necessary for visual responsiveness, but they are not *sufficient*. Connections are required to regions of the brain that lie outside the visually specialized centers themselves for visual responsiveness and, I would postulate, for visual awareness to arise. However, in no sense can we conclude that area 46 is a 'consciousness center'. It is part of a complex system, of which area 46 may just be the tip of the iceberg. We are dealing with major dynamic shifts between dorsal and subcortical when we shift from performance with awareness and without awareness.

SUMMING UP

It is time to pull some strings together. First, in virtually every area of cognitive neuropsychology there are residual functions of good capacity that continue in the absence of the subject's awareness. Secondly, by comparing aware with unaware modes, with matched performance levels, we have a route to brain imaging of these two modes. Thirdly, in order to determine whether the subject is aware or not aware, it cannot be done by studying the discriminative capacity alone—it can be good in the absence of awareness. To go back to an earlier distinction, we have to go 'off-line' to do this. In operational terms, within the blindsight mode, but in similar terms for all of the syndromes, we have to use something like the 'commentary key' in parallel with the ongoing discrimination, or (as in the animal experiments) obtain an independent classification of the events being discriminated. Fourthly, wherever the brain capacity for making the commentary exists, it is certainly outside the specialized visual processing areas, and may involve several different systems.

To have, not to hold: but gripping.

REFERENCES

Azzopardi, P. and Cowey, A. (1997) Is blindsight like normal, near-threshold vision? *Proceedings of the National Academy of Sciences of the United States of America*, 94, 14190–14194.

Barbur, J.L. (1995) A study of pupil response components in human vision. In: Robbins, J.G., Djamgoz, M.B.A. and Taylor, A. (eds), *Basic and Clinical Perspectives in Vision Research*. Plenum Press, New York, pp. 3–18

Barbur, J.L. and Forsyth, P.M. (1986) Can the pupil response be used as a measure of the visual input associated with the geniculo-striate pathway? *Clinical Vision Sciences*, 1, 107–111.

Barbur, J.L. and Thomson, W.D. (1987) Pupil response as an objective measure of visual acuity. *Ophthalmic and Physiological Optics*, 7, 425–429.

Barbur, J.L., Harlow, A.J. and Sahraie, A. (1992) Pupillary responses to stimulus structure, colour, and movement. *Ophthalmic and Physiological Optics*, 235, 137–141.

Barbur, J.L., Harlow, J.A. and Weiskrantz, L. (1994a) Spatial and temporal response properties of residual vision in a case of hemianopia. *Philosophical Transactions of the Royal Society of London, Series B*, 343, 157–166.

Barbur, J.L., Harlow, J.A., Sahraie, A., Stoerig, P. and Weiskrantz, L. (1994b) Responses to chromatic stimuli in the absence of V1: pupillometric and psychophysical studies. In: Vision science and its applications. *Optical Society of America Technical Digest*, 2, 312–315.

Barbur, J.L., Sahraie, A., Simmons, A., Weiskrantz, L. and Williams, S.C.R. (1998) Residual processing of chromatic signals in the absence of a geniculostriate projection. *Vision Research*, 38, 3447–3453.

Bauer, R.M. (1984) Autonomic recognition of names and faces in prosopagnosia: a neuropsychological application of the guilty knowledge test. *Neuropsychologia*, 22, 457–469.

Berti, A and Rizzolatti, G. (1992) Visual processing without awareness: evidence from unilateral neglect. *Journal of Cognitive Neuroscience*, 4, 345–351.

Bisiach, E. (1992) Understanding consciousness: clues from unilateral neglect and related disorders. In: Milner, A.D. and Rugg, M.D. (eds), *The Neuropsychology of Consciousness*. Academic Press, London, pp. 113–137.

Brent, P.J., Kennard, C. and Ruddock, K.H. (1994) Residual colour vision in a human hemianope: spectral responses and colour discrimination. *Proceedings of the Royal Society of London, Series B*, 256, 219–225.

Brooks, D.N. and Baddeley, A.D. (1976) What can amnesic patients learn? *Neuropsychologia* 14, 111–122.

Claparède, E. (1911) Recognition et moite. *Archives de Psychologie Geneva*, 11, 79–90.

Corkin, S. (1968) Acquisition of motor skill after bilateral medial temporal lobe excision. *Neuropsychologia* 6, 255–265.

Cowey, A. and Stoerig, P. (1991) The neurobiology of blindsight. *Trends in Neurosciences*, 29, 65–80.

Cowey, A. and Stoerig, P. (1995) Blindsight in monkeys. *Nature*, 1995, 373, 247–249.

Cowey, A. and Stoerig, P. (1997) Visual detection in monkeys with blindsight. *Neuropsychologia*, 35, 929–1997.

Delay, J. and Brion, S. (1969) *Le Syndrome de Korsakoff*. Massoon, Paris.

Dennett, D.C. (1991) *Consciousness Explained*. Penguin Press, London.

Frederici, A.D. (1982) Syntactic and semantic processes in aphasic deficits: the availability of prepositions. *Brain and Language*, 15, 245–258.

Gabrieli, J.D.E., Milberg, W., Keane, M.M. and Corkin, S. (1990) Intact priming of patterns despite impaired memory. *Neuropsychologia* 28, 417–428.

Gazzaniga, M.S. (1966) Visuomotor integration in split-brain monkeys with other cerebral lesions. *Experimental Neurology*, 16, 289–298.

Gross, C.G. (1991) Contribution of striate cortex and the superior colliculus to visual function in area MT, the superior temporal polysensory area, and inferior temporal cortex. *Neuropsychologia*, 29, 497–515.

Heywood, C.A., Cowey, A. and Newcombe, F. (1991) Chromatic discrimination in a cortically colour blind observer. *European Journal of Neuroscience*, 3, 802–912.

Horn, G. (1985) *Memory, Imprinting, and the Brain*. Clarendon Press, Oxford.

Horn, G. (1990) Neural bases of recognition memory investigated through an analysis of imprinting. *Philosophical Transactions of the Royal Society of London, Series B*, 329, 133–142.

Horn, G. (1998) Visual imprinting and the neural mechanisms of recognition memory. *Trends in Neurosciences*, 21, 300–305.

Humphrey, N.K. (1970) What the frog's eye tells the monkey's brain. *Brain, Behavior and Evolution*, 3, 324–337.

Humphrey, N.K. (1974) Vision in a monkey without striate cortex: a case study. *Perception*, 3, 241–255.

Humphrey, N. and Weiskrantz, L. (1967) Vision in monkeys after removal of the striate cortex. *Nature*, 215, 595–597.

James, W. (1890) *Principles of Psychology*. Macmillan and Co., London.

Kentridge, R.W., Heywood, C.A. and Weiskrantz, L. (1997) Residual vision in multiple retinal locations within a scotoma: implications for blindsight. *Journal of Cognitive Neuroscience*, 9, 191–202.

Kasten, E. and Sabel, B.A. (1995) Visual field enlargement after computer training in brain-damaged patients with homonymous deficits: an open pilot trial. *Restorative Neurology and Neuroscience*, 8, 113–127.

Kerkhoff, G., Munsinger, U. and Meier, E. (1994) Neurovisual rehabilitation in cerebral blindness. *Archives of Neurology*, 51, 474–481.

Knowlton, B.J., Ramus, S.J. and Squire, L.R. (1992) Intact artificial grammar learning in amnesias: dissociation of abstract knowledge and memory for specific instances. *Psychological Science*, 3, 172–179.

Ladavas, E., Paladini, R. and Cubelli, R. (1993) Implicit associative priming in a patient with left visual neglect. *Neuropsychologia*, 31, 1307–1320.

Linebarger, M.C., Schwartz, M.F. and Saffran, E.M. (1983) Sensitivity to grammatical structure in so-called agrammatic aphasics. *Cognition*, 13, 361–392.

Marcel, A.J. (1998) Blindsight and shape perception: deficit of visual consciousness or of visual function? *Brain*, 121, 1565–1588.

Marshall, J. and Halligan, P. (1988) Blindsight and insight in visuo-spatial neglect. *Nature*, 335, 766–777.

Marzi, C.A., Tassinari, G., Aglioti, S. and Lutzemberger, L. (1986) Spatial summation across the vertical meridian in hemianopics: a test of blindsight. *Neuropsychologia*, 30, 783–795.

McAndrews, M.P., Glisky, E.L. and Schacter, D.L. (1987) When priming persists: long-lasting implicit memory for a single episode in amnesic patients. *Neuropsychologia*, 25, 297–506.

McLeod, P., Dittrich, W., Driver, J., Perrett, D. and Zihl, J. (1997) Preserved and impaired detection of structure from motion by a 'motion-blind' patient. *Visual Cognition*, 3, 363–391.

Milner, A.D. and Goodale, M.A. (1995) *The Visual Brain in Action*. Oxford University Press, Oxford.

Mohler, C.W. and Wurtz, R.H. (1977) Role of striate cortex and superior colliculus in visual guidance of saccadic eye movements in monkeys. *Journal of Neurophysiology*, 43, 74–94.

Nakamura, R.K. and Mishkin, M. (1980) Blindness in monkeys following non-visual cortical lesions. *Brain Research*, 188, 572–577.

Nakamura, R.K. and Mishkin, M. (1986) Chronic blindness following lesions of nonvisual cortex in the monkey. *Experimental Brain Research*, 62, 173–184.

Nakamura, R.K., Schein, S.J. and Desimone, R. (1986) Visual responses from cells in striate cortex of monkeys rendered chronically 'blind' by lesions of nonvisual cortex. *Experimental Brain Research*, 63, 185–190.

Paillard, J., Michel, F. and Stelmach, G. (1983) Localization without content: a tactile analogue of 'blind sight'. *Archives of Neurology*, 40, 548–551.

Pasik, P. and Pasik, T. (1982) Visual functions in monkeys after total removal of visual cerebral cortex. *Contributions to Sensory Physiology*, 7, 147–200.

Pöppel, E., Held, R. and Frost, D. (1973) Residual visual function after brain wounds involving the central visual pathways in man. *Nature*, 243, 295–296.

Rodman, H.T., Gross, C.G. and Albright, T.D. (1989) Afferent basis of visual response properties in area MT of the macaque. I. Effects of striate cortex removal. *Journal of Neuroscience*, 9, 2033–2050.

Rossetti, Y., Rode, G. and Boisson, D. (1995) Implicit processing of somaesthetic information: a dissociation between where and how? *NeuroReport*, 6, 506–510

Rossetti, Y., Rode, G., Perenin, M. and Boisson, D. (1996) No memory for implicit perception in blindsight and numbsense. Presented at: *Towards a Science of Consciousness 1996 'Tucson II'*, held at Tucson, Arizona.

Sahraie, A., Weiskrantz, L., Barbur, J.L., Simmons, A., Williams, S.C.R. and Brammer, M.L. (1997) Pattern of neuronal activity associated with conscious and unconscious processing of visual signals. *Proceedings of the National Academy of Sciences of the United States of America*, 94, 9406–9411.

Schacter, D.L. (1992) Consciousness and awareness in memory and amnesia: critical issues. In: Milner, A.D. and Rugg, M.D. (eds), *The Neuropsychology of Consciousness*. Academic Press, London, pp. 179–200.

Schacter D.L., Cooper, L.A., Tharan, M. and Rubens, A. (1991) Preserved priming of novel objects in patients with memory disorders. *Journal of Cognitive Neuroscience*, 3, 118–131.

Scoville, W.B. and Milner, B. (1957) Loss of recent memory after bilateral hippocampal lesions. *Journal of Neurology, Neurosurgery and Psychiatry*, 20, 11–21.

Shallice, T. and Saffran, E. (1986) Lexical processing in the absence of explicit word identification: evidence from a letter-by-letter reader. *Cognitive Neuropsychology*, 3, 429–458.

Sperry, R.W. (1974) Lateral specialization in the surgically separated hemispheres. In: Schmitt, F.O. and Worden, F.G. (eds), *The Neurosciences: Third Study Program*. MIT Press, Cambridge, Massachusetts, pp.

Sperry, R.W., Myers, R.E. and Schrier, A.M. (1960) Perceptual capacity in the isolated visual cortex in the cat. *Quarterly Journal of Experimental Psychology*, 12, 65–71.

Stoerig, P. and Cowey, A. (1991) Increment threshold spectral sensitivity in blindsight: evidence for colour opponency. *Brain*, 114, 1487–1512.

Stoerig, P. and Cowey, A. (1992) Wavelength sensitivity in blindsight. *Brain*, 115, 425–444.

Torjussen, T. (1976) Residual function in cortically blind hemifields. *Scandinavian Journal of Psychology*, 17, 320–322.

Torjussen, T. (1978) Visual processing in cortically blind hemifields. *Neuropsychologia*, 16, 15–21.

Tranel, D. and Damasio, A.R. (1985) Knowledge without awareness: an autonomic index of facial recognition by prosopagnosics. *Science*, 228, 1453–1455.

Tyler, L.K. (1988) Spoken language comprehension in a fluent aphasic patient. *Cognitive Neuropsychology*, 5, 375–400.

Tyler, L.K. (1992) The distinction between implicit and explicit language function: evidence from aphasia. In: Milner, A.D. and Rugg, M.D. (eds), *The Neuropsychology of Consciousness*. Academic Press, London, pp. 159–179.

Warrington, E.K. and Weiskrantz, L. (1968) New method of testing long-term retention with special reference to amnesic patients. *Nature*, 217, 972–974.

Weiskrantz, L. (1961) Encephalisation and the scotoma. In: Thorpe, W.H. and Zangwill, O.L. (eds), *Current Problems in Animal Behaviour*. Cambridge University Press, Cambridge, pp. 30–58.

Weiskrantz, L. (1986, update, 1998) *Blindsight. A Case Study and Implications*. Oxford University Press, Oxford.

Weiskrantz, L. (1987) Neuroanatomy of memory and amnesia: a case for multiple memory systems. *Human Neurobiology*, 6, 93–105.

Weiskrantz L. (1990a) Outlooks for blindsight: explicit methodologies for implicit processes. The Ferrier Lecture. *Proceedings of the Royal Society of London, Series B*, 239, 247–278.

Weiskrantz, L. (1990b) Problems of learning and memory: one or multiple systems? *Philosophical Transactions of the Royal Society of London, Series B*, 329, 99–108.

Weiskrantz, L. (1996) Blindsight revisited. *Current Opinions in Neurobiology*, 6, 215–220.

Weiskrantz, L. (1997) *Consciousness Lost and Found. A Neuropsychological Exploration*. Oxford University Press, Oxford.

Weiskrantz, L. and Warrington, E.K. (1970) Verbal learning and retention by amnesic patients using partial information. *Psychonomic Science*, 20, 210–211.

Weiskrantz, L. and Warrington, E.K. (1979) Conditioning in amnesic patients. *Neuropsychologia*, 17, 187–194.

Weiskrantz, L., Warrington, E.K., Sanders, M.D. and Marshall, J. (1974) Visual capacity in the hemianopic field following a restricted occipital ablation. *Brain*, 97, 709–728.

Weiskrantz, L., Barbur, J.L. and Sahraie, A. (1995) Parameters affecting conscious versus unconscious visual discrimination without V1. *Proceedings of the National Academy of Sciences of the United States of America*, 92, 6122–6126.

Weiskrantz, L., Cowey, A. and LeMare, C. (1998) Learning from the pupil: a spatial visual channel in the absence of V1 in monkey and human. *Brain*, 121, 1065–1072.

Young, A.W. and De Haan, E.H.F. (1992) Face recognition and awareness after brain injury. In: Milner, A.D. and Rugg, M.D. (eds), *The Neuropsychology of Consciousness*. Academic Press, London, pp. 69–90.

Young, A.W., De Haan, E.H.F. and Newcombe, F. (1990) Unawareness of impaired face recognition. *Brain and Cognition*, 14, 1–18.

Young, M.P. (1992) Objective analysis of the topological organization of the primate cortical visual system. *Nature*, 358, 152–155.

Young, M.P. (1993) The organization of neural systems in the primate cerebral cortex. *Proceedings of the Royal Society of London, Series B*, 252, 13–18.

Zihl, J. and von Cramon, D. (1985) Visual field recovery from scotoma in patients with postgeniculate damage: a review of 55 cases. *Brain*, 108, 335–365.

Zihl, J., von Cramon, D. and Mai, N. (1983) Selective disturbance of movement vision after bilateral brain damage. *Brain*, 106, 313–340.

PART FOUR EPILOGUE

19   IN MEMORY

Gabriel Horn

The major objective of cognitive neuroscience is to understand the neural mechanisms of thought processes. It is difficult to conceive of these processes taking place solely in the present continuous, without any reference to the past. Past experience may influence future behaviour and the interpretation of current events; and the information contained in memory may occupy our current thoughts. Although the neural bases of memory in particular and of thought processes in general have been the subjects of speculation for many centuries the field of cognitive neuroscience is a relatively new one. Why is this so, what specific issues do cognitive neuroscientists address and how is it that these issues have begun to be addressed only relatively recently?

LAYING THE FOUNDATIONS OF COGNITIVE NEUROSCIENCE

During the first half of the twentieth century much of the effort of neurophysiologists was directed towards understanding spinal reflexes, the cable properties of cell membranes, the ionic basis of the nerve impulse, synaptic transmission, the physiological properties of peripheral sensory and motor structures and the organization of the autonomic nervous system. The general organization of the cerebral cortex was known from anatomical studies and from knowledge of the clinical effects of brain lesions. The use of evoked potentials and methods of electrical stimulation disclosed the orderly projection of the sensory surfaces of the body on to the primary sensory areas of the cortex as well as the topographic organization of the sensorimotor cortex. But in primates, and especially in humans these areas are slender strips of cortex bounding huge 'association areas' about which relatively little was known. Certainly damage to these areas had profound effects on behaviour, for example on attention (posterior parietal lobes; see Denny-Brown and Chambers, 1958), visual recognition (infer-ior temporal lobes; Kluver and Bucy, 1939) planning, decision making and complex aspects of personality (prefrontal lobes; see Fulton, 1949). But knowledge of the anatomy and physiology of the brain was not advanced enough to make any real impact on our understanding of the neural mechanisms underlying these aspects of thought processes.

Sensory inputs to the cerebral cortex were thought to exercise control over action via intracortical pathways which directly link sensory to motor areas, or indirectly do so through the association areas. It was also assumed that the cortex must be engaged if a sensory stimulus is to evoke a conscious response. It therefore came as a surprise when, in the late 1930s and early 1940s, it was found that patients with small lesions in the brainstem/diencephalon were deeply, and often irreversibly comatose (Jefferson, 1944; Penfield, 1952), findings that were replicated in the cat and monkey (Lindsley *et al.*, 1950; French and Magoun, 1952). Soon after the clinical observations had been made, it was shown that electrical stimulation of structures in the diencephalon or in the brainstem reticular formation led to changes in the electroencephalogram (EEG) of widespread areas of the cerebral cortex (Morrison and Dempsey, 1942; Moruzzi and Magoun, 1949; Jasper, 1949). The anatomical pathways that might mediate these affects remained mysterious until 1963 when Shute and Lewis demonstrated just such a route from brainstem to cerebral cortex. The brainstem reticular formation receives input from all sensory modalities as well as from the cerebral cortex. Taken together, the evidence suggested that the reticular formation played an important role in modulating cortical activity and that it is implicated in sleep and wakefulness, arousal, attention and consciousness – all aspects of cognitive functions. Further analysis of these functions had to await the development and application of new techniques, especially the microelectrode, the ability to record neuronal activity from behaving animals, and the use of powerful computers to analyse that activity and to relate it to behaviour.

The use of the microelectrode had a major impact on the study of neuron physiology, and especially of transmission at synaptic and neuromuscular junctions (Eccles, 1964; Katz, 1966). The microelectrode also led to major developments in sensory physiology. Kuffler (1952) plotted the receptive fields of cat retinal ganglion cells. Soon afterwards Mountcastle and his colleagues studied the receptive field organization of the somatic sensory relay nuclei in the thalamus, and of neurons in the sensorimotor cortex of the cat and monkey (Mountcastle, 1957; Powell and Mountcastle, 1959; Poggio and Mountcastle, 1963). This work, which demonstrated the columnar organization of that area of cortex, was followed up by the studies of Hubel and Wiesel (1961, 1962, 1965b). They analysed the way in which visual receptive fields are transformed within the visual pathways. All this work set the foundations not only for a detailed analysis of sensory processing, but also for the analysis of a 'higher' or cognitive level of sensory processing, especially of visual perception.

The world in which we live is rarely composed of stimuli that are unimodal. We may see an object and touch it, hear it rattle or move, and perhaps detect its odour. We may reach out to pick it up and do so accurately whether we are standing up or lying down, whether the head is vertical or bent to one side. Signals in the different sensory pathways must somehow be integrated to give a coherent construct of that world, and to allow us to act appropriately. Studies of the neural bases of this integration flourished in the second half of the 20th century, and some of that work is described in this volume.

Whilst all these aspects of the physiology of perception were being investigated, there was increasing interest in the physiological basis of *selective* perception, or attention. Some physiological correlates of attention had been observed by Berger (1930) in his pioneering work on the EEG, work that was confirmed by Adrian and Matthews in 1934. They showed that in humans the occipital alpha rhythm is present when the eyes are closed. The rhythm is abolished when the eyes are open during pattern vision. Adrian (1944) went on to show that the alpha rhythm returns if the subject, with open eyes, listens to the ticking of a watch. Adrian considered that the alpha rhythm is not abolished by visual input *per se*; disruption only occurs if we attend to the visual stimulus. He postulated that the alpha rhythm reflects the synchronous discharge of cortical neurons. Afferent input to the visual cortex disrupts this synchrony and

hence disrupts the alpha rhythm. From these considerations he inferred that during attention to an auditory stimulus, signals in the visual pathways are blocked before reaching the visual cortex. Recent evidence confirms that signals in the retino-thalamic-striate pathway are modulated by attentiveness, but that the first point of modulation is at the postsynaptic level in the striate cortex (Horn and Wiesenfeld, 1974; Horn, 1976; Motter, 1993; Hillyard, 1995; Roelfsema *et al.*, 1998). Interest in attention was further stimulated by studies of the brainstem reticular formation and the diencephalon referred to above. These systems have reciprocal connections with the sensory pathways and the cerebral cortex. These connections made them plausible systems to be engaged, on the one hand in attenuating sensory inputs from unattended stimuli and, on the other hand, in enhancing the activity of those parts of the cerebral cortex which are involved in focal attention. Jung (1954) was interested in this latter aspect of attention and he compared attention to a searchlight illuminating details of cerebral function (cf. Crick, 1984). All these experiments and speculations created a climate of interest in attention, an interest that was further stimulated by the psychological studies of Broadbent (1958) in humans. With the development of techniques for recording neuronal activity in behaving animals, and of imaging techniques for studying the brain of humans engaged in mental tasks, the stage was set for a detailed analysis of selective perception at both the physiological and psychological levels of analysis (see for example, Bushnell *et al.*, 1981; Näätänen, 1992; Humphreys *et al.*, 1999 and Chapter 4).

Selective attention is at the heart of awareness and awareness is at the heart of consciousness. We select for response only a limited number of the constellation of sensory events that impinge on us, or of the messages in memory that are recalled. Some responses may be 'automatic', as when the experienced motorist drives a car, constantly adjusting his/her activity to changing conditions of the road, but without 'noticing', or 'being aware' of having done so. Other responses are 'noticed' in the sense that we are aware of them. We say of these responses that we 'attend' to them or that we are 'conscious' of them. The motorist may be 'preoccupied with', or 'attending to' or 'thinking about' a painting or a piece of music, without being aware of the highly skilled motor acts he/she is performing whilst negotiating a bend in the highway. With the explosion of interest in cognitive neuroscience it is hardly surprising that there has been a corresponding explosion of interest in the neuro-biological nature of consciousness (Marcel and Bisiach, 1988; Dennett, 1991; Searle, 1992; Crick, 1994). Many neuroscientists rejoiced when Ryle (1949) exorcised the ghost from the machine, but the rejoicing was not universal (Eccles, 1953; Popper, 1972; Thorpe, 1978). Discussions in this field tend to generate more heat than light: even to refer to 'the neurobiological nature' of consciousness is to adopt a stance that many would argue is more philosophical than biological. Never-theless, changes in the state of the brain have subtle, or even profound affects on consciousness, as dis-cussed above in reference to the brainstem reticular formation. Furthermore, the work of Weiskrantz (1997 and Chapter 18 this volume) gives a firm empirical foundation for the analysis at the neural level of the state to which the term 'conscious' is given.

Through the process of learning an animal acquires information about the world, and its efficiency in doing so is influenced by many factors, for example, its motivational state, its level of alertness and its attentiveness to the task. The ways in which animals learn, and some of the rules governing learning had been studied at the behavioural level since the latter part of the nineteenth century, and these studies were to prove crucial to the neural analyses that were to follow later. For example, classical conditioning was characterized by Pavlov (1927), instrumental con-ditioning by Konorski (1948) and by Konorski and Miller (1937), habituation by Humphrey (1933), imprinting by Spalding (1873), Heinroth (1911), Lorenz (1937), Hinde (1962), Bateson (1966), and bird-song learning by Thorpe (1958).

Information acquired through learning is stored as memory. Memory gives individuals their personal, psychological/behavioural identity. Without memory we have no past: rather than being reflective beings we become reflexive beings. It is only necessary to examine patients with advanced Alzheimer's disease to see how damaging to an individual's identity severe memory impairment or loss may be. Yet important as memory is to both human and non-human animals, virtually nothing was known of its neural basis in the first part of the 20th century. Neurophysiological events had time-courses that were measured in milliseconds, with the exception of post-tetanic potentiation of monosynaptic spinal reflexes where the potentiation might last for several hours (Lloyd, 1949; Eccles and McIntyre, 1951). But the relevance of this form of potentiation to memory was

a matter of speculation. Whilst neural processes which are long-lasting are candidate mechanisms, persistence *per se* is not a sufficient condition for a process to be implicated in memory. To give a crude example, the gliosis that follows a penetrating injury of the brain is, in some sense at least, a memory of that injury; but it does not follow that gliosis is involved in the storage of information acquired through learning. Much more than persistence is required for a physiological change to be a serious candidate for the storage of learned material. Long-term potentiation (LTP) has many of the presumed properties of a neural mechanism for this kind of memory, but it is proving frustratingly difficult to determine whether or not it is such a mechanism (Bolhuis and Reid, 1992; Bannerman *et al.*, 1995; Saucier and Cain, 1995; see also p. 353).

Attempts to localize and identify the trace, or the engram left in the brain by learning had been made by Lashley in a series of experiments that extended over much of his life-time in research. In a much-quoted paragraph referring to that work Lashley (1950) wrote:

'I sometimes feel, in reviewing the evidence on the localisa-tion of the memory trace, that the necessary conclusion is that learning just is not possible.'

Developments since that time give cause for opti-mism. Some of that work is described below and in other chapters of this volume. The first sign of a breakthrough came from the study habituation, which Thorpe (1956) strongly promoted as the most perva-sive, simple form of learning in the animal kingdom.

A MEMORY NOT TO RESPOND

Some unconditioned behavioural responses, evoked without prior training experience, may cease to be evoked if the eliciting stimulus is repeatedly pre-sented without either reward or punishment. How-ever, if a novel stimulus is substituted for the repeated stimulus, the response may again be elicited. This behaviour is consistent with a mechanism whereby the repeated presentation of a stimulus leads to a functional closure of the neural pathway linking the sensory input to the motor output. By implication, the memory of habituation is a memory not to respond to the repeated, unreinforced stimulus.

Habituation has a number of relatively well-defined characteristics. If, after a behavioural response has waned, the stimulus is withdrawn for some time and then re-presented, the response may return. Within limits, response attenuation is specific to the stimulus. For example, a 500 Hz tone was found to wake a sleeping cat and did so again after the cat had been allowed to fall asleep. When this cycle was repeated 20–30 times, the stimulus gradually became ineffective. The cat woke up when a 100 Hz tone was substituted for the 500 Hz tone. Once the arousal response to the 500 Hz tone had been established, smaller shifts in frequency, as from 500 Hz to 600 Hz, were usually found to be ineffective in arousing the animal (Sharpless and Jasper, 1956). That is, one of the features of habituation is that there is stimulus generalization – the failure to respond to the repeated stimulus is extended to include a failure to respond to stimuli that, in the naïve animal, are capable of eliciting the response.

In a resting mammal, a novel visual stimulus may elicit a 'visual orientation response,' the animal directing its gaze to the source of the stimulus. The superior colliculus, or optic tectum is involved in this response. The structure is a major target of optic tract axons which terminate there in an orderly array so that the visual fields are represented systematically across the tectal surface. Given this link with the visual system it initially came as a surprise to find that neurons in the *optic* tectum of the rabbit responded not only visual stimuli, but also to auditory and to somatic sensory stimuli (Horn and Hill, 1964; 1966). These findings were soon confirmed in other species, and extended to show that the projection to the optic tectum of these non-visual inputs is also topographically arranged (Jassik-Gerschenfeld, 1965; Gordon, 1973; Drager and Hubel, 1976). With the benefit of hindsight this kind of multisensory afferent organization of the optic tectum makes perfectly good sense. The orientation response is not only elicited by visual stimuli; it may also be elicited by novel auditory and somatic sensory stimuli. Presumably when, in the behaving animal, such a stimulus evokes impulse activity in a focus in the optic tectum, the animal directs its gaze to the part of its sensory space which corresponds to that focus, and so to the stimulus (Mohler and Wurtz, 1977; Stryker and Schiller, 1975; Jay and Sparks, 1987; Stein *et al.*, Chapter 2).

Since repeated, or iterated presentation of an un-reinforced stimulus results in the habituation of the orientation response, some insight into the neural changes underlying the habituation process might be gained by studying the responses of neurons in the

optic tectum to repeated sensory stimulation. When visual, auditory or somatic sensory stimuli are presented at intervals of a few seconds the responses of many neurons in the optic tectum of the rabbit were found to wane (Horn and Hill, 1964, 1966). The number of stimuli required to bring about a marked attenuation of the response varied from neuron to neuron, although in a majority of them attenuation was quite marked by the fifteenth presentation. There was a variable degree of recovery of the response if the stimulus was withdrawn for some 20 seconds or so. When, as a result of repeated presentation of a given stimulus the response had waned, the neuron usually responded to another stimulus. For example, the response of a neuron to 1kHz tone gradually declined as the stimulus was presented at intervals of approximately 1.5 seconds; by the twenty-eighth presentation the neuron responded barely or not at all to this stimulus. A 1.5kHz tone was then substituted without breaking the rhythm of stimulus presentation. The neuron responded briskly to this stimulus – as briskly indeed as it had done in a test given before the 'habituating' sequence had been delivered. Although the neuron responded to a 950 Hz tone before the habituating sequence had been given, it did not do so immediately afterwards. These results demonstrate that response attenuation is stimulus-specific, although this specificity is imprecise because there is some stimulus generalization. The failure to respond to the 1kHz tone cannot be attributed to inhibition of the recorded neuron because the pathway for the 1.5kHz stimulus was 'open.' This finding was a general one for habituating neurons, implying that the breakdown in transmission of signals was presynaptic to them.

The results described above show, collectively, that there is a relatively close, parametric similarity in the changes that characterize the (behavioural) habituation of the orientation response and those which characterize the habituation of neurons in a pathway involved in that response. It seemed possible, therefore, that the neural changes could account for the behavioural changes (Horn, 1965, 1967, 1970; Horn and Hill 1964). A similar proposal was made by Spencer *et al.* (1966*a*, *b*, *c*) and Thompson and Spencer (1966) on the basis of their elegant experiments on the habituation of the flexor reflex in the cat spinal cord (see also Bell *et al.*, 1964).

A characteristic of behavioural habituation is that it is sometimes possible to re-establish the response to the repeated stimulus by presenting an intense or noxious intercurrent stimulus (Humphrey, 1933); Prosser and Hunter, 1936). Prosser and Hunter showed that an extinguished spinal reflex response recovered if the animal became generally excited. At the neuronal level, Bell *et al.* (1964) recorded the responses of neurons in the midbrain reticular formation to the repeated movements of an object in the visual field. When the response had waned to a low level, it returned immediately after a somatic or an acoustic stimulus had been delivered. Similar effects of intercurrent stimulation have been shown for neurons in the mammalian spinal cord (Spencer *et al.*, 1966a, b, c) as well as in other nervous systems (Bruner and Tauc, 1966; Rowell and Horn, 1967, 1968; Castellucci *et al.*, 1970). These experiments demonstrated that the effects of neuronal habituation may be reversed rapidly. Because an intercurrent stimulus may reverse habituation in neurons in many parts of the nervous system, the effects of the stimulus must be mediated by regions that have widespread connections to other parts of the brain and spinal cord. Such widely connected systems in mammals originate in the brainstem and diencephalon (Scheibel and Scheibel, 1958; Shute and Lewis, 1963; Dahlström and Fuxe, 1964) and probably have their counterparts in other nervous systems (Rowell, 1970; Bruner and Tauc, 1966; Carew *et al.*, 1979; Mackey *et al.*, 1989).

The reversal of habituation is referred to as 'dishabituation,' both at the behavioural and the neuronal levels (Horn and Hinde, 1970). Where the intercurrent stimulus enhances non-habituated responses the term 'sensitization' is used. Sensitization also occurs at both levels and may involve different processes from those involved in dishabituation (see Hinde, 1970). At the behavioural level sensitization is sometimes referred to as 'pseudoconditioning' (Hilgard and Marquis, 1961). At the neuronal level there is evidence that the facilitation of a decremented neuronal response (dishabituation) involves different intracellular signalling pathways from those involved in facilitating a non-decremented response (sensitization) although the two biochemical pathways may interact (Fitzgerald *et al.*, 1990; Byrne and Kandel, 1996).

What mechanisms underlie neuronal habituation? Hints came through the use of extracellular and intracellular microelectrodes, respectively to record the activity of single neurons in the mammalian CNS. A common finding, using extracellular microelectrodes, was that a novel stimulus was capable of evoking a response in a neuron after the response to a repeated stimulus had waned; and the magnitude of the

response to the novel stimulus was unaffected by prior habituation to the repeated stimulus. Furthermore, the firing rate of the recorded neuron was usually unaffected by habituation (Bell *et al.*, 1964; Horn and Hill, 1964, 1966; Segundo *et al.*, 1967a; Vinogradova, 1970). These observations implied that the recorded neuron was not itself inhibited as the response to the repeated stimulus waned. Direct support for this implication came through the use of intracellular recording microelectrodes. Spencer *et al.* (1966c) and Segundo *et al.* (1967b) found that during habituation there was a decline in the amplitude of the postsynaptic potential but no detectable changes in the postsynaptic neuron. Since the site of change during habituation was always presynaptic, the mechanism might be a depression of synaptic transmission somewhere in the pathway activated by the stimulus and the recorded neuron. Nonetheless, the possibility remained that inhibitory mechanisms shut off the input to the recorded neuron, and these mechanisms were operated by small neurons that were not detected by either extracellular or intracellular recording microelectrodes.

It is not easy to clarify these issues in the tangled network of the mammalian CNS. Hope of further advances came from studies of a synapse in which there are no interneurons (see below) and from a nervous system with relatively few neurons, some of which have large cell bodies. These may easily be penetrated by microelectrodes and recordings made over many hours. The marine gastropod *Aplysia* possess such a nervous system (Arvanitaki and Chalazonitis, 1958) and this sea snail became the focus of intense study in the context of habituation, beginning with the pioneering work of Bruner and Tauc (1966).

Bruner and Tauc (1966) observed that when a drop of water fell on a head tentacle of *Aplysia* the tentacle was withdrawn. If the drop was applied repeatedly at intervals of some 10 seconds the tentacular response gradually declined. Bruner and Tauc recorded from a giant neuron in the left pleural ganglion in *Aplysia* and recorded a large excitatory postsynaptic potential (EPSP) whenever a drop of water evoked a tentacular contraction. As this response declined so too did the EPSP. Their evidence suggested that the breakdown in transmission involved presynaptic rather than postsynaptic changes, and pointed to a diminution in the amount of transmitter released by successive impulses in the presynaptic nerve fibre. Bruner and Tauc's proposal was based on the assumption that the effects they observed were recorded at a mono-synaptic junction. They were cautious as to whether this assumption was met in their experiments.

Such a monosynaptic junction is contained within the stellate ganglion of the squid, *Loligo vulgaris* (Young, 1939; Llinas, 1999). Does transmission across this synapse fail on repeated, intermittent stimulation of the presynaptic fibre? Horn and Wright (1970) showed that it did and, drawing on earlier work on this synapse by Bullock and Hagiwara (1957) and Bryant, (1959), suggested that stimulus repetition brings about an uncoupling of the action potential in the membrane of the presynaptic terminal from the release of transmitter from that terminal. Since this release is calcium-dependent (Katz and Miledi, 1967; Miledi, 1973), it seemed plausible to suppose that transmission failure involved changes in the presynaptic terminal that affected the movement of calcium ions into it (Horn and Wright, 1970; Horn, 1970).

Kandel and his colleagues, in an impressive series of experiment have further advanced our understanding of the cellular mechanisms of habituation, dishabituation and sensitization in *Aplysia*, concentrating on the neural pathways mediating the gill-withdrawal reflex (Hawkins *et al.*, 1987; Byrne and Kandel, 1996). First they identified this pathway and the synapses at which habituation occurs (Kupferman and Kandel, 1969). They showed that a tactile stimulus applied to the sensory surface, located on the siphon, activates a sensory neuron that synapses directly onto motor neurons controlling gill withdrawal. The sensory neuron also synapses on interneurons that in turn activate the motor neurons. When the tactile stimulus to the siphon is repeatedly applied the synaptic potentials recorded in the motor neurons and the interneurons become progressively smaller. This change is brought about by a gradual reduction in the release of neurotransmitter (Klein *et al.*, 1980). The change occurs during a training trial of some 10 presentation of the tactile stimulus. This form of habituation lasts for minutes rather than hours. However, Castellucci *et al.* (1978) went on to demonstrate that, by giving four sets of these trials spaced over time, response attenuation might last for several weeks. This long-term behavioural change is accompanied by a reduction in the functional connections between sensory neurons and motor neurons and by a reduction in the number of active zones at the terminals of the sensory neurons (Bailey and Chen, 1983).

An intense or noxious stimulus may often restore a response that has waned. As discussed above, such findings suggest that the effects of this stimulus are mediated by a diffusely connected system of neurons (see Figure 19.1A). The findings also imply that reversal of the waned response must entail a restoration of synaptic transmission as a result of the activity of neurons in this system, which might mobilize transmitter in the depressed terminals. So much was guessed from early work (Horn, 1967, 1970). But the cellular mechanism for enhancing transmission in the depressed pathway was not then well understood. Carew *et al.* (1979) restored the gill-withdrawal reflex, both at the behavioural and neuronal levels, by delivering an electrical stimulus to the neck region in a single training trial. This noxious stimulus is thought to activate a group of facilitatory neurons that make synaptic contact with the terminals of the sensory neurons (Mackey *et al.*, 1989). Some of the facilitatory neurons release serotonin that enhances transmitter release from the terminals of the sensory neuron. The biochemical cascade initiated by serotonin leads, amongst other changes, to a prolongation of the action potential in the sensory neuron. This prolongation allows more calcium to enter its terminals and so enhances the release of neurotransmitter (see Figure 19.1B).

Several training trials lead to behavioural sensitization that may persist for days or even weeks. At the cellular level sensitization is associated with presynaptic facilitation mediated by serotonin through its action on the release of neurotransmitter. Serotonin also promotes structural changes, but to be effective this neuromodulator must bind to receptors in both the cell body and terminals of the sensory neuron (Sun and Schacher, 1998).

In the 1960s, when the microelectrode was first extensively used to analyse the neuronal basis of habituation, little was known of the basis of intracellular signalling. This knowledge, applied to the study of cellular mechanisms of this simple form of learning has proved immensely fruitful. And there is a very good accord between the experimental observations and theoretical models made over thirty years ago, and the findings of much more recent work.

A MEMORY FOR OBJECTS: THE CASE OF IMPRINTING

Whereas habituation involves the waning of a response, many other forms of learning involve the elaboration, modification, or shaping of a response to

A　　　　　　　　　　　　　　**B**

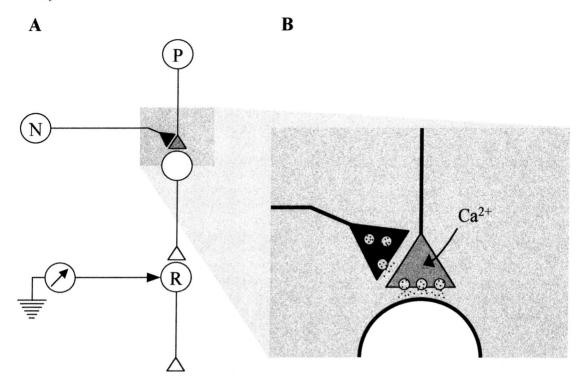

Figure 19.1. Mechanism of dishabituation. (**A**) A stimulus excites a burst of impulses in neuron P. This response is transmitted to neuron R. The activity of neuron R is recorded through the microelectrode. Repeated presentations of the stimulus are associated with consistent discharges in neuron P, but with a progressive reduction in the response of neuron R. The block in transmission was assumed to result from synaptic depression in the terminals of neuron P secondary to an imbalance between the processes of transmitter mobilization and release. This imbalance was thought to result from changes in the movement of calcium ions into the terminals (Horn, 1970). An intense intercurrent stimulus re-establishes transmission.The effect was thought to be mediated by neurons (see neuron N) which have widespread connection and which make axo-axonic connections. Transmission was thought to be restored by the activity of N-type neurons that enhance the mobilization of transmitter in the depressed synapse. (**B**) Serotonin released at a depressed sensory terminal of *Aplysia* restores transmission in the gill-withdrawal reflex pathway. Restoration is associated with a broadening of the action potential in the sensory nerve terminal, an increase in the influx of calcium ions and the mobilization of transmitter substance (see Kandel and Schwartz 1982). Serotonin may effect the mobilization of transmitter in other ways (Byrne and Kandel, 1996). (**A**, after Horn, 1967, **B**, based on Klein *et al.*, 1980).

a particular stimulus, event or set of events. Such learning implies that the stimulus is recognized and is distinguished from other stimuli or event(s) and is associated with a response. The response may be expressed, it may be covert and/or it may influence the way in which the animal responds to future experiences, by for example learning to perform a new task more rapidly than it might otherwise have done. These considerations suggest that the subject stores as memory the information it has learned about the stimulus or event(s), incorporates that information into other memory systems and is able to use the

stored information to modify its behaviour. The work that is described below was undertaken to investigate the nature of the trace left in the nervous system by an object which, through learning, an animal comes to recognize and to respond to selectively.

A major impediment to analysing the neural composition of memory's trace — what is *in* memory — is that the site or sites of information storage have proved to be elusive. Following the demonstration that, in patients, the hippocampal region is crucial for the formation of certain kinds of memory (Scoville and Milner, 1957; Milner, 1966; Warrington and Weiskrantz,

1982; Squire, 1987) this region has been the target of intense experimental analysis. However, even where the hippocampus can be shown to be crucial for memory, it does not follow that the region is itself a site of storage. Whether it is a store at all, whether it serves as a comparator matching stored information with incoming sensory information (see Vinogradova, 1970), whether it serves as part of a novelty detection network (Vinogradova, 1970; Eichenbaum 1999), whether it plays a role in attentive behaviour or whether it has still other functions, there are issues which still remain to be resolved (Warrington and Weiskrantz, 1982; Gaffan, 1993; Bolhuis *et al.*, 1994; Maguire *et al.*, 1996; Teng and Squire, 1999; Bontempi *et al.*, 1999).

The problem of identifying a region in which information acquired through learning is stored has largely been overcome in the case of imprinting. Since the problem of localization has loomed so large in memory research it is necessary to justify this claim in detail; for if it is justified the way is open for an *experimental* analysis of the neural changes that comprise the basis of memory.

The young of certain animals show co-ordinated locomotor activity soon after birth or hatching. These are precocial animals and include the young of guinea pigs, ducks and domestic chickens. Precocial animals quickly learn to recognize their mother and become socially attached to her. The learning process is known as imprinting (Lorenz, 1937; Hinde, 1962; Bateson, 1966; Sluckin, 1972; Bolhuis 1991). Domestic chicks, for example, learn the visual characteristics of their mother; if she moves about the chicks follow her and they also respond to her calls. If reared without the mother visually naïve chicks approach a wide range of conspicuous objects, and if exposed to one of them long enough approach it in preference to others. The fact that artificial objects are effective in eliciting this behaviour has made it possible to study imprinting in the laboratory.

But ease of studying imprinting in the laboratory is not a sufficient condition for using domestic chicks as the animal of choice for analysing the neural mechanisms of memory. There are many other reasons. Eggs may be incubated in the laboratory under controlled conditions (e.g. of temperature, humidity, darkness). Young chicks sleep for much of the first few hours after hatching and so can be reared in darkness in a warm incubator. If chicks are taken out of the incubator when they are approximately 18–26h, and exposed to a visually conspicuous object (the training stimu-

lus, see for example Fig 19.4A and B) they quickly learn its characteristics and subsequently approach it in preference to other objects. The period of exposure varies according to the properties of the stimulus. For example, moving objects are more effective than stationary objects, red more effective than green (Kovach, 1971; Bolhuis, 1991). In my laboratory the period of exposure to the training object is commonly between 0.5–2 hours. Thus a major attraction of studying imprinting in chicks for the analysis of memory is that prior to exposure to the training stimulus the chick has not received any visual experience. A further attraction is that chicks have a yolk sac that is adequate to support their dietary needs for at least three days after hatching; accordingly there is no need to subject them to the extraneous visual stimulation that feeding entails. What is more, when the dark-reared chick is first exposed to an object it rapidly learns its characteristics. Because the memory systems of the brain have not previously been engaged in storing information about the visual world they are like blank sheets upon which that information is inscribed; such a memory system offered hope that the nature of that inscription could be elucidated.

Correlative studies

Does exposure to a training stimulus lead to neural changes?

In formulating a strategy to answer this question it was assumed that the 'trace' left in the nervous system by an item to be stored involves the formation of new connections, or the strengthening of pre-existing connections (Cajal, 1911; Hebb, 1949). Such changes are likely to involve protein synthesis and to changes in the metabolism of RNA.

In the first series of experiments designed to answer the question we took advantage of previous work which demonstrated that the readiness with which birds can be imprinted is dependent on maturational age (Bateson, 1966; Gottlieb, 1961); early hatching chicks having the advantage in this respect over late hatching chicks. Exposure to an imprinting stimulus led to an increase in protein synthesis in one of three large brain samples, the dorsal part (roof) of the cerebral hemispheres. The effect was found only in the brains of early hatching chicks—not in those of late hatching chicks nor in those of untrained control chicks which had been exposed to the light of an over head bulb (Bateson *et al.*, 1969). In this and in all subsequent experiments measurement of neural changes were, whenever possible, made without knowledge of the behavioural experience of the chicks. In this respect the experiments were conducted 'blind'.

In a subsequent experiment net RNA synthesis into the three brain samples was determined by measuring the incorporation of radioactive uracil into the acid-insoluble components of these samples. After chicks had been trained by exposing them to an imprinting stimulus, net RNA synthesis was higher in trained chicks than in chicks which had simply been exposed to an overhead light. The effect was found only in the roof of the forebrain. Net synthesis was higher in chicks which had been exposed to the stimulus long enough for them to have formed a preference for it, than in chicks exposed to the stimulus for a shorter time and which were unlikely to have formed such a preference (Bateson *et al.*, 1972; Bateson, 1974).

Are the biochemical changes related to learning?
The controls used in the two sets of experiments suggest that they might be. But when a chick is trained it is handled, exposed to a moving flashing light, it may approach that stimulus, emit various calls, and so on—'side effects' of the procedure of training the bird. All may bring about neural changes. If some of these effects differ between the groups of chicks used in an experiment (for example, one group of chicks being more active than another) the neural changes observed may have more to do with the side-effects of training than with changes that may comprise the trace of memory. We therefore embarked on a series of experiments to clarify these issues.

If handling and behavioural excitement lead to changes in brain biochemistry the changes are likely to occur in both hemispheres. This presumption is particularly plausible if the mediating factors (for example, hormones such as corticosterone, biogenic amines) are carried in the systemic circulation. The presumption is also plausible if the biochemical effects of training result from differences between trained and untrained chicks in the extent to which the two groups move. For example, motor neurons in the cerebral hemispheres of the trained chicks may discharge at a higher rate, or even develop more connections than motor neurons of untrained chicks, if these move about less than the trained birds. Such neuronal changes could account for the biochemical differences between the two groups of chicks.

These ambiguities would be resolved if it were possible to train chicks in such a way as to 'train' one hemisphere by restricting visual input to it. If net RNA synthesis proved to be the same in the 'trained' hemisphere as in the 'untrained' hemisphere, then the biochemical changes found in the experiments of Bateson *et al.* (1969; 1972) could be accounted for by these side-effects of training. In the event, when visual input was restricted to one hemisphere, net RNA synthesis was higher in the forebrain roof of the 'trained' hemisphere than in that of the 'untrained' hemisphere (Horn *et al.*, 1973). These results suggest that these particular side-effects are implausible explanations for the findings of Bateson *et al.* (1969; 1972).

In the experiments of Horn *et al.* (1973) visual input was restricted to one hemisphere by occluding one eye of chicks in which a cerebral commissure had previously been divided. After training, chicks were given a preference test. In this test they were shown the training stimulus and a novel stimulus. Chicks tested with the eye which had been open during training preferred the training object, and were therefore imprinted (Sluckin, 1972). In contrast, chicks tested with the eye that had been occluded during training failed to show a preference. An implication of these findings is that the visually experienced hemisphere was capable of supporting the preference whereas the visually naïve hemisphere was not.

It does not, however, follow that the higher level of net RNA synthesis in the 'trained' hemisphere reflected a memory-specific change. The stimulus used for imprinting the chicks, a rotating flashing light, is likely to have activated more vigorously the visual pathways of the trained chicks than those of their controls which were not exposed to the stimulus. This activation by, for example, mobilizing transmitter substances in the visual pathways, may have increased protein and RNA synthesis in the imprinted chicks. Such ambiguities were addressed in two further sets of experiments.

In the first of these, day-old chicks were trained by exposing them for 240 minutes to an orange flashing rotating light. They developed a stronger preference for that stimulus than chicks trained for only 20 minutes (Bateson *et al.*, 1973). We reasoned that if the two groups were exposed again to the stimulus for an hour on the following day (day 2), those trained for the shorter time on day 1 ('undertrained') would have more to learn about the training object than those trained for the longer period ('overtrained'). Accordingly, if the increase in net RNA synthesis in the forebrain roof is related to learning, synthesis measured on day 2 should be higher in the undertrained chicks than in the overtrained chicks. In contrast, if sensory stimulation *per se* is responsible for the increased level of RNA synthesis it should not differ between the two groups of chicks since they were trained for the same length of time on day 2. We found that RNA synthesis on day 2 was inversely related to the duration of training on day 1.

In the following experiment we took advantage of the variation in the strength of preferences exhibited by chicks trained for a fixed period of time. All chicks were exposed to the training object for 72 minutes. The preference of each chick was then measured in a test in which it was allowed to approach that object and one it had not seen before. There was a positive correlation between preference for the training object and net RNA synthesis in the anterior part of the forebrain roof. No other measure of behaviour was correlated with this biochemical change nor was there a significant correlation between preference and net RNA synthesis in the other brain regions studied (Bateson *et al.* 1975).

Taking the results of all the control procedures together it seemed reasonable to suppose that the biochemical changes in the forebrain roof were closely linked to the learning process.

Are the biochemical changes localized?

To address this issue an autoradiographic technique was developed which reliably reflected the incorporation of radioactive uracil into acid-insoluble substances in the brain (Horn and McCabe, 1978). The experimental design was similar to the 'undertrained/overtrained' experiment described above (Bateson *et al.*, 1973). Serial sections were cut off the brains of the two groups of chicks, each of which had received injections of radioactive uracil. Autoradiographs were prepared and the optical density of various brain regions was measured (Horn *et al.*, 1979). Optical density varied with incorporation; on visual inspection of the autoradiographs brain regions with high levels of incorporation appeared darker than regions with relatively lower levels of incorporation.

There were quite serious constraints to this procedure. The method, which was manual, was very time-consuming so that it was not realistic to measure the optical density of all brain regions. Accordingly a pilot experiment was conducted to provide some guidance in deciding which regions to select for measurement. The autoradiographs of five pairs of over-

trained and undertrained chicks were coded and inspected without knowledge of the prior experience of the chicks: the objective was to predict each chick's prior training experience on the basis of this inspection. The training schedule was correctly predicted for four of the pairs on the basis of differences in optical density in the medial part of the hyperstriatum ventrale, especially its intermediate region. Although this prediction (four out of five correct) was not statistically significant, it was suggestive. For this reason, in the definitive experiment, the optical density of this region was measured along with that of a number of other regions, including certain sensory and motor areas. After the measurements had been taken ('blind'), and the code broken only measurements from one region differed significantly between the two sets of brains. The region was indeed the intermediate and medial part of the hyperstriatum ventrale, and has come to be known by the acronym IMHV (Horn *et al.*, 1979; Horn, 1981). It extends some 2.4 mm in the antero-posterior plane of the cerebral hemispheres, themselves approximately 10mm long (Figure 19.2). The lateral boundary of the region was not determined in these experiments, though Jones *et al.* (1999), using another technique have provided evidence of its lateral extent. The IMHV is slender, being about 0.5 mm wide. This region, on the basis of its embryology (Horn, 1985) and connections (Bradley *et al.* 1985; Metzger *et al.*, 1998) appears to be homologous to part or parts of the mammalian cerebral cortex, but to which part is a matter of speculation. It certainly does not correspond to the mammalian striate cortex as some have suggested (Daisley *et al.*, 1998). The striate cortex is the primary projection area of the thalamic lateral geniculate nucleus. The retina is the major source of afferents to this nucleus. The avian equivalent of the lateral geniculate nucleus projects to a laminated structure, the visual wulst, not to IMHV (Hunt and Webster, 1972; Karten *et al.*, 1973; Medina and Reiner, 2000). On the basis of its connections IMHV has been compared to the prefrontal and anterior cingulate areas of primate cerebral cortex (Horn 1985). Whilst the comparison is a tentative one, it is of interest that both of these regions have been implicated in long-term memory functions in mammals, including humans (Horn, 1985; Fink *et al.*, 1996; Bontempi *et al.*, 1999).

Invasive studies

All of the above studies were correlative: a change in a biochemical measure was related to a change in behaviour. As the series of experiments proceeded a

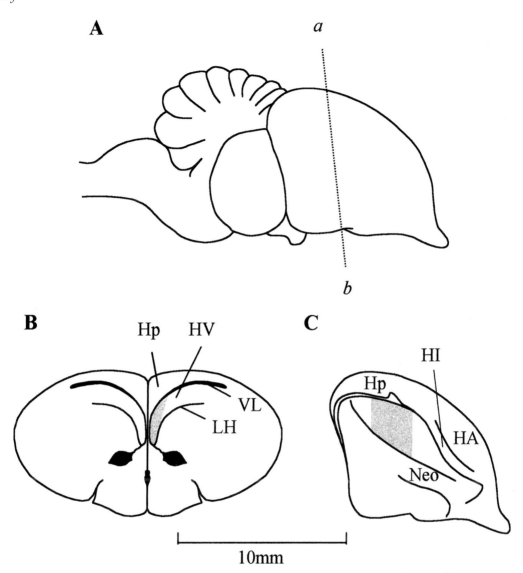

Figure 19.2. Diagrammatic views of the brain of a 2-day-old chick. (**A**) Side view. (**B**) Coronal section through the plane a … b of **A**. (**C**) Parasagittal section. The shaded areas in **B** and **C** represent the intermediate and medial part of the hyperstriatum ventrale (IMHV). Abbreviations: HA, hyperstriatum accessorium; HI, intercalated nucleus of the hyperstriatum accessorium; Hp, hippocampus; HV, hyperstriatum ventrale; LH, lamina hyperstriatica; Neo, neostriatum; VL, ventriculus lateralis. HA and HI are components of the visual wulst.

variety of factors that might have accounted for the biochemical changes were successively eliminated; and the possibility that the changes were specifically related to learning became progressively stronger. Nevertheless, correlation is not causation, and the evidence that IMHV was specifically involved in imprinting needed to be subjected to some invasive investigations. One such investigation is to observe the consequences on imprinting of placing lesions in

the IMHV. This kind of intervention inevitably has its own shortcomings such as, for example, changing sensory thresholds or impairing locomotor activity. But used as a method for studying a particular brain region the function of which had been predicted through the use of other techniques, lesioning is a valuable part of the neuroscientist's armoury.

Chicks with bilateral lesions of IMHV would not be expected to acquire a preference for a stimulus through imprinting if the region is crucial for this form of learning. To test this expectation, chicks with such lesions, and sham-operated controls, were placed individually in running wheels and trained by exposing them to a rotating, illuminated object. The running wheel rotated as the chick attempted to approach the object. After training each chick was given a preference test. The chick, in the running wheel, was exposed to the training stimulus and, successively, to an alternative stimulus that it had not previously seen. A preference score was calculated as the activity (rotations of the running wheel) directed to the training stimulus expressed as a per cent of the total activity in the test. Sham-operated control chicks acquired a strong preference for the training object. Birds with IMHV lesions failed to develop a preference for the training object: they approached each object with similar vigour, achieving a preference score that was not significantly different from the chance level of 50 per cent (McCabe *et al.*, 1981).

If the IMHV serves as a *storage* site for information acquired through learning, then chicks should be amnesic if the area is lesioned after they have been trained. To examine this prediction, trained chicks were given a preference test, anaesthetized and lesions made in the IMHV of both right and left hemispheres. When the chicks had recovered from the anaesthetic each was given a second preference test. In the first preference test the trained, intact chicks strongly preferred the training object; in the second, postoperative test they showed no such preference. This finding contrasted with the results for three other groups of chicks, those that had simply been anaesthetized and those that had received bilateral lesions in one or other of two brain areas outwith IMHV. These groups selectively approached the training object in both the pre- and postoperative tests (McCabe *et al.*, 1982). These two experiments lent support to the biochemical studies, which suggested that IMHV played an important role in learning. Indeed, all of the results are consistent with the hypothesis that IMHV stores information—that it is a memory system. If this suggestion is correct it should, in principle, be possible to introduce information into IMHV by artificial means and so influence the chick's preferences. This possibility is not as bizarre as it might at first appear to be. Chicks are able to distinguish between lights flashing at 4.5 Hz and 1.5 Hz, if exposed to one or other of them for long enough (five hours). If trains of electric pulses are delivered to

IMHV of untrained chicks at say 4.5 Hz, are the chicks' preferences subsequently biased towards a light flashing at that frequency?

To address this question, electrodes were implanted into the right and left IMHV of two groups of visually naive chicks (McCabe *et al.*, 1979). One group received trains of pulses at 4.5 Hz and the other group received trains at 1.5 Hz. There were no overt behavioural signs of this stimulation at the time the trains were being delivered. After five hours stimulation ceased and each chick was given a preference test. In this test lights flashing at either 4.5 Hz or 1.5 Hz were presented simultaneously and the chick allowed to express its choice. Those chicks that had received pulse trains at 4.5 Hz preferred the light flashing at that frequency; those which had received pulse trains at 1.5 Hz preferred the light flashing at this frequency.

Such biasing of preferences did not occur if the pulse trains were delivered to two other brain regions, suggesting that the effects of stimulating IMHV were regionally selective. The two ineffective brain regions were the hyperstriatum accessorium and the ectostriatum, respectively. Both are major visual areas of the forebrain, which were later shown to project directly or indirectly to IMHV (Bradley *et al.*, 1985; Metzger *et al.*, 1998). Thus the results of the stimulation experiments suggested two things: (i) that input to the IMHV from the visual pathways alone is not sufficient for chicks to use, in subsequent behavioural tests, the temporal information contained within that input, and therefore (ii) for the temporal information to be used in this way, input to IMHV from at least one other source is necessary.

These suggestions are consistent with Young's (1963) proposal that for certain kinds of learning, 'registration in memory' is dependent on the conjunction of sensory input and input from a reinforcing system. Crow (1968) and Kety (1970, 1972) suggested that noradrenergic neurons may comprise one such system. In mammals and in birds noradrenaline-containing neurons are clustered in the locus ceoruleus in the midbrain. These neurons project to wide areas of the central nervous system, including the cerebral hemispheres. Hence many regions in the forebrain which receive inputs from sensory pathways also receive an input from the noradrenergic system.

If activation of the noradrenergic system is necessary for information to be registered in memory, then drugs which deplete or block the action of this transmitter should prevent learning (Kety, 1970). Do drugs of this kind impair imprinting? One such drug, DSP4, when administered systemically to rats lowers noradrenaline levels in the cerebral cortex (Jaim-Etcheverry and Zeiher, 1980) and, when administered in the same way to chicks, lowers noradrenaline levels in the forebrain (Davies *et al.*, 1985). To study the effects of the drug on imprinting, chicks were trained by exposing them to a rotating red box. When subsequently tested their preference for the box was impaired. In contrast, chicks that had received injections of distilled water and were then trained on the red box subsequently preferred it to an alternative object. After the test had been given a region of the brain composed mainly of IMHV was removed from DSP4 treated and from control chicks. There was a positive correlation between the amount of noradrenaline in this brain sample and the strength of the preference for the training stimulus: the higher the level of noradrenaline the stronger the preference. A variety of other measures of the chicks' behaviour were taken (for example, approach activity in the preference test, latency of the first approach count of the running wheel during training, time accurately to peck a rocking bead). In none of these measures did DSP4 treated chicks differ significantly from the controls.

The results of this study give some support for the involvement of noradrenaline in the process by which chicks learn the characteristics of an artificial object. The support is necessarily qualified. For example, the drug may exert its effects on imprinting not through its actions on noradrenaline, but through physiological changes that co-vary with noradrenaline concentrations. Nonetheless the findings of the study are consistent with the notion that sensory inputs to IMHV are not alone sufficient for the information those inputs carry to be stored in a memory system. Electrical stimulation of the two visual projection areas, hyperstriatum accessorium and ectostriatum are unlikely to have activated noradrenergic axons in IMHV; but electrical stimulation of IMHV directly is likely to have excited axons non-specifically. Such stimulation is likely to have activated noradrenergic terminals and the terminals of other pathways activity of which may be a necessary ('enabling') condition for sensory information to be stored.

A memory system outwith IMHV

Bilateral lesions of IMHV placed before training impair the acquisition of a preference through imprinting (McCabe *et al.*, 1981). Similar lesions placed shortly after training impair retention (McCabe *et al.*, 1982). However if the lesions are made the day after training, chicks continue to prefer the training object (Cipolla-Neto *et al.*, 1982). These findings implied that a long-term storage system exists outwith IMHV, and it was referred to as S′ (S-dash); and whilst IMHV is necessary for the *acquisition* of a preference its role in *storage*, with the discovery of S′, became unclear. For example, IMHV might serve as a temporary store until S′ becomes functional some hours after training; or IMHV might serve as a permanent store, in parallel with S′.

These issues were clarified by a series of experiments in which lesions were placed in a two-stage procedure. The right IMHV was lesioned before training. After recovery the chicks were trained and their preference measured. These chicks, with the left IMHV intact, selectively approached the training object: they had learned its characteristics. The left IMHV of these chicks was then lesioned, and the chicks' preferences again measured. The chicks failed to show a preference, behaving as if they were amnesic. These results, considered in the context of all the preceding experiments, suggested that the left IMHV is a long-term store.

This experiment left open questions relating to the formation of S′. These issues became clearer in an experiment in which the left IMHV was lesioned before training. These chicks, with the right IMHV intact, acquired a preference through exposure to the training stimulus. After completion of the preference test the right IMHV of these chicks was lesioned. On the following day their preferences were again tested. They preferred the training object. This result implied the existence of a store outwith IMHV that supported the continuing preference (see Figure 19.3).

We inferred from the lesion studies, particularly from the two sets of sequential lesion experiments, that (i) the presence of the right IMHV was necessary for the formation of S′, but that (ii) the left IMHV was not so involved. The right IMHV might serve as a temporary, or buffer store until S′ became fully functional; or the right IMHV might be a permanent store, lying in parallel with S′. Evidence from studies referred to below (Nicol *et al.*, 1995; Solomonia *et al.*, 2000) suggest that the latter possibility is the correct one.

The results of other lesion studies implied that S′ becomes functional between 6–8 hours after the begining of training (Davey *et al.*, 1987; Honey *et al.*, 1995; Bolhuis and Honey, 1998). It is, perhaps worth

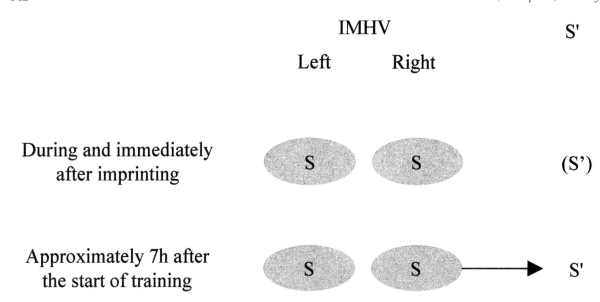

Figure 19.3.   Model of memory systems for imprinting. Information necessary for the recognition of a familiar object is stored in the left and right IMHV (S). By approximately 7 hours after the beginning of training an additional store, S', beyond the confines of IMHV is able to support a preference for the imprinted object. It is possible that memories are formed in S' during and immediately after imprinting, but the information in the store only becomes available through the subsequent activity of the right IMHV. For these reasons S' is initially shown bracketed (information not available), and later unbracketed (information available). For further discussion see pp. 341–342 and pp. 353–356.

emphasizing that the existence of S' is inferred from behaviour; its location is not known so it has not been possible to study the neural changes that take place there as memories are established. Such changes have been studied in the IMHV.

Exploration of IMHV

It is implicit in the preceding sections that no single experiment can provide convincing evidence that a particular region of the brain stores information. However, the results of all the experiments taken together provide converging evidence that IMHV is such a storage site. The experiments described below lend further support for this view and have made it possible to study the formation of the elusive engram.

Neurophysiological
The IMHV is a polysensory region anatomically connected to visual, auditory and somatic sensory projection areas of the telencephalon (Bradley *et al.*, 1985; Metzger *et al.*, 1998; Horn 1985). In the pigeon the region also receives an input from the olfactory bulb (Rieke and Wenzel, 1978). Responses to sensory stimuli may be recorded from neurons in IMHV using

microelectrodes. In anaesthetized chicks such responses are rare and relatively weak (Brown and Horn, 1979; McLennan and Horn, 1992). In contrast, in unanaesthetized, behaving chicks, many neurons in the region respond briskly to visual and/or to auditory stimuli (Brown and Horn, 1994; Nicol *et al.*, 1995). Responses to stimuli of other modalities have not been tested.

The proportion of recording sites in the left IMHV that respond to a visual stimulus depends on whether or not the chicks are imprinted on that stimulus (Brown and Horn, 1994). Thus the proportion of sites responding to a rotating red box in chicks which are imprinted to that object is more than double that found in untrained chicks (Figure 19.4A, B). Overall a similar pattern of change is found in the right IMHV (Nicol *et al.*, 1995). The responses of some 30 per cent of recording sites in these regions are highly selective for the imprinted stimulus (Figure 19.4C). Other neurons generalize across colour or shape (Figure 19.4D) much as imprinted chicks generalize behaviourally under the appropriate test conditions (Bolhuis and Horn, 1992). These effects of imprinting are regionally specific; they are not observed in the hippocampus, which projects to the IMHV (Nicol *et al.*, 1998a).

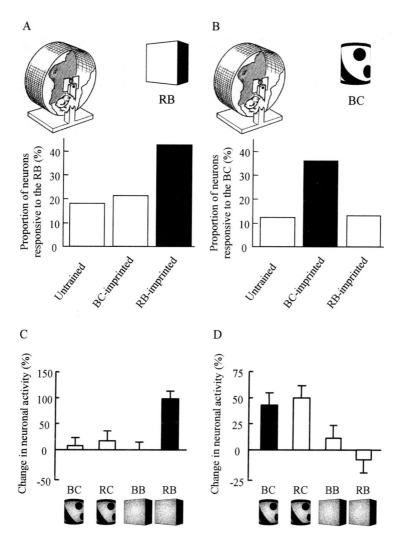

Figure 19.4. Learning-related changes in IMHV neuronal responsiveness. Three groups of chicks were reared in darkness. Chicks in two of these groups were trained when they were ~24 h old. Chicks in these groups were placed individually in a running wheel and exposed to either a rotating red box (RB) or to a rotating blue cylinder (BC). After training the chicks were given a preference test. Those exposed to say the RB preferred it to another object, say the BC. After the preference test a micro-electrode assembly was attached to the skull under anaesthesia. The following day chicks were placed in the running wheel and recordings were made from small groups of neuron in single microelectrode penetration through the left IMHV. Control chicks were treated similarly to the imprinted chicks but was not trained. At each recording site a stimulus, say the RB was switched on for two revolutions. The RB was presented in this way ~10 times. Another stimulus was then presented in a similar way. Stimulus presentations were only accepted if the chick looked at the stimulus. The procedure was repeated at each recording site. A site was considered to be responsive if the mean number of action potential over the ~10 presentations, was significantly greater than the mean number recorded immediately before these presentation (spontaneous activity). (**A, B**) Mean percentage of sites responsive to the RB (**A**) or the BC (**B**) in the three groups of chicks. The training experience of each group is indicated below each histogram bar. Filled bars represent the percentage of sites responding to the familiar stimulus. The open bars represent the percentage of sites responsive to a stimulus that was not the one to which the chicks had been trained. The percentage of sites responsive to a familiar stimulus (for example, RB to an RB-trained chick) were significantly (P< 0.001) higher than (i) the percentage of sites responsive to the alternative stimulus (for example, RB to a BC-trained chick) (ii) the percentage of sites responding in the untrained chicks. (**C**) Response selectivity in a RB-imprinted chick. Responses are expressed as a percentage change from the mean level of spontaneous activity (error bars show standard errors of the means). Test stimulus is shown below each histogram bar. There was a significant response only to the imprinted stimulus (P< 0.001). (**D**) Generalization of response in a BC-imprinted chick. The response to the imprinted stimulus did not differ significantly from that to a rotating red cylinder, but both responses differed significantly from the from those to the two other stimuli. At this recording site there was thus a generalization of shape. (Data from Brown and Horn, 1994).

When the distance between the chick and an object is varied, the response of some neurons in IMHV also varies: the responses of some neurons decrease and those of others increase linearly with distance. The responses of still other neurons may change in a non-linear fashion. Such neurons respond when the object is at one distance but not when it is at another, for example when an object is 1 m away, but not when it is 0.5 or 2 m away from the chick. Another group of neurons in IMHV respond similarly to the object placed at each of these distances. These neurons exhibit 'distance-invariance' or 'size-constancy' (Nicol *et al.*, 1998b).

In contrast to the learning-dependent changes in the responses of IMHV neurons described above, the distance-related responses are not dependent on learning. These responses are elicited by objects of which the bird has had little prior experience, and occur in birds that have had no opportunity to explore these objects in a spatially extended environment (Nicol *et al.*, 1999a). Contrary to what has long been supposed (Berkeley, 1709), a neural mechanism for size constancy thus exists in the virtual absence of these kinds of visual/locomotor experience.

The neurophysiological studies of Brown and Horn (1994) and Nicol *et al* (1995) demonstrated that the responses of some IMHV neurons are modified profoundly by imprinting, and signal the presence of the familiar object. What changes in neuronal structure and function might underlie these modifications?

Synaptic changes

Postsynaptic

The effects of imprinting training on the morphology of IMHV synapses were examined in study that involved the use of an electron microscope (Bradley *et al.*, 1981; Horn *et al.*, 1985). Training was without effect on (i) the mean number of synapses per unit volume of tissue, (ii) the mean size of synaptic boutons, or (iii) the mean size of dendritic spine heads. However, in the left IMHV, but not in the right, the mean length of the postsynaptic density (PSD) of dendritic spines was greater by 17 per cent in chicks trained for 140 minutes than in untrained chicks or in chicks trained for only 20 minutes. The PSD contains receptors for L-glutamate (Fagg and Matus, 1984) and the PSDs of excitatory synapses are mainly on dendritic spines (Harris and Kater, 1994). Consistent with the increase in PSD length on spines there is, after training, a learning-related increase in the mean number of L-glutamate receptors of the NMDA type in the left IMHV, but not in the right (McCabe and Horn, 1988; Johnston *et al.*, 1993, 1995). When activated by glutamic acid, NMDA receptors might serve to amplify the current flow into the dendritic spine (Daw *et al.*, 1993). An upregulation of NMDA receptor numbers is likely to lead to a corresponding enhancement of this amplification and thus to an increase in the efficacy of synaptic transmission. The enhanced influx of calcium ions into the spine through the NMDA channels might activate second messenger-dependent kinases and so have diverse effects on the structure and function of the spine (Lynch and Baudry, 1984; Horn, 1985; Daw *et al.*, 1993).

There is a temporal discontinuity between the timing of the increase in the mean PSD length and of the increase in NMDA receptor number. The increase in the number of NMDA receptors was present at ~11 hours, but not at ~8 hours or earlier after the beginning of training (McCabe and Horn, 1991), whereas the morphological changes were in place earlier, ~6.5 hours from that starting point. The morphological studies did not exclude the possibility that the changes in PSD length were present earlier than this since such changes may occur very quickly. For example, increases in PSD length have been observed in synapses of the rat dentate gyrus two minutes after termination of high frequency stimulation which established LTP (Desmond and Levy, 1986; Bradley *et al.*, 1991). The rapidity of this change implies that PSD length is controlled locally, in the region of the synapse (Shashoua, 1985) or in the dendritic spine: protein-synthetic machinery in the form of polyribosomes and membranous cisterns is present at the base of dendritic spines (Steward and Reeves, 1988; Steward *et al.*, 1998). By contrast, the increase in NMDA numbers is relatively slow and may involve nuclear gene expression. The PSD of spine synapses is a 'target' for NMDA receptor proteins (Harris and Kater, 1994). Accordingly, no special signalling to the nucleus is required for these receptors to reach the modified synapse: the newly extended area of PSD 'flags up' the spine to which the receptors are to be directed (Horn, 1985; 1990; McCabe and Horn, 1991). This hypothesis receives support from recent work and has been termed 'synaptic tagging' (Frey and Morris, 1998; Dudai and Morris, Chapter 9).

The temporal discontinuity between changes in PSD length and the changes in NMDA receptor number creates a problem: if both of these changes are involved in memory, what is the basis of the memory in the hours that follow training, but before the up-regulation of NMDA receptor number has occurred? One possibility (but see also p. 345, below) is that the early changes may have LTP-like characteristics (Horn and McCabe, 1990), with changes in PSD length initially associated with a correspondingly rapid change in the function and/or number of AMPA subtype of glutamate receptors (Malenka and Nicoll, 1999; for further discussion of LTP see Winder and Kandel (Chapter 10) and Dudai and Morris (Chapter 9)).

Presynaptic

So far the discussion of synaptic change associated with imprinting has focused on postsynaptic elements. There are, however, a number of experimental results that suggest that imprinting also leads to changes in presynaptic elements. Clathrin proteins are involved in recycling the membrane of synaptic vesicles (Morris and Schmid, 1995). The amount of clathrin heavy-chain proteins present in the IMHV region is increased 25 hours after the beginning of training, the increase being related to the strength of learning (Figure 19.5A). The effects were more pronounced in the left than in the right IMHV. These results would predict an increase in the number of vesicles in synaptic boutons, especially in the left IMHV. Such data are not available for imprinting, but they are available for passive avoidance learning in the chick. Twenty four hours after training the mean number of vesicles per synapse is higher in trained chicks than in controls; the increase occurs in both left and right IMHV, but is much greater in the left (Stewart *et al.*, 1984).

Other evidence pointing to an enhancement in the release of neurotransmitters comes from studies of auditory imprinting in chicks. The medial hyperstriatum ventrale and the anterior hyperstriatum ventrale are involved in this form of learning (Scheich, 1987). Using an *in vivo* microdialysis technique and studying tone-imprinted chicks two days after training, an enhanced glutamate response to the familiar tone was found in the region (Gruss and Braun, 1996).

These presynaptic changes are present a day or more after training, but such changes may occur before this time. Synaptic vesicles are present in synaptic terminals in two pools: a reserve pool and a readily available pool. Vesicles in the reserve pool are held in place by crosslinkage to actin filaments by synapsin I. When synapsin I is phosphorylated by calcium-calmodulin-dependent kinase II (CaM kinase II) it dissociates from both actin filaments and synaptic vesicles. The vesicles are then free to move and

become available for release. This movement is likely to be facilitated by partial disassembly of the actin filament network (Trifaro and Vitale, 1993). The myristolated alanine-rich protein kinase C substrate (MARCKS) is a membrane-bound protein that is found in high concentrations in presynaptic terminals. Membrane bound MARCKS crosslinks actin filaments and also binds calmodulin in the presence of calcium. When membrane bound MARCKS is phosphorylated it ceases to crosslink actin filaments (Aderem, 1992). It also releases calcium-calmodulin which, by activating CaM kinase II is likely to lead to the phosphorylation of synapsin I. These consequences of MARCKS phosphorylation would result in the mobilization of synaptic vesicles from the reserve pool. Within ~3 hours after the beginning of training there is, in the left IMHV but not in other brain regions sampled, a significant increase in the phosphorylation of MARCKS, the magnitude of the increase being correlated with the strength of learning (Figure 19.5B).

These considerations lead to the prediction of an early effect of imprinting on the release of neurotransmitters from IMHV neurons. This prediction was examined in a study in which slices of the left and right IMHV were removed from the brains of chicks ~5 hours after the beginning of training. Potassium stimulated, calcium-dependent (presumed synaptic) release of putative amino acid neurotransmitters was measured. The release of the inhibitory neurotransmitter gamma-aminobutyric acid (GABA), and taurine of from the left but not from the right IMHV was correlated with the strength of the chicks' preference for the training stimulus. The higher the preference score the greater was the release of these amino acids (McCabe *et al.*, 1998). The role of taurine in the CNS is not clear (Saransaari and Oja, 1992), but the amino acid may be implicated in modulating synaptic transmission (Galaretta *et al.*, 1996).

Additional evidence points to a role in imprinting for neurons which are immunopositive for these amino acids. Activation of certain neurons by a number of procedures may influence the expression of immediate early genes such as *c-fos* in the mammalian and chick CNS (Hunt *et al.*, 1987; Anokhin and Rose, 1991; see also Clayton, Chapter 7). Imprinting is associated with an increase in the number of neurons in IMHV that are immunopositive for Fos, the protein product of *c-fos*. The increase, which is present within 2 hours of the start of training, is correlated with preference score and occurs in both right and left IMHV (Figure 19.5C). No such increases were found in other

346

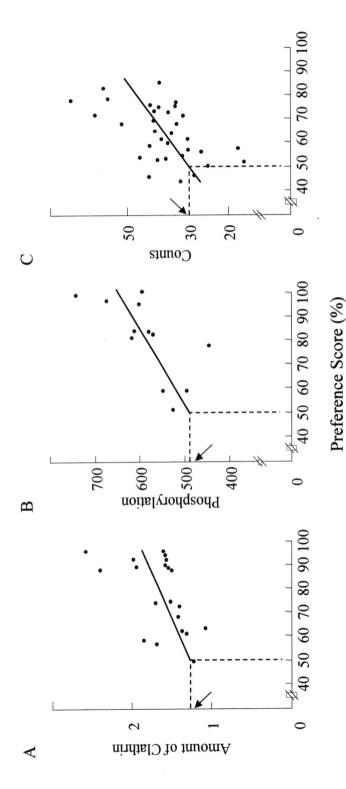

Figure 19.5. Relationship between measures of neuronal change and of learning. Chicks were trained by exposure for 60–90 min to an imprinting stimulus. In the three experiments that generated the data for the three scattergrams, chicks with different preference scores were matched for approach to the imprinting object during training. Measures of neural change (Y-axes) are plotted against a measure of the strength of learning, preference score (X-axes). For a given neural change, the mean value for untrained chicks is indicated by an arrow. The broken line gives the expected value for the change in trained chicks with a preference score of 50%, that is 'no preference', or chance performance. All chicks were reared in darkness but the trained chicks differed from the untrained chicks in having been handled, placed and allowed to run in the wheel (see Figure 19.4 A, B), exposed to the imprinting stimulus and given a preference test. A, B, C. In all experiments the expected value for trained chicks performing at chance was close to the mean value for untrained chicks. This finding, together with the significant, positive correlations with preference score implies that the changes found in IMHV are not 'side-effects' of the training procedure (resulting for example, from arousal, visual stimulation, movement during training), but are specifically related to learning/retention. (**A**) Left IMHV. Relationship between a measure of amounts of clathrin heavy chain proteins and preference score (r = 0.53; P < 0.015). (Modified from Solomonia *et al.,* 1997). (**B**) Left IMHV. Relationship between phosphorylation of MARCKS protein in arbitrary units of optical density and preference score (r = 0.67; P < 0.017). (Data from Sheu *et al.,* 1993). C Left and right IMHV combined. Fos-immunopositive nuclei in IMHV. Counts were made in two sampling frames (0.3 mm by 0.9 mm) within the right and left IMHV. There were no significant differences between counts from the two sides. The correlation coefficient between counts and preference score was significant (r = 0.52; P<0.01). (Modified from McCabe and Horn, 1994).

brain regions that were sampled. The changes found in IMHV occur in Fos-positive neurons that are also immunopositive for GABA and taurine (McCabe and Horn, 1994; Ambalavanar *et al.*, 1999; Potter *et al.*, 1998).

The finding that chicks with higher preference scores have higher counts of Fos-positive neurons than chicks with lower preference scores might arise out of a selection process: chicks hatched with higher counts of this kind of neuron learn more efficiently than those with lower counts. This view is unlikely to be correct (Horn and Johnson, 1989; McCabe and Horn, 1994). Instead, the evidence strongly suggests that the observed increase in the number of Fos-positive neurons in IMHV is a consequence of learning (McCabe and Horn, 1994).

The studies described above indicate that, in the early stages of imprinting, inhibitory neurons are specifically engaged in memory formation. The *in vitro* release experiments suggest that this engagement may take the form of an increase in the amount of inhibitory transmitter available for release by an impulse in GABA-positive neurons. As learning proceeds this increased inhibitory activity might serve to 'shape' the response of IMHV neurons (see Figure 19.4C), just as inhibitory activity is involved in shaping the receptive fields of neurons in the visual cortex (Hubel and Wiesel, 1959, 1965a; Horn, 1962; Sillito, 1977). However, the neural microcircuitry that might be involved in such shaping of responses of IMHV neurons is not known. In the IMHV neurons that are immunopositive for GABA synapse onto neurons that are also GABA-positive, as well as onto neurons which are not (Watson *et al.*, 1991). Accordingly, the excitability of IMHV neurons may be controlled by a withdrawal of inhibition (inhibition of inhibition), as well as by direct inhibition.

Whether inhibitory systems continue to be engaged in the long-term, as they are engaged in the short term is not clear. There is a hint that they may not be. Thus, in the left IMHV, the *in vitro* release of GABA is correlated with preference scores up to ~11 hours after the beginning of training, but ceases to be so correlated ~25 hours after this start time (Meredith *et al.*, 2000). In addition, the amount of the GABA$_A$ receptor γ4-subunit transcript is decreased in IMHV, as well as in several other brain regions, ~14 hours after the beginning of training. The decrease, relative to untrained controls, is not in place ~5 hours earlier (Harvey *et al.*, 1998). These two sets of findings suggest that there may be a decreasing involvement

of the inhibitory system in memory processes as time passes from the start of training.

Nevertheless, the studies of changes in clathrin proteins, synaptic vesicle numbers, *in vivo* glutamate release, NMDA receptor number and of PSD length described above, and which are related to the learning experience, all point to the continuing involvement of pre- and postsynaptic elements in memory.

Synaptic specificity

Memories are often highly specific, even allowing for a degree of generalization. Many theories of the neural basis of memory suppose that particular neural pathways are established through learning and that these pathways correspond to particular memories (Tanzi, 1893; Cajal, 1911; Konorski, 1948; Hebb, 1949). As an aside, these theories implicitly predict that if these pathways become partially disconnected at some stage after they have been formed, then the specificity of recall will be impaired—the more so if any reconnections that are made are aberrant.

In all of these theories the key to establishing a specific neural pathway is the synapse. Hebb (1949) proposed that synapses would be strengthened if, under certain conditions, there is repeated conjoint activation of pre- and postsynaptic elements. Stent (1973) added the complementary proposal that there would be a reduction in efficacy at synapses between a presynaptic axon and the postsynaptic neuron, if the postsynaptic neuron is driven by another input.

It is not too difficult to see how particular synapses could be strengthened on the postsynaptic side. In the discussion of changes in PSD length and NMDA receptor number that occur after imprinting, a relatively simple mechanism was proposed for just such strengthening. In essence it is that at affected synapses the length of the PSD increases very quickly, possibly within minutes after the triggering event. This length change may be the sufficient condition for additional receptors to be channelled into that particular synapse (see p. 344 above). But how is synapse specificity to be achieved if memory also involves presynaptic changes, and in particular an increase in the amount of transmitter released from presynaptic terminals?

Synapse specificity could be achieved if the triggering event for synaptic change leads to the release from the postsynaptic spine to the presynaptic bouton a retrograde signal (Griffith, 1966; 1967). Such a signal might enhance the influx into that terminal of calcium ions. These ions, by activating calmodulin may initiate the cascade of events that leads to the enhancement of release of neurotransmitter from that particular terminal (see p. 345 above). Another possibility is that learning leads to an increase in the amount of neurotransmitter synthesized in the presynaptic neuron. If that were to happen more transmitter would be available to all terminals of that neuron. Since a single neuron may be connected to many other neurons (Sholl, 1956), how could an increase in transmitter availability be restricted to a subset of the terminals of that neuron? One possibility is that, through imprinting, the length of the presynaptic density (PreSD) of some synapses increases along with the PSD. If the added PreSD contains the presynaptic vesicular grid that provides vesicles with specialized areas of plasma membrane at which synaptic vesicles are docked (Akert *et al.*, 1972; Südhof, 1995) there would be additional sites for the release of transmitter. Hence a general upregulation of the neurotransmitter synthesis in the presynaptic neuron would lead to an increase in transmitter release only at these modified synapses. In this model the primary change at a synapse is cytoskeletal—a change in length of the PreSD and of the PSD of that synapse. These changes would signal to the pre- and postsynaptic neurons the set of synapses into which the additional vesicles/receptors, respectively are to be channelled.

Synaptic stability

Memories may last for many weeks, months, or years. Yet the shape and size of neurons in the CNS are not stable. The extent of branching of the dendritic tree, the numbers of synaptic terminals, and of dendritic spines all vary. The variation is perhaps most marked during development, where a controlling factor is the level of thyroid hormone (Eayrs, 1960; Eayrs and Horn, 1955). But other factors also play a part in shaping neuronal architecture: the level of nutrition (Horn, 1955; Eayrs and Horn, 1955; Balázs, 1977), the degree of environmental enrichment/impoverishment (Diamond *et al.*, 1964) and of sensory experience/deprivation (Valverde, 1971). Changes in cortical representation also occur under physiological conditions. When monkeys are trained to use particular fingers to obtain food, the area of somatosensory cortex representing the tips of these fingers is enlarged (Jenkins *et al.*, 1990). In the face of such seemingly continuous changes of neuronal architecture, how may specific neuronal connections be maintained?

The idea that neurons are interconnected by fine fibrils gave way to the view that the terminal of an axon is not continuous with, but is merely in contact with the neuron on which it impinges. Recent work, however, suggests that pre- and postsynaptic elements are interlinked by neural cell adhesion molecules (NCAMs). The NCAM family in adult animals consists of three major isoforms with molecular masses of 180, 140 and 120 kDa (Edelman and Crossin, 1991; Fields and Itoh, 1996). Both NCAM 180 and NCAM 140 are transmembrane proteins. In mice, NCAM 140 is expressed in both pre- and postsynaptic membranes; NCAM 180 is restricted to postsynaptic sites, the NCAM 180-specific epitope being localized to the PSD (Persohn *et al.*, 1989). The cytoplasmic domains of some NCAMs, NCAM 180 in particular, are associated with cytoskeletal proteins (Persohn *et al.*, 1989; Fields and Itoh, 1996). Through homophilic binding in the extracellular domain, the pre- and postsynaptic elements of a synapse, and hence the respective cytoskeletons of the parent neurons, become linked together. The synapse then becomes more than a functional entity; it becomes a structurally interlocked unit.

The amounts of the three major isoforms of NCAM in the IMHV are increased ~25 hours, but not ~10.5 hours after the start of imprinting training. When the data were analysed according to hemisphere, the major impact of imprinting was found to be in the left IMHV. Here, but not in the right IMHV or in other brain regions sampled, the increases were related to the strength of learning (Solomonia *et al.*, 1998). By the following day, however, ~50 hours after the start of training, a learning-related increase in the amount of NCAM 180 was found in the right IMHV (Solomonia *et al.*, 2000).

The changes in the amounts of NCAMs present in the right and left IMHV are likely to strengthen pre- to postsynaptic adhesion and more effectively interconnect the cytoskeletal frameworks of the two elements of those synapses which are modified by learning. Such a structural change could provide the stability of neuronal connectivity needed in a memory system in which the architecture of neurons is subject to dynamic remodelling. If NCAMs have such a function it follows that memory is likely to be impaired by, for example, a reduction in the adhesiveness of NCAMs, uncoupling the intracellular domains of these molecules from the cytoskeleton or by a down-regulation of these proteins (Fields and Itoh, 1996).

If a change is correlated with learning/memory then prevention of that change should impair these processes. Ideally, the preventive method should target specifically those synapses which have been, or are to be modified, conditions which are difficult to meet. However, if the interference *fails* to have any effect on memory, that would be evidence that the changes are not necessary for memory. Scholey *et al.* (1993), studying passive avoidance learning in chicks injected anti-NCAM antibodies into their brains 6 hours after training. Scholey *et al.* found that retention was impaired when measured 18 hours later. It is likely that the antibodies reached many areas of the brain (Davis *et al.*, 1979; Rose and Jork, 1987) so that these studies (Scholey *et al.*) alone do not provide evidence of a selective role of IMHV NCAMs in memory. However, if the findings of Scholey *et al.* are considered with the those of Solomonia *et al.* (1998, 2000), the combined evidence is consistent with the view that changes in IMHV NCAMs are not only correlated with, but are also necessary for memory formation.

The learning-related changes in NCAMs may have a function beyond that of stabilizing synapses. Doherty *et al.* (1995) have shown that NCAMs may regulate neurite outgrowth. If they have this effect in IMHV these proteins may further strengthen the connections between the neurons that are involved in imprinting.

The development of the engrams

Neurophysiological studies

It has proved possible in behaving chicks to record for many hours the activity of individual neurons (Cipolla-Neto *et al.*, 1979; Brown and Horn, 1994; Nicol *et al.*, 1995). Using this technique, Nicol *et al.*, (1999*b*; Horn *et al.*, 2000*a*) recorded neuronal activity simultaneously from the right and left IMHV. Each chick, which was free to move in the running wheel, was trained by exposing it either to a rotating red box (RB) or a rotating blue cylinder BC (see Figure 19.4A and B respectively). The responsiveness of the recorded neuron to each of these stimuli was measured before training (Test T1), after the first hour of training (T2), after the second hour of training (T3), approximately four hours later (T4), and on the following day (T5). Software sorting techniques were used to identify action potentials on the basis of their waveforms. In this way it was possible to track the activity of individual neurons from T1 through T3. At T4, the microelectrodes were advanced to new recording positions, a procedure that was repeated at T5, in order to sample a different population of neurons within each IMHV.

In untrained chicks the proportion of neurons responding to either stimulus showed no systematic changes over the course of the experiment (see Figure 19.6, open squares). The pattern was similar in trained chicks for neurons that responded to the alternative visual stimulus, but not to the training stimulus (Figure 19.6 filled squares). In contrast to this stability in responsiveness, the proportion of neurons responding to the training stimulus increased significantly over the period of training (Figure 19.6 filled circles). As in previous studies (Nicol *et al.*, 1995), no hemispheric asymmetries in the magnitude of this increase were found. The change in the proportion of neurons responding to the training stimulus was not linear. The proportion responding at T1 (26/230; 11%) increased to 57/230 (25%) at T2, and then dropped slightly at T3 (50/230; 22%). The electrode was then moved and at T4, ~8 hours after the beginning of training, the proportion responding to the training stimulus fell significantly from the peak at T2, to 74/451 (16%), and was no longer significantly different from the proportion responding at T1, before training had begun. After T4 the chicks were returned to the incubator and left there overnight. Next morning the electrodes were advanced a further ~100 μm. The proportion of neurons now responding to the training stimulus, ~25 hours after the start of training, was 90/251 (36%).

The dip in the proportion of neurons responding to the training stimulus at T4 was not associated with any obvious change in the behaviour of the birds. For example, their approach activity to the training stimulus did not change significantly between T3 and T4. It is possible that the dip in responsiveness was an artefact of moving the microelectrode. There is no evidence from previous recordings from IMHV of such an effect (Nicol *et al.*, 1995). Nor is there such evidence from within the study itself. The electrode was moved immediately prior to T5, when the proportion of neurons responding to the training stimulus was at its maximum.

Assuming that these fluctuations in the percentages of neurons responding to the training stimulus reflect physiological processes, what might these processes be? One possibility is that a population of neurons becomes responsive to the training stimulus, then permanently ceases to do so as another population becomes engaged, and so on, with a dearth of them at T4. In this view, for example, the population of neurons responding at T5 would be a completely different population from that which responded at say

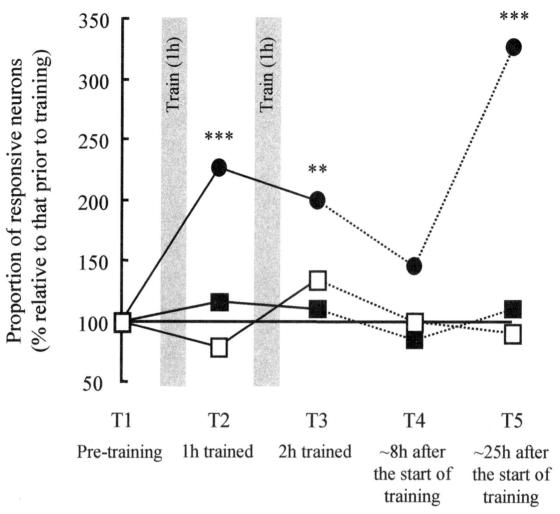

Figure 19.6. Evolution of changes in neuronal responsiveness during the formation of engrams in left and right IMHV. On the day of hatching a microelectrode assembly was attached to the skull of each chick under general anaesthesia. The following day the chick was exposed to a training stimulus for two periods each of 1 hour. Before training microelectrodes were advanced into both left and right IMHV to record the activity of individual neurons. Neurons were then tested, at test 1 (T1) for responses when the chick was exposed to a rotating red box (RB) and to a rotating blue cylinder (BC); 15–20 presentations were made of each stimulus (for other details see legend to Figure 19.4). The order of presentation was varied from chick to chick. After the first training period the second test of neuronal responsiveness was given (T2). The third test (T3) was given after the second period of training. All these tests were given while the recording electrodes remained at the same site (indicated by the continuous line linking the points on the curves). The activity of the same neurons, identified on the basis of their waveform, was tracked throughout this period. The microelectrode was then advanced to a new recording position in IMHV and the fourth test (T4) given, ~8 hours after the beginning of training. The chick was then returned to the dark incubator and ~25 hours after the start of training the microelectrodes again advanced in IMHV, and the fifth test of neuronal responsiveness (T5) was given. Broken line connect symbols representing data from these tests. The proportion of neurons responding at T1 is given the value of 100%. The proportions of neurons responding at other tests are compared with that at T1 and are shown as the percentage change from that proportion. (Significance levels: ***, P< 0.001; **, P< 0.01). Results from trained chicks are shown as filled symbols, those from untrained chicks as shown as open symbols (at T1 all chicks were untrained). Filled circles represent the percentage change in the proportion of neurons responsive to the training stimulus, filled squares the percentage change in the proportion of neurons responsive to the alternative stimulus. There were no significant differences between left and right IMHV and the data from both sides have been combined. (Based on Nicol *et al.*, 1999*b*).

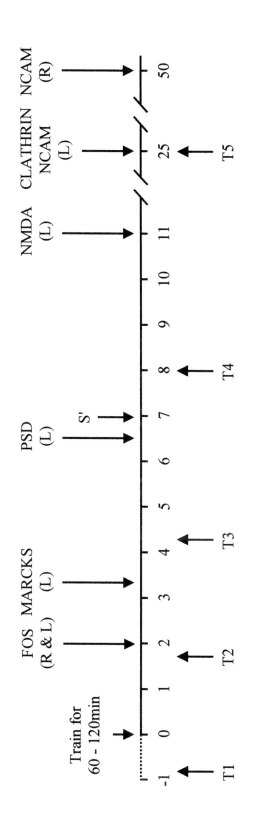

Figure 19.7. Timing of events before and after imprinting. All are mean times and are given in hours before or after the start of training. The mean timings of the tests of neuronal responsiveness (T1 ... T5) before and after training are indicated on by the arrows below the horizontal line. Abbreviations: L, left IMHV; R, right IMHV; S', the storage system outside the confines of IMHV. All other terms are defined in the text.

T2. Another possibility is that individual neurons become responsive and that responsiveness wanes and waxes again through time.

One way of examining these possibilities is to ask whether the proportions responding at T5 and T4 can be predicted from the proportions responding at earlier tests. Because individual neurons (230 of them) were tracked from T1 to T3, it is possible to state whether or not they responded at one or more of these times; and in particular whether they responded after each period of training, that is at T2 and T3.

Fifty-seven neurons responded to the training stimulus at T2. Of these only 22 also responded at T3. At this time 50 neurons responded, the deficit of *28* neurons being recruited from the neurons that at T2 were unresponsive. Thus, the number of neurons that responded once after the first or the second training period is the sum of the numbers given in italics, that is 85. Assuming that, after the interval of some 17 hours between T4 and T5, these neurons respond again, then the expected per cent responding at T5 is 37% (85/230). The observed per cent of neurons responding to the training stimulus at T5 was 36% (90/251); and these two percentages correspond closely to the values derived from two previous in studies (Brown and Horn, 1994; Nicol *et al.*, 1995).

It is also possible to predict the proportion of the neurons responding to the training stimulus at T4 from the patterns of responsive/unresponsive neurons observed at T2 and T3 if certain assumptions are made. One assumption is that those neurons that were responsive/unresponsive at T2 and T3 remain in these respective states at T4. Another assumption is that, of those neurons that were responsive/unresponsive at T2 or T3, the pattern of change from T3 to T4 is similar to that from T2 to T3 (for details, see Horn *et al.* 2000a). The predicted per cent responding at T4 on the basis of these assumptions is 17% (39/230); the observed per cent was 16% (74/451).

The match between the predicted values and observed values of the per cent neurons responding to the training stimulus at T4 and T5, suggests that the decline and subsequent recovery occurs in the same neurons, and so supports the second possibility referred to above.

At T4 the proportion of neurons in IMHV which respond to the training stimulus is similar to the proportion that responded to it before training. If neurons in IMHV are crucial for signalling the presence of the familiar stimulus then at T4 chicks would not be expected to show a preference for that stimulus. That is, there should be a decline in retention matching this decline in neuronal responsiveness to the imprinted stimulus. This issue was examined in a separate study in which the preferences of chicks were measured at various times after the start of training. In one group the preference test was given at the time corresponding to T2. In another group of chicks the test was given at the times corresponding to T4 and to T5 (see Figure 19.7). The mean preference score of each group was significantly above the chance level of 50%, and there were no significant differences between the means. In other words, chicks strongly preferred the imprinted stimulus at a time when the proportion of neurons in IMHV that responded to the training stimulus was at the pre-training level.

These results might imply that neurons in IMHV do not provide the signals necessary for the training stimulus to be recognized. However, at the time of T4, ~8 hours after the start of training, S' is already formed (see Figure 19.7). This system is able to sustain an imprinted preference in the absence of IMHV (Cipolla-Neto *et al.*, 1982; Davey *et al.*, 1987; Honey *et al.* 1995), and so would be expected do so when IMHV neuron cannot provide the information necessary for recognition. If the kind of variation in neuronal responsiveness found in IMHV occurs in other memory systems, they may well incorporate some additional store such as S'- a store which is in parallel with, but formed after the storage process has begun in the equivalent structure to IMHV (see p. 355 below).

Cellular mechanisms

What cellular mechanisms might underlie such changes in responsiveness? It is possible, as discussed above (p. 345), that memory over the first few hours following imprinting training depends on changes occurring locally, at the modified synapses. This form of memory could be dependent on processes which characterize the early phase of LTP, such as an up-regulation of AMPA (Malenka and Nicoll, 1999). Over the longer term, mechanisms are engaged that depend on changes in gene expression, probably in both pre- and postsynaptic neurons. That changes in gene expression occur is inferred from the findings that imprinting leads to increases within IMHV in: (i) RNA synthesis (see pp. 336–338), (ii) the number neurons expressing the protein product of the immediate early gene *c-fos* , (iii) the number of NMDA receptors, (iv) the amounts of NCAMs and (v) of clathrin proteins. The reasons for supposing that both pre- and postsynaptic perikaryal nuclei are involved are, on the one hand, that clathrin proteins are involved in recycling the membrane of synaptic vesicles (p. 345) and, on the other hand, that NCAM 180 is restricted to the postsynaptic density. NCAM 140 is expressed in both pre- and postsynaptic membranes (see p. 348). The intracellular signals that are initiated by imprinting, and which activate gene expression in IMHV neurons have not been investigated systematically.

It is unlikely that the learning-related changes in IMHV are simply activity-dependent—that the repeated activity of a synapse generated by impulse activity in the presynaptic axon is sufficient to initiate these changes (McCabe *et al.*, 1979; Davies *et al.*, 1985; and pp. 340–341). The experiments of Davies *et al.* (1983, 1985) suggest that noradrenaline is involved in memory formation, perhaps by 'enabling' the learning-related neural changes to take place. If noradrenaline is such an enabling substance it is unlikely to be the only one: even excitatory amino-acid neurotransmitters may exercise such a function by regulating trophic factor gene expression (Mount *et al.*, 1993).

It was suggested (p. 352) that the responsiveness of individual IMHV neurons to the training stimulus waxes, wanes and waxes again. The cell mechanisms that underlie these oscillations are not known. It is possible that the first phase is controlled by factors operating locally, at synapses modified by learning. The third phase could be mediated by gene expression and specifically by the increased number of NMDA receptors. This increase occurs ~11 hours after the beginning of training, in the interval between T4 and T5 (Figure 19.7). What is surprising is that the two phases of responsiveness are separated by an interval of several hours in which the responsiveness of a high proportion of neurons is reduced. It is as if the early, synaptically local changes, are supplemented by changes involving gene expression, but that the two sets of change do not permit a smooth transition in synaptic efficacy. The temporal mismatch is unlikely to be due to the time taken for axon-/dendritic transport: IMHV neurons are relatively small, the distal tips of dendrites rarely being greater than 200 μm from the soma (Bradley and Horn, 1982; Tömböl *et al.*, 1990) whilst fast anterograde transport is in the region of 250 μm/min (Grafstein and Forman, 1980; Bunge, 1986).

Long-term potentiation, the late phases of which may require gene transcription and protein synthesis, has often been proposed as a mechanism for memory (Teyler and DiScenna, 1987). Could the above kind of variation in responsiveness found in IMHV be understood in terms of LTP? Hippocampal LTP as measured by the amplitude of the field potentials evoked by perforant path to dentate granule cell synapses, once established is stable for long periods of time (Bliss and Gardner-Medwin, 1973). There have been no reports of a reduction in the field potential at the time corresponding to T4, after LTP has been induced. The absence of such evidence may simply be because no- one appears to have looked at the relevant time (C. Abraham, T.V.P. Bliss and S. Laroche, personal communication). However, the changes occurring at T2 and T3 are unlikely to be revealed by field potential studies. The percentage of neurons responding at each of the tests was very similar (25% and 22% respectively) so the amplitude of a field potential if evoked at these test times (T2 andT3) would also be very similar. Such amplitude stability might be interpreted as implying stability in the population of neurons responding at each time. In fact less than half of neurons responding at T3 also responded at T2. The shortfall was met by recruiting neurons that has not responded to the imprinting stimulus at T2.

The role of hippocampal LTP in spatial memory is already in doubt (Bolhuis and Reid, 1992; Bannerman *et al.*, 1997; Saucier and Cain, 1997) and until the issues raised by the results described above are resolved any judgement about the role of LTP in real memory systems must be suspended.

Are some neurons specialized for memory functions?
In discussing the neural basis of habituation attention was focused on neurons which exhibit synaptic depression when these neurons are repeatedly activated. However, many synapses continue to transmit when others have long since ceased to do so. Such functional differences imply biochemical differences and raise the question of whether, even for such a simple form of learning as habituation, neurons are specialized for memory functions. A similar question arises in the case of imprinting.

Imprinting is associated with an increase, in IMHV, in the number of Fos-positive neurons that are immunopositive for GABA and for the calcium-binding protein parvalbumin (McCabe and Horn, 1994; Ambalavanar *et al.*, 1999). Imprinting is not associated with changes in the number of Fos-positive neurons that are also immunopositive for the calcium-binding protein Calbindin-D28k (Ambalavanar *et al.*,

1999). These findings demonstrate that only a sub-population of IMHV neurons are modified by learning. The neurophysiological evidence concerning distance-sensitive and distance-invariant neurons points to the same conclusion. Furthermore, different measures of behaviour correlate with different biochemical changes. For example, there is a learning-related increase in the phosphorylation of the protein kinase C (PKC) substrate protein MARCKS soon after imprinting (p. 345). This increase is independent of training approach activity. In contrast the phosphorylation of another PKC substrate protein, F1 (GAP-43 or neuromodulin) is not correlated with the strength of learning, but is significantly correlated with training approach activity (Sheu *et al.*, 1993).

These diverse results suggest that a population of neurons with a particular molecular profile is involved in memory functions. If this view is supported by further evidence it raises a number of issues. For example, the evidence given above indicates that learning, in the case of imprinting, is accompanied by changes in perikaryal gene expression in both pre- and postsynaptic neurons (pp. 345–349). One mechanism for signalling to the respective nuclei arises from alterations at the modified synapses. Because such alterations may be very rapid they are unlikely to involve, although they may initiate changes in perikaryal gene expression (see p. 344). In the case of the presynaptic neuron such a signal could involve retrograde axonal transport, but not necessarily so. Changes in gene expression in both pre- and post-synaptic neurons may occur as a result of signals impinging on the dendrites and/or on the respective perikarya. Such a route may be used to mediate fast changes in immediate early gene expression, such as those found in drug induced seizures when the levels of mRNA encoded by *c-fos* are increased within minutes of application of the agent (Morgan *et al.*, 1987; Safan *et al.*, 1988). It is therefore possible that changes in perikaryal gene expression occur in neurons which are presynaptic, as well as in neurons which are post-synaptic to a modified synapse. Changes in neurons specialized for memory functions may be initiated in these neurons by the repeated conjunction of activity impinging on them from axons conducting the sensory signals and from axons arising from a re-inforcing system, releasing enabling substances such as serotonin or noradrenaline. Hebb's (1949) postulate would also imply the additional conjunction of activity in the postsynaptic neuron. Such conjunctive activity would not be expected to modify the structure or function of neurons that are not specialized for memory functions.

The idea that some neurons may be specialized for memory is not one of instant appeal, although that is no reason why it should not be considered. The idea is perhaps only an extension to the cellular level of that which exists at the more macroscopic level: the accessory olfactory bulb (Brennan and Keverne, Chapter 6), the perirhinal cortex (Brown, Chapter 11) and the IMHV. And if there are neurons specialized for memory functions it might be possible to characterize them at the molecular level, identify them using immunocytochemical methods, and ultimately to visualize an engram. It should also prove possible to analyse at the cellular level as well as at the level of neural circuitry, the changes that underlie disorders of memory and so to devise a strategy for reversing or mitigating these dysfunctions.

Three memory systems

The electrophysiological changes which occur during and after training are quite similar in left and right IMHV (Brown and Horn, 1994; Nicol *et al.*, 1995, 1999b; Horn *et al.*, 2000a); and changes in the numbers of Fos-positive neurons are not significantly different between the two sides. In contrast there are, for some biochemical measures, asymmetries between left and right IMHV. Thus, there may a significant correlation between preference score and a biochemical change in the left IMHV but not with the change in the right IMHV. This is the case for example for NMDA receptors, MARCKS phosphorylation and the amounts of NCAM and clathrin proteins. However, in each of these instances the value of the correlation coefficient for the right IMHV was not significantly different from that for the left. A clue as to what might be happening comes from data on NCAMs. Approximately 25 hours after the start of training the effects of imprinting are expressed mainly in the left IMHV; but at ~50 hours the effects are expressed mainly in the right IMHV (Solomonia *et al.*, 1998; 2000). The findings taken together suggest that imprinting brings about learning-related changes in both right and left IMHV, but that the two regions are out of phase with each other: the reasons for the putative phase difference are not clear. It is possible that the left IMHV is developmentally more advanced than the right. Nevertheless there are operational differences between the two sides: the right IMHV is necessary for the functioning of S' but the left is not (Cipolla-Neto *et al.*, 1982).

The existence of the third memory system, S' is inferred from lesion studies (see pp. 341–342), and some aspects of its role in memory have been studied by Honey *et al.* (1995). Little else about S' is known. Can any light be thrown on its location from the study of memory systems in other animals? The development of non-invasive brain imaging techniques have made it possible in human subjects to enquire whether particular brain regions are activated during the performance of tasks that require recall of information from memory. Certainly the evolutionary gap that separates humans from birds is wide. But information about the organization of normal brain function, both in humans and in animals has often come from studies of human patients. For example, Hughlings Jackson in the 19th century was the first to appreciate that the sequence of involuntary movements that characterizes an epileptic seizure reflects the spatial layout of the motor cortex (Nathan 1988). Jackson's clinical observations led to a flurry of research, that is still continuing, and which demonstrates the existence of orderly representations of sensory as well as motor systems in the cerebral hemispheres of vertebrates. A more recent example of the importance of human neuropathology for posing questions of general neurobiological interest is the case of H.M. He was subject to a bilateral medial temporal lobectomy (Scoville and Milner, 1957). The operation resulted in a profound anterograde amnesia and initiated an intense research effort to understand the functions of the hippocampus in man and in other vertebrates. So it is perhaps entirely legitimate to examine the results of work on human cerebral function in the hope that it might clarify some conundrums in animal neurobiology.

A number of studies have investigated changes of regional cerebral blood flow in human subjects asked to recall visual images from memory. There is general agreement that there is activation of the prefrontal areas and extrastriate visual areas, including those adjacent to the striate cortex, V2 and V3 (Roland and Freiburg, 1985; Maguire *et al.*, 1996). If the retrieved memory was of words the visual areas were not engaged, but the auditory association areas were (Roland and Freiburg, 1985). These observations suggest that the recall of visual images involves the visual association areas selectively, in addition to the prefrontal cortex.

In birds the visual wulst, which includes the hyperstriatum accessorium (Figure 19.2, HA) and the intercalated nucleus of the hyperstriatum accessorium (Figure 19.2. HI) are considered to correspond to the mam-

malian visual cortex. HI receives input from thalamic nuclei that are targets of termination for axons in the optic tract. HI projects to the overlying HA (Karten *et al.*, 1973; Shimizu *et al.*, 1995; Medina and Reiner, 2000). However, Shimizu *et al.* (1995) urge caution in making simplistic comparisons between the mammalian striate cortex and the visual wulst. Indeed, it is possible that this area of the avian brain incorporates functions that are more a characteristic of the mammalian extrastriate visual cortex than of the striate cortex. Thus amongst the more superficially placed neurons in the HA of the barn owl, Pettigrew and Konishi (1976) demonstrated the existence of sharply tuned disparity-selective neurons. Whilst such neurons have been recorded in the primate striate cortex (Poggio, 1984), they also occur in an orderly array in the adjacent area 18, or V2 (Hubel and Livingstone, 1987).

Whilst disparity-selective neurons may be an adaptation to the frontal vision found in the barn owl, the finding of these cells in HA hints that this region may combine some of the features of both striate and adjacent visual cortex of mammals. If so then, by analogy with the human data, HA may play a role in visual learning and memory (Payne *et al.*, 1984) and so be a plausible candidate for serving the functions of S'. Is there any evidence linking HA to memory function in the chick? As controls for studying learning- related changes in IMHV, various other brain regions have been investigated, including the hippocampus, the posterior neostriatum, the lateral aspect of the cerebral hemispheres and the visual wulst. Only in the latter, and only in some instances, have changes been observed that correlate with preference score: the phosphorylation of the growth-associated protein, F1 (Sheu *et al.*, 1993), the number of Fos-positive cells (McCabe and Horn, 1994) and the amount of NCAM 180 (Solomonia *et al.*, 2000). The changes in F1 and in Fos-positive neurons occur soon after imprinting (see p. 345–347); yet S' is not able to support a preference for the familiar object until several hours have elapsed after the beginning of training (see Figure 19.7). If these biochemical events in HA are related to the formation of S', the cellular changes that they reflect must await a signal from the right IMHV for them to function as a memory store (see pp. 341–342).

The studies of human brain function referred to above suggest that when recall involves the retrieval of modality-specific items from memory, the relevant association cortex, in addition to the prefrontal cortex are engaged. An extensively used form of learning in the chick requires the bird to associate a coloured bead with a bitter-tasting substance, methylanthranilate, which also has a powerful smell. It is therefore of interest that this form of learning in chicks involves the IMHV region and the lobus paraolfactorius, LPO (Rose and Csillag, 1985; Patterson and Rose, 1992). In pigeons LPO receives a projection from the olfactory bulb (Rieke and Wenzel, 1978). It is conceivable therefore that, for learning that involves a powerful gustatory/olfactory negative reinforcer, S' is contained within LPO, the forebrain nucleus of the olfactory pathway; and that for the visual learning of imprinting S' is located in the visual HA. IMHV is involved in both kinds of learning and, as has been suggested on the basis of its anatomical connections, may correspond to the prefrontal cortex (Horn, 1985). These issues are likely to be active areas of research in the years ahead.

CONCLUDING REMARKS

The latter part of the 20th century was an exciting period in the history of the neurosciences. Techniques became available that made it possible to answer questions about the role of the brain in thought processes, questions which, easy to formulate, could not previously be resolved. Many are still not resolved so that the present century is likely to be even more exciting than the century that has closed. There have of course been dangers in the past, and it is likely similar dangers will emerge in the future. In an understandable desire to advance knowledge, assumptions are occasionally made that an experimental model of a phenomenon *is* the phenomenon. For example, many scientists working on hippocampal LTP are cautious as to whether it has a role to play in memory. But anecdotally it is not rare to hear students, and scientists outside the field of neurobiology identifying hippocampal LTP with memory. In a rather different case certain rules have been proposed by which synaptic strengthening (Hebb, 1949) and weakening (Stent, 1973) may occur during learning (see p. 347). The changes in synaptic connections that occur during development (Hubel and Wiesel, 1965a) may follow these rules. But more evidence is required in order to determine whether or not they apply widely in determining synaptic strength in memory systems. Indeed there is evidence that Stent's rule does not apply to the formation of the memory trace in imprinting (Horn *et al.*, 2000b), and that the synaptic facilitation observed during the classical conditioning of a defensive withdrawal reflex in *Aplysia* does not follow Hebb's rule (Carew *et al.*, 1984). These examples may be exceptional, and one or other or both rules may be shown to operate in other real memory systems. The examples do, however, single out the dangers of reification, of identifying the hypothesis with the substantive phenomenon. This is not to deny the importance of formulating hypotheses and of being imaginative in interpreting results. Only by doing so may new ideas be generated, subjected to the rigour of experimental analysis, and our knowledge of neural function in cognition built on the firm foundation of natural science.

ACKNOWLEDGEMENTS

The work on habituation and the early work on imprinting were supported by grants from the US Public Health Service. The SRC and the BBSRC in the UK have given generous financial support over the many years that followed, as has the Wellcome Trust. I am greatly indebted to all of them. But most of all I would like to express my gratitude to my students, colleagues and to the wider scientific community for their intellectual stimulation and for the many friendships I have formed.

REFERENCES

Aderem A. (1992) Signal transduction and the actin cytoskeleton: the roles of MARCKS and profilin. *Trends in Biochemical Sciences*, **17**, 438–443.

Adrian, E.D. (1944) Brain rhythms. *Nature*, **153**, 360–362.

Adrian, E.D., and Matthews, B.H.C. (1934) Berger rhythm: potential changes from the occipital lobes in man. *Brain*, **57**, 355–385.

Akert, K., Pfenninger, K., Sandi, C., and Moor, H. (1972) Freezing etching and cytochemistry of vesicles and membrane complexes in synapses of the central nervous system. In *Structure and Function of Synapses* (ed. G.D. Pappas and D.P. Purpura) pp. 67–86. Raven press, New York.

Ambalavanar, R., McCabe, B.J., Potter, K.N., and Horn, G. (1999) Learning-related Fos-like immunoreactivity in the chick brain: time course and co-localization with GABA and parvalbumin. *Neuroscience*, **93**, 1515–1534.

Anokhin, K.V., and Rose, S.P.R. (1991) Learning-induced increase of immediate early gene messenger RNA in the chick forebrain. *European Journal of Neuroscience*, **3**, 162–167.

Arvanitaki, A., and Chalazonitis, N. (1958) Configuration modales de l'activité propres a differents neurons d'un meme centre. *Journal de Physiologie Paris*, **50**, 122–125.

Bailey, C.H., and Chen, M. (1983) Morphological basis of long-term habituation and sensitization in Aplysia. *Science*, **220**, 91–93.

Balázs, R. (1977) Effect of thyroid hormone and under-nutrition on cell acquisition in the rat brain. In *Thyroid Hormones and Brain Development* (ed. G.D. Grave). pp. 287–302. Raven Press, New York.

Bannerman, D.M., Good, M.A., Butcher, S.P., Ramsay, M., and Morris, R.G. (1995) Distinct components of spatial learning revealed by prior training and NMDA receptor blockade. *Nature*, **378**, 182–186.

Bateson, P.P.G. (1966) The characteristics and context of imprinting. *Biological Reviews*, **41**, 177–220.

Bateson, P.P.G. (1974) Length of training, opportunities for comparison, and imprinting in chicks. *Journal of Comparative and Physiological Psychology*, **86**, 586–589.

Bateson, P.P.G., Horn, G., and Rose, S.P.R. (1969) Effects of an imprinting procedure on regional incorporation of tritiated lysine into protein of chick brain. *Nature*, **223**, 534–535.

Bateson, P.P.G., Horn, G., and Rose, S.P.R. (1972). Effects of early experience on regional incorporation of precursors into RNA and protein in the chick brain. *Brain Research*, **39**, 449–465.

Bateson, P.P.G., Rose, S.P.R., and Horn, G. (1973) Imprinting: lasting effects on uracil incorporation into chick brain. *Science*, **181**, 576–578.

Bateson, P.P.G., Horn, G. and Rose, S.P.R. (1975) Imprinting: correlations between behaviour and incorporation of [^{14}C]uracil into chick brain. *Brain Research*, **84**, 207–220.

Bell, C., Sierra, G., Buendia, N., and Segundo, J.P. (1964) Sensory properties of neurons in the mesencephalic reticular formation. *Journal of Neurophysiology*, **27**, 961–987.

Berger, H. (1930) Über das Elektroenkephalogram des Menschen. II. *Journal für Psychologie und Neurologie* (Leipzig), **40**, 160–179.

Berkeley, G. (1709) *An Essay Towards a New Theory of Vision*. J. Pepyat, Dublin.

Bliss, T.V.P., and Gardner-Medwin, A.R. (1973) Long-lasting potentiation of synaptic transmission in the dentate area of unanaesthetised rabbit following stimulation of the perforant path. *Journal of Physiology*, **232**, 357–374.

Bolhuis, J.J. (1991) Mechanisms of avian imprinting: A review. *Biological Reviews*, **66**, 303–345.

Bolhuis, J.J., and Honey, R.C. (1998) Imprinting, learning and development: from behaviour to brain and back. *Trends in Neurosciences*, **21**, 306–311.

Bolhuis, J.J., and Horn, G. (1992) Generalization of learned preferences in filial imprinting. *Animal Behaviour*, **44**, 185–187.

Bolhuis, J.J. and Reid, I.C. (1992) Effects of intraventricular infusion of the N-methyl-D-aspartate (NMDA) receptor antagonist AP5 on spatial memory of rats in a radial arm maze. *Behavioural Brain Research*, **47**, 151–157.

Bolhuis, J.J., Stewart, C.A., and Forrest, E.M. (1994) Retrograde amnesia and memory reactivation in rats with ibotenate lesions to the hippocampus or subiculum. *Quarterly Journal of Experimental Psychology*, **47B**, 129–150.

Bontempi, B., Laurent-Demir, C., Destrade, C., and Jaffard, R. (1999) Time-dependent reorganization of brain circuitry underlying long-term memory storage. *Nature*, **400**, 671–675.

Bradley, P., and Horn, G. (1982) A Golgi analysis of the hyperstriatum ventrale of the chick. *Journal of Anatomy*, **134**, 599–600.

Bradley, P., Davies, D.C., and Horn, G. (1985) Connections of the hyperstriatum ventrale of the domestic chick (*Gallus domesticus*) *Journal of Anatomy*, **140**, 577–589.

Bradley, P., Horn, G., and Bateson, P.P.G. (1981) Imprinting: an electron microscopic study of chick hyperstriatum ventrale. *Experimental Brain Research*, **41**, 115–120.

Bradley, P.M., Burrows, B.D., Titmuss, J., and Webb, A.C. (1991) Morphological correlates of persistent potentiation in the chick brain slice. *NeuroReport*, **2**, 197–200.

Broadbent, D.E. (1958) *Perception and Communication*. Pergamon Press, London.

Brown, M.W., and Horn, G. (1979) Neuronal plasticity in the chick brain: electrophysiological effects of visual experience on hyperstriatal neurons. *Brain Research*, **162**, 142–147.

Brown, M.W., and Horn, G. (1994) Learning-related alterations in the visual responsiveness of neurons in a memory system of the chick brain. *European Journal of Neuroscience*, **6**, 1479–1490.

Brunelli, M., Castellucci, V., and Kandel, E.R. (1976) Synaptic facilitation and behavioral sensitization in *Aplysia*: possible role of serotonin and cyclic AMP. *Science*, **194**, 1178–1181.

Bruner, J., and Tauc, L. (1966) Habituation at the synaptic level in *Aplysia*. *Nature*, **210**, 37–39.

Bryant, S.H. (1959) The function of the proximal synapse of the squid stellate ganglion. *Journal of General Physiology*, **42**, 609–616.

Bullock, T.H., and Hagiwara, S. (1957) Intracellular recording from the giant synapse of the squid. *Journal of General Physiology*, **40**, 565–577.

Bunge, M.B. (1986) The axonal cytoskeleton: its role in generating and maintaining cell form. *Trends in Neurosciences*, **9**, 477–482.

Bushnell, M.C., Goldberg, M.E., and Robinson, D.L. (1981) Behavioral enhancement of visual responses in cerebral cortex. I. Modulation in posterior parietal cortex related to visual attention. *Journal of Neurophysiology*, **46**, 755–772.

Byrne, J.H., and Kandel, E.R. (1996) Presynaptic facilitation revisited: state and time dependence. *Journal of Neuroscience*, **16**, 425–435.

Cajal, S.R. (1911) *Histologie du système nerveux de l'homme et des vértébrés*. Maloine, Paris.

Carew, T.C., Castelluci, V.F., and Kandel, E.R. (1979) Sensitization in *Aplysia*: restoration of transmission in synapses inactivated by long-term habituation. *Science*, **205**, 417–419.

Carew, T.J., Hawkins, R.D., Abrams, T.W., and Kandel, E.R. (1984) A test of Hebb's postulate at identified synapses which mediate classical conditioning in *Aplysia*. *Journal of Neuroscience*, **4**, 1217–1224.

Castellucci, V.F., Kupfermann, I., Pinsker, H. and Kandel, E.R. (1970) Neuronal mechanisms of habituation and dishabituation of the gill withdrawal reflex in *Aplysia*. *Science*, **167**, 1445–1448.

Castelluci, V.F., Carew, T.J. and Kandel, E.R. (1978) Cellular analysis of long-term habituation of the gill-withdrawn reflex of *Aplysia californica*. *Science*, **202**, 1306–1308.

Cipolla-Neto, J., Horn, G., and McCabe, B.J. (1979) A method for recording unit activity from the brain of the freely moving chick. *Journal of Physiology*, **295**, 8–9P.

Cipolla-Neto, J., Horn, G., and McCabe, B.J. (1982) Hemispheric asymmetry and imprinting: The effects of sequential lesions to the hyperstriatum ventrale. *Experimental Brain Research*, **48**, 22–27.

Crick, F. (1984) Function of the thalamic ventricular complex: the searchlight hypothesis. *Proceedings of the National Academy of Sciences of the USA*, **81**, 4586–4590.

Crick, F. (1994) *The Astonishing Hypothesis*. Macmillan, New York.

Crow, T.J. (1968) Cortical synapses and reinforcement: an hypothesis. *Nature*, **219**, 736–737.

Dahlström, A., and Fuxe, K. (1964) Evidence for the existence of monoamine-containing neurons in the central nervous system. *Acta Physiologica Scandanavica, Supplement*, **232**, 1–55.

Daisley, J.N., Gruss, M., Rose, S.P.R., and Braun, K. (1998) Passive avoidance training and recall are associated with increased glutamate levels in the intermediate and medial hyperstriatum ventrale of the 2 day-old chick. *Neural Plasticity*, **6**, 53–61.

Davey, J.E., McCabe, B.J., and Horn, G. (1987) Mechanisms of information storage after imprinting in the domestic chick. *Behavioural Brain Research*, **26**, 209–210.

Davies, D.C., Horn, G. and McCabe, B.J. (1983) Changes in telencephalic catecholamine levels in the domestic chick. Effects of age and visual experience. *Developmental Brain Research*, **10**, 251–255.

Davies, D.C., Horn, G., and McCabe, B.J. (1985) Noradrenaline and learning: the effects of the noradrenergic neurotoxin in DSP4 on imprinting in the domestic chick. *Behavioral Neuroscience*, **99**, 652–660.

Davis, J.L., Masuoka, D.T., Gerbrandt, L.K., and Cherkin, A. (1979) Autradiographic distribution of L-proline in chicks after intracerebral injection. *Physiology & Behavior*, **22**, 693–695.

Daw, N.W., Stein, P.S.G., and Fox, K. (1993) The role of NMDA receptors in information processing. *Annual Review of Neuroscience*, **16**, 207–222.

Dennett, D. (1991) *Consciousness Explained*. Little, Brown, New York.

Denny-Brown, D., and Chambers, R.A. (1958) The parietal lobe and behavior. *Research Publications of the Association for Research into Nervous and Mental Diseases*, **36**, 35–117.

Desmond, N.L., and Levy, W.B. (1986) Changes in the postsynaptic density with long-term potentiation in the dentate gyrus. *Journal of Comparative Neurology*, **253**, 476–482.

Diamond, M.C., Krech, D. and Rosenzweig, M.R. (1964) The effect of an enriched environment on the histology of the rat cerebral cortex. *Journal of Comparative Neurology*. **123**, 111–120.

Doherty, P., Fazeli, M.S., and Walsh, F.S. (1995) The neural cell-adhesion molecule and synaptic plasticity. *Journal of Neurobiology*, **26**, 437–446.

Drager, V.C., and Hubel, D.H. (1976) Topography of visual and somatosensory projections to mouse superior colliculus. *Journal of Neurophysiology*, **39**, 91–101.

Eayrs, J.T. (1960) Influence of the thyroid on the central nervous system. *British Medical Bulletin*, **16**, 122–127.

Eayrs, J.T., and Horn, G. (1955) The development of the cerebral cortex in hypothyroid and starved rats. *Anatomical Record*, **121**, 53–62.

Eccles, J.C. (1953) *The Neurophysiological Basis of Mind*. Clarendon Press, Oxford.

Eccles, J.C. (1964) *The Physiology of Synapses*. Springer, Berlin.

Eccles, J.C., and McIntyre, A.K. (1951) Plasticity of mammalian monosynaptic reflexes. *Nature*, **167**, 466–468.

Edelman, G.M., and Crossin, K.L. (1991) Cell adhesion molecules: implications for a molecular biology. *Annual Review of Biochemistry*, **60**, 155–190.

Eichenbaum, H. (1999) The hippocampus: the shock of the new. *Current Biology*, **9**, R482–R484.

Fagg, G.E., and Matus, A. (1984) Selective association of N-methyl-D-aspartate and quisqualate types of L-glutamate receptor with postsynaptic densities. *Proceedings of the National Academy of Sciences of the USA*, **81**, 6876–6880.

Fields, R.D., and Itoh, K. (1996) Neural cell adhesion molecules in activity dependent development and synaptic plasticity. *Trends in Neurosciences*, **19**, 473–480.

Fink, G.R., Markowitsch, H.J., Reinkemeier, M., Bruckbauer, T., Kessler, J., and Heiss, W-D. (1996) Cerebral representation of one's own past: neural networks involved in autobiographical memory. *Journal of Neuroscience*, **16**, 4275–4282.

Fitzgerald, K., Wright, W.G., Marcus, E.A., and Carew, T.J. (1990) Multiple forms of non-associative plasticity in *Aplysia*—a behavioural, cellular and pharmacological analysis. *Philosophical Transactions of the Royal Society of London, B*, **329**, 171–178.

French, J.D., and Magoun, H.W. (1952) Effects of chronic lesions in central cephalic brain stem of monkeys. *Archives of Neurology and Psychiatry (Chicago)*, **68**, 591–604.

Frey, U., and Morris, R.G.M. (1998) Synaptic tagging; Implications for late maintenance of hippocampal long-term potentiation. *Trends in Neurosciences*, **21**, 181–187.

Fulton, J.F. (1949) *Functional Localization in the Frontal Lobes and Cerebellum*. Clarendon Press, Oxford.

Gaffan, D. (1993) Additive effects of forgetting and fornix transection in the temporal gradient of retrograde amnesia. *Neuropsychologia*, **31**, 1055–1066.

Galarreta, M., Bustamente, J., del Rio, R.M., and Solis, J.M. (1996) Taurine induces a long lasting increase of synaptic efficacy and axon excitability in the hippocampus. *Journal of Neuroscience*, **16**, 92–102.

Gordon, B. (1973) Receptive fields in deep layers of cat superior colliculus. *Journal of Neurophysiology*, **36**, 157–178.

Gottlieb, G. (1961) Developmental age as a baseline for determination of the critical period in imprinting. *Journal of Comparative and Physiological Psychology*, **54**, 422–427.

Grafstein, B., and Forman, D.S. (1980) Intracellular transport in neurons. *Physiological Reviews*, **60**, 1167–1283.

Griffith, J.S. (1966) A theory of the nature of memory. *Nature*, **211**, 11160–1163.

Griffith, J.S. (1967) *A View of the Brain*. Clarendon Press, Oxford.

Gruss, M., and Braun, K. (1996) Stimulus-evoked increase of glutamate in mediorostral neostriatum/hyperstriatum ventrale of domestic chick after auditory filial imprinting: an *in vivo* microdialysis study. *Journal of Neurochemistry*, **66**, 1167–1173.

Harris, K.M., and Kater, S.B. (1994) Dendritic spines–cellular specializations imparting both stability and flexibility to synaptic function. *Annual Review of Neuroscience*, **17**, 341–371.

Harvey, R.J., McCabe, B.J., Solomonia, R.O., Horn, G., and Darlison, M.G. (1998) Expression of the GABA$_A$ receptor γ4-subunit gene: anatomical distribution of the corresponding mRNA in the domestic chick forebrain and the effect of imprinting training. *European Journal of Neuroscience*, **10**, 3024–3028.

Hawkins, R.D., Clark, G.A. and Kandel, E.R. (1987) Cell biological studies of learning in simple vertebrate and invertebrate systems. In *Handbook of Physiology. Part I, Higher functions of the nervous system* (ed. F. Plum), Vol. 6, pp. 25–83. American Physiological Society, Bethesda.

Hebb, D.O. (1949) *The Organization of Behavior*. John Wiley & Sons, New York.

Heinroth, O. (1911) Beiträge zur biologie, namentlich Ethologie und Psychologie der Anatiden. *Proceedings of the 5th International Ornithological Congress*, 589–702.

Hilgard, E.R., and Marquis, D.G. (1961) *Conditioning and Learning*, Methuen, London.

Hillyard, S.A., Mangun, G.R., Woldorff, M.G., and Luck, S. (1995) Neural systems mediating attention. In *The Cognitive Neurosciences* (ed. M.S. Gazzaniga), pp. 665–681. The M.I.T. Press, Cambridge Massachusetts.

Hinde, R.A. (1962) Some aspects of the imprinting problem. *Symposium of the Zoological Society of London*, **8**, 129–138.

Hinde, R.A. (1970) *Animal Behaviour*. McGraw Hill, New York.

Honey, R.C., Horn, G., Bateson, P., and Walpole, M. (1995) Functionally distinct memories for imprinting stimuli: behavioral and neural dissociations. *Behavioral Neuroscience*, **109**, 689–698.

Horn, G. (1955) Thyroid deficiency and inanition: the effects of replacement therapy on the development of the cerebral cortex of young albino rats. *Anatomical Record*, **121**, 63–80.

Horn, G. (1962) Some neural correlates of perception. In *Viewpoints in biology* (ed. J.D. Carthy and C.L. Duddington), Vol. 1, pp. 242–285.

Horn, G. (1965) Physiological and psychological aspects of selective perception. In *Advances in the Study of Animal Bbehaviour* (ed. D.S. Lehrman, R.A. Hinde and E. Shaw), pp. 155–215.

Horn, G. (1967) Neuronal mechanisms of habituation. *Nature*, **215**, 707–711.

Horn, G. (1970) Changes in neuronal activity and their relationship to behaviour. In *Short-term Changes in Neural Activity and Behaviour*, (ed. G. Horn and R.A. Hinde), pp. 567–606. Cambridge University Press, Cambridge.

Horn, G. (1976) Physiological studies of attention and arousal. In *Mechanisms in Transmission of Signals for Conscious Behaviour*, (ed. T. Desiraju), pp. 285–299. Elsevier, Amsterdam.

Horn, G. (1981) Neural mechanisms of learning: an analyses of imprinting in the domestic chick. *Proceedings of the Royal Society of London, B*, **213**, 101–137.

Horn, G. (1985) *Memory, Imprinting, and the Brain*. Clarendon Press, Oxford.

Horn, G. (1990) Neural bases of recognition memory investigated through an analysis of imprinting. *Philosophical Transactions of the Royal Society of London, B*, **1329**. 133–142.

Horn, G., and Hill, R.M. (1964) Habituation of the response to sensory stimuli of neurons in the brain stem of rabbits. *Nature*, **202**, 296–298.

Horn, G., and Hill, R.M. (1966) Responsiveness to sensory stimulation of units in the superior colliculus and subjacent tectotegmental regions of the rabbit. *Experimental Neurology*, **14**, 199–223.

Horn, G., and Hinde, R.A. (ed.) (1970) *Short-term Changes in Neural Activity and Behaviour*. Cambridge University Press, Cambridge.

Horn, G., and Johnson, M.H. (1989) Memory systems in the chick: dissociations and neuronal analysis. *Neuropsychologia*, **27**, 1–22.

Horn, G., and McCabe, B.J. (1978) An autoradiographic method for studying the incorporation of uracil into acid-insoluble compounds in the brain. *Journal of Physiology*, **275**, 2–3P.

Horn, G., and McCabe, B.J. (1990) Learning by seeing: N-methyl-D-aspartate receptors and recognition memory. In *Excitatory Amino acids and Neural Plasticity*, (ed. Y-Ben Ari), pp. 187–96. Plennum Press, New York.

Horn, G., and Wiesenfeld, Z. (1974) Attention in the cat: electrophysiological and behavioural studies. *Experimental Brain Research*, **21**, 67–82.

Horn, G., and Wright, M.J. (1970) Characteristics of transmission failure in the squid stellate ganglion: a study of a simple habituating system. *Journal of Experimental Biology*, **52**, 217–231.

Horn, G., Bradley, P., and McCabe, B.J. (1985) Changes in the structure of synapses associated with learning. *Journal of Neuroscience*, **5**, 3161–3168.

Horn, G., McCabe, B.J., and Bateson, P.P.G. (1979) An autoradiographic study of the chick brain after imprinting. *Brain Research*, **168**, 361–373.

Horn, G., Nicol, A.U., and Brown, M.W. (2000a) Tracking memory's trace – the engram. *In preparation*.

Horn, G., Nicol, A.U., and Brown, M.W. (2000b) Evidence against synaptic competition in memory formation. *European Journal of Neuroscience*, **11**, in press.

Horn, G., Rose, S.P.R., and Bateson, P.P.G. (1973) Monocular imprinting and regional incorporation of tritiated uracil into the brains of intact and 'split-brain' chicks. *Brain Research*, **56**, 227–237.

Hubel, D.H., and Livingstone, M.S. (1987) Segregation of form, color and stereopsis in primate area 18. *Journal of Neuroscience*, **7**, 3387–3415.

Hubel, D.H., and Wiesel, T.N. (1959) Receptive fields of single neurons in the cat's striate cortex. *Journal of Physiology*, **148**, 574–591.

Hubel, D.H., and Wiesel, T.N. (1961) Integrative action in the cat's lateral geniculate body. *Journal of Physiology*, **155**, 385–398.

Hubel, D.H., and Wiesel, T.N. (1962) Receptive fields binocular interaction and functional architecture in the cat's visual cortex. *Journal of Physiology*, **160**, 105–154.

Hubel, D.H., and Wiesel, T.N. (1965a) Binocular interaction in striate cortex of kittens reared with artificial squint. *Journal of Neurophysiology*, **28**, 1041–1059.

Hubel, D.H., and Wiesel, T.N. (1965b) Receptive fields and functional architecture in two nonstriate visual areas (18 and 19) of the cat. *Journal of Neurophysiology*, **28**, 229–289.

Humphrey, G. (1933) *The Nature of Learning*. Routledge and Kegan Paul, London.

Humphreys, G., Duncan, J., and Treisman, A. (1999) *Attention, Space and Action*. Oxford University Press, Oxford.

Hunt, S.P. and Webster, K.E. (1972) Thalamo-hyperstriate interrelations in the pigeon. *Brain Research*, **44**, 647–651.

Hunt, S.P., Pini, A., and Evan, G. (1987) Induction of *c-fos*-like protein in spinal cord neurons following sensory stimulation. *Nature*, **328**, 632–634.

Jaim-Etcheverry, G., and Zieher, L.M. (1980) DSP4: a novel compound with neuro-toxic effects on noradrenergic neurons of adult and developing rats. *Brain Research*, **188**, 513–523.

Jasper, H.H. (1949) Diffuse projection systems: the integrative action of the thalamic reticular system. *Electroencephalography and Clinical Neurophysiology*, **1**, 405–419.

Jassik-Gerschenfeld, D. (1965) Somesthetic and visual responses of superior colliculus neurons. *Nature*, **208**, 898–900.

Jay, M.F., and Sparks, D.L. (1987) Sensorimotor integration in the primate superior colliculus: II coordinates of auditory signals. *Journal of Neurophysiology*, **57**, 35–55.

Jefferson, G. (1944) The nature of consciousness. *British Medical Journal*, **1**, 1–5.

Jenkins, W.M., Merzenich, M.M., Ochs, U.T., Allard, T., and Guic-Robles, E. (1990) Functional reorganization of primary somatosensory cortex in adult owl monkeys after behaviorally controlled tactile stimulation. *Journal of Neurophysiology*, **63**, 82–104.

Johnston, A.N., Rogers, L.J., and Dodd, P.R. (1995) [H-3] MK-801 binding asymmetry in the IMHV region of dark-reared chicks is reversed by imprinting. *Brain Research Bulletin*, **37**, 5–8.

Johnston, A.N., Rogers, L.J., and Johnston, G.A.R. (1993) Glutamate and imprinting–the role of glutamate receptors in the encoding of imprinting memory. *Behavioural Brain Research*, **54**, 137–143.

Jones, H.J.E., Marsden, R.M., and McCabe, B.J. (1999) Fos expression in the hyperstriatum ventrale and neostriatum of the chick forebrain after visual imprinting. *Neural Plasticity*, Supplement 1, 128.

Jung, R. (1954) Correlation of bioelectrical and autonomic phenomena with alternations of consciousness and arousal in man. In *Brain Mechanisms and Consciousness*, (ed. E.D. Adrian, F. Bremer, H. Jasper and J.F. Delafresnaye), pp. 310–44. Blackwell, Oxford.

Kandel, E.R., and Schwartz, H. (1982) Molecular biology of learning: modulation of transmitter release. *Science*, **218**, 433–443.

Karten, H.J., Hodos, W., Nauta, W.J.H., and Revzin, A.M. (1973) Neural connections of the 'visual Wulst' of the avian telencephalon. Experimental studies in the pigeon (*Columbia livia*) and owl (*Speotyto cunicularia*) *Journal of Comparative Neurology*, **150**, 253–278.

Katz, B. (1966) *Nerve, Muscle and Synapse*. McGraw-Hill, New York.

Katz, B., and Miledi, R. (1967) The timing of calcium action during neuromuscular transmission. *Journal of Physiology*, **189**, 535–544.

Kety, S.S. (1970) The biogenic amines in the central nervous system: their possible roles in arousal, emotion and learning. In *The neurosciences: Second Study Program* (ed. F.O. Schmitt), pp. 324–336. Rockefeller University Press, New York.

Kety, S.S. (1972) The possible role of the adrenergic systems of the cortex in learning. *Research Publications of the Association for Research into Nervous and Mental Disorders*, **50**, 376–386.

Klein, M., Shapiro, E., and Kandel, E.R. (1980) Synaptic plasticity and the modulation of the Ca^{2+} current. *Journal of Experimental Biology*, **89**, 117–157.

Klüver, H., and Bucy, P.C. (1939) Preliminary analysis of functions of the temporal lobes in monkeys. *Archives of Neurology and Psychiatry (Chicago)*, **42**, 979–1000.

Konorski, J. (1948) *Conditional Reflexes and Neuron Organization*. Cambridge University Press, Cambridge.

Konorski, J., and Miller, S. (1937) On two types of conditional reflex. *Journal of General Psychology*, **16**, 264–272.

Kovach, J.K. (1971) Effectiveness of different colours in the elicitation and development of approach behaviour in chicks. *Behaviour*, **38**, 154–168.

Kuffler, S.W. (1952) Neurons in the retina: organization, inhibition and excitation problems. *Cold Spring Harbor Symposium of Quantitative Biology*, **17**, 281–292.

Kupferman, I, and Kandel, E.R. (1969) Neural controls of a behavioral response mediated by the abdominal ganglion of *Aplysia*, *Science*, **154**, 917–919.

Lashley, K.S. (1950) In search of the engram. *Symposia of the Society for Experimental Biology*, **4**, 454–482.

Lindsley, D.B., Scheiner, L.H., Knowles, W.B., and Magoun, H.W. (1950) Behavioral and EEG changes following chronic brain stem lesions in the cat. *Electroencephalography and Clinical Neurophysiology*, **2**, 483–498.

Llinas, R. (1999) *The Squid Giant Synapse*. Oxford University Press, Oxford.

Lloyd, D.P.C. (1949) Post-tetanic potentiation of response in monosynaptic reflex pathways of the spinal cord. *Journal of General Physiology*, **33**, 147–170.

Lorenz, K. (1937) The companion in the birds world. *Auk*, **54**, 245–273.

Lynch, G., and Baudry, M. (1984) The biochemistry of memory: a new and specific hypothesis. *Science*, **224**, 1057–1063.

Mackey, S.L., Kandel, E.R., and Hawkins, R.D. (1989) Identified serotonergic neurons LCB1 and RCB1 in the cerebral ganglia of *Aplysia* produce presynaptic facilitation of siphon sensory neurons. *Journal of Neuroscience*, **9**, 4227–4235.

Maguire, E.A., Frackowiak, R.S.J., and Frith, C.D. (1996) Learning to find your way: a role for the human hippocampal formation. *Proceedings of the Royal Society of London, B*, **263**, 1745–1750.

Malenka, R.C., and Nicoll, R.A. (1999) Long-term potentiation–a decade of progress? *Science*, **285**, 1870–1874.

Marcel, A.J., and Bisiach, E. (1988) *Consciousness in Contemporary Science*. Clarendon Press, Oxford.

McCabe, B.J., and Horn, G. (1988) Learning and memory: regional changes in N-methyl-D-aspartate receptors in the chick brain after imprinting. *Proceedings of the National Academy of Sciences of the USA*, **85**, 2849–2853.

McCabe, B.J., and Horn, G. (1991) Synaptic transmission and recognition memory: time course of changes in N-Methyl-D-aspartate receptors after imprinting. *Behavioral Neuroscience*, **105**, 289–294.

McCabe, B.J., Cipolla-Neto, J., Horn, G., and Bateson, P.P.G. (1982) Amnesic effects of bilateral lesions placed in the hyperstriatum ventrale of the chick after imprinting. *Experimental Brain Research*, **48**, 13–21.

McCabe, B.J., Horn, G., and Bateson, P.P.G. (1979) Effects of rhythmic hyperstriatal stimulation in chicks' preferences for visual flicker. *Physiology & Behavior*, **23**, 137–140.

McCabe, B.J., Horn, G., and Bateson, P.P.G. (1981) Effects of restricted lesions of the chick forebrain on the acquisition of preferences during imprinting. *Brain Research*, **205**, 29–37.

McCabe, B.J., Kendrick, K.M., and Horn, G. (1998) Release of putative amino acid neurotransmitters in the brain of the domestic chick following exposure learning (imprinting). *Journal of Physiology*, **505P**, 60.

McCabe, B.J., and Horn, G. (1994) Learning-related changes in Fos-like immunoreactivity in the chick forebrain after imprinting. *Proceedings of the National Academy of Sciences of the USA*, **91**, 417–421.

McLennan, J.G., and Horn, G. (1992) Learning-dependent changes in the responses to visual stimuli of neurons in a recognition memory system. *European Journal of Neuroscience*, **4**, 1112–1122.

Medina, L., and Reiner, A. (2000) Do birds possess homologues of mammalian primary visual somatosensory and motor cortices? *Trends in Neurosciences*, **23**, 1–12.

Meredith, R.M., McCabe, B.J., Kendrick, K. and Horn, G. (2000) Learning-related release of GABA and taurine in chick brain: a transient correlation following imprinting. *European Journal of Neuroscience*, **11**, in press.

Metzger, J., Jiang, S.C., and Braun, K. (1998) Organization of the dorsocaudal neostriatal complex: a retrograde and anterograde tracing study in the domestic chick with special emphasis on pathways relevant to imprinting. *Journal of Comparative Neurology*, **395**, 380–404.

Miledi, R. (1973) Transmitter release induced by injection of calcium ions into nerve terminals. *Proceedings of the Royal Society of London*, Series B, **183**, 473–498.

Milner, B. (1966) Amnesia following operation on the temporal lobes. In *Amnesia* (ed. C.W.M. Whitty and O.L. Zangwill), pp. 109–133. Butterworth, London.

Mohler, C.N., and Wurtz, R.H. (1977) Role of striate cortex and superior colliculus in visual guidance of saccadic eye movements in monkeys. *Journal of Neurophysiology*, **40**, 74–94.

Morgan, J.I., Cohen, D.R., Hempstead, J.L. and Curran, T. (1987) Mapping patterns of *c-fos* expression in the central nervous after seizure. *Science*, 237, 192–197.

Morison, R.S., and Dempsey, E.W. (1942) A study of thalamic cortical relations. *American Journal of Physiology*, **135**, 281–292.

Moruzzi, G., and Magoun, H.W. (1949) Brainstem reticular formation and activation of the EEG. *Electroencephalography and Clinical Neurophysiology*, **1**, 455–473.

Morris, S.A., and Schmid, S. (1995) The Ferrari of endocytosis? *Current Biology*, **5**, 113–115.

Motter, B.C. (1993) Focal attention produces spatially selective processing in visual cortical areas V1, V2 and V4 in the presence of competing stimuli. *Journal of Neurophysiology*, **70**, 909–919.

Mount, H.J., Dreyfuss, C.F., and Black, I.B. (1993) Purkinje cell survival is differentially regulated by metabotropic and ionotropic excitatory amino acid receptors. *Journal of Neuroscience*, **13**, 317–379.

Mountcastle, V.B. (1957) Modality and topographic properties of single neurons of cat's somatic sensory cortex. *Journal of Neurophysiology*, **20**, 408–434.

Näätänen, R. (1992) *Attention and Brain Function*, Lawrence Erlbaum, Hillsdale, NJ.

Nathan, P. (1988) *The Nervous System*. Oxford University Press, Oxford.

Nicol, A.U., Brown, M.W., and Horn, G. (1995) Neurophysiological investigations of a recognition memory system for imprinting in the domestic chick. *European Journal of Neuroscience*, **7**, 766–776.

Nicol, A.U., Brown, M.W., and Horn, G. (1998a) Hippocampal neuronal activity and imprinting in the behaving chick. *European Journal of Neuroscience*, **10**, 2738–2741.

Nicol, A.U., Brown, M.W., and Horn, G. (1998b) Neural encoding of subject-object distance in a visual recognition system. *European Journal of Neuroscience*, **10**,, 34–44.

Nicol, A.U., Brown, M.W., and Horn, S. (1999a) Is neuronal encoding of subject-object distance dependent on learning? *NeuroReport*, **10**, 1671–1675.

Nicol, A.U., Brown, M.W., and Horn, G. (1999b) The development of learning-related changes in responsiveness of neurons in a visual recognition system. *Journal of Physiology*, **520**, 79.

Patterson, T.A, and Rose, S.P.R. (1992) Memory in the chick: multiple cues, distinct brain locations. *Behavioral Neuroscience*, **106**, 465–470.

Pavlov, I.P. (1927) *Conditioned Reflexes*. Oxford University Press, Oxford.

Payne, J.K., Horn, G., and Brown, M.W. (1984) Modifiability of responsiveness in a visual projection area of the chick brain: visual experience is only one of several factors involved. *Behavioural Brain Research*, **13**, 163–172.

Penfield, W. (1952) Epileptic automatism and the centrencephalic integrating system. *Research Publications of the Association for Nervous and Mental Diseases*, **30**, 513–528.

Persohn, E., Pollerberg, E., and Schachner, M. (1989) Immunoelectron microscopic localization of the 180kD component of the neural cell adhesion molecule N-CAM in post-synaptic membranes. *Journal of Comparative Neurology*, **288**, 92–100.

Pettigrew, J.D., and Konishi, M. (1976) Neurons selective for orientation and binocular disparity in the visual Wulst of the Barn owl (*Tyto alba*) *Nature*, **193**, 675–678.

Poggio, G.F. (1984) Processing of stereoscopic information in primate visual cortex. In *Dynamic Aspects of Neocortical function* (ed. G.M. Edelman, W.E. Gall and W.M. Cowan) pp. 613–635. Wiley, New York.

Poggio, G.F., and Mountcastle, V.B. (1963) The functional properties of ventrobasal thalamic neurons studies in unaneasthetized monkeys. *Journal of Neurophysiology*, **26**, 775–806.

Popper, K. (1972) *Objective Knowledge: an Evolutionary Approach*. Clarendon Press, Oxford.

Potter, K.N., McCabe, B.J. and Horn, G. (1998) Co-expression of Fos, Fra-2, Jun and egr-1 with gamma-aminobutyric acid (GABA) and taurine in a chick forebrain region involved in visual imprinting. *European Journal of Neuroscience*, **10**, 145.

Powell, T.P.S. and Mountcastle, V.B. (1959) Some aspects of the functional organization of the postcentral gyrus of the monkey: a correlation of findings obtained in a single unit analysis with cytoarchitecture. *Bulletin of Johns Hopkins Hospital*, **105**, 133–162.

Prosser, C., and Hunter, W.S. (1936) The extinction of startle responses and spinal reflexes in the white rat. *American Journal of Physiology*, **117**, 609–618.

Rieke, G.K., and Wenzel, B.M. (1978) Forebrain projections of the pigeon olfactory bulb. *Journal of Morphology*, **158**, 41–56.

Roelfsema, P.R., Lamme, V.A.F., and Spekreijse, H. (1998) Object-based attention in the primary visual cortex of the macaque monkey. *Nature*, **395**, 376–381.

Roland, P.E., and Friberg, L. (1985) Localization of cortical areas activated by thinking. *Journal of Neurophysiology*, **53**, 1219–1243.

Rose, S.P.R., and Csillag, A. (1985) Passive avoidance training results in lasting changes in deoxyglucose metabolism in left hemisphere regions of chick brain. *Behavioral and Neural Biology*, **44**, 315–324.

Rose, S.P.R., and Jork, R. (1987) Long-term memory formations blocked by 2-deoxygalactose, a fucose analog. *Behavioral and Neural Biology*, **48**, 246–258.

Rowell, C.H.F. (1970) Incremental and decremental processes in the insect central nervous system. In *Short-term Changes in Neural Activity and Behaviour* (ed. G. Horn and R.A. Hinde), pp. 237–280. Cambridge University Press, Cambridge.

Rowell, C.H.F., and Horn, G. (1967) Response characteristics of neurons in an insect brain. *Nature*, **216**, 702–703.

Rowell, C.H.F., and Horn, G. (1968) Dishabituation and arousal in the response of single nerve cells in an insect brain. *Journal of Experimental Biology*, **49**, 171–183.

Ryle, G. (1949) *The Concept of Mind*. Hutchinson, London.

Saffen, D.W., Cole, A.J., Worley, P.F., Christy, P., Ryder, K. and Baraban, J.M. (1988) Convulsant-induced increase in transcription factor messenger RNAs in rat brain. *Proceedings of the National Academy of Sciences of the U.S.A.*, **85**, 7795–7799.

Saransaart, P., and Oja, S.S. (1992) Release of GABA and taurine from brain slices. *Progress in Neurobiology*, **38**, 455–482.

Saucier, D., and Cain, D.P. (1995) Spatial learning without NMDA receptor-dependent long-term potentiation. *Nature*, **378**, 186–9.

Scheibel, M.E., and Scheibel, A.B. (1958) Structural substrates of integrative patterns in the brain stem reticular core. In *Reticular Formation of the Brain*, (ed. H.H. Jasper and L.D. Proctor), pp. 31–55. Little Brown, Boston.

Scheich, H. (1987) Neural correlates of auditory filial imprinting. *Journal of Comparative Physiology, A*, **161**, 605–619.

Scholey, A.B., Rose, S.P.R., Samani, M.R., Bock, E., and Schachner, M. (1993) A role for the neural cell-adhesion molecule in a late, consolidating phase of glycoprotein-synthesis 6 hours following passive-avoidance training of the young chick. *Neuroscience*, **55**, 499–509.

Scoville, W.B., and Milner, B. (1957) Loss of recent memory after bilateral hippocampal lesions. *Journal of Neurology, Neurosurgery and Psychiatry*, **20**, 11–21.

Searle, J. (1992) *The Rediscovery of the Mind*. MIT Press, Cambridge, Mass.

Segundo, J.P., Takenaka, T., and Encabo, H. (1967a) Somatic sensory properties of bulbar reticular neurons. *Journal of Neurophysiology*, **30**, 1221–1238.

Segundo, J.P., Takenaka, T., and Encabo, H. (1967b) Electrophysiology of bulbar reticular neurons. *Journal of Neurophysiology*, **30**, 1194–1220.

Sharpless, S., and Jasper, H. (1956) Habituation of the arousal reaction. *Brain*, **79**, 655–680.

Shashoua, V.E. (1985) The role of extracellular proteins in neuroplasticity and learning. *Cell and Molecular Neurobiology*, **5**, 183–207.

Sheu, F.S., McCabe, B.J., Horn, G. and Routtenberg, A. (1993) Learning selectively increases protein kinase C substrate phosphorylation in specific regions of the chick brain. *Proceedings of the National Academy of Sciences of the U.S.A.*, **90**, 2705–2709.

Shimizu, T., Cox, K., and Karten, H.J. (1995) Intratelencephalic projections of the visual Wulst in pigeons. (*Columba livia*) *Journal of Comparative Neurology*, **359**, 551–572.

Sholl, D.A. (1956) *The Organization of the Cerebral Cortex*. Methuen, London.

Shute, C.C.D., and Lewis, P.R. (1963) Cholinesterase-containing systems of the brain of the rat. *Nature*, **119**, 1160–1164.

Sillito, A.M. (1977) Inhibitory processes underlying the directional specificity of simple, complex and hypercomplex cells in the cat's visual cortex. *Journal of Physiology*, **271**, 699–720.

Sluckin, W. (1972) *Imprinting and Early Learning*. Methuen, London.

Solomonia, R.O., Kiguradze, T., McCabe, B.J. and Horn, G. (2000) Neural cell adhesion molecules, the α-subunit of calcium calmodulin dependent protein kinase and long-term memory in domestic chicks, Neuro Report, in press.

Solomonia, R.O., McCabe, B.J., and Horn, G. (1998) Neural cell adhesion molecules, learning and memory in the domestic chick. *Behavioral Neuroscience*, **112**, 646–655.

Spalding, D.A. (1873) Instinct with original observations on young animals. *Macmillans Magazine*, **27**, 282–293 reprinted *British Journal of Animal Behaviour*, 1954, **2**, 2–11.

Spencer, W.A., Thompson, R.F., and Neilson, D.R. Jr. (1966a) Response decrement of the flexion reflex in the acute spinal cat and transient restoration by strong stimuli. *Journal of Neurophysiology*, **29**, 221–239.

Spencer, W.A., Thompson, R.F., and Neilson, D.R. Jr. (1966b) Alterations in responsiveness of ascending and reflex pathways activated by iterated cutaneous afferent volleys. *Journal of Neurophysiology*, **29**, 240–252.

Spencer, W.A., Thompson, R.F., and Neilson, D.R. Jr. (1966c) Decrement of ventral root electrotonus and intracellularly recorded PSPs produced by iterated cutaneous afferent volleys. *Journal of Neurophysiology*, **29**, 253–274.

Squire, L.R. (1987) *Memory and Brain*. Oxford University Press, Oxford.

Stent, G.S. (1973) A physiological mechanisms for Hebb's postulate of learning. *Proceedings of the National Academy of Sciences of the USA*, **70**, 997–1001.

Steward, O., and Reeves, T.M. (1988) Protein-synthetic machinery beneath postsynaptic sites on CNS neurons: association between polyribosomes and other organelles at the synaptic site. *Journal of Neuroscience*, **8**, 176–184.

Steward, O., Wallace, C.S., Lyford, G.L., and Worley, P.F. (1998) Synaptic activation causes the mRNA for the IEG *Arc* to localize selectively near activated postsynaptic sites on dendrites. *Neuron*, **21**, 741–751.

Stewart, M.G., Rose, S.P.R., King, T.S., Gabbott, P.L.A., and Bourne, R. (1984) Hemispheric asymmetry of synapses in chick medial hyperstriatum ventrale following passive avoidance learning: a stereological investigation. *Developmental Brain Research*, **12**, 261–269.

Stryker, M.P., and Schiller, P.H. (1975) Eye and head movements evolved by electrical stimulation of monkey superior colliculus. *Experimental Brain Research*, **23**, 103–112.

Südhof, T.C. (1995) The synaptic vesicle cycle: a cascade of protein-interactions. *Nature*, **375**, 645–653.

Sun, Z-Y., and Schacher, S. (1998) Binding of serotonin to receptors at multiple sites is required for structural plasticity accompanying long-term facilitation of *Aplysia*. *Journal of Neuroscience*, **18**, 3991–4000.

Tanzi, E. (1893) I fatti e le induzioni nell' odierna istologia del systema nervoso. *Riv. Sper. Freniat. Med. Leg. Alien. Ment.*, **19**, 419–472.

Teng, E., and Squire, L.R. (1999) Memory for places learned long ago is intact after hippocampal damage. *Nature*, **400**, 675–677.

Teyler, T.J. and Discenna, P. (1987) Long-term potentiation. *Annual Review of Neuroscience*, **10**, 131–161.

Thompson, R.F. and Spencer, W.A. (1966) Habituation: a model phenomenon for the study of neuronal substrates of behavior. *Psychological Review*, **173**, 16–43.

Thorpe, W.H. (1956) *Learning and Instinct in Animals*. Methuen, London.

Thorpe, W.H. (1958) The learning of song pattern by birds, with especial reference to the song of the chaffinch, *Fringilla coelebs. Ibis*, **100**, 535–570.

Thorpe, W.H. (1978) *Purpose in a World of Chance*. Oxford University press, Oxford.

Tömböl, T., Csillag, A. and Stewart, M.G. (1990) Cell types of the hyperstriatum ventrale of the domestic chicken *Gallus domesticus*. A Golgi study. *Journal für Hirnforschung*, **29**, 319–334.

Trifaro, J.M., and Vitale, M.L. (1993) Cytoskeleton dynamics during neurotransmitter release. *Trends in Neurosciences*, **16**, 466–472.

Valverde, F. (1971) Rate and extent of recovery from dark rearing in the visual cortex of the mouse. *Brain Research*, **33**, 1–11.

Vinogradova, O.S. (1970) Registration of information and the limbic system. In *Short-term Changes in Neural Activity and Behaviour*, (ed. G. Horn and R.A. Hinde), pp. 95–140. Cambridge University Press, Cambridge.

Warrington, E.K., and Weiskrantz, L. (1982) Amnesia: a disconnection syndrome? *Neuropsychologia*, **20**, 233–248.

Watson, A.H.D., McCabe, B.J., and Horn, G. (1991) Quantitative analysis of the ultrastructural distribution of GABA-like immunoreactivity in the intermediate and medial part of hyperstriatum ventrale of the chick. *Journal of Neurocytology*, **20**, 145–156.

Weiskrantz, L. (1997) *Concsciousness Lost and Found*. Oxford University Press, Oxford.

Young, J.Z. (1939) Fused neurons and synaptic contacts in the giant nerve fibres of cephalopods. *Philosophical Transactions of the Royal Society of London*, B., **229**, 465–503.

Young, J.Z. (1963) Some essentials of neural memory systems. Paired centers that regulate and address the signals of the results of action. *Nature*, **198**, 626–630.

INDEX